Handbook of Experimental Pharmacology

Volume 91

Microbial Resistance to Drugs

Contributors

A. Böck · L.E. Bryan · S. Chamberland · E. Cundliffe
C.A. Currie-McCumber · L.P. Elwell · M.E. Fling · I.Y. Gluzman
H. Hummel · D.J. Krogstad · A.G.W. Leslie · A.A. Medeiros
H. Nikaido · L.J.V. Piddock · C.C. Sanders · P.H. Schlesinger
F.D. Schoenknecht · W.V. Shaw · D.M. Shlaes · B.G. Spratt
D.E. Taylor · R.L. Then

Editor

L.E. Bryan

Springer-Verlag
Berlin Heidelberg New York
London Paris Tokyo

Professor LAWRENCE E. BRYAN
M.D., Ph.D., F.R.C.P. (C.)
Head, Department of Microbiology
and Infectious Diseases
Faculty of Medicine
University of Calgary
Health Sciences Centre
3330 Hospital Drive N.W.
Calgary, Alberta, Canada T2N 4N1

With 39 Figures

ISBN-13:978-3-642-74097-8 e-ISBN-13:978-3-642-74095-4
DOI: 10.1007/978-3-642-74095-4

Library of Congress Cataloging-in-Publication Data. Microbial resistance to drugs / contributors, A. Böck ... [et al.]; editor, L. E. Bryan. p. cm. – (Handbook of experimental pharmacology; v. 91) Includes index. ISBN-13:978-3-642-74097-8 (U.S.: alk. paper) 1. Drug resistance in microorganisms. I. Böck, A. II. Bryan, L. E. III. Series. QP905. H3 vol. 91 [QR177] 615'.1 s – dc19 [615'.329] 88-35480 CIP

Softcover reprint of the hardcover 1st edition 1989

2122/3130-543210 – Printed on acid-free paper

List of Contributors

A. Böck, Lehrstuhl für Mikrobiologie der Universität München, Maria-Ward-Str. 1a, D-8000 München 19

L. E. Bryan, Department of Microbiology and Infectious Diseases, University of Calgary, Health Sciences Center, Faculty of Medicine, 3330 Hospital Drive, N.W., Calgary, Alberta, Canada T2N 4N1

S. Chamberland, Lilly Research Laboratory, Lilly Corporate Center, MC 539–98A/2nd Floor, Indianapolis, IN 46285-0438, USA

E. Cundliffe, Leicester Biocentre and Department of Biochemistry, University of Leicester, Adrian Building, University Road, Leicester LE1 7RH, Great Britain

C. A. Currie-McCumber, Veterans Administration Medical Centre 1110-W, 10701 East Boulevard, Cleveland, OH 44106, USA

L. P. Elwell, Department of Microbiology, Wellcome Research Laboratory, Burroughs Wellcome Co., 3030 Cornwallis Road, Research Triangle Park, NC 27709, USA

M. E. Fling, Department of Microbiology, Wellcome Research Laboratory, Burroughs Wellcome Co., 3030 Cornwallis Road, Research Triangle Park, NC 27709, USA

I. Y. Gluzman, Departments of Medicine and Pathology, Washington University School of Medicine, Box 8118, 660 South Euclid Avenue, St. Louis, MO 63110, USA

H. Hummel, Abteilung für Mikrobiologie der Universität München, Maria-Ward-Str. 1a, D-8000 München 19

D. J. Krogstad, Department of Medicine and Pathology, Washington University School of Medicine, Box 8118, 660 South Euclid Avenue, St. Louis, MO 63110, USA

A. G. W. Leslie, Blackett Laboratory, Imperial College, London SW7 2BZ, Great Britain

A. A. Medeiros, Division of Infectious Disease and the Clinical Microbiology Laboratory, The Miriam Hospital, 164 Summit Avenue, Providence, RI 02906, USA

H. Nikaido, Department of Microbiology and Immunology, University of California, Berkeley, CA 94720, USA

L. J. V. Piddock, Department of Medical Microbiology, The Medical School, The University of Birmingham, Birmingham B15 2TJ, Great Britain

C. C. Sanders, Creighton University, Department of Medical Microbiology, 2500 California St., Omaha, NB 68178, USA

P. H. Schlesinger, Department of Biomedical Research, Washington University School of Dental Medicine, Box 8118, South Euclid Avenue, St. Louis, MO 63110, USA

F. D. Schoenknecht, Departments of Laboratory Medicine and Microbiology, University of Washington, University Hospital SB-10, Seattle, WA 98195, USA

W. V. Shaw, Department of Biochemistry, University of Leicester, Adrian Building, University Road, Leicester LE1 7RH, Great Britain

D. M. Shlaes, Veterans Administration Medical Center 1110-W, 10701 East Boulevard, Cleveland, OH 44106, USA

B. G. Spratt, The University of Sussex, School of Biological Sciences, Biology Building, Falmer, Brighton BN1 9QG, Great Britain

D. E. Taylor, Department of Medical Microbiology and Infectious Diseases, University of Alberta, 1-41 Medical Sciences Building, Edmonton, Alberta, Canada T6G 2H7

R. L. Then, Pharmaceutical Research Department, F. Hoffmann-La Roche & Co., Ltd., CH-4002 Basel

Preface

Most often when the subject of antimicrobial resistance is discussed, the organizational emphasis is on individual antimicrobial agents or groups of agents. Thus we tend to see discussion of resistance to β-lactams, tetracyclines, aminoglycosides etc. In this book many of the authors were asked to emphasize the mechanism of resistance in their discussion and from that to show how susceptibility to various agents was affected. In part this was done to help emphasize the enormous contribution that the study of antimicrobial resistance has made to our understanding of fundamental physiologic and genetic processes in bacteria. When one looks back over the study of antimicrobial resistance, it is clear that it has been the birthplace of many fundamental advances in molecular biology and of an appreciation of the role of many key functions in the life of a bacterium. In addition, and hopefully to an increasing extent in the future, such study has also contributed to advances in antimicrobial chemotherapy. Throughout the book resistance mechanisms have been placed in perspective as to their significance as causes of resistance to key drugs or groups of drugs. Some are of much greater significance than others in terms of the prevalence or the degree of resistance produced. Whatever their numerical significance, however, each of the mechanisms, without question, throws light on fundamental cellular processes and the way in which they interact with antimicrobial agents. Thus they also tell us much about how antibiotics act – as well as why they don't. Sections of the book also are designed to place the exciting biological advances in the context of the everyday world of detection of these problems, their spread, their distribution in different bacteria and how they contribute to persistence of bacteria in some modern-day clinical circumstances.

As the study of resistance has progressed, it has become possible in some instances to actually predict susceptibility levels with a surprising degree of accuracy, such as with the minimal inhibitory concentrations of β-lactams in cells of measured permeability and β-lactamase content. A victory for rationality. Another observation of interest is the communality that exists between prokaryotic and eukaryotic approaches to resistance to noxious agents. It is quite possible that both groups of organisms use efflux systems to reduce concentrations of antimicrobial compounds, including antimalarial and anticancer drugs, below toxic levels in the cell. In spite of wonderful advances in our understanding of the mechanisms of antimicrobial resistance – described throughout this volume – it is remarkable how much more there is to learn. For example, recently we have seen the introduction of the fluoroquinolone agents, derivatives of the older quinolones. The actual target of these drugs still has not been defined with finality, and increasing evidence suggests it involves direct binding to DNA rather than to the DNA gyrase proteins. This is a story reminiscent of the interaction of many drugs with ribosomes, in which it took a long time to finally show that it was the nucleic acid component which was the key to drug binding, not the protein. As outlined in this book, it took studies of resistance to help unravel this topic. Furthermore, if we ever do start feeling smug about our vast knowledge in the field, we only need to watch the remarkable modifications microbes make as seemingly highly armoured drugs are introduced into clinical use. The wide diversity of β-lactamases and the facility with which very poorly hydrolyzed drugs can be be attacked by microbially restructured enzymes are examples that should rapidly destroy any overconfidence of our superior knowledge. On the other hand, there is also no reason to be unduly pessimistic. Our knowledge base has broadened tremendously, and the pharmaceutical industry has shown a capability to introduce new and improved drugs with a skill that should be greatly admired.

Having watched the scene of antimicrobial resistance from the viewpoints of investigator, author and editor, I realize that no book will ever cover the entire subject with a depth, content or perspective that will satisfy everyone. In this volume a group of people from many parts of the world and with unusual expertise have brought together data and views that I hope many will find informative and, interesting and that may imbue another generation of investigators with interest in this fascinating group of topics.

Calgary L. E. BRYAN

Contents

CHAPTER 5

Plasmid-Determined Beta-Lactamases

CHAPTER 6

The Chromosomal Beta-Lactamases

CHAPTER 7

CHAPTER 8

Resistance to Quinolones and Fluoroquinolones

CHAPTER 11

Resistance to Trimethoprim

CHAPTER 12

Resistance to Sulfonamides

CHAPTER 13

Chloramphenicol Acetyltransferases
W. V. SHAW and A. G. W. LESLIE. With 5 Figures 313

CHAPTER 14

General Properties of Resistance Plasmids
D. E. TAYLOR. With 5 Figures 325

CHAPTER 17

Microbial Persistence or Phenotypic Adaptation to Antimicrobial Agents: Cystic Fibrosis as an Illustrative Case

CHAPTER 18

Microbes Causing Problems of Antimicrobial Resistance

CHAPTER 1

Role of the Outer Membrane of Gram-Negative Bacteria in Antimicrobial Resistance

H. NIKAIDO

A. Introduction

The extensive use of antibiotics in recent years has been very effective in combating infections caused by "classical" pathogenic bacteria, but at the same time it produced an increase in infections, often hospital-acquired, by antibiotic-resistant gram-negative bacteria of moderate or even marginal pathogenicity (MCGOWAN 1985). The general resistance to antibiotics, often encountered in such gram-negative bacteria, is largely due to the presence of an extra membrane layer on the surface of these organisms: the outer membrane of these bacteria acts as an effective permeation barrier and retards the influx of antibiotic molecules into the bacterial cell.

The barrier property of the outer membrane can be most clearly analyzed for the penetration of β-lactams, because the barrier effect is enhanced by the nearly ubiquitous presence of β-lactamase in the periplasmic space, the space in between the outer and inner cytoplasmic membranes (SYKES and MATTHEW 1976). Because of this reason, much of this chapter will analyze the role of the outer membrane in β-lactam resistance. The penetration of other agents will then be discussed, although the amount of available quantitative information is rather small. Architecture and functions of the outer membrane have been reviewed (LUGTENBERG and VAN ALPHEN 1983; NIKAIDO and VAARA 1985), and the diffusion of β-lactams has been discussed in detail (NIKAIDO 1985). Earlier studies have been summarized by PARR and BRYAN (1984).

B. The Outer Membrane Barrier

I. The Lipid Bilayer

The basic continuum of the bacterial outer membrane is a lipid bilayer, as in most other biological membranes (NIKAIDO and VAARA 1985). Lipid bilayers are usually very permeable to lipophilic solutes (STEIN 1967). However, many gram-negative bacteria, including Enterobacteriaceae, are quite resistant to hydrophobic antibiotics and inhibitory agents, such as actinomycin D, novobiocin, rifamycin SV, macrolides, and various dyes and detergents. Furthermore, this resistance is due to the barrier property of the outer membrane, because the resistance is decreased drastically when the structure of its bilayer region is modified, either by mutational alteration (NIKAIDO 1976), or transient removal (LEIVE 1974), of its

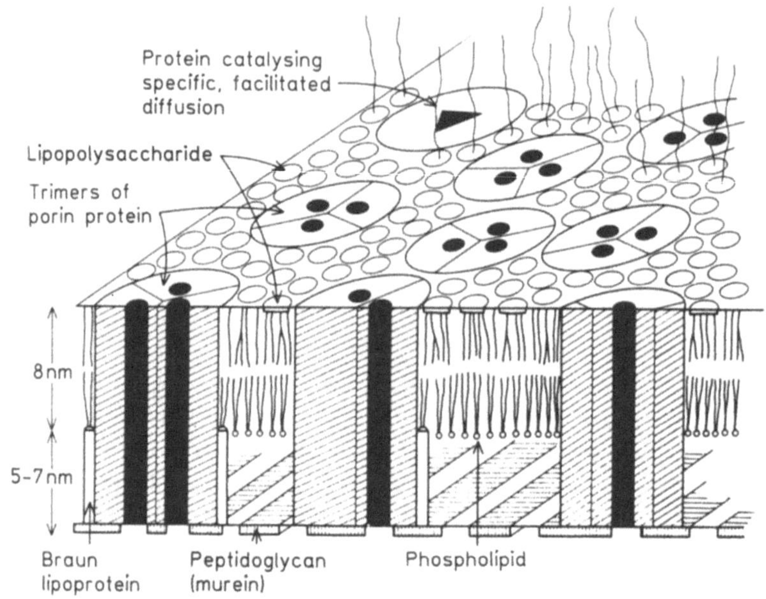

Fig. 1. A schematic model of the *E. coli* and *S. typhimurium* outer membrane. Note the asymmetric distribution of lipids in the bilayer continuum. Some features, such as the length of the saccharide chain of LPS, are not drawn to scale. Although peptidoglycan layer is shown as a monolayer, it may exist as a cross-linked gel-like matrix (HOBOT et al. 1984). The specific-channel protein is drawn as a monomer for simplicity; LamB protein, for example, is known to exist as a trimer. From NIKAIDO and NAKAE (1979) with permission from Academic Press

lipopolysaccharide component. Thus the lipid bilayer of the outer membrane usually has a very low permeability toward lipophilic or hydrophobic solutes.

Why is the permeability of the lipid bilayer region of the outer membrane so low? Electron microscopic (MÜHLRADT and GOLECKI 1974) and enzyme modification (FUNAHARA and NIKAIDO 1980) studies showed that practically all of the lipopolysaccharide molecules are located in the outer leaflet of the bilayer. Moreover, covalent labeling and enzyme digestion studies showed that glycerophospholipid molecules are located all in the inner leaflet of the bilayer, at least in *S. typhimurium* (KAMIO and NIKAIDO 1976). Thus the bilayer region of the outer membrane is highly asymmetric (Fig. 1), and one can assume that the outer leaflet, consisting essentially only of lipopolysaccharide, may act as an effective barrier, because a lipopolysaccharide molecule contains up to 7 covalently linked hydrocarbon chains, which are all saturated, and produces a much less fluid, nearly crystalline structure (NIKAIDO et al. 1977 a; LABISCHINSKI et al. 1985) in comparison with phospholipids. Furthermore, the region of head group close to the membrane surface contains many, mostly negatively charged residues, which could produce a strong meshwork structure when bridged by divalent cations (NIKAIDO and VAARA 1985). The negatively charged groups, however, can become the target of attack by polycationic antibiotics (Sect. G).

The barrier property of the lipopolysaccharide/phospholipid bilayer can be compromised, as was alluded to earlier. The best understood case is the "deep rough" mutants of *E. coli* and *Salmonella*. These mutants produce lipopolysaccharide molecules with incomplete saccharide chains, but experimental evidence suggests that what is responsible for the increased permeability is not the shortening of the saccharide chains per se, but the decreased incorporation of outer membrane proteins and the consequent relocation of significant fraction of phospholipid molecules into the outer leaflet (KAMIO and NIKAIDO 1976). This creates the conventional glycerophospholipid bilayer domains in the outer membrane, which should allow a rapid permeation of lipophilic molecules. Such phospholipid domains are probably also created by the removal of lipopolysaccharide molecules via the EDTA treatment of the bacteria (LEIVE 1974). In addition there are other types of mutations that increase the outer membrane permeability by mechanisms not clearly understood at the present time (see Sect. F).

II. The Porin Pathway

Gram-negative bacteria must take in nutrients from the media and excrete waste products in the presence of the outer membrane, the bilayer region of which has very low permeability for hydrophobic solutes and presumably for hydrophilic solutes as well. This requirement apparently led to the development of porins, a class of proteins that produce water-filled, non-specific, transmembrane diffusion channels (NIKAIDO and VAARA 1985; BENZ 1985). Porins are usually produced in a very large number of copies: in *E. coli* it is one of the most abundant proteins, being present in approximately 100,000 copies per cell. They usually have molecular weights between 30,000 and 40,000, and are known to contain a very large fraction of β-sheets (where investigated), in contrast to other membrane-spanning proteins known to be rich in α-helices. The significance of porin pathway for antibiotic resistance is briefly summarized by GUTMANN et al. (1984).

In enteric bacteria, porins form very stable trimeric structures. However, in *Paracoccus denitrificans* (ZALMAN and NIKAIDO 1985) and *Rhodobacter sphaeroides* (YAN and NIKAIDO, to be published), organisms related in their evolutionary origin, porins form stable dimers. Porins from some non-enteric organisms can be purified as monomers, which are able to form channels upon reconstitution (for example see YOSHIMURA et al. 1983).

An important property of enteric bateria, except those belonging to the *Proteus-Morganella-Providencia* group (MITSUYAMA et al. 1987), is that they usually produce a family of porins that share extensive sequence homology (see NIKAIDO and VAARA 1985). Thus *E. coli* K12 produces two species, OmpF (*o*uter *m*embrane *p*rotein F) and OmpC. When cultured in media deficient in phosphate, they produce another porin, PhoE. However, body fluids and tissues of higher animals contain high levels of inorganic phosphate, and therefore the production of PhoE does not seem to have any clinical relevance. *S. typhimurium* LT2 produces OmpF, OmpC, and in addition OmpD porin. The synthesis of these proteins is regulated by environmental conditions. Those mimicking the situation inside the body of higher animals, i.e. osmotic strength of 300 mosM or higher and temperature of 37 °C or higher, tend to favor the production of OmpC porin over

OmpF, and the conditions prevailing in natural waters, i.e. low osmolality and low temperature, favor the production of OmpF over OmpC. Furthermore, the production of OmpD, as well as the third porin often present in clinical strains of *E. coli*, is controlled by catabolite repression.

Most of the antibiotics that are effective against *E. coli* appear to diffuse through the porin channels, and this has been shown directly for many cephalosporins by measuring the rate of diffusion across the outer membrane, by coupling it to their hydrolysis in the periplasmic space, using the method introduced by ZIMMERMANN and ROSSELET (1977). These studies (cited in YOSHIMURA and NIKAIDO 1985) showed that porins were responsible for at least 90% of the penetration, through the outer membrane, of cephaloridine, cephamandole, cephalothin, ampicillin, and 6-aminopenicillanic acid, although very recently β-lactams have been designed to penetrate the outer membrane by utilizing specific pathways (Sect. F).

Although the porin channels are totally non-specific, the rate of penetration of solutes is greatly influenced by the gross physicochemical properties of the solute, because the channels are very narrow, with estimated diameters of 1.2 and 1.1 nm for OmpF and OmpC porins of *E. coli*, respectively. Thus even small molecules pass through the porin channel with some difficulty; it is only the large number of porins per cell that counteracts this hindrance and creates a significant degree of permeability. These considerations suggest that one should always measure the *rates* of penetration of various solutes, in other words, *permeability coefficients* of the outer membrane. Qualitative measurements and statements on whether a compound is "permeable" or "not permeable" across the outer membrane mean very little, and are often very misleading (see below).

III. The Specific Pathways

Gram-negative bacteria often produce specific diffusion pathways for nutrients that diffuse with insufficient rates through the non-specific porin channel. For example, maltodextrins, vitamin B_{12}, and iron-chelator complexes are all too large for the small diameters of *E. coli* porin channels described above, and *E. coli* produces LamB, BtuB, and a large number of iron-chelator "receptor" proteins for the uptake of these compounds (NIKAIDO and VAARA 1985). Similarly, *P. aeruginosa* produces a glucose-specific channel protein, D1 (HANCOCK and CAREY 1980) and presumably siderophore receptors. Although these channels are usually too specific for allowing the diffusion of antibiotics, there are some exceptions that are discussed in Sect. F.

C. The Measurement of Outer Membrane Permeability

I. Measurement in Intact Cells

One method can be used to get precise values of permeability coefficients of the outer membrane for β-lactams. It was proposed independently by SAWAI et al. (1977) and by ZIMMERMANN and ROSSELET (1977), and involves the measurement of the rate of β-lactam hydrolysis by intact cells. The rate of entry of β-lactam across the outer membrane, V_{entry}, is described by Fick's first law of diffusion,

$$V_{entry} = P \times A \times (C_o - C_p) \quad (1)$$

where P, A, C_o, and C_p denote permeability coefficient, area of the outer membrane, drug concentration in the outside medium, and drug concentration in the periplasm, respectively. On the other hand, the rate of hydrolysis of β-lactam by the periplasmic β-lactamase molecules, $V_{hydrolysis}$, follows the Michaelis-Menten relationship,

$$V_{hydrolysis} = C_p \times V_{max}/(C_p + K_m) \quad (2)$$

where V_{max} and K_m describe the well-known kinetic constants of the enzyme (measured obviously in cell extracts, where there is no barrier for access of the substrate molecules). C_p can thus be calculated from Eq. 2, and can be compared with C_o.

ZIMMERMANN and ROSSELET (1977) realized further that at steady state, V_{entry} must equal $V_{hydrolysis}$, and thus the two equations can be combined and could be solved for $P \times A$, which they called "permeability parameter." Since the area of outer membrane per unit weight of cells is expected to be reasonably similar among closely related organisms, it is a simple matter to calculate the permeability coefficient from these equations (NIKAIDO 1985).

In practice, several precautions are necessary. For example, the determination of C_p becomes imprecise if assays are done under the conditions in which C_p is well above the K_m of the enzyme. It is also extremely important, especially for slowly penetrating compounds and for organisms with low outer membrane permeability, to prevent cell lysis and damage to the outer membrane, because hydrolysis by enzymes released from, or located in, lysing or damaged cells will make relatively large contributions to the hydrolysis rates observed. With *E. coli* and *S. typhimurium*, addition of Mg^{2+} to growth media, wash buffer, and the assay mixture helps to minimize this problem (NIKAIDO et al. 1977b). The contribution from the released enzyme can and must be evaluated by carrying out an assay with the supernatant of cell suspension, but that from the enzyme still associated with the damaged or leaky cells is impossible to correct for. HEWINSON et al. (1986) measured the permeability of *P. aeruginosa* outer membrane to cephalosporin C by using the Zimmermann-Rosselet method, and found that the permeability was about 100-fold higher than that reported earlier for other cephalosporins (ANGUS et al. 1982; YOSHIMURA and NIKAIDO 1982) and that it varied with the external concentration of the drug. Both of these results, however, may be explained if some of the β-lactamase molecules were exposed on the surface of the outer membrane. This example suggests that Zimmermann-Rosselet assays should be performed at different external concentrations of the substrate, in order to make certain that the values of the permeability coefficients remain constant. In our experience, this has always been the case at least for zwitterionic β-lactams, but it seems possible that some of the clinical isolates, such as the one used by HEWINSON et al. (1986), may have an unusually fragile outer membrane or have different localization pattern for the β-lactamase. Another point that should be kept in mind is that the permeation rates of compounds with net charges will vary according to the magnitude of the Donnan potential across the outer membrane (STOCK et al. 1977); this point will be discussed more fully in the next section.

A major problem with the Zimmermann-Rosselet assay is that the β-lactams must be susceptible to enzymatic hydrolysis. KOJO et al. (1980a, b) proposed a modification applicable to β-lactamase-resistant compounds. This involves the measurement, in intact cells, of the hydrolysis rates of easily hydrolyzed compounds such as cephaloridine in the presence of a β-lactamase-resistant compound that acts as an inhibitor of β-lactamase. Unfortunately, the published data (KOJO et al. 1980b) are internally inconsistent. Perhaps the system is too complex and the precision of the measurement is not sufficient for the extensive manipulation of data required (NIKAIDO 1985).

With β-lactams that form long-lived complexes with β-lactamases, we can assess, semiquantitatively, their rates of penetration into the periplasm by treatment of intact cells with these drugs, followed by breaking of cells and assay of the extent of inactivation of the periplasmic enzyme (BUSH et al. 1985). Although this appears to be a useful method, one drawback is that even the β-lactams that were once believed to be totally β-lactamase-resistant are now known to be hydrolyzed at significant rates (LIVERMORE 1983; VU and NIKAIDO 1985), and thus the steady-state periplasmic concentration of these drugs is influenced not only by the outer membrane permeability but also by the action of β-lactamases (see below). Another point is that often it is assumed that every interaction between the enzyme and the β-lactam produces the long-lived, inactivated enzyme, but in many cases only a fraction of the enzyme-substrate complex becomes converted into this form [$E'S^*$ in the terminology of FRÈRE and JORIS (1985)].

Binding of β-lactams to the penicillin-binding proteins was also used to assess the penetration rates in a similar way (ZIMMERMANN 1980; RODRIGUEZ-TÉBAR et al. 1982). Intact cells are incubated with β-lactams, which are allowed to penetrate through the outer membrane and then bind covalently to the penicillin-binding proteins. Radioactively labeled β-lactam is also added either simultaneously, or after the breaking open of the cells. Again the weakness of the method is that the periplasmic concentration of the drugs is not determined by the outer membrane permeability alone, but by the balance between that and the rate of hydrolysis in the periplasm, which is rarely negligible. However, the method may produce results roughly reflective of the outer membrane permeability when the compound used is degraded very slowly and its periplasmic concentration is affected much more by its slow penetration through the outer membrane, e.g. in organisms producing outer membranes of exceptionally low permeability such as *P. aeruginosa*.

Several other methods have been proposed for the measurement of outer membrane permeability, especially of β-lactams, but their validity is questionable (see NIKAIDO 1985 for detailed discussion). The ratio of β-lactam hydrolysis rates in broken cell preparations and in intact cells, called "crypticity" or "permeability index" (SMITH et al. 1964; RICHMOND and SYKES 1973), is misleading as a quantitative indicator because the magnitude of this index changes drastically depending on the substrate concentration used for assay (NIKAIDO 1985). Comparison of MICs in test strains and in "hypersensitive" strains is again often very useful as a qualitative indicator. However, even the "hypersensitive" strains do maintain an outer membrane barrier, and the extent of increase in the permeability is likely to be quite different depending on the nature of solutes. Similar problems exist for methods that use transiently permeabilized cells (NIKAIDO 1985). Practical details of methods for measuring outer membrane permeability in general have been described (NIKAIDO 1986).

II. Measurement in Reconstituted Vesicles

Since most antibiotics active against gram-negative bacteria are likely to cross the outer membrane via porin channels (see above), their outer membrane permeability can be deduced from their penetration rate through porin channels, conveniently measured in reconstituted vesicles. Early reconstitution studies involved the measurement of the extent of efflux of solutes initially trapped within the intravesicular space. Such an approach, however, had a rather poor time resolution, and was not suitable for the precise measurement of diffusion rates.

The preferred method at present is the "liposome swelling" method, originally developed for measurement of diffusion rates of sugars (LUCKEY and NIKAIDO 1980a, b; NIKAIDO 1983; NIKAIDO and ROSENBERG 1983). We make phospholipid liposomes that contain porin molecules within the bilayer membrane, and impermeable solutes such as dextran in the intravesicular space. When these liposomes are diluted into an isoosmotic solution of the test solute, the test solute diffuses into the liposome through the porin channel, following its concentration gradient. This causes the water to flow into the vesicles, and the liposomes swell. The swelling of the liposomes decreases their average refractive index, and can be followed by the decrease of the turbidity of the suspension. The diffusion process can be slowed to an easily observable range by using a porin/lipid ratio of, for example, 1/1000 (w/w) (NIKAIDO and ROSENBERG 1983), in contrast to the nearly 1/1 (w(w) ratio found in the outer membrane (SMIT et al. 1975).

In the original procedure, liposomes were made in dextran. These liposomes, however, exhibited anomalous behavior in solutions of electrolytes such as β-lactams, presumably owing to the Donnan potential created by the presence of charged groups on the dextran molecule. Furthermore, the diffusion rate of anionic solutes should ideally be determined in liposomes containing anions that are too large to diffuse through the porin channel, such as NAD; otherwise the influx of positive counterions following their own concentration gradient creates membrane potential, which then produces unpredictable fluxes of the diffusible cations as well as anions. On the other hand, we would like to have a single liposome preparation that is usable for the measurement of permeability of both zwitterionic and anionic solutes. Thus as a compromise we use liposomes containing both neutral (12 m*M* stachyose) and anionic (4 m*M* Na-NAD) solutes, and use a buffer containing NAD as its anionic component (NIKAIDO and ROSENBERG 1983). This system worked reasonably well for the assay of the permeability of zwitterionic, monoanionic, and dianionic β-lactams (YOSHIMURA and NIKAIDO 1985), but we must emphasize that the system is a compromise and the values obtained cannot be of the highest precision.

The advantage of the liposome swelling method is its simplicity. However, the movement of *any* solute molecule across the liposome membrane can produce the swelling or shrinking of the liposomes. For this reason, one should be extremely careful in the planning and execution of swelling experiments. The limitations of the swelling assay are described below.

(a) The solutes must cross the membrane through the porin channels. With nonelectrolytes, this point can be established easily by using porin-free vesicles as a control. However, the situation becomes more complicated with salts of organic acids (as with most β-lactams). With the porin-containing liposomes, the protonated form of such organic acids can cross the lipid bilayer part of the membrane, and the intravesicular proton can be exchanged with external alkali cation that rapidly flows in through the porin channel. Yet in the porin-free "control" liposome the flux of the protonated organic acid will stop nearly instantaneously because of the buildup of pH gradient, thus creating a false impression that the compound does not diffuse through the bilayer. This possibility can be checked by using liposomes containing, instead of porin, gramicidin A, which allows the diffusion of alkali cations but not of β-lactams (NIKAIDO and ROSENBERG 1983). Use of this control showed that many of the penicillins are indeed too hydrophobic for this assay of porin function. Similarly, many other agents, such as tetracyclines and chloramphenicol, appear to be too hydrophobic for this assay. Although it has been claimed that this difficulty can be overcome by the use of phospholipids with high melting points (KOBAYASHI et al. 1982), this conclusion is based on the use of liposomes not containing any cation carrier such as gramicidin A, and therefore its validity is questionable.

(b) The method currently available cannot be used for compounds with net positive charges, such as aminoglycosides. Although it has been used for such compounds (NAKAE and NAKAE 1982), the relationship between the swelling rate and the permeability of tested cationic drugs is very remote, since the influx of permeable, negative counterion is predicted to produce complex fluxes of permeable buffer ions.

(c) Since NAD and most β-lactams diffuse through *P. aeruginosa* porin F channel with rather similar rates, this method is not applicable for such porins producing large diameter channels.

The swelling assay measures the rate of penetration of solutes in the absence of significant electric potential, but in the intact cell, Donnan potential, inside negative, always exists across the outer membrane (STOCK et al. 1977). This slows down the diffusion of compounds with net negative charge, as was recently shown by measurement in cells with Donnan potentials spanning a wide range (SEN et al. 1988). In fact, although cephacetrile, a monoanionic compound, diffuses at 60% of the rate of cephaloridine, a zwitterionic compound, through OmpF porin channels in reconstituted liposomes (YOSHIMURA and NIKAIDO 1985), in intact cells suspended in 10 m*M* sodium phosphate buffer-5 m*M* $MgCl_2$ the cephacetrile diffusion rate was only 15% of that of cephaloridine (NIKAIDO et al. 1983). Similarly, the permeation rate through OmpF porin channel of SCE-20, a dianionic compound, was 19% and 3.6% of that of cephacetrile in liposomes (NIKAIDO and ROSENBERG 1983) and in intact cells (NIKAIDO et al. 1983), respectively. Thus the influx of molecules carrying net negative charges is very significantly decreased in intact cells, especially in media of low ionic strength, which increases the Donnan potential across the membrane. In this connection, YAMAGUCHI et al. (1986) noted that the penetration rate of cefazolin, a monoanionic compound, through the outer membrane of intact cells of *E. coli* was influenced by the ionic strength of the suspending medium, and that $MgSO_4$ was far more effective than NaCl in increasing the penetration rate. They, however, came to a wrong conclusion that this was due to the neutralization of the anionic groups on the walls of the porin channel, apparently because they were unaware of the fact that 10 m*M* $MgSO_4$ is as effective as 150 m*M* NaCl in collapsing the Donnan potential.

D. Permeability of Bacterial Outer Membranes to β-Lactam Antibiotics

I. Penetration Rates in *E. coli*

1. Effect of Hydrophobicity

There have been many suggestions that increased hydrophobicity decreases the efficacy of β-lactam compounds against gram-negative bacteria, especially *E. coli*. For example BIAGI et al. (1970) showed that the hydrophobicity of various β-lactams, as determined by the *R*m values in reverse-phase thin-layer chromatography, correlated negatively with their efficacy in *E. coli*, whereas positive correlation was observed for efficacy in *Staphylococcus aureus*, a gram-positive organism. However, this simple correlation tended to disappear when compounds of wider range were compared (e.g. BIRD and NAYLER 1971), an observation which is now understandable because we know that the efficacy is a complex parameter, and is strongly affected not only by permeability but also by the susceptibility of drug to β-lactamases and by its affinity to the target (NIKAIDO and NORMARK 1987).

Outer membrane permeation rates of β-lactams of varying hydrophobicity were first measured by ZIMMERMANN and ROSSELET (1977), using their method that combines outer membrane permeation with periplasmic hydrolysis (Sect. C.I.), and an inverse correlation between hydrophobicity and permeation rate was established. This work was further extended by NIKAIDO et al. (1983). By using the octanol/water partition coefficient of the *uncharged form* of β-lactams, rather than their apparent partition coefficient, as the indicator of hydrophobicity, a very good inverse correlation between hydrophobicity and the permeation rate through *E. coli* outer membrane was seen among the first-generation cephalosporins, a tenfold increase in the partition coefficient producing about a fivefold decrease in permeation rate through the OmpF porin channel (Fig. 2). These results were also confirmed by the swelling experiments with purified OmpF porin (YOSHIMURA and NIKAIDO 1985). Some of the compounds in Fig. 2, however, do not follow this simple pattern (see the next section).

These results are also consistent with similar experiments of MURAKAMI and YOSHIDA (1982), carried out with fewer compounds. These workers found that the relative permeation rate of cephalothin was 13% of that of cefazolin; this is close to our value of 15% (NIKAIDO et al. 1983). Furthermore, they found that the replacement of the ring sulfur atom with oxygen in cephalothin and cephamandole decreased the hydrophobicity and also increased the penetration rate.

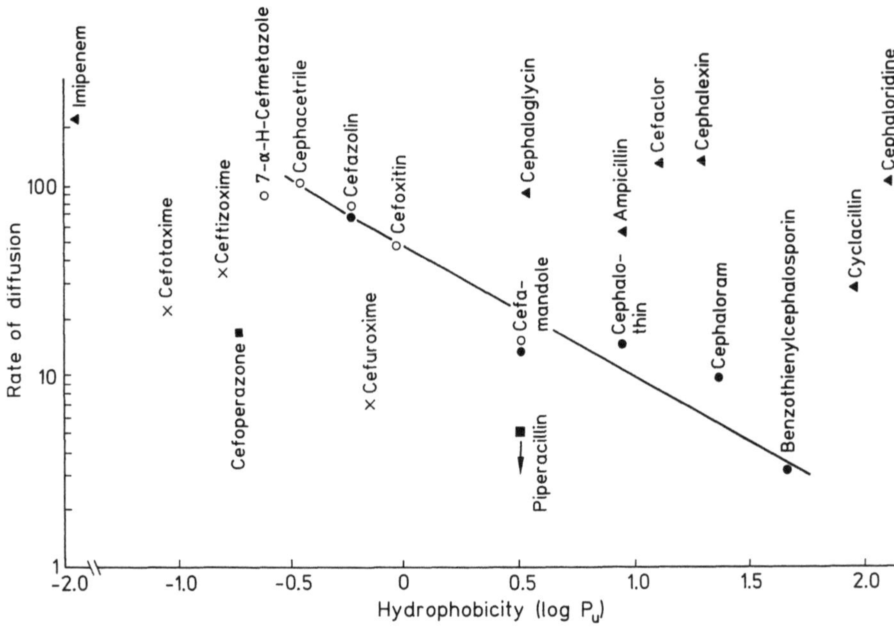

Fig. 2. Rates of penetration of β-lactams through *E. coli* OmpF porin channel. Note that the rates were measured in reconstituted liposomes except as indicated below, and that the electrical charges on the β-lactam molecule will have a stronger effect on the diffusion rate in intact cells because of the presence of Donnan potential. ▲, zwitterionic compounds; ○, "classical" monoanionic compounds; ×, monoanionic compounds with substituted oxime side chains; ■, monoanionic compounds with bulky side chains; ●, monoanionic compounds measured in intact cells. The relative permeation rates are expressed as percentage of the rate for cephacetrile. Redrawn from YOSHIMURA and NIKAIDO (1985)

As mentioned earlier in Sect. B.II, *E. coli* K-12 produces two porin species, OmpF and OmpC, in ordinary media. In proteoliposome swelling studies, we showed that hydrophobicity exerted a much stronger influence on the penetration rate of peptides through the narrower OmpC channel than on the rate through the wider OmpF channel (NIKAIDO and ROSENBERG 1983). It seems reasonable that the same holds true for penetration in intact cells. Although our assay in intact cells (NIKAIDO et al. 1983) appeared to show that the effect of hydrophobicity was similar in OmpF- and OmpC-containing cells, the data points with OmpC-containing cells had very low values and were probably not accurate.

Because most of the penicillins are too hydrophobic to be tested with the proteoliposome assay, direct comparison between penicillins and cephalosporins is difficult. We can however compare ampicillin with its cephalosporin analogs, cephaloglycin and cephalexin (Table 1), and find that cephalosporins permeate two- to threefold faster. This is to be expected from the difference in hydrophobicity, as penicillins have about four times higher partition coefficients in octanol/water than the corresponding cephalosporins (YOSHIMURA and NIKAIDO 1985).

It was concluded that penicillins are somehow more efficient than cephalosporins in diffusing through lipid bilayers, because ampicillin permeated through li-

Table 1. Penetration rates of some β-lactams through the porin channels of *E. coli*[a]

β-Lactam	M_r	Relative diffusion rate through:	
		OmpF channel	OmpC channel
Monoanionic compounds			
Cephacetrile	338	(100)	(100)[b]
Cefazolin	453	77	
Cefoxitin	426	46	
Ceftizoxime	382	35	19
Cefotaxime	454	22	8
Cefoperazone	644	16	
Cefamandole	461	14	
Cefuroxime	410	7	
Piperacillin	516	< 5	
Zwitterionic compounds			
Imipenem	299	216	280
Cephaloridine	415	167	
Cephalexin	347	129	
Cephaloglycin	405	87	
Ampicillin	333	46	
Dianionic compounds			
Moxalactam	518	34	10
Azthreonam	433	22	12
Ceftriaxone	552	20	< 4
Sulbenicillin	412	5	
Carbenicillin	376	6	
Compounds with one positive and two negative charges			
Cephalosporin C	414	72	
Penicillin N	358	56	
Cefsulodin	531	37	
Ceftazidime	545	12	< 4

[a] The data show the relative rates of diffusion of β-lactam molecules through the porin channels in reconstituted liposomes. It should be emphasized that compounds with net negative charges, especially dianionic compounds, are retarded much more severely in their diffusion through the porin channels of intact cells, because of the presence of interior-negative Donnan potential across the outer membrane (see Sect. C.II). The data are taken from YOSHIMURA and NIKAIDO (1985)

[b] The rates were normalized to that for cephacetrile. The actual permeation rate of cephacetrile through the OmpC channel was 25%–30% of the rate found with the OmpF channel

posome membranes relatively rapidly in comparison with cefazolin and cephaloridine (YAMAGUCHI et al. 1982). But these data are what is expected from the nature of substituents, and do not necessarily show that penicillins are fundamentally different from cephalosporins. Thus a small but significant fraction of ampicillin molecules should exist in the uncharged form, which can cross the bilayer. In contrast, cefazolin cannot cross the bilayer without the simultaneous influx of alkali metal counterion, to which phospholipid bilayers are essentially impermeable. Similarly, cephaloridine is expected to penetrate lipid bilayers very poorly, because it cannot exist in an uncharged form.

2. Effect of Size

When solutes of widely different sizes are used in liposome swelling experiments, the strong effect of solute size on penetration rates is clearly seen (Fig. 3). But many β-lactams fall into the molecular weight range of 350–450, and the effect of size was not usually apparent in the comparison of their diffusion rates. There are exceptions, however. Those compounds with unusually large size (for example piperacillin and cefoperazone) diffused through OmpF channel only with marginal rates (Fig. 2). Another example is the group of compounds with oxyimino substituents on the α carbon of the 7-substituent, such as cefotaxime, ceftizoxime, and cefuroxime (Fig. 2), which penetrate nearly an order of magnitude more slowly than predicted from their hydrophobicity alone. Apparently these substituents jut out of the main plane of the cephalosporin nucleus, and produce significant steric hindrance at the entrance of the pore (YOSHIMURA and NIKAIDO 1985).

3. Effect of Charge

The OmpF and OmpC porin channels prefer cations as shown by black lipid film experiment (reviewed in BENZ 1985) or by liposome swelling experiments (NIKAIDO and ROSENBERG 1983). This is also clearly seen with β-lactams, zwitterionic compounds diffusing more rapidly, and dianionic compounds more slowly, than monoanionic ones (Table 1; Fig. 2). Moreover the effect of charge may become further magnified in intact cells because of the presence of Donnan potential across the outer membrane (see Sect. C.II).

II. Permeation Rate and Efficacy in *E. coli*

1. The β-Lactamase Barrier

Even when the β-lactam molecule successfully penetrates through the outer membrane barrier, it may get degraded by the periplasmic β-lactamase before it reaches the target, penicillin-binding proteins. Practically every gram-negative bacteria seems to produce endogenous, presumably chromosomally coded β-lactamase (class C enzyme of AMBLER 1980; SYKES and MATTHEW 1976), and many resistant strains contain plasmids that code for class A enzymes, represented by the TEM enzyme. The properties of various β-lactamases have been studied extensively, but a few pertinent points must be emphasized here.

(a) Because the affinity of various β-lactam substrates toward the enzymes can be very different, with *Km* values ranging from less than 0.05 μ*M* to more than 30000 μ*M*, reports of activities determined at a single substrate concentration do not indicate the real specificity of the enzyme, especially in view of the importance of the activity at low concentrations (see below).

(b) Assays are usually carried out at substrate concentrations of 0.1 m*M* or higher. However, penicillin-binding proteins are irreversibly inactivated by very low concentrations of β-lactams (Frère and Joris 1985). We may assume, as a first approximation, that such concentrations are close to the I_{50}, or the concentration that inhibits, by 50%, the binding of the penicillin G to one of the "essential" penicillin-binding proteins, i.e. 1B, 2, and 3. This assumption is justified by the observation that the lowest I_{50} value among these three (c_{inh} of Table 2) usually corresponds rather well with the MIC of that particular β-lactam with mutants defective either in the outer membrane barrier (Curtis et al. 1979) or in the β-lactamase barrier (Nikaido and Normark 1987). The values of c_{inh} are usually in the range of 0.1–6 μ*M* (Curtis et al. 1979) (see also Table 2), and the behavior of β-lactamase at these low substrate concentrations is extremely important (Livermore 1983; Vu and Nikaido 1985), because the bacteria will have been killed a long time ago if the periplasmic concentration rises to levels much higher than c_{inh}.

2. The Synergism Between the Two Barriers

Because the β-lactam molecules must pass through the outer membrane barrier and the β-lactamase barrier in succession, the effects of these barriers must be synergistic. If we consider the probability of any β lactam molecule reaching the

Table 2. Target access index in several *E. coli* strains[a]

	Perm. coeff.	c_{inh}	Target access index (TAI)[b] in strains producing				
			Chromosomal (AmpC) enzyme[c]				TEM enzyme
			SN03	LA5	LA51	TE18	JF701(R_{471a})
	(nm/s)	(μ*M*)					
Penicillin G	20	3	0.2	0.02	0.0008	0.0002	0.00006
Ampicillin	980	2	67	5.5	0.23	0.053	0.001
Cephalothin	110	2	1.6	0.13	0.005	0.001	0.028
Cephaloridine	3570	6	850	70	2.9	0.67	0.26
Cefazolin	620	10	215	17.5	0.73	0.17	0.26
Cefoxitin	370	10	3460	281	11.8	2.71	270
Cefotaxime	180	0.1	120	9.7	0.4	0.09	5.7
Ceftazidime	96	0.1	690	56	2.4	0.54	55.2
Azthreonam	33	0.1	920	75	3.1	0.72	10

[a] The data in this table are from Nikaido and Normark (1987)
[b] Target access index, reflecting the probability of β-lactam molecule reaching the target without getting hydrolyzed. See text for definition
[c] LA5 was the wild type strain, whereas LA51 and TE18 overproduced the chromosomal enzyme to different extents. SN03 was an underproducer

target at the far end of the periplasm, this should then be proportional to the product of the probability of passage across the outer membrane and the probability of diffusing unhydrolyzed through the periplasm. We recently defined an index, target access index (TAI), which reflects the probability mentioned above (NIKAIDO and NORMARK 1987):

$$TAI = (P \cdot A) \cdot [V_{max}/(Km + c_{inh})]^{-1} \qquad (3)$$

Clearly the first term $(P \cdot A)$ reflects the probability of passage through the outer membrane, and the second term $[V_{max}/(Km + c_{inh})]^{-1}$ is inversely related to the rate of hydrolysis at the β-lactam concentration just sufficient to inhibit the target, i.e. c_{inh}. [Our definition of TAI was aided greatly by the theoretical treatment proposed by WALEY (1987) in order to analyze the interaction between the outer membrane barrier and β-lactamase-catalyzed degradation].

Target access index allows one to predict MICs in any organism, as long as one knows how permeable the outer membrane is to the drug, and how sensitive the drug is to the β-lactamase. We assume that the cells will be killed when the steady state concentration of the drug in the periplasm reaches c_{inh}, and that at steady state the net influx across the outer membrane is balanced by the hydrolytic degradation in the periplasm (see Sect. C.I). Then the external concentration of the drug that will bring about this situation, i.e. the MIC, can be predicted by a simple equation derived from Zimmermann-Rosselet Eq. 1 and 2 (NIKAIDO and NORMARK 1987):

$$MIC = (TAI^{-1} + 1)\, c_{inh}\,. \qquad (4)$$

Calculation of this type was carried out for five strains of *E. coli* producing widely different levels of two types of β-lactamases, for 13 different β-lactams (NIKAIDO and NORMARK 1987). In $5 \times 13 = 65$ such predictive attempts, the predicted MIC values were within plus-minus 1 tube of the value obtained in serial twofold dilution assay in 44 cases. Furthermore, two compounds, cefsulodin and carbenicillin, consistently gave observed MICs that are widely different from the predicted ones, and we suspect that some of the parameters used for these compounds must be in error. If we exclude these two compounds, the rate of success of this quantitative MIC prediction approach was 43/55, i.e. 78%. These results suggest that the theoretical model is a correct one, and further indicate that the data used in the calculation, such as the kinetic parameters of the enzymes and c_{inh} values, were not far off.

Target access index reflects the probability with which β-lactam molecules reach the target, given the presence of the two successive barriers. However, sometimes we would like to know the relative importance of each of the barriers. We can get an appreciation of this by calculating how effective each of the barriers will be in the absence of the other. When we have only the outer membrane barrier, the decrease in the periplasmic concentration will occur mainly by the dilution due to the increase in cellular volume during growth. Analysis of the β-lactamase only situation can be carried out by assuming that the β-lactamase molecules would exist at exactly the same location as in the real cell but the cell would be totally devoid of the outer membrane barrier. These theoretical analyses (NIKAIDO and GEHRING 1987) led to the predictions shown in Table 3, indicating that

Table 3. Calculated steady-state β-lactam concentration at the target under various conditions

	C at target (μg/ml)
JF701(R_{471a}) (producing TEM enzyme) in 4096 μg/ml penicillin G:	
With both barriers (real cell)	0.8
With no outer membrane (hypothetical)	4013
With no β-lactamase barrier (hypothetical)	4092
TE18 (chromosomal enzyme overproducer) in 1024 μg/ml cephalothin:	
With both barriers (real cell)	1
With no outer membrane (hypothetical)	1020
With no β-lactamase barrier (hypothetical)	1024

each of the barriers alone is nearly completely useless, and that the synergism between the two is absolutely necessary for the production of an effective barrier. Thus although it is possible to evaluate each of the barriers in a quantitative manner (NIKAIDO and GEHRING 1987), such an analysis does not seem to contribute much toward our understanding of the resistance of gram-negative bacteria. Similarly, although either the outer membrane or the β-lactamase barrier can act as a "limiting step" in determining the *flux* of β-lactams, there is no such limiting step when we consider the *steady-state concentration* of β-lactam at the target, increases in the outer membrane permeability for a drug being as effective as increases in its β-lactamase resistance in improving its overall access to the target, and therefore its efficacy, as seen from Eq. 3.

3. The Effect of Loss of Porins on β-Lactam Susceptibility

Decrease in outer membrane permeability (P) caused by the physiological repression or mutational loss of porin(s) should increase the MICs for β-lactams. However, the quantitative relationship between the two is complex. First, the portion of the outer membrane other than the porin channels, including the bilayer region, must allow a slow penetration of any solutes (see also Sect. F), and this "baseline" or "leakage" permeability can become more significant for compounds with very low permeability through porins, or in organisms with a porin pathway of generally low permeability, such as *P. aeruginosa* (Sect. D.IV). Second, although a decrease in permeability decreases TAI according to Eq. 3, a decrease in TAI does not always produce large changes in the resistance level. This is due to the form of Eq. 4. When the TAI is much larger than 1, then even severalfold changes in the values of P and therefore of TAI are unlikely to produce more than minimal changes of MIC. In contrast, very large changes of MIC accompany the alterations of P when TAI is much smaller than 1.

In Table 4, we calculated expected changes in MIC by assuming that the "porin-deficient" mutants have lost 99.9% of the porin molecules present in the parent strain. The observed changes in MICs are fairly similar to those predicted,

Table 4. Predicted and observed changes in MIC in "porin-deficient" mutants of *E. coli*[a]

β-Lactam	MIC (porinless strain)/MIC (wild type)					
	Observed				Predicted[b]	
	A	B	C	D	Without "leakage"	With "leakage"
Cephaloridine	16	8	16	8	8	7
Cefazolin	8	8	16	16	28	7
Cephalothin	ND	8	32	16	442	21
Penicillin G	2	ND	ND	2	490	5
Cefotaxime	ND	2	2	ND	48	4
Azthreonam	ND	2	4	ND	8	1

[a] This table shows the extent of increase of MIC observed in porinless (OmpF-OmpC-) mutants of *E. coli*. Sources of observed values are: A, HARDER et al. (1981); B, JAFFÉ et al. (1983); C, CURTIS et al. (1985); and D, SAWAI et al. (1982). ND stands for "not determined"
[b] Predicted change in MIC was calculated from TAI values according to equation [4], by assuming that the porin content decreases to 0.1% of that in the wild type strain. This is not an unreasonable assumption because one of the less leaky porin mutants we studied (BAVOIL et al. 1977) contained less than 1% of the amount present in the wild type. The column on the left ("without leakage") lists values obtained by using permeability coefficients of the porin channels alone (NIKAIDO and NORMARK 1987). The column on the right lists values obtained by assuming that "leakage" corresponding to the permeability coefficient of 0.5×10^{-6} cm s^{-1} (i.e. approximately 5% of the rate of diffusion of cephalothin through the porin channels) occurs for all compounds in both the wild type and the mutant strain

if the presence of the non-porin "leakage" pathway is assumed. The absence of a large increase in the MIC for penicillin G becomes understandable as a result of leakage. The relative contribution of leakage is expected to be significant because penicillin G penetrates only very slowly through porin channels. The MICs for cefotaxime and azthreonam do not increase much either, but in part because of a different reason. Since their TAI values are much larger than 1 in the parent strain, decreases in TAI do not produce a proportionately large effect on the MICs, as expected from theoretical considerations described above.

4. Can "Trapping" Produce Significant Resistance?

When it was discovered that overproduction of chromosomally coded β-lactamase made strains of *Enterobacter*, *Serratia*, and *Pseudomonas* highly resistant to a wide range of expanded spectrum β-lactams, it was proposed that the resistance was due to the non-hydrolytic binding (or "trapping") of the drug molecules by the enzymes (e.g. SANDERS 1983). This proposal was made largely because at that time the significance of β-lactamase activity at low substrate concentrations was not appreciated, and because it was mistakenly believed that most expanded spectrum β-lactams were absolutely resistant to hydrolysis by commonly found enzymes. Quantitative analysis (VU and NIKAIDO 1985; NIKAIDO 1985) showed that trapping alone can produce only extremely low levels of resistance, whereas the hydrolysis kinetics by the enzyme can largely explain the high level of resistance observed, at least for *E. cloacae*.

III. Outer Membrane Permeability in Other Enteric Bacteria

Salmonella typhimurium LT2 produces three porins in ordinary laboratory media, OmpF, OmpC, and OmpD. Our recent study with OmpF and OmpC porins from a clinical isolate showed that OmpF produced a larger channel than OmpC (MEDEIROS et al. 1987), a situation similar to *E. coli*. The properties of the OmpD channel have not yet been properly investigated.

Enterobacter cloacae strain 206 was reported to produce two porin species, 37K and "39K–40K" (SAWAI et al. 1982). Swelling assays with reconstituted liposomes showed 39K–40K porin(s) produced a larger channel with the estimated diameter of 1.6 nm, whereas the 37K porin produced a channel of 1.2 nm (KANEKO et al. 1984). However, this strain was apparently *K. pneumoniae*, rather than *E. cloacae* (SAWAI et al. 1987).

Our recent studies with several true *E. cloacae* strains produced results different from the data of the Sawai group (OYA and NIKAIDO, to be published). Our data suggest the presence of three porin species. The fastest migrating one seems to be OmpF, because its synthesis is repressed in high osmolality media. The bands with intermediate and the lowest mobility probably correspond to OmpD and OmpC, respectively, on the basis of their response to catabolite and salt repression. In contrast to the results of KANEKO et al. (1984), liposome swelling experiments showed that the OmpF or 37K protein produced a much wider pore than 40K or OmpC. When grown in low osmolality media, OmpF was largely responsible for influx of β-lactams, which took place at rates comparable to that in *E. coli*. When the cells were grown in high osmolality media, OmpF production was totally repressed, yet unlike in *E. coli* the synthesis of OmpC porin was not drastically increased. This may explain the observed low outer membrane permeability of *E. cloacae*, grown in a high osmolality medium (VU and NIKAIDO 1985).

Porin-deficient mutants of *K. pneumoniae* and *E. cloacae* show moderate resistance to cephalosporins and to some other antibiotics, as expected (SAWAI et al. 1982; WERNER et al. 1985; THEN and ANGEHRN 1986). One of the mutants of the latter authors may have a deep-rough defect in lipopolysaccharide because it is hypersusceptible to hydrophobic agents.

GOLDSTEIN et al. (1983) reported that treatment of a patient with *Serratia marcescens* bacteremia with cefotaxime and amikacin resulted in the emergence of resistant mutants with severely decreased levels of a major outer membrane protein with the size expected for porins (41 kilodaltons). Altered protein pattern was detected in similar clinical isolates by TRAUB and BAUER (1987). Furthermore, GUTMANN and CHABBERT (1984) found similar outer membrane alterations in resistant mutants of *Serratia marcescens* isolated from a patient receiving moxalactam therapy. Although the altered proteins have not yet been rigorously characterized, they are very likely to be the major porin(s) in this species.

Species belonging to *Proteus*, *Morganella*, and *Providencia* apparently produce only one major porin species, and mutants lacking these major porin species were isolated by using their low level resistance to cefoxitin (MITSUYAMA et al. 1987).

IV. Outer Membrane Permeability in *P. aeruginosa* and Other "Intrinsically Resistant" Organisms

It has been suspected for a long time that the intrinsic resistance of *P. aeruginosa* was largely due to the poor permeability of its outer membrane, but it was only in recent years that this hypothesis was confirmed by direct experimental results (reviewed in NIKAIDO and HANCOCK 1986). Briefly, ANGUS et al. (1982) found that the outer membrane permeability for nitrocefin, measured by the Zimmermann-Rosselet method (Sect. C.I), was two orders of magnitude lower than the permeability of *E. coli* outer membrane to other β-lactams. Direct comparison us-

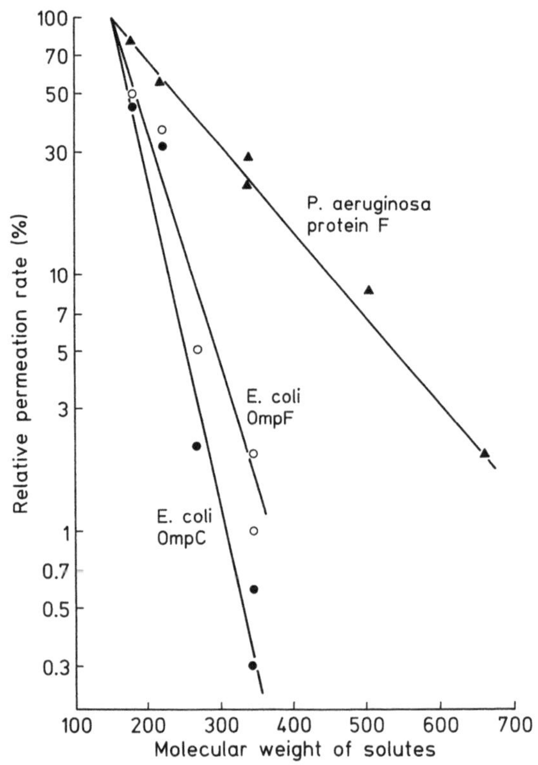

Fig. 3. Rates of penetration of various sugars through porin channels. *E. coli* OmpF (○), *E. coli* OmpC (●), and *P. aeruginosa* F (▲) porins were used in reconstitution of liposomes. The rates are expressed as percentage of the rate of penetration of L-arabinose. The sugars used are: M_r 180 (D-glucose), 221 (*N*-acetyl-D-glucosamine), 262 (2,3-diacetamido-2,3-dideoxy-D-glucose), 342 (sucrose and lactose), 504 (raffinose), and 666 (stachyose). The data were taken from NIKAIDO and ROSENBERG (1983) and YOSHIMURA et al. (1983)

ing cephacetrile and cephaloridine showed permeability coefficients of around 10^{-6} cm/s in *P. aeruginosa* (YOSHIMURA and NIKAIDO 1982), 100- to 500-fold lower than the values for *E. coli* (NIKAIDO et al. 1983). Permeability to glucose 6-phosphate and *p*-nitrophenylphosphate was also at least 100-fold lower than that of *E. coli* (YOSHIMURA and NIKAIDO 1982).

Search for proteins with porin activity in reconstituted systems led to the identification of the major porin, protein F (HANCOCK et al. 1979; YOSHIMURA et al. 1983). Its large channel size (estimated diameter: 2 nm) at first appeared incompatible with the low permeability coefficient of the outer membrane. However, reconstitution with purified porin produced very low permeability both in black lipid systems (BENZ and HANCOCK 1981) and liposomes (YOSHIMURA et al. 1983), and it was proposed that only a small fraction of the porin molecules form open channels. More recently, this hypothesis was proven to be true in black lipid film experiments, in which the majority of porins was confirmed to produce extremely small step increase in conductance (WOODRUFF et al. 1986); thus most of the porin channels are "closed" or nonfunctional in the physiological context, yet are not completely closed physically. The major role of protein F in β-lactam penetration was confirmed by a sixfold decrease in nitrocefin permeability in a mutant lacking protein F (NICAS and HANCOCK 1983).

Recently, however, these conclusions were questioned by two laboratories. CAULCOTT et al. (1984) concluded, from study of the efflux of radiolabeled sugars from the periplasm of intact cells, that disaccharides are the largest molecules that could penetrate through porin channel. YONEYAMA et al. (1986) and YONEYAMA and NAKAE (1986) concluded, mainly on the basis of the extent of penetration of solutes into periplasmic space, that only the solutes of the size of monosaccharides or smaller could rapidly penetrate through the porin channel. These studies unfortunately suffer from the lack of appreciation of the effect of solute size on penetration *rates*. As seen in Fig. 3, larger solutes penetrate more slowly than smaller solutes even when the channel diameter is relatively large. Thus it is expected that, when the extent of penetration into the periplasm is determined after a fixed period of incubation, smaller compounds would have penetrated more extensively than larger solutes.[1] Furthermore, unbiased plotting of the data in Fig. 3 of YONEYAMA and NAKAE (1986) shows that sugars larger than disaccharides are indeed penetrating into the periplasm, and Fig. 2 of YONEYAMA et al. (1986) shows also very significant penetration of large sugars into the periplasm. Thus smaller solutes may penetrate more efficiently because of the inherent property of the F porin channel, and possibly because of the involvement of minor channels (for example the D1 channel, see Sect. F), but the results so far do not seem to justify their conclusion that even disaccharides cannot penetrate through the *P. aeruginosa* outer membrane.

Because the F channel is large, the diffusion rates of solutes are affected somewhat less severely by small changes in their size, hydrophobicity, etc. Thus in

[1] Since YONEYAMA and NAKAE (1986) acknowledge the "generous comments" from the present author, it may appear unethical for him to criticize the paper after its publication. It should be stated here that the manuscript of this paper was not made available to the present author in spite of his request, so that he was unable to comment on this paper before its publication.

E. coli, a relatively hydrophobic compound, nitrocefin, penetrates four times more slowly than cephacetrile, yet in *P. aeruginosa* there is only 30% difference between the penetration rates of these two compounds (HELLMAN and NIKAIDO, unpublished data). This apparent indifference to the structural details of the solute is another strong piece of evidence that a large channel is responsible for the penetration of most β-lactams and probably most other antibiotics.

Because of the low permeability of the F porin channel, any other mechanism of penetration tends to acquire a large relative significance in *P. aeruginosa*. These "non-porin" pathways will be described in Sect. F.

It seems likely that other "intrinsically resistant" gram-negative bacteria also produce outer membranes of low general permeability. In some of these organisms, porins with exceptionally narrow channel diameters have been found. *Alcaligenes faecalis* and *Sphaerotilus natans* were found to produce porins that barely allow the passage of pentoses (ZALMAN 1982). The results on *A. faecalis* agree with recent independent study by ISHII and NAKAE (1988). Black lipid film reconstitution has shown that *Pseudomonas cepacia* also produces a porin with a very narrow channel (PARR et al. 1987). Although the narrowness of these channels is consistent with the antibiotic resistance of these organisms, it is not yet clear how larger solutes (such as sugars) penetrate their outer membrane.

V. Gram-Negative Bacteria with Very High Sensitivity to β-Lactams

Some gram-negative bacteria show very high sensitivity to β-lactams. For example, *Rhodobacter capsulatum* strains are reported to have MICs of 0.006–0.06 μg/ml for benzylpenicillin (WEAVER et al. 1975). Although it is tempting to attribute this to a large (1.6 nm diameter) size of the porin channel of this organism (FLAMMANN and WECKESSER 1984), a related species, *R. sphaeroides*, shows an MIC of 60 μg/ml in spite of the presence of only slightly smaller porin channels (1.3 nm diameter) (WECKESSER et al. 1984). Possibly the activity of β-lactamase plays a more important role in determining the susceptibility of these organisms (see Sect. D.II).

Some strains of *Haemophilus influenzae* are also very sensitive to penicillin G, with MICs as low as 0.06 μg/ml (COULTON et al. 1983). Outer membrane permeability for penicillin G, measured by the Zimmermann-Rosselet method, was at least tenfold higher than that of *E. coli* (COULTON et al. 1983), and the diameter of the porin channel appeared to be much larger than that of *E. coli* (VACHON et al. 1985).

Neisseria gonorrhoeae is also very sensitive to benzylpenicillin, and MICs were between 0.002 and 0.02 μg/ml when the agent was first introduced (SPARLING 1977). The anion preference of the porin channel (YOUNG et al. 1983) may accelerate the diffusion of most β-lactams, and possibly the lipid bilayer region of the outer membrane is more permeable in this species. However, again the low level of endogenous β-lactamase (SPARLING 1977; SYKES and MATTHEW 1976) may be even more important. Mutations that appear to affect the lipid bilayer region of the outer membrane of this organism will be discussed in Sect. F.

E. Permeation of Some Other Agents Through Porin Channels

Common tetracycline derivatives and chloramphenicol are assumed to cross the outer membrane mostly via porin channels, because porin-deficient mutants are slightly more resistant to these compounds (PUGSLEY and SCHNAITMAN 1978). "Deep rough" lipopolysaccharide mutants, with their increased permeability of the lipid bilayer region (NIKAIDO 1976), also show increased resistance to these compounds, suggesting that they utilize the porin channels which are produced in smaller numbers in these mutants (SMIT et al. 1975). Increased hydrophobicity of tetracycline derivatives resulted in decreased efficacy against wild type *E. coli*, but not against deep rough mutants, suggesting again that tetracyclines mainly utilize the porin channel at least in wild type cells (LEIVE et al. 1984). However, an extremely hydrophobic tetracycline derivative minocycline may utilize the lipid bilayer part of the outer membrane for penetration, because it appears to diffuse across the outer membrane quite rapidly in spite of its hydrophobicity, and because absence of OmpF porin does not increase the resistance of *E. coli* to this compound (MCMURRY et al. 1982).

Many of the chloramphenicol-resistant mutants isolated in the laboratory belong to the porin-deficient class, as shown by the fact that one of the "classical" chloramphenicol-resistant mutant class in *E. coli*, *cmlB*, turned out to be mutants in the structural gene of the wider channel porin OmpF (REEVE and DOUGHERTY 1968). BURNS et al. (1985) described a chloramphenicol-resistant clinical isolate of *Haemophilus influenzae* lacking an 40,000 dalton outer membrane protein, which corresponds in its size to the protein identified as porin by COULTON et al. (1985).

An *E. coli* K12 mutant lacking the OmpF porin was shown to be more resistant to most quinolone compounds (HIRAI et al. 1986a), although no such resistance was found for another "porin-deficient" mutant (PIDDOCK and WISE 1986). The passage of these compounds through the porin channels seems reasonable, because they are rather hydrophilic (ASHBY et al. 1985; HIRAI et al. 1986a). Many mutants resistant to new quinolones are also moderately more resistant to other agents such as β-lactams, chloramphenicol, and trimethoprim (SANDERS et al. 1984; GUTMANN et al. 1985; MOUTON and MULDERS 1987), and at least some of them appear to lack porin as judged by the pattern of outer membrane proteins (SANDERS et al. 1984; GUTMANN et al. 1985). In some cases the missing protein was identified as the OmpF porin (HOOPER et al. 1986; HIRAI et al. 1986b). However, the situation may be rather complicated here, because HIRAI et al. (1986b) found that the mutation maps near *marA* (GEORGE and LEVY 1983), a gene that produces a pleiotropic resistance to several antibiotics.

Recently PIDDOCK et al. (1987) reported on the emergence of *P. aeruginosa* mutant in a patient treated with enoxacin. It showed increased resistance to not only quinolones but also a wide range of β-lactams, and produced only undetectable levels of porin F.

Aminoglycosides also seem to use the porin channel in enteric bacteria, and these agents will be discussed in Sect. G.

F. Contribution of Non-porin Pathways

Although the lipid bilayer region of the enterobacterial outer membrane shows very low permeability toward hydrophobic solutes (Sect. B.I), this does not mean that the bilayer is totally impermeable. Thus the permeation through the bilayer can become significant especially for agents that are unable to use the porin pathway, or for agents that are not degraded or inactivated rapidly once they cross the outer membrane. In fact we saw that the penetration of β-lactams could not be explained fully unless we hypothesized the existence of non-porin "leakage" pathway (Sect. D.II.3), which can at least partially correspond to the passage through the bilayer.

Under certain conditions the diffusion through the lipid bilayer region can become accelerated. Glycerophospholipid bilayers are generated in "deep rough" lipopolysaccharide mutants or in wild type cells treated with EDTA, and this explains the enhanced permeability of the outer membrane toward hydrophobic agents (Sect. B.I). In addition, there are many mutations that produce lipophile-permeable outer membrane in enteric organisms, via poorly understood mechanisms. These include the *acrA*, *envA*, and *tolC* mutations, as well as the mutation(s) present in the widely used antibiotic-hypersensitive *E. coli* mutants DC2 and DC3 of RICHMOND et al. (1976) (see NIKAIDO and VAARA 1985 for review). An antibiotic hypersensitive mutant of *Pseudomonas aeruginosa* was once believed to be altered in the permeability of porin channel (see below) as a result of alteration in the structure of lipopolysaccharide (ANGUS et al. 1982), but this now seems unlikely because the *P. aeruginosa* porin synthesized in the presence of *E. coli* lipopolysaccharide was fully functional (WOODRUFF et al. 1986). GODFREY et al. (1984) described mutants of *P. aeruginosa* that are altered in their lipopolysaccharide and are more resistant to β-lactams. If we assume that the permeability of the porin channels is not affected by the lipopolysaccharides, this observation suggests that a significant fraction of β-lactam molecules penetrates through the lipopolysaccharide/phospholipid bilayer region in the wild type organisms.

Recently CHAPMAN and GEORGOPAPADAKOU (1988) showed that Mg^{2+} strongly inhibits the uptake of some quinolones, and that quinolones perturbed the organization of the lipid bilayer region of the outer membrane most probably by chelating Mg^{2+} and Ca^{2+} in the membrane. They suggest that quinolones, especially hydrophobic quinolones, also penetrate the outer membrane by utilizing this second pathway, i.e. by disorganizing the lipid bilayer region and then by dissolving into the interior of the newly created phospholipid bilayer patches.

MANESS and SPARLING (1973) showed, among various gonococcal isolates, that there was a good correlation between the resistance to benzylpenicillin and that to other hydrophobic antibiotics and dyes. Genetic analysis led to the discovery that resistance was conferred by two mutations, *mtr* and *penB*, and that another mutation, *env*, made the strains hypersensitive (SPARLING 1977). Furthermore, these mutations were shown to affect the outer membrane permeability by a direct assay of crystal violet penetration (GUYMON and SPARLING 1975). Although the molecular mechanisms that alter the outer membrane permeability in these mutants are not understood, the *mtr* mutants contain an extra protein in the outer membrane (GUYMON et al. 1978), and *env* mutants are reported to have an increased phospholipid/protein ratio in this membrane (LYSKO and MORSE 1981). Thus considered together with the phenotype of these mutants, it seems likely that these mutations affect the structure of the lipopolysaccharide/phospholipid bilayer.

There are antibiotics that utilize specific diffusion pathways (Sect. B.III) for crossing the outer membrane. First, there are antibiotics intentionally designed to utilize these pathways, for example cephalosporins containing catechol or similar substituents for diffusion through the iron-chelator pathways (KATSU et al. 1982; BREUER et al. 1985; OHI et al. 1986). One of these compounds was shown to be much less effective in *tonB* mutants, which are defective in siderophore transport, a result confirming the utilization of the siderophore pathways in the uptake of these β-lactam compounds (WATANABE et al. 1987). As expected, utilization of this non-porin pathway of diffusion makes these compounds especially effective against *P. aeruginosa*, in which the major porin pathway is very inefficient. Second, some antibiotics may be able to use specific pathways presumably because they can fortuitously take conformations that allow them to bind to the binding site of the channel. Again this will become significant especially in such organisms as *P. aeruginosa*. QUINN et al. (1986) showed that several clinical isolates of *P. aeruginosa*, which are moderately resistant to imipenem but not to other β-lactams, lacked an outer membrane protein of apparent molecular weight 45000. The β-lactamase activity and the penicillin-binding proteins were unaltered. Similar mutants were isolated in the laboratory by BÜSCHER et al. (1987), who suggested, on the basis of the electrophoretic mobility of the outer membrane protein found to be missing in the mutants, that it may be protein D1, which was earlier suggested to function as a glucose channel (HANCOCK and CAREY 1980), or protein D2. We have confirmed that D1 indeed produces a glucose-specific channel. Although the purified protein allows the diffusion of imipenem, the activity of this protein may not be enough to explain the imipenem resistance of the mutants (TRIAS et al. 1988).

Finally, some outer membrane proteins other than the major porin species have been implicated in the diffusion of antibiotics and chemotherapeutic agents. HIRAI et al. (1987) showed that one class of norfloxacin-resistant mutants of *P. aeruginosa* contained one additional outer membrane protein of apparently 54000 daltons. The mutant showed a slower rate of uptake of norfloxacin, but it is not yet clear how the presence of a new protein can decrease the influx of this drug. BURNS et al. (1986) cloned the chloramphenicol resistance gene from transposon Tn*1696*. This gene is expressed in *E. coli*, and decreases the influx of chloramphenicol without inactivating it enzymatically. It was also found to decrease the amount of a minor outer membrane protein of 50000 daltons. Since chloramphenicol appears to penetrate mainly through the major porin channel in *E. coli*, it is unexpected that the loss of another minor protein could have a major effect on its diffusion, and this interesting finding seems to warrant further study.

G. Outer Membrane Permeability to Polycationic Agents

I. Polymyxin and Related Antibiotics

Polymyxin B is a cyclic peptide antibiotic with a fatty acid "tail" and with five positively charged groups (STORM et al. 1977). Its ultimate lethal target is thought to be the cytoplasmic membrane, but it has to traverse the outer membrane before it reaches this target. It is too large to go through the narrow porin channels of enteric bacteria, but apparently it can cross the outer membrane by disorganizing and disrupting it. Thus polymyxin binds to the outer membrane (TEUBER and BADER 1976), causes electron microscopically visible alterations in this membrane (LOUNATMAA et al. 1976), and disrupts the outer membrane barrier as judged by increased permeability to hydrophobic antibiotics (ROSENTHAL and STORM 1977) and lysozyme (TEUBER 1970).

Genetic studies of polymyxin-resistant, *pmrA*, mutants of *S. typhimurium* confirmed the notion that polymyxin acts first by binding to and disorganizing the outer membrane. Such mutants are altered in their lipopolysaccharide, which contains four- to sixfold larger amounts of a cationic component, 4-aminoarabinose, than the wild type lipopolysaccharide (VAARA et al. 1981). This makes the lipopolysaccharide less anionic, and decreases the binding of polycationic polymyxin B to the outer membrane.

VAARA and VAARA (1983a, b) studied the action of hydrophilic polycationic agents upon gram-negative bacteria, and showed that both a oligolysine (Lys_{20}) and "polymyxin B nonapeptide" (PMBN, polymyxin B from which the N-terminal diaminobutyric acid residue was removed together with the fatty acid tail) had little antibacterial activity by itself yet made *E. coli* and *S. typhimurium* cells much more sensitive to hydrophobic antibiotics such as novobiocin, fusidic acid, erythromycin, rifampin, and actinomycin D. It appears that binding of PMBN expands the molecular area occupied by lipopolysaccharide, thereby increasing the permeability of the lipopolysaccharide monolayer half of the outer membrane, whereas Lys_{20} acts mainly by releasing lipopolysaccharide molecules from the outer membrane (VAARA and VAARA 1983b).

As was discussed earlier, the intrinsic resistance of *P. aeruginosa* to most antibiotics is due to the low permeability of its outer membrane (Sect. D.IV). Polymyxin is effective against this organism, presumably because it uses a disruptive mechanism to cross the outer membrane. Low-level polymyxin-resistant mutants of *P. aeruginosa* were found to overproduce an outer membrane protein H1 (NICAS and HANCOCK 1980). This protein is also overproduced by wild type cells under conditions of Mg^{2+} starvation. Since the mutant outer membrane contained lower amounts of Mg^{2+} than that of the wild type, it was suggested that H1 substitutes for Mg^{2+} in the mutant outer membrane, thereby making it more difficult for polymyxin to bind to the lipopolysaccharides by displacing the Mg^{2+} ions. These results suggest that different organisms use different strategies in order to develop resistance against polymyxin. Since the *P. aeruginosa* lipopolysaccharide is known to contain much larger amounts of phosphate residues than that of *Enterobacteriaceae* (NIKAIDO and HANCOCK 1986), it may be that significantly decreasing the net negative charge of lipopolysaccharide is not possible without the complete disruption of the architecture of the outer membrane. *P.*

aeruginosa can also be "adapted" to grow in very high concentrations (about 1 mg/ml or higher) of polymyxin, but alterations in such strains are very complex and difficult to analyze. Interestingly, one of the changes often encountered appears to be the loss of porin (GILLELAND and LYLE 1979).

II. Aminoglycosides

1. *E. coli* and Other Enteric Bacteria

Porin channels of *E. coli* and probably most other members of *Enterobacteriaceae* have such narrow diameters that we can barely show the penetration of neutral trisaccharides through them (DECAD and NIKAIDO 1976). Many aminoglycosides are equivalent to trisaccharides in size, but they should diffuse through the porin channels quite rapidly when one considers that porin channels prefer cations, and that the penetration rates of aminoglycosides, with three or more positive charges, will be speeded up 100-fold or more by the presence of Donnan potential alone (Sect. C.II; see also NICHOLS et al. 1985; SEN et al. 1988). A few aminoglycosides are larger, up to the pentasaccharide size of lividomycin A, yet it seems likely that they penetrate through the porin channels because these molecules are flexible.

The inhibition of aminoglycoside action by salts in the medium was described in 1943 (FOSTER and WOODRUFF 1943), and since then has been "rediscovered" by numerous investigators. PLOTZ et al. (1961) showed that the inhibition was due to decreased uptake of aminoglycosides. In a thorough study, DONOVICK et al. (1948) established that divalent cations (Ba^{2+}, Mg^{2+}, Ca^{2+}) were far more inhibitory than monovalent cations, and that multivalent anions (phosphate, tartrate, citrate, and sulfate) were more inhibitory than monovalent anions such as nitrate and chloride. Since both multivalent cations and multivalent anions are more effective in collapsing Donnan potential than are monovalent cations and anions (Sect. C.II; SEN et al. 1987), we can hypothesize that the "salt effect" is mainly due to the collapse of Donnan potential which will lead to decreased penetration rates and decreased equilibrium concentration of the drug in the periplasm.

Porin-deficient mutants do not usually show significantly increased resistance to aminoglycosides (PUGSLEY and SCHNAITMAN 1978), although one report showed that the loss of the wider channel porin OmpF made *E. coli* more resistant to kanamycin and gentamicin (FOULDS and CHAI 1978). The absence of a large effect is understandable because the values of TAI (Sect. D.II.2) will be very large for aminoglycosides in wild-type strains as a consequence of the presumed high rate of permeation and the virtual absence of inactivating mechanism in the periplasm; as emphasized in Sect. D.II.3, the absence of effect on MIC cannot be taken as the evidence that aminoglycosides utilize nonporin pathways for crossing the outer membrane.

2. *P. aeruginosa*

In spite of the very low permeability of *P. aeruginosa* outer membrane, some aminoglycoside antibiotics are quite effective against this organism. HANCOCK et al.

(1981) proposed that this is due to the binding of aminoglycoside to the highly negatively charged lipopolysaccharides of the outer membrane, resulting in the disorganization and disruption of outer membrane barrier, finally followed by the influx of the drug following the Donnan potential gradient, in a way similar to the permeation pathway of polymyxin B. In fact the treatment of *P. aeruginosa* with aminoglycosides permeabilizes the outer membrane for the influx of lysozyme (HANCOCK et al. 1981) and a hydrophobic fluorescent probe 1-*N*-phenylnaphthylamine (LOH et al. 1984). This hypothesis is also supported by the study of salt effect on aminoglycoside efficacy. As described earlier, with enteric bacteria the salt effect can be explained nearly completely by the collapse of Donnan potential. In contrast, the action of aminoglycosides on *P. aeruginosa* is inhibited specifically by low concentrations of divalent cations in addition to the general salt effect seen in enteric bacteria (MEDEIROS et al. 1971; BEGGS and ANDREWS 1976). Most probably divalent cations compete with aminoglycoside in binding to the lipopolysaccharide, a first step in aminoglycoside penetration in *P. aeruginosa*.

H. Conclusions

The rate of outer membrane penetration of various β-lactams may vary nearly one hundredfold, and this observation at first gives an impression that the permeability is not a major factor in determining the efficacy of the antibiotic. Yet theoretical analysis (Sect. D.II) shows that the outer membrane permeability is equally important as the resistance to enzymatic degradation (and the affinity to the target site) in all cases.

In fact the emergence of bacteria such as *P. aeruginosa* and *E. cloacae* as serious infectious agents in recent years owes much to the intrinsically low permeability of the outer membrane of these organisms. In contrast, acquired resistance in normally susceptible gram-negative bacteria has so far involved mostly the production of periplasmic β-lactamases, aminoglycoside- and chloramphenicol-modifying enzymes, tetracycline pump-out systems, etc. This is understandable because the decrease in outer membrane permeability will impair the ability of the organisms to accumulate nutrients. However, in recent years, the widespread use of antibiotics resistant to inactivation, such as the third-generation cephalosporins, semisynthetic aminoglycosides, and newer quinolones, appears to have initiated the selection of mutant bacterial strains with decreased porin content. It is difficult at present to assess the importance of the resistance of this type in clinical situations. However, we should note that such mutants are readily isolated in the laboratory (for example HARDER et al. 1981; JAFFE et al. 1982; SANDERS et al. 1984; GUTMANN et al. 1985; WERNER et al. 1985; GUTMANN et al. 1988). There is no reason to suspect that the occurrence of the mutants of this type is restricted to the laboratory, and such mutants were isolated during treatment of patients with β-lactams (GUTMANN and CHABBERT 1984; MEDEIROS et al. 1987), β-lactam/aminoglycoside combinations (GOLDSTEIN et al. 1983; SANDERS and WATANAKUNAKORN 1986), quinolones (AOYAMA et al. 1987; PIDDOCK et al. 1987), or presumably chloramphenicol (BURNS et al. 1985). We suspect that the relatively small number of reported porin-deficient strains of clinical origin is simply due to the fact that most clinical microbiology laboratories are not equipped to perform the analysis of outer membrane proteins. Interestingly, β-lactam therapy seems to select permeability mutants especially frequently in *Serratia marcescens* (GOLDSTEIN et al. 1983; GUTMANN et al. 1984; SANDERS and WATANAKUNAKORN 1986), probably because *Serratia* cannot survive the attack by third-generation cephalosporins through the overproduction of its chromosomal β-lactamase, which happens to be rather inefficient in hydrolyzing these agents (JORIS et al. 1986). If this reasoning is correct, "better" antibiotics and chemotherapeutic agents that are able to overcome most other resistance mechanisms are precisely those that are likely to select out the porin mutants, which unfortunately show a wide cross-resistance to a large number of agents.

Finally there is a possibility that decrease in porin content could be caused by some R plasmids. IYER et al. (1978) found that plasmid rRM98, when transferred into *E. coli* B/r, often caused the disappearance of the porin, although the molecular mechanisms involved are not clear. NAGAI and MITSUHASHI (1972) identified several R plasmids that caused chloramphenicol resistance in *E. coli* presumably through lowered permeability, although it is not clear whether the alteration involves the outer membrane or the cytoplasmic membrane.

It is often argued that decrease in outer membrane permeability is unlikely to occur because it will be deleterious for the survival of the mutants. However, gram-negative bacteria can survive well with a much fewer number of porin molecules than are normally present, provided that the environment contains high concentrations of nutrients (NIKAIDO and VAARA 1985), and in some mutants porins necessary for survival in nutrient-poor environments are left intact (MEDEIROS et al. 1987). Thus possibly the disadvantages of having porin mutations may not be exorbitantly high, in comparison with the extra "load" for making enormous amounts of β-lactamases.

References

Ambler RP (1980) The structure of β-lactamases. Philos Trans R Soc (Lond) [Biol] 289B:321–331

Angus BL, Carey AM, Canon DA, Kropinski AMB, Hancock REW (1982) Outer membrane permeability of *Pseudomonas aeruginosa*: comparison of a wild type with an antibiotic-supersusceptible mutant. Antimicrob Agents Chemother 21:299–308

Aoyama H, Sato K, Kato T, Hirai K, Mitsuhashi S (1987) Norfloxacin resistance in a clinical isolate of *Escherichia coli*. Antimicrob Agents Chemother 31:1640–1641

Ashby J, Piddock LJV, Wise R (1985) An investigation of the hydrophobicity of the quinolones. J Antimicrob Chemother 16:805–810

Bavoil P, Nikaido H, von Meyenburg K (1977) Pleiotropic transport mutants of *Escherichia coli* lack porin, a major outer membrane protein. Mol Gen Genet 158:23–33

Beggs WH, Andrews FA (1976) Role of ionic strength in salt antagonism of aminoglycoside action on *Escherichia coli* and *Pseudomonas aeruginosa*. J Infect Dis 134:500–504

Benz R (1985) Porin from bacterial and mitochondrial outer membranes. CRC Crit Rev Biochem 19:145–190

Benz R, Hancock REW (1981) Properties of the large ion-permeable pores formed from protein F of *Pseudomonas aeruginosa* in lipid bilayer membranes. Biochim Biophys Acta 646:298–308

Biagi GL, Guerra MC, Barbaro AM, Gamba MF (1970) Influence of lipophilic character on the antibacterial activity of cephalosporins and penicillins. J Med Chem 13:511–515

Bird AE, Nayler JHC (1971) Design of penicillins. In: Ariens EJ (ed) Drug design, vol 2. Academic, New York, pp 277–318

Breuer H, Bisacchi GS, Drossard JM, Ermann P, Koster WH, Kronenthal D, Kuester P et al. (1985) Structure-activity relationships among sulfonylaminocarbonyl activated monobactams leading to SQ 83,360 (Abstr). 25th Interscience Conference on Antimicrobial Agents Chemotherapy, Minneapolis

Burns JL, Mendelman PM, Levy J, Stull TL, Smith AL (1985) A permeability barrier as a mechanism of chloramphenicol resistance in *Haemophilus influenzae*. Antimicrob Agents Chemother 27:46–54

Burns JL, Rubens CE, Mendelman PM, Smith AL (1986) Cloning and expression in *Escherichia coli* of a gene encoding nonenzymatic chloramphenicol resistance from *Pseudomonas aeruginosa*. Antimicrob Agents Chemother 29:445–450

Büscher K-H, Cullman W, Dick W, Opferkuch W (1987) Imipenem resistance in *Pseudomonas aeruginosa* resulting from diminished expression of an outer membrane protein. Antimicrob Agents Chemother 31:703–708

Bush K, Tanaka SK, Bonner DP, Sykes RB (1985) Resistance caused by decreased penetration of β-lactam antibiotics into *Enterobacter cloacae*. Antimicrob Agents Chemother 27:555–560

Caulcott CA, Brown MRW, Gonda I (1984) Evidence for small pores in the outer membrane of *Pseudomonas aeruginosa*. FEMS Microbiol Lett 21:119–123

Chapman JS, Georgopapadakou NH (1988) Routes of quinolone permeation in *Escherichia coli*. Antimicrob Agents Chemother 32:438–442

Coulton JW, Mason P, Dorrance D (1983) The permeability barrier of *Haemophilus influenzae* type b against β-lactam antibiotics. J Antimicrob Chemother 12:435–449

Curtis NAC, Orr D, Ross GW, Boulton MG (1979) Affinities of penicillins and cephalosporins for the penicillin-binding proteins of *Escherichia coli* K-12 and their antibacterial activity. Antimicrob Agents Chemother 16:533–539

Curtis NAC, Eisenstadt RL, Turner KA, White AJ (1985) Porin-mediated cephalosporin resistance in *Escherichia coli* K-12. J Antimicrob Chemother 15:642–644

Decad GM, Nikaido H (1976) Outer membrane of gram-negative bacteria. XII. Molecular-sieving function of cell wall. J Bacteriol 128:325–336

Donovick R, Bayan AP, Canales P, Pansy F (1948) The influence of certain substances on the activity of streptomycin. III. Differential effects of various electrolytes on the action of streptomycin. J Bacteriol 56:125–137

Flammann HT, Weckesser J (1984) Porin isolated from the cell envelope of *Rhodopseudomonas capsulata*. J Bacteriol 159:410–412

Foster JW, Woodruff HB (1943) Microbiological aspects of streptothricin. II. Antibiotic activity of streptothricin. Arch Biochem 3:241–255

Foulds J, Chai T-J (1978) New major outer membrane protein found in an *Escherichia coli tolF* mutant resistant to bacteriophage TuIb. J Bacteriol 133:1478–1483

Frère J-M, Joris B (1985) Penicillin-sensitive enzymes in peptidoglycan biosynthesis. CRC Crit Rev Microbiol 4:299–396

Funahara Y, Nikaido H (1980) Asymmetric localization of lipopolysaccharides on the outer membrane of *Salmonella typhimurium*. J Bacteriol 141:1463–1465

George AM, Levy SB (1983) Gene in the major cotransduction gap of the *Escherichia coli* K-12 linkage map required for the expression of chromosomal resistance to tetracycline and other antibiotics. J Bacteriol 155:541–548

Gilleland HE Jr, Lyle RD (1979) Chemical alterations in cell envelopes of polymyxin-resistant *Pseudomonas aeruginosa* isolates. J Bacteriol 138:839–845

Godfrey AJ, Hatlelid L, Bryan LE (1984) Correlation between lipopolysaccharide structure and permeability resistance in β-lactam-resistant *Pseudomonas aeruginosa*. Antimicrob Agents Chemother 26:181–186

Goldstein FW, Gutmann L, Williamson R, Collatz E, Acar JF (1983) In vivo and in vitro emergence of simultaneous resistance to both β-lactam and aminoglycoside antibiotics in a strain of *Serratia marcescens*. Ann Microbiol (Paris) 134:329–337

Gutmann L, Chabbert YA (1984) Different mechanisms of resistance to latamoxef (moxalactam) in *Serratia marcescens*. J Antimicrob Chemother 13:15–22

Gutmann L, Williamson R, Collatz E (1984) The possible role of porins in bacterial antibiotic resistance. Ann Intern Med 101:554–557

Gutmann L, Williamson R, Moreau N, Kitzis M-D, Collatz E, Acar JF, Goldstein FW (1985) Cross-resistance to nalidixic acid, trimethoprim, and chloramphenicol associated with alterations in outer membrane proteins of *Klebsiella*, *Enterobacter*, and *Serratia*. J Infect Dis 151:501–507

Gutmann L, Billot-Klein D, Williamson R, Goldstein FW, Mounier J, Acar JF, Collatz E (1988) Mutation of *Salmonella paratyphi* A conferring cross-resistance to several groups of antibiotics by decreased permeability and loss of invasiveness. Antimicrob Agents Chemother 32:195–201

Guymon LF, Sparling PF (1975) Altered crystal violet permeability and lytic behavior in antibiotic-resistant and -sensitive mutants of *Neisseria gonorrhoeae*. J Bacteriol 124:757–763

Guymon LF, Walstad DL, Sparling PF (1978) Cell envelope alterations in antibiotic-sensitive and -resistant strains of *Neisseria gonorrhoeae*. J Bacteriol 136:391–401

Hancock REW, Carey AM (1980) Protein D1: a glucose-inducible, pore-forming protein from the outer membrane of *Pseudomonas aeruginosa*. FEMS Microbiol Lett 8:105–109

Hancock REW, Decad GM, Nikaido H (1979) Identification of the protein producing transmembrane diffusion pores in the outer membrane of *Pseudomonas aeruginosa*. Biochim Biophys Acta 554:323–331

Hancock REW, Raffle VJ, Nicas TI (1981) Involvement of the outer membrane in gentamicin and streptomycin uptake and killing in *Pseudomonas aeruginosa*. Antimicrob Agents Chemother 19:777–785

Harder KJ, Nikaido H, Matsuhashi M (1981) Mutants of *Escherichia coli* that are resistant to certain beta-lactam compounds lack the *ompF* porin. Antimicrob Agents Chemother 20:549–552

Hewinson RG, Lane DC, Slack MPE, Nichols WW (1986) The permeability parameter of the outer membrane of *Pseudomonas aeruginosa* varies with the concentration of a test substrate, cephalosporin C. J Gen Microbiol 132:27–33

Hirai K, Aoyama H, Irikura T, Iyobe S, Mitsuhashi S (1986 a) Differences in susceptibility to quinolones of outer membrane mutants of *Salmonella typhimurium* and *Escherichia coli*. Antimicrob Agents Chemother 29:535–538

Hirai K, Aoyama H, Suzue S, Irikura T, Iyobe S, Mitsuhashi S (1986 b) Isolation and characterization of norfloxacin-resistant mutants of *Escherichia coli* K-12. Antimicrob Agents Chemother 30:248–253

Hirai S, Suzue S, Irikura T, Iyobe S, Mitsuhashi S (1987) Mutations producing resistance to norfloxacin in *Pseudomonas aeruginosa*. Antimicrob Agents Chemother 31:582–586

Hobot JA, Carlmalm E, Villiger W, Kellenberger E (1984) Periplasmic gel: new concept resulting from the reinvestigation of bacterial cell envelope ultrastructure by new methods. J Bacteriol 160:143–152

Hooper DC, Wolfson JS, Souza KS, Tung C, McHugh GL, Swartz MN (1986) Genetic and biochemical characterization of norfloxacin resistance in *Escherichia coli*. Antimicrob Agents Chemother 29:639–644

Ishii J, Nakae T (1988) Size of diffusion pore of *Alcaligenes faecalis*. Antimicrob Agents Chemother 32:378–384

Iyer R, Darby V, Holland IB (1978) Alterations in the outer membrane proteins of *Escherichia coli* B/r associated with the presence of the R plasmid rRM98. FEBS Lett 85:127–132

Jaffé A, Chabbert YA, Derlot E (1983) Selection and characterization of β-lactam-resistant *Escherichia coli* K-12 mutants. Antimicrob Agents Chemother 23:622–625

Joris B, De Meester F, Galleni M, Masson S, Dussart J, Frère J-M, Van Beeumen J, Bush K, Sykes R (1986) Properties of a class C β-lactamase from *Serratia marcescens*. Biochem J 239:581–586

Kamio Y, Nikaido H (1976) Outer membrane of *Salmonella typhimurium*: accessibility of phospholipid head groups to phospholipase C and cyanogen bromide activated dextran in the external medium. Biochemistry 15:2561–2570
Kaneko M, Yamaguchi A, Sawai T (1985) Purification and characterization of two kinds of porins from the *Enterobacter cloacae* outer membrane. J Bacteriol 158:1179–1181
Katsu K, Inoue M, Mitsuhashi S (1982) In vitro antibacterial activity of E-0702, a new semisynthetic cephalosporin. Antimicrob Agents Chemother 22:181–185
Kobayashi Y, Takahashi I, Nakae T (1982) Diffusion of β-lactam antibiotics through liposome membranes containing purified porins. Antimicrob Agents Chemother 2:775–780
Kojo H, Shigi Y, Nishida M (1980a) A novel method for evaluating the outer membrane permeability to β-lactamase-stable β-lactam antibiotics. J Antibiot (Tokyo) 33:310–316
Kojo H, Shigi Y, Nishida M (1980b) *Enterobacter cloacae* outer membrane permeability to ceftizoxime (FK749) and five other cephalosporin derivatives. J Antibiot (Tokyo) 33:317–321
Labischinski H, Barnickel G, Bradaczek H, Naumann D, Rietschel ET; Giesbrecht P (1985) High state of order of isolated bacterial lipopolysaccharide and its possible contribution to the permeation barrier property of the outer membrane. J Bacteriol 162:9–20
Leive L (1974) The barrier function of the gram-negative envelope. Ann NY Acad Sci 235:109–127
Leive L, Telesetsky S, Coleman WG Jr, Carr D (1984) Tetracyclines of various hydrophobicities as a probe for permeability of *Escherichia coli* outer membranes. Antimicrob Agents Chemother 25:539–544
Livermore DM (1983) Kinetics and significance of the activity of the Sabbath and Abraham's β-lactamase of *Pseudomonas aeruginosa* against cefotaxime and cefsulodin. J Antimicrob Chemother 11:169–179
Loh B, Grant C, Hancock REW (1984) Use of the fluorescent probe 1-*N*-phenylnaphthylamine to study the interaction of aminoglycoside antibiotics with the outer membrane of *Pseudomonas aeruginosa*. Antimicrob Agents Chemother 26:546–551
Lounatmaa K, Mäkelä PH, Sarvas M (1976) The effect of polymyxin on the outer membrane of *Salmonella*: ultrastructure of wild-type and polymyxin-resistant strains. J Bacteriol 127:1900–1907
Luckey M, Nikaido H (1980a) Specificity of diffusion channels produced by phage receptor protein of *Escherichia coli*. Proc Natl Acad Sci USA 77:167–171
Luckey M, Nikaido H (1980b) Diffusion of solutes through channels produced by phage lambda receptor protein of *Escherichia coli*: inhibition by higher oligosaccharides of maltose series. Biochem Biophys Res Commun 93:166–171
Lugtenberg B, van Alphen L (1983) Molecular architecture and functioning of the outer membrane of *Escherichia coli* and other gram-negative bacteria. Biochim Biophys Acta 737:51–115
Lysko PG, Morse SA (1981) *Neisseria gonorrhoeae* cell envelope: permeability to hydrophobic molecules. J Bacteriol 145:946–952
Maness MJ, Sparling PF (1973) Multiple antibiotic resistance due to a single mutation in *Neisseria gonorrhoeae*. J Infect Dis 128:321–330
McGowan JE Jr (1985) Changing etiology of nosocomial bacteremia and fungemia and other hospital-acquired infections. Rev Infect Dis [Suppl 3] 7:S357–S370
McMurry LM, Cullinane JC, Levy SB (1982) Transport of the lipophilic analog minocycline differs from that of tetracycline in susceptible and resistant *Escherichia coli* strains. Antimicrob Agents Chemother 22:791–799
Medeiros AA, O'Brien TF, Wacker WEC, Yulug NF (1971) Effect of salt concentration on the apparent in vitro susceptibility of *Pseudomonas* and other gram-negative bacilli to gentamicin. J Infect Dis [Suppl] 124:S59–S64
Medeiros AA, O'Brien TF, Rosenberg EY, Nikaido H (1987) Loss of OmpC porin in a strain of *Salmonella typhimurium* causes increased resistance to cephalosporins during therapy. J Infect Dis 156:751–757

Mitsuyama J, Hiruma R, Yamaguchi A, Sawai T (1987) Identification of porins in outer membrane of *Proteus, Morganella,* and *Providencia* spp. and their role in outer membrane permeation of β-lactams. Antimicrob Agents Chemother 31:379–384

Mouton RP, Mulders LTA (1987) Combined resistance to quinolones and beta-lactams after in vitro transfer on single drugs. Chemotherapy 33:189–196

Mühlradt PF, Golecki JR (1975) Asymmetrical distribution and artifactual reorientation of lipopolysaccharide in the outer membrane bilayer of *Salmonella typhimurium.* Eur J Biochem 51:343–352

Murakami K, Yoshida T (1982) Penetration of cephalosporins and corresponding 1-oxacephalosporins through the outer layer of gram-negative bacteria and its contribution to antibacterial activity. Antimicrob Agents Chemother 21:254–258

Nagai Y, Mitsuhashi S (1972) New type of R factors incapable of inactivating chloramphenicol. J Bacteriol 109:1–7

Nakae R, Nakae T (1982) Diffusion of aminoglycoside antibiotics across the outer membrane of *Escherichia coli.* Antimicrob Agents Chemother 22:554–559

Nicas TI, Hancock REW (1980) Outer membrane H1 of *Pseudomonas aeruginosa*: involvement in adoptive and mutational resistance to ethylenediamine-tetraacetate, polymyxin B, and gentamicin. J Bacteriol 143:872–878

Nicas TI, Hancock REW (1983) Outer membrane permeability in *Pseudomonas aeruginosa*: isolation of a porin protein F-deficient mutant. J Bacteriol 153:281–285

Nichols WW, Hewinson RG, Slack MPE, Walsmley HL (1985) Estimation of the permeability parameter (C) for the flux of a charged molecule across the gram-negative bacterial outer membrane. Biochem Soc Trans 13:697–698

Nikaido H (1976) Outer membrane of *Salmonella typhimurium.* Transmembrane diffusion of some hydrophobic compounds. Biochim Biophys Acta 433:118–132

Nikaido H (1983) Proteins forming large channels from bacterial and mitochondrial outer membranes: porins and phage lambda receptor protein. Methods Enzymol 97:85–100

Nikaido H (1985) Role of permeability barriers in resistance to β-lactam antibiotics. Pharmacol Ther 27:197–231

Nikaido H (1986) Transport through the outer membrane of bacteria. Methods Enzymol 125:265–278

Nikaido H, Gehring K (1987) Significance of outer membrane barrier in β-lactam resistance. In: Shockman GD (ed) Antibiotic inhibition of bacterial cell surface assembly and function. American Society for Microbiology, Washington

Nikaido H, Hancock REW (1986) Outer membrane permeability of *Pseudomonas aeruginosa.* In: Sokatch JR (ed) The bacteria, vol 10. Academic, Orlando, pp 145–193

Nikaido H, Nakae T (1979) The outer membrane of gram-negative bacteria. Adv Microb Physiol 20:163–250

Nikaido H, Normark S (1987) Sensitivity of *Escherichia coli* to various β-lactams is determined by the interplay of outer membrane permeability and degradation by periplasmic β-lactamases: a quantitative predictive treatment. Mol Microbiol 1:29–36

Nikaido H, Rosenberg EY (1983) Porin channels in *Escherichia coli*: studies with liposomes reconstituted from purified proteins. J Bacteriol 153:241–252

Nikaido H, Vaara M (1985) Molecular basis of bacterial outer membrane permeability. Microbiol Rev 45:1–32

Nikaido H, Takeuchi Y, Ohnishi S, Nakae T (1977a) Outer membrane of *Salmonella typhimurium.* Electron spin resonance studies. Biochim Biophys Acta 465:152–164

Nikaido H, Bavoil P, Hirota Y (1977b) Outer membranes of gram-negative bacteria. XV. Transmembrane diffusion rates in lipoprotein-deficient mutants of *Escherichia coli.* J Bacteriol 132:1045–1047

Nikaido H, Rosenberg EY, Foulds J (1983) Porin channels in *Escherichia coli*: studies with β-lactams in intact cells. J Bacteriol 153:232–240

Ohi N, Aoki B, Shinozaki T, Moro K, Noto T, Nehashi T, Okazaki H, Matsunaga I (1986) Semisynthetic β-lactam antibiotics. I. Synthesis and antibacterial activity of new ureidopenicillin derivatives having catechol moieties. J Antibiot (Tokyo) 39:230–241

Parr TR Jr, Bryan LE (1984) Nonenzymatic resistance to β-lactam antibiotics and resistance to other cell wall synthesis inhibitors. In: Bryan LE (ed) Antimicrobial drug resistance. Academic, Orlando, pp 81–111
Parr TR Jr, Moore RA, Moore LV, Hancock REW (1987) Role of porins in intrinsic antibiotic resistance of *Pseudomonas cepacia*. Antimicrob Agents Chemother 31:121–123
Piddock LJV, Wise R (1986) The effect of altered porin expression in *Escherichia coli* upon susceptibility to 4-quinolones. J Antimicrob Chemother 18:547–552
Piddock LJV, Wijnands WJA, Wise R (1987) Quinolone/ureidopenicillin cross-resistance. Lancet 2:907
Plotz PH, Dubin DT, Davis BD (1961) Influence of salts on the uptake of streptomycin by *Escherichia coli*. Nature 191:1324–1325
Pugsley AP, Schnaitman C (1978) Outer membrane proteins of *Escherichia coli*. VII. Evidence that bacteriophage-directed protein 2 functions as a porin. J Bacteriol 133:1181–1189
Quinn JP, Dudek EJ, DiVincenzo CA, Lucks DA, Lerner SA (1986) Emergence of resistance to imipenem during therapy for *Pseudomonas aeruginosa* infections. J Infect Dis 154:289–294
Reeve ECR, Dougherty P (1968) Linkage relationships of two genes causing partial resistance to chloramphenicol in *Escherichia coli*. J Bacteriol 96:1450–1451
Richmond MH, Sykes RB (1973) The β-lactamases of gram-negative bacteria and their possible physiological role. Adv Microb Physiol 9:31–85
Richmond MH, Clark DC, Wotton S (1976) Indirect method for assessing the penetration of beta-lactamase-non-susceptible penicillins and cephalosporins in *Escherichia coli* strains. Antimicrob Agents Chemother 10:215–218
Rodriguez-Tébar A, Rojo F, Montilla JC, Vazquez D (1982) Interaction of β-lactam antibiotics with penicillin-binding proteins from *Pseudomonas aeruginosa*. FEMS Microbiol Lett 14:295–298
Rosenthal K, Storm DB (1977) Disruption of the *Escherichia coli* outer membrane permeability barrier by immobilized polymyxin B. J Antibiot (Tokyo) 30:1087–1092
Sanders CC (1983) Novel resistance selected by the new expanded-spectrum cephalosporins: a concern. J Infect Dis 147:585–589
Sanders CC, Watanakunakorn C (1986) Emergence of resistance to β-lactams, aminoglycosides, and quinolones during combination therapy for infection due to *Serratia marcescens*. J Inf Dis 153:617–619
Sanders CC, Sanders WE Jr, Goering RV, Werner V (1984) Selection of multiple antibiotic resistance by quinolones, β-lactams, and aminoglycosides with special reference to cross-resistance between unrelated drug classes. Antimicrob Agents Chemother 26:797–801
Sawai T, Matsuba K, Yamagishi S (1977) A method for measuring the outer membrane permeability of β-lactam antibiotics in gram-negative bacteria. J Antibiot (Tokyo) 30:1134–1136
Sawai T, Hiruma R, Kawana N, Kaneko M, Taniyasu F, Inami A (1982) Outer membrane permeation of β-lactam antibiotics in *Escherichia coli*, *Proteus mirabilis*, and *Enterobacter cloacae*. Antimicrob Agents Chemother 22:585–592
Sawai T, Hirano S, Yamaguchi A (1987) Repression of porin synthesis by salicylate in *Escherichia coli*, *Klebsiella pneumoniae*, and *Serratia marcescens*. FEMS Microbiol Lett 40:233–237
Sen K, Hellman J, Nikaido H (1988) Porin channels in intact cells of *Escherichia coli* are not affected by Donnan potentials across the outer membrane. J Biol Chem 263:1182–1187
Shimizu K, Kuroda T, Hsieh W-C, Chung H-Y, Chong Y, Hare RS, Miller GH et al. (1985) Comparison of aminoglycoside resistance patterns in Japan, Formosa, and Korea, Chile, and the United States. Antimicrob Agents Chemother 28:282–288
Smit J, Kamio Y, Nikaido H (1975) Outer membrane of *Salmonella typhimurium*: chemical analysis and freeze-fracture studies with lipopolysaccharide mutants. J Bacteriol 124:942–958
Smith JT, Hamilton-Miller JMT, Knox R (1964) Quinacillin: a comparison with other penicillinase-resistant penicillins. Nature 203:1148–1150

Sparling PF (1977) Antibiotic resistance in the gonococcus. In: Roberts RB (ed) The gonococcus. Wiley, New York, pp 111–135
Stein WD (1967) The movement of molecules across cell membranes. Academic, New York
Stock JB, Rauch B, Roseman S (1977) Periplasmic space in *Salmonella typhimurium* and *Escherichia coli*. J Biol Chem 252:7850–7861
Storm DR, Rosenthal KS, Swanson PE (1977) Polymyxin and related peptide antibiotics. Annu Rev Biochem 46:723–763
Sykes RB, Matthew M (1976) The β-lactamases of gram-negative bacteria and their role in resistance to β-lactam antibiotics. J Antimicrob Chemother 2:115–157
Teuber M (1970) Lysozyme-dependent production of spheroplasts-like bodies from polymyxin B treated *Salmonella typhimurium*. Arch Mikrobiol 70:139–146
Teuber M, Bader J (1976) Action of polymyxin on bacterial membranes. Binding capacities for polymyxin B of inner and outer membranes isolated from *Salmonella typhimurium* G30. Arch Microbiol 109:51–58
Then RL, Angehrn P (1986) Multiply resistant mutants of *Enterobacter cloacae* selected by β-lactam antibiotics. Antimicrob Agents Chemother 30:684–688
Traub WH, Bauer D (1987) Outer membrane protein alterations in *Serratia marcescens* resistant against aminoglycoside and β-lactam antibiotics. Chemotherapy 33:172–176
Trias J, Rosenberg EY, Nikaido H (1988) Specificity of the glucose channel formed by protein D1 of *Pseudomonas aeruginosa*. Biochim Biophys Acta 938:493–496
Vaara M, Vaara T (1983a) Polycations sensitizes enteric bacteria to antibiotics. Antimicrob Agents Chemother 24:107–113
Vaara M, Vaara T (1983b) Polycations as outer membrane disorganizing agents. Antimicrob Agents Chemother 24:114–122
Vaara M, Vaara T, Jensen M, Helander I, Nurminen M, Rietschel ET, Mäkelä PH (1981) Characterization of the lipopolysaccharide from the polymyxin-resistant *pmrA* mutants of *Salmonella typhimurium*. FEBS Lett 129:145–149
Vachon V, Lyew DJ, Coulton JW (1985) Transmembrane permeability channels across the outer membrane of *Haemophilus influenzae* type b. J Bacteriol 162:918–924
Vu H, Nikaido H (1985) Role of β-lactam hydrolysis in the mechanism of resistance of a β-lactamase-constitutive *Enterobacter cloacae* strain to expanded-spectrum β-lactams. Antimicrob Agents Chemother 27:393–398
Waley SG (1987) An explicit model for bacterial resistance: application to β-lactam antibiotics. Microbiol Sci 4:143–146
Watanabe N, Nagasu T, Katsu K, Kitoh K (1987) E-0702, a new cephalosporin, is incorporated into *Escherichia coli* cells via the *tonB*-dependent iron transport system. Antimicrob Agents Chemother 31:497–504
Weaver PF, Wall JD, Gest H (1975) Characterization of *Rhodopseudomonas capsulata*. Arch Microbiol 105:207–216
Weckesser J, Zalman LS, Nikaido H (1984) Porin from *Rhodopseudomonas sphaeroides*. J Bacteriol 159:199–205
Werner V, Sanders CC, Sanders WE Jr, Goering RV (1985) Role of β-lactamases and outer membrane proteins in multiple β-lactam resistance of *Enterobacter cloacae*. Antimicrob Agents Chemother 27:455–459
Woodruff WA, Parr TR Jr, Hancock REW, Hanne L, Nicas TI, Iglewski B (1986) Expression in *Escherichia coli* and function of porin protein F of *Pseudomonas aeruginosa*. J Bacteriol 167:473–479
Yamaguchi A, Hiruma R, Sawai T (1982) Phospholipid bilayer permeability of beta-lactam antibiotics. J Antibiot (Tokyo) 35:1692–1699
Yamaguchi A, Yanai M, Tomiyama N, Sawai T (1986) Effects of magnesium and sodium ions on the outer membrane permeability of cephalosporins in *Escherichia coli*. FEBS Lett 208:43–47
Yoneyama H, Nakae T (1986) A small diffusion pore in the outer membrane of *Pseudomonas aeruginosa*. Eur J Biochem 157:33–38
Yoneyama H, Akatsuka A, Nakae T (1986) The outer membrane of *Pseudomonas aeruginosa* is a barrier against the penetration of disaccharides. Biochem Biophys Res Commun 134:106–112

Yoshimura F, Nikaido H (1982) Permeability of *Pseudomonas aeruginosa* outer membrane to hydrophilic solutes. J Bacteriol 152:636–642
Yoshimura F, Nikaido H (1985) Diffusion of β-lactam antibiotics through the porin channels of *Escherichia coli* K-12. Antimicrob Agents Chemother 27:84–92
Yoshimura F, Zalman LS, Nikaido H (1983) Purification and properties of *Pseudomonas aeruginosa* porin. J Biol Chem 258:2308–2314
Young JDE, Blake M, Mauro A, Cohn ZA (1983) Properties of the major outer membrane protein from *Neisseria gonorrhoeae* incorporated into model lipid membranes. Proc Natl Acad Sci USA 80:3831–3835
Zalman LS (1982) Pore-forming proteins of bacterial and mitochondrial outer membranes. PhD thesis, University of California, Berkeley
Zalman LS, Nikaido H (1985) Dimeric porin from *Paracoccus denitrificans*. J Bacteriol 162:430–433
Zimmermann W (1980) Penetration of β-lactam antibiotics into their target enzymes in *Pseudomonas aeruginosa*: comparison of a highly sensitive mutant with its parental strain. Antimicrob Agents Chemother 18:94–100
Zimmermann W, Rosselet A (1977) Function of the outer membrane of *Escherichia coli* as a permeability barrier to beta-lactam antibiotics. Antimicrob Agents Chemother 12:368–372

CHAPTER 2

Cytoplasmic Membrane Transport and Antimicrobial Resistance

L. E. BRYAN

A. Summary of Transport Systems

In general compounds enter bacterial cells by means of either diffusion or active transport.

I. Diffusional

1. Passive Diffusion

Passive diffusion represents that system where a compound moves across the membrane by virtue of a concentration gradient. The rate of diffusion is directly proportional to the concentration gradient.

2. Facilitated Diffusion

In this process a substance enters a cell through the existence of a concentration gradient. However, in contrast to passive diffusion a carrier protein is involved. Generally speaking, rates of facilitated diffusion are more rapid than those of simple diffusion at equivalent concentrations. However, facilitated diffusion systems exhibit saturation kinetics.

II. Active Transport

In these systems a substance may be moved into a cell against a concentration gradient and energy will be expended to complete the process. Although aminoglycoside antibiotics are an exception, active transport systems involve a carrier mechanism and show saturation kinetics. Active transport may be driven by chemiosmosis and may be divided into symport, antiport and uniport mechanisms describing the processes of ion cotransport. Symport is a system for translocating two substrates at the same time in one direction utilizing one carrier. Antiports represent those circumstances where two substrates are translocated simultaneously by the carrier in opposite directions. Uniport systems represent those situations where the substrate is charged and moves in response to a membrane potential. Thus, cations may be accumulated with a negative electrical potential inside the cell or anions may be extruded. If the substance also exists in an uncharged state, an uniport system operates as a facilitated diffusion mechanisms.

The driving force for active transport associated with chemiosmosis is one or other of the components of the proton motive force. Simply put these represent either a proton gradient in that under normal circumstances the external environment is more acidic than the interior of a cell. The second component is an electrical potential such that under usual circumstances the inside of the cell is electrically negative so that a charge gradient exists across the membrane (ROSEN and KASHKET 1978).

Another group of transport systems are linked directly to phosphate bond energy rather than through the effect of ATP on ion and proton gradients. Generally speaking these systems contain components which are lost from the cell by the process of osmotic shock and do not function as membrane vesicle accumulation systems.

III. Group Translocation

Group translocation is another form of energy coupled transport. However unlike active transport systems the compound which undergoes transport is chemically altered during passage through the membrane. A well described example of this type of system is the phosphotransferase system. In this mechanism enzyme 1 located in the cytoplasm transfers phosphate from phospho-enolpyruvate to HPr. The latter is a protein of approximately 9000 molecular weight which is located in the cytoplasm. The sugar in question is transported with a sugar-specific, membrane bound enzyme (enzyme II). The high energy phosphate is transferred from HPr to one of various sugar specific enzymes (enzyme III) which phosphorylate the sugar bound to the membrane bound enzyme and the phosphorylated sugar is transported to the inner surface of the membrane.

B. Antimicrobial Resistance Associated with Antimicrobial Transport

I. Introduction

A large number of antimicrobial agents exert their principal inhibitory activities within the bacterial cytoplasm. To reach their target sites, antimicrobial agents may pass through the cytoplasmic membrane by the use of diffusional mechanisms, the use of existing transport systems for which the antimicrobial agent has affinity or by the use of apparently special systems. In terms of cytoplasmic membrane transport, resistance can arise through alteration of existing transport systems or of those components associated with the special systems that function with certain antibiotics. Unfortunately in the case of many antibiotics there are few data as to how they transverse the cytoplasmic membrane.

II. Use of Existing Transport Systems

1. D-Cycloserine

D-Cycloserine is transported across the cytoplasmic membrane by use of the D-alanine-glycine transport system (WARGEL et al. 1971). Mutations affecting a gene which specifies this system (*cyc*A) are defective in the accumulation of D-glycine, D-alanine and D-cycloserine (ANRAKU 1978).

2. Fosfomycin (Phosphonomycin)

Fosfomycin has an intracellular target, the enzyme phosphoenolpyruvate: UDP-Glc-NAc-3-enolpyruvyltransferase. It is transported by the sn-glycerol-3-phosphate and hexose phosphate transport systems. Mutants resistant to fosfomycin are most frequently defective in either of these two transport systems. Cells grown in medium containing glucose and phosphate also are more resistant to phosphonomycin apparently through "repression" of the glycerol-3-phosphate transport system.

Fosfomycin accumulation results in only a 4- to 20-fold concentration in *E. coli* and *Salmonella typhimurium* respectively. This concentration gradient is significantly below that seen for the natural substrates and suggests that fosfomycin may be entering by virtue of facilitated diffusion (KAHAN et al. 1974; TSURUOKA et al. 1978).

When MICs of fosfomycin were determined in media with and without glucose-6-phosphate, which induces the hexose phosphate transport system, little or no difference was reported. However transport was not studied under these circumstances (DETTE et al. 1983).

3. Peptide Antibiotics

Transport systems exist within bacterial cytoplasmic membranes which are capable of the transport of dipeptides and oligopeptides. The relatively broad substrate specificity seen with such transport systems has enabled them to be used as carriers of peptides containing naturally occurring and other amino acid analogs. Subsequent to transport intracellular hydrolysis liberates an amino acid which is toxic to the bacterial cell. The agent alafosfalin is an example of a dipeptide antibiotic which is hydrolzyed to release -1-aminoethylphosphonic acid, which inhibits peptidoglycan synthesis. This compound is concentrated 100- to 1000-fold within the cell where it inhibits alanine racemase and secondarily UDP-*N*-acetylmuramyl-L-alanine synthetase (ATHERTON et al. 1979, 1983).

In general peptide transport systems can be divided into those which will transfer dipeptides and those which transport oligopeptides. It seems likely that more than one transport system exists for both dipeptides and oligopeptides (PAYNE and GILVARG 1978).

A recent study of alafosfalin transport showed complex kinetics, suggesting multiple transport proteins with differing affinities for the phosphonodipeptide. Thus multiple dipeptide transport permeases are utilized. In contrast a trianaline derivative of this antibiotic was transported by classical Michaelis-Menten kinetics, suggesting the use of a single saturable oligopeptide system. Thus although a number of oligopeptide transport systems have been identified, it may be that one is used predominately for the uptake of a given oligopeptide antibiotic.

It has been reported that mutants defective in a oligopeptide transport system may become resistant to certain tripeptide antibiotics. For example, the compound plumbermycin B. Dipeptide antibiotics remain active on mutants defective in oligopeptide transport. However, as noted above, in some circumstances oligopeptides remain active in mutants with a defective oligopeptide transport system because of the use of an alternative oligopeptide permease.

Dipeptide permeases appear to be specific for L-residues. In oligopeptide transport, mixtures of L and D residues may occur.

Therefore, resistance to dipeptide antibiotics, based on the studies of alafosfalin, are unlikely to be accomplished by mutations affecting a single dipeptide transport system. Alternatively, resistance to oligopeptide antibiotics may occur if a mutation occurs in the specific oligopeptide transport system used by that compound. Another important mechanism for resistance to these compounds is in the endopeptidases which cleave the substance within the cell to release the toxic product (ATHERTON et al. 1983).

The peptide systems described above require ATP for energy. It has been stated that the activity of alafosfalin decreases when the cells are grown anaerobically because of a decrease in transport. However, it has recently been shown that anaerobes are susceptible to this compound (GRAPPEL et al. 1985).

4. Sideromycins

These are compounds which occur naturally or are semisynthetic in that an antibiotic moiety has been linked with a naturally occurring siderophore. Albomycin and ferrimycin A_1 are synthesized by streptomycetes and use siderophore-binding proteins to be transported into the cell (NUESCH and KNUSEL 1967). In the case of albomycin this involves a protein specified by the *fhu*A (formerly *ton*A) gene locus. The *ton*B gene product is also required for proper function of this protein and is assumed to be involved in "energy coupling." The *fhu*A specified protein is necessary for the uptake of ferrichrome and albomycin binds to that protein in the outer membrane of bacterial cells. Thereafter by a process which is not understood the compound is cleaved into the iron carrier moiety and the aminoacyl-thioribosyl pyrimidine part. Cleavage of the latter moiety, which stays inside the cell along with iron, is brought about by one or more peptidases depending upon the bacterial species. The iron carrier component is excreted (KADNER and BASSFORD 1978; BRAUN et al. 1983; HARTMANN et al. 1979; NIKAIDO and VAARA 1985).

Mutants which are resistant to albomycin result from impairment of transport and map in the *fhu*A gene and the closely linked *fhu*B, *fhu*C and *fhu*D genes. However, another class of mutations resistant to this compound also occur which are indirectly related to the transport process and are associated with a reduction of peptidase activity. Ferrimycin A_1 contains the iron carrier ferrioxamine B and competes for the same transport system. Likely this compound is activated as albomycin by means of a peptidase (BRAUN et al. 1983).

The synthesis of compounds with antimicrobial activity to iron carrier moieties has been used to produce semisynthetic antimicrobial agents. These include, for example, sulphanilamido-nicotinic acid ferricrocinyl ester, sulphanilamido-nicotinic acid, ferrioxamine B, sulphanilamido-carbonic acid ferricrocinyl ester and sulphanilamido-carbonyl ferrioxamine B. The last two compounds have not been reported to have antimicrobial activity and probably this lack of activity results from a failure to split off the antibiotically active group within the cell. Based on competition by the siderophores ferricrocin and ferrioxamine B, it is likely the first two compounds utilize a similar type of transport mechanism as described for albomycin. Mutations may therefore presumably arise from modification of the transport system or of the peptidase activity needed to split the compound (Chopra and Ball 1982).

5. Other Agents

A variety of other compounds which have antimicrobial activity but which are not clinically used are of interest because of the transport systems they use. One of these is showdomycin, a structural analog of uridine. The principal target and additional targets of this drug are intracellular. Although a variety of enzymes are inhibited probably the most important one is uridine monophosphate kinase.

In strains of *E. coli* which were showdomycin resistant, there was not appreciable accumulation of either the uracil or ribosyl moiety of uridine. Although the transport processes utilized for accumulation of uridine and its components are complex, it seems that there is one transport system which recognizes uridine and showdomycin (Komatsu and Tanaka 1972, 1973).

Several other agents with weak antimicrobial activity are also likely transported by existing transport systems. These would include: 3,4-dihydroxybutyl-1-phosphonate, which is transported by the *sn*-glycerol-3-phosphate system, streptozotocin transported by the phosphoenolpyruvate:phosphotransferase system and norjirimycin also transferred by the phosphoenolpyruvate:phosphotransferase system. Mutants defective in either enzyme I or the HPr components or in enzyme II are streptozotocin-resistant. Sodium cyanide and dinitrophenol inhibits uptake of streptozotocin as well as *N*-acetyl-D-glucosamine, which streptozotocin is an analog of. In general this is inconsistent with transport by the PTS, suggesting that possibly more than a single transport system may be involved (Chopra and Ball 1982).

III. Use of Special Transport Systems

1. Aminoglycoside Antibiotics

a) Uptake

Aminoglycoside antibiotics are an important group of antimicrobial agents which possess positive charges. They contain a cyclic alcohol in glycosidic linkage with amino-substituted sugars. The most common aminocyclitol is deoxystreptamine, which may exist either with 4,5 disubstitutions or with 4,6 disubstitutions. Other aminocyclitols include streptidine (streptomycin) and actinamine. The latter is found in spectinomycin, which is an aminocyclitol in that it does not contain an amino sugar.

The most extensive study of aminoglycoside transport has been carried out with streptomycin or dihydrostreptomycin and gentamicin. Additional studies have also been performed with kanamycin and to a lesser extent amikacin.

In gram-negative bacteria aminoglycosides diffuse through outer membrane pores. In certain bacteria such as *Pseudomonas aeruginosa* it also appears that these compounds may bind to phosphate residues, disorganize the outer membrane and facilitate their own entry to the cytoplasmic membrane (LOH et al. 1984). Recently pictorial evidence of "holes in the outer membrane" has been shown in *Pseudomonas aeruginosa*. Under highly specific conditions holes can also be seen developing in the cytoplasmic membrane. The latter situation appears to occur under conditions of potassium cyanide treatment where the internalization of the aminoglycoside does not occur and where cell repair mechanisms are inhibited (MARTIN and BEVERIDGE 1986).

In gram-positive and gram-negative bacteria there appears to be a common process by which aminoglycosides are transported across the cytoplasmic membrane. This process and the affinity for ribosomal binding are the major determinants in determining activity of these compounds.

The process of transport of aminoglycosides has been extensively refined in the past several years although some details are not yet clear. The highly charged (3–6 positive charges at neutral pH) compounds bind to anionic groups at the surface of the cytoplasmic membrane. This binding process can be inhibited by divalent cations and at higher concentrations monovalent cations. It is likely therefore that most of the binding is to phosphate residues of phospholipids and perhaps other polar groupings on the exterior surface of the cytoplasmic membrane such as might be found in terminal electron transport, for example, with respiratory quinones.

Aminoglycosides move across the cytoplasmic membrane in response to an internally negative electrical potential ($\Delta\psi$). The concept that aminoglycoside transport rates might reflect the cross-membrane proton motive force was first proposed by BRYAN and VAN DEN ELZEN (1977). Evidence for the membrane potential ($\Delta\psi$) in transport was provided by BRYAN et al. (1980). Subsequently DAMPER and EPSTEIN (1981) pointed out the role of membrane potential to the activity of aminoglycosides. The demonstration of the requirement for a threshold electrical potential was reported almost simultaneously through the work of MILLER et al. (1980) and from our own laboratory (MATES et al. 1982; BRYAN and KWAN 1981). Subsequently BRYAN and KWAN (1983) showed that the quantity of streptomycin taken up increased with increasing electrical potential at certain concentrations (100 µg/ml) but not at lower concentrations (25 µg/ml). In the latter instance once the threshold electrical potential had been achieved it appeared that the uptake of streptomycin was maximal. Thereafter EISENBERG et al. (1984) showed a quantitative association between electrical potential and early gentamicin uptake. Thus, both these laboratories were able to show the requirement for a threshold electrical potential and that at least at certain concentrations of streptomycin or gentamicin there was a relationship between the amount of drug taken up and the electrical potential of the cell.

Uptake of gentamicin or streptomycin when done with extreme care and under very sensitive uptake conditions can be divided into three phases (BRYAN and VAN DEN ELZEN 1976). The first of these is termed the energy independent phase and represents binding to the cytoplasmic membrane or in gram-negative bacteria to both outer membrane and cytoplasmic membrane. In gram-positive bacteria additional binding might occur also to anionic cell surface components. Thereafter, another phase of uptake occurs which has been termed energy dependent uptake phase I (EDP-I). Although some workers have not been able to detect this phase of uptake, it can be consistently demonstrated particularly under conditions of low ionic strength such that occur with the use of some types of nutrient both (Bryan and Van den Elzen 1975, 1976). Following this phase of uptake, energy dependent phase II (EDP-II) occurs. This uptake phase is much accelerated and its onset is simultaneous with the first evidence of inhibition of incorporation of amino acids as shown by Bryan and Van den Elzen (1977). Anand and Davis (1960) showed biphasic uptake of streptomycin which corresponds to the energy independent phase and energy dependent phase II. Their work did not demonstrate EDPI, considered by the author to be energy driven uptake needed for initial transport of the aminoglycoside to the ribosomal component.

In the examination of streptomycin uptake the use of ribosomally resistant mutants eliminates energy dependent phase II uptake under most circumstances. A similar situation can also be achieved by the use of streptomycin modifying enzymes which, for example, convert streptomycin to streptomycin adenylate (Dickie et al. 1978).

Kinetic analysis demonstrated that EDP-II uptake is not saturable and shows diffusion characteristics. The same conclusion can be made for EDP-I uptake except at extremely high concentration (2 mg/ml streptomycin) in ribosomally resistant mutants where saturation may be obtainable (Bryan and Van den Elzen 1977). Thus the process acts like one of diffusion driven by an electrical potential. However, as pointed out in 1978 by Dickie et al. and shown more recently by Nichols and Young (1985), the vast majority of streptomycin taken up by the cell is not released. In the presence of energy inhibitors although a large percentage of the cell associated dihydrostreptomycin is retained there is very slow release (Dickie et al. 1978).

The dependence of streptomycin and gentamicin on electrical potential for uptake led us to propose that uptake was a uniport following which the aminoglycoside became associated with an intracellular sink. Streptomycin uptake cannot be demonstrated by the use of conventional membrane vesicles from *E. coli* (Bryan and Kwan 1983; Nichols and Young 1985). [A description of dihydromycin uptake by vesicles of *Pseudomonas putida* has however been reported (Thomson et al. 1985)]. However, some gentamicin uptake could be demonstrated in vesicles which apparently contain functional protein synthesis (Bryan and Kwan 1983).

Consideration of the failure of transport to occur in vesicles, the requirement for streptomycin susceptible ribosomes to show EDP-II under normal conditions and the failure to lose aminoglycoside to the external medium caused us to propose that binding occurred to ribosomes and other nucleic acids within the cell. This would represent a sink. It has been known for some time that the use of toluene can cause a release of streptomycin from the cell. This has been used to argue that a sink is not an effective explanation for the retention of streptomycin (or gentamicin). However, it seems perfectly reasonable that the highly hydrophobic environment produced with toluene or butanol may disturb the binding characteristics and/or the structure of the nucleic acids involved in ribosomes and of

DNA so that the drugs are released. Our view has always been that the binding sink did not represent simply binding to the high affinity ribosomal binding site but rather to any of a series of negative charges associated with nucleic acids or ribosomes or DNA.

The process by which gentamicin or streptomycin passed through the cytoplasmic membrane has not been finally determined. No convincing evidence for a carrier has been provided although HOLTJE (1979) proposed that a polyamine transport system could serve as a carrier. It remains possible that a series of carriers could serve or that some other membraneous structure which allowed an aminoglycoside to bind to it such as a respiratory quinone or components of terminal electron transport could be used. Evidence has been advanced for and against this proposal and the jury is still out (MUIR et al. 1981; BRYAN and KWAN 1983; MCENROE and TABER 1984).

Another perplexing aspect of aminoglycoside uptake has been the stimulation of the rate of accumulation which occurs at the onset of EDP-II. As noted above this is coincident with the first evidence of inhibition of protein synthesis (BRYAN and VAN DEN ELZEN 1977). It has been our view that this results from modification of the ribosomal cycle and the subsequent gradual disorganization of the membrane because of the transfer of the aminoglycosides to specific and nonspecific nucleic acid binding sites. Removal of aminoglycosides would leave pore-like defects in the membrane. It is important to emphasize that ribosomal binding of streptomycin to the high affinity site is needed only to initiate perturbation of the ribosomal cycle (although puromycin can do the same thing). As a direct result the number or frequency or affinity of additional binding sites is significantly increased. According to this proposal the rate limiting step for uptake is the removal of streptomycin from the membrane to the complex of nucleic acid associated with ribosomes, messenger RNA as well as perhaps DNA. Firm binding to nucleic acid would account for intracellular retention of the drug. Alternative views recently proposed have been that of DAVIS et al. (1986), who has proposed that misread or incomplete polypeptide chains can be incorporated into the membrane, creating abnormal channels. These channels would allow for increased streptomycin uptake and further misreading or inhibition of protein synthesis. Another similar view is that polysomes at the membrane may be involved in the formation of transient pores for nasent protein. These could become magnified when the rate of formation of initiation complexes and short peptide is increased (SCHLESSINGER, personal communication). Our studies have shown that the accelerated rate of streptomycin uptake remains dependent upon the electrical potential and cannot be explained by an increase in electrical potential (BRYAN and KWAN 1983). It seems likely also that an accelerated uptake which occurs in certain mutants which are uncoupled for oxidative phosphorylation and electron transport cannot be explained by an increase of electrical potential (BRYAN and VAN DEN ELZEN 1977).

Our proposal (BRYAN and KWAN 1983), and those of DAVIS et al. (1986) and Schlessinger, all contain a requirement for pore formation. The process by which the pore comes about differs somewhat. In our proposal we believe that modification of the ribosomal cycle increased the rate of removal of the aminoglycoside from a membrane and in so doing leaves a pore structure. In that of Davis it would appear that short polypeptides are inserted into the membrane due the consequences of the effect of streptomycin on protein synthesis and creates the pores. In the third proposal pores would result because of a normal function of ribosomes in creating pores for protein secretion and this process is accelerated by the effects of streptomycin. In our view it is still difficult to explain in any of these hypotheses how the streptomycin accumulation process remains dependent on an electrical potential. Surely pores which allow the release of small and later larger molecular materials would also destroy the membrane potential. In addition the enhanced uptake of streptomycin seen with uncoupled mutants would presumably not involve protein synthesis at all.

In summary several aspects of streptomycin and gentamicin transport are clear. Binding occurs to the cell surface through an energy independent process. Thereafter a small quantity of streptomycin or gentamicin is moved across the cell by a process which is dependent upon at the very least a membrane potential and possibly terminal electron transport. Streptomycin or gentamicin bind to ribosomes and initiate misreading and/or protein inhibition. The effects on the ribosomal cycle and protein synthesis are associated with accelerated aminoglycoside transport which is dependent upon membrane potential but does not require an elevation of membrane potential. In our view EDP-II transport is most likely associated with modification of the ribosomal cycle and either a direct effect of that (as proposed by Schlessinger) on pore formation or through the action of aminoglycosides themselves in disorganizing membrane regions to produce pores. We feel that pores created through insertion of misread polypeptides is also a feasible proposal.

b) Resistance and Uptake

α) Aminoglycoside Modifying Enzymes. The mechanism by which these enzymes achieve resistance is associated with transport. In the vast majority of cases aminoglycoside modifying enzymes do not result in significant detoxification of drug external to the cell. It is therefore only that drug which is being accumulated which undergoes modification. A process of rate competition exists whereby the rate of modification competes with the rate of aminoglycoside entry. Modifying enzymes are located intimately related to the cytoplasmic membrane and if they possess a low *Km* for a given aminoglycoside they modify all drug which enters the cell. The drug therefore fails to interact effectively with ribosomes and does not produce a modification of ribosomal cycle and protein synthesis. The failure to induce the change in the ribosomal cycle also prevents the accelerated phase of uptake. Under circumstances where an enzyme has a relatively high *Km* or possibly but less likely a very low V_{max}, transport may result in unmodified drugs within the cell and the interaction with ribosome and pertubation of ribosomal cycle and protein synthesis occurs (DICKIE et al. 1978). GARCIA-RIESTRA et al. (1985) have shown adenylylated streptomycin is not accumulated.

The rate competition explanation of the mechanism of action of aminoglycoside modifying enzymes predicts that conditions which enhance transport, for example, high concentrations of the drug or in hypersensitive mutants, the effect of modifying enzymes will be reduced or eliminated. Alternatively conditions which increase or decrease enzyme efficiency with no change in transport will respectively increase or decrease resistance. In general these predictions have been met (HOLTJE 1979; VASTOLA et al. 1980).

β) Phenotypic Resistance. In general reduced susceptibility to aminoglycosides is manifest under a series of sets of conditions which are associated with reduction in transport.

Antagonism exhibited by divalent cations for aminoglycosides in all bacteria but particularly pronounced in *Pseudomonas aeruginosa* is due to interference with the primary binding or energy independent phase of uptake. Aminoglycosides bind to anionic residues within the outer membrane of gram-negative bacteria and the cytoplasmic membrane of all bacteria. The principle binding site is phosphate residues as part of lipopolysaccharide or phospholipids. In the case of the outer membrane phosphate residues occur within the deeper portion of lipopolysaccharide and the general view is that such residues are cross-linked between two molecules by particularly the divalent cation magnesium. Hancock and his colleagues have studied this interaction extensively particularly in *Pseudomonas aeruginosa* (HANCOCK et al. 1981). They have shown that the binding of, for example, gentamicin to phosphate residues cannot be accommodated within the normal structure of lipopolysaccharide and disorganization of outer membrane occurs. This is referred to as self promoted uptake and seems to be a general property of cationic antimicrobial agents. Apparently due to lower concentration of phosphate residues in other gram-negative bacteria such as *E. coli*, the self promoted uptake pathway is much less active. Recently, electron microscopic evidence of holes in the outer membrane has been shown by Beveridge and colleagues (MARTIN and BEVERIDGE 1986).

As the concentrations of particularly magnesium or calcium increase, there is competition with the aminoglycosides for binding to the phosphate residues. This interferes with the initial binding phase which is a prelude to all transport and contributes to higher MIC value.

γ) pH. The major driving force for aminoglycoside uptake is the magnitude of electrical potential. The size of $\Delta\psi$ is inversely related to the other component of the proton motive force, Δ pH (FELLE et al. 1980). Over the pH range 5 to 7.5 Δ pH is maximal when the external pH is 5 and minimal when the external pH is 7.5. The inverse situation holds for $\Delta\psi$. Therefore $\Delta\psi$ is higher at pH 7.5 than 5 and results in a more extensive entry of aminoglycosides into the cell. As pointed out by BRYAN et al. (1980), transport of gentamicin and streptomycin decline with falling pH. This results in greater resistance.

Aminoglycosides are more active at pH 9 than pH 8 and it is difficult to account for this difference in activity entirely through the effect on $\Delta\psi$ as there is little change in it over this pH range. It is also possible that pH changes result in a different amount of ionization of aminoglycosides or of ionic cell surface binding sites, helping to explain the effect of higher pHs.

Therefore it would be anticipated that aminoglycosides are less active under conditions of low pH such as, for example, those which occur in many abscesses (BRYANT 1984).

δ) *Anaerobiosis*. It has been known for some time that the action of streptomycin was impaired under anaerobic conditions (KOGUT et al. 1965). Uptake of streptomycin is impaired anaerobically (HANCOCK 1962). So-called anaerobic bacteria are also generally resistant to aminoglycosides unless they carry out a significant level of electron transport usually to nitrate as a terminal acceptor. BRYAN et al. (1979) showed that *Clostridium perfringens* and *Bacteroides fragilis* had protein synthesis mechanisms which were susceptible to the action of streptomycin and gentamicin but that they did not accumulate the drug in batch culture over 1 hour uptake periods. However, at relatively high dihydrostreptomycin concentrations the inclusion of hemin, fumarate and menadione in the growth medium with *Bacteroides fragilis* did allow uptake to occur. No aminoglycoside inactivation could be demonstrated in these anaerobic bacteria. Other studies on *E. coli* growing anaerobically also showed impaired uptake in batch culture and a marked delay in uptake in chemostat cultures (MUIR et al. 1985). BRYAN and KWAN (1981) showed that uptake of gentamicin could be achieved under anaerobic conditions by the inclusion of phenazine metholsulphate (PMS) and ascorbate in the uptake mixture. Some uptake was also achieved in *Clostridium perfringens* by these same conditions. These studies suggested that either PMS ascorbate was being used as an electron transport system and acting as the proposed transporter or the PMS ascorbate was able to achieve an adequate $\Delta\psi$ such the transport would occur. Work done by MANDEL et al. (1983) showed that uptake could be stimulated in *Staphylococcus aureus* grown anaerobically by the use of DCCD or nigericin, which in turn increased electrical potential.

Recent work by MUIR et al. (1985) has shown that although anaerobic uptake is significantly delayed using chemostat uptake conditions compared to aerobic uptake of streptomycin, when uptake does occur it occurs at a rate equal to that of aerobic cells providing growth rates were equal. Uptake under anaerobic conditions could be prevented by the use of CCCP indicating that it was dependent upon proton motive force. Information on the value of $\Delta\psi$ under anaerobic conditions has been conflicting. This might be partially explained by growth circumstances or the rate of growth being examined.

BRYAN and KWAN (1981) have proposed that resistance of anaerobic bacteria is due to impairment of aminoglycoside transport. Whether this is due to the lack of a component of electron transport used as a transporter or an impaired electrical potential has not been clear. It seems reasonable at this time to conclude that the weight of evidence would suggest that resistance is most likely due to an impaired electrical potential. The role of respiratory activity would seem most likely to be involved in more effectively creating a threshold electrical potential needed for transport. However, the requirement for a transporter complex cannot be excluded by any of these studies.

ε) *Transport-Mediated Resistance Due to Modified Cellular Energetics or Modified Cell Binding*. Anaerobic resistance to aminoglycosides has been discussed under phenotypic resistance above. However, it could equally well be discussed in this section because of its clear relationship to cellular energetics. In addition, however, there have been the isolation of a series of bacteria which are associated with aminoglycoside resistance and have a wide variety of "energy" deficiencies associated either with electron transport or the maintenance of a proton motive force. Isolates of this type from clinical or animal infections have been reported by several authors including Annear (1975), Gerber et al. (1982), Miller et al. (1980), Musher et al. (1977, 1979), Pelletier et al. (1979) and Spagna et al. (1978). These strains and others have been shown to have such defects as deficiency in respiratory quinone content (Bryan and Van den Elzen 1977; Miller et al. 1980; Acar et al. 1978), deficiency in terminal cytochromes (Bryan et al. 1980; Bryan and Kwan 1981), hemin deficiency (Bryan and Van den Elzen 1977), increased proton leakiness (Adler and Rosen 1976) and reduced NADH and D-lactate oxidases with demethylmenaquinone and a structural analog of ubiquinone in place of ubiquinone (Muir et al. 1981).

In those circumstances where such isolates have been isolated from clinical circumstances or animal models, these colonies have regularly shown a small colony phenotype. In comparison of similar isolates derived by mutagenesis (Bryan et al. 1980; Bryan and Kwan 1981) growth rates were slower for the mutant. The commonality of these mutations is that most of them have impaired electron transport. In some, however, electron transport was normal and there was only defectiveness of proton motive force. Two interpretations of the cause of resistance in these mutants have been made. One is that there is a need for electron transport and the component of the electron transport to act as a transporter for aminoglycosides. However, it seems more likely that the explanation for resistance in all or most of these is that there is an impaired electrical potential such that the threshold value is not achieved or achieved at a much slower rate.

These mutations are probably of considerable clinical significance. They occur frequently and produce resistance levels which are often the 4- to 8-fold less susceptible. Because of their slow growth they may be readily overgrown by revertants and are not easily detected by conventional susceptibility testing methodologies. They likely explain slow responses to aminoglycosides or clinical failure in an individual case. They are unlikely to persist as stable causes of resistance and therefore there significance has, in my view, been underestimated.

Another form of resistance associated with reduced aminoglycoside transport has been found particularly in clinical isolates of *Pseudomonas aeruginosa*. It is possible in some of these that there is overproduction of the H_1 protein (Nicas and Hancock 1980). However, in another set that were studied, there was a conversion from smooth to rough LPS phenotype (loss of ladder pattern of LPS) (Bryan et al. 1984). Whether this phenomenon accounts for the aminoglycoside resistance directly or is an associated finding is not clear. More recent studies on LPS from some of these isolates show that they have a reduced content of phosphate residues (McGroarty and Bryan, unpublished). It is therefore possible that the amount of aminoglycoside binding to the lipopolysaccharide is reduced. However, studies of this type have not been finalized at this time. In some instances very low levels of modifying enzyme activity have been found associated with strains that show the loss of the ladder pattern of LPS and have significantly higher levels of resistance. Strains without enzymatic activity and lacking the ladder pattern of LPS tend to show low to moderate levels of aminoglycoside resistance (Bryan et al. 1984). Kono and O'Hara (1977) have also described strains of *Pseudomonas aeruginosa* that are not associated with detectable enzymes and which show aminoglycoside resistance. Unlike other accumulation deficient strains these isolates have a narrow aminoglycoside resistance spectrum involving kanamycin or streptomycin as well as non-aminoglycoside antibiotics. No detectable modifying enzymes have been found but the mechanism by which the lack of accumulation of aminoglycosides would operate in these strains is not understood (KONO and O'HARA 1976, 1977).

2. Tetracyclines

a) Uptake

Most studies of tetracycline uptake have been done with tetracycline with a lesser number of studies using chlortetracycline and minocycline. Current evidence would indicate that tetracyclines cross the outer membranes by means of passive diffusion through outer membrane pores. Somewhat surprisingly although minocycline is considerably more hydrophobic than tetracycline, the outer membrane of *E. coli* does not appear to constitute a major permeability barrier relative to tetracycline. Minocycline in general is more active on gram-positive bacteria. This is in keeping with the general observation of a trend towards greater activity for hydrophobic derivatives of antimicrobial agents than hydrophilic derivatives for gram-positive bacteria. This trend apparently results from greater opportunity of hydrophobic compounds to solubilize within the cytoplasmic membrane. It is not the purpose of this chapter to discuss the role of the outer membrane but it is important to note briefly that mutations producing deficiency in the F porin of *E. coli* were associated with reduced tetracycline activity and a minimal reduction of minocycline activity. Thus, tetracycline would appear to use a hydrophilic pore route whereas minocycline mainly uses the hydrophobic pathway (CHOPRA and ECCLES 1978). Lipophilic derivatives of a series of tetracyclines showed some increase in activity in mutations affecting lipopolysaccharide (LEIVE et al. 1984). Removal of lipopolysaccharide by EDTA increases the uptake of minocycline and to a lesser extent tetracycline (MCMURRY et al. 1982).

Levy and colleagues have also indicated that the rate of penetration through the outer membrane may vary depending upon growth of organisms in complex versus minimal medium. Cells grown in minimal medium accumulated more tetracycline than those grown in L-broth "rich" medium. In view of the fact that both an influx and efflux system apparently exists at the cytoplasmic membrane, the rate of entry through the outer membrane is important to determination of the final susceptibility level (MCMURRY et al. 1983).

The process of transport of tetracyclines through the inner membrane is a complex one. It is likely that there is more than one transport system responsible. Studies have shown that there is an energy independent phase of uptake which is rapid and obvious in the early phase of uptake. This type of uptake has been shown in *E. coli* (MCMURRY and LEVY 1978; ARGAST and BECK 1985) and in *Bacteroides fragilis* (FAYOLLE et al. 1980). In addition energy dependent uptake also occurs. Evidence indicates that there is both an influx transport system and an efflux transport system in tetracycline-susceptible bacteria. Evidence for the efflux system has been provided using inverted membrane vesicles (MCMURRY et al. 1983). It is not yet clear whether a carrier is involved in the efflux system. The efflux appears to be more effective for minocycline than for tetracycline and becomes of greater significance when entry through the outer membrane is limited such as occurs in rich medium.

There is also evidence for energy mediated influx. Although kinetics consistent with a carrier mediated process have been described (DOCKTER and MAGNUSON 1974; SAMRA et al. 1977; LINDLEY et al. 1984), it is likely that this is a reflection of the fluorescent assay used rather than demonstration of a saturable carrier. SMITH and CHOPRA (1983) showed that tetracycline fluorescence does not necessarily reflect true internal drug concentrations. This was due in part to fluorescence quenching at high fluor concentrations, undeterminable and changing divalent cation concentration and an inability to measure local internal pH. Studies performed with radiolabelled tetracycline have not provided good evidence for a carrier. Therefore if a carrier mediated system is involved it may well involve more than one carrier.

Active accumulation of tetracycline can utilize both phosphate bond hydrolysis and the proton motive force, again supporting the probability of more than one carrier type for tetracycline (SMITH and CHOPRA 1984). The presence of more than one carrier is also consistent with the failure to isolate chromosomal mutants resistant to a high level of tetracycline. MCMURRY et al. (1981) have used right-side-out inner membrane vesicles from susceptible *E. coli* cells and have shown that tetracycline and minocycline (unpublished studies) are accumulated in vesicles. Inhibitors of electron transport, ATPase and of the proton gradient all interfered with tetracycline uptake. In summary, therefore, it would appear that tetracycline crosses the inner membrane utilizing active uptake systems energized either by proton motive force or phosphate bond energy hydrolysis and by simple diffusion. A competing active efflux system of lower activity which is stronger for minocycline than tetracycline limits net active uptake (LEVY 1984).

b) Resistance and Uptake

Once again the situation with respect to tetracycline resistance is complex. At least in some instances it involves tetracycline accumulation. Most investigations have been done relating to plasmid mediated tetracycline resistance. In gram-negative bacteria at least four genetic classes of tetracycline resistance determinants have been found among various plasmids. The examples are class A, plasmid RP1 and Tn*1721*; class B, Tn*10*; class C, pBR322 and class D, RA1. It would appear that some or all of these encode a tetracycline efflux system which is of higher affinity and greater activity than the intrinsic cellular efflux system (LEVY 1984). However, it should be noted that in gram-positive bacteria alternative mechanisms for tetracycline resistance have been shown which are independent of tetracycline efflux.

BURDETT et al. (1982) identified 3 genetically distinct tetracycline resistance determinants in streptococci. These are designated *tet*L, *tet*M and *tet*N. BURDETT (1986) has shown that tetracycline resistance is associated with reduced tetracycline accumulation in *tet*L but not in *tet*M or *tet*N. In the latter two groups protein synthesis in cellular extracts was resistant to tetracycline. A similar situation has been shown in *Streptomyces rimosus*. OHNUKI et al. (1985) cloned the *tet*A and *tet*B genes from *S. rimosus* into *S. griseus*. The *tet*A gene specified tetracycline resistance through a cytoplasmic factor which was ribosomally associated and made protein synthesis resistant to tetracycline. *Tet*B was associated with reduced accumulation of intracellular tetracycline. Both genes were inducible.

For some time there has been a concern that small differences in the drug accumulated by resistant versus sensitive cells did not correlate with the large differences in MIC of tetracycline (AVTALION et al. 1981; REYNARD et al. 1971; LEVY et al. 1977). LEVY (1984) has pointed out some of the inconsistencies with the explanation of resistance being only based on reduced accumulation. The possibility of a cytoplasmic factor which associates with ribosomes preventing tetracycline binding still exists but there is no good evidence for this in gram-negative bacteria at the present time. However, as noted there is good evidence for a similar type of picture in gram-positive bacteria.

Therefore at this time it would be appear that efflux of tetracycline is the major reason for tetracycline resistance in gram-negative bacteria. Genetic determinants specifying tetracycline resistance have in general been shown to encode for a tetracycline inducible membrane protein turned TET. The nucleotide sequence (HILLEN and SCHOLLMEIER 1983; POSTLE et al. 1984), organization (WRAY et al. 1981) and regulation of expression (HILLEN et al. 1983) from Tn*10* (class B) have been reported. TET protein appears to contain two genetically defined domains, is membrane bound, is needed for efflux, probably binds tetracycline and does not block the host active uptake system. Class A and C determinants also produce inner membrane proteins similar to the TET protein (summarized in LEVY 1984). In addition to the TET protein, studies of the Tn*10* determinant have demonstrated that a repressor of approximately 23000 to 25000 daltons is also coded. Tetracycline resistance is "inducible" with Tn*10* and in most plasmid specified tetracycline resistance studied to date (YANG et al. 1976; WRAY et al. 1981; BECK et al. 1982; HILLEN et al. 1982).

In summary there are two protein products expressed from the three tetracycline resistance determinants studied in depth to date. These include a repressor at 23000 to 25000 molecular weight and the TET protein at 34000 to 43000 molecular weight.

Recently DOSCH et al. (1984) have shown that the tetracycline resistance element of pBR322 complements the potassium transport defect of *Escherichia coli* K12 mutants, having markedly impaired potassium transport. Therefore the plasmid mediates potassium transport. Interestingly, the Tn*10* element did not do this showing that such an effect is not a general property of genetic elements specifying resistance to tetracycline. KANEKO et al. (1985) have provided evidence using inverted membrane vesicles that the plasmid encoded tetracycline transport was mainly due to an electrically neutral proton/tetracycline antiport system. Therefore the major driving force would be the proton gradient.

The TET protein structural gene consists of two domains which complement each other intracistonically (CURIALE and LEVY 1982). The significance of this in turns of function of the protein is not apparently understood at the present time.

In summary, plasmid mediated tetracycline resistance is associated with the production of a membrane associated TET protein which is presumed to mediate tetracycline transport. A repressor protein has also been demonstrated accounting for the inducibility of tetracycline resistance. Resistance is achieved through an active efflux system which at least in Tn*10* is driven by Δ pH. Tetracycline resistance can be achieved in certain bacteria through protection of protein synthesis machinery. Whether this contributes to resistance in gram-negative bacteria has not been finalized to date.

IV. Diffusional Systems

1. Fluoroquinolone and Quinolone Antibiotics

It is generally agreed that the major target of action of this large group of antimicrobial agents termed "quinolones" and more recent derivatives generally referred to as "fluoroquinolones" is DNA gyrase which is an intracellular target. Therefore these compounds must penetrate the cytoplasmic membrane in both gram-positive and gram-negative bacteria and the outer membrane in gram-negative bacteria. Recent studies (BEDARD et al. 1987) have shown that the whole cell uptake of enoxacin is a diffusional process. Uptake studies utilizing radiolabelled drug or a bioassay method of measuring unlabelled drug have shown a rapid association of the drug with cells and only limited additional accumulation with time. Uptake is not saturable and is not influenced by inhibitors of a electron transport, glycolytically derived energy, membrane ATPase activity or agents which collapse the proton gradient. Therefore there seems to be no energy requirements for enoxacin uptake. The rate of accumulation was reduced at 4 °C but this is an observation consistent with diffusion. Similar results have been reported utilizing norfloxacin (HOOPER et al. 1986a), and for ciprofloxacin, pefloxacin, amifloxacin and norfloxacin (DIVER et al. 1986).

Recently in our own laboratory and as reported by COHEN et al. (1987) and by HOOPER et al. (1987) there appears to be an energy dependent efflux system. Work by COHEN et al. (1987) using everted membrane vesicles has shown a saturable efflux system which is inhibited by dinitrophenol and CCCP. HOOPER et al. (1987) have also reported that norfloxacin resistant mutants had greater increase in accumulation of norfloxacin than did wild type bacteria. The significance of this finding is not yet clear.

Our own laboratory has also findings consistent with an energy dependent efflux system. However, the significance of the efflux system to the activity of fluoroquinolones remains unclear. Our own investigations have not been able to establish that there is any increase in killing associated with greater accumulation as a result of inhibiting efflux. The efflux system is markedly less active in nutrient broth as compared to brain heart infusion broth and this does not correlate clearly with differential activity of fluoroquinolones.

Our results are consistent with the view that fluoroquinolones diffuse through outer membrane porins, which is rate limiting with respect to diffusion. Thereafter they rapidly diffuse across the cytoplasmic membrane and an equilibrium is set up. The intracellular concentration of the drug depends upon the rate of diffusion in and the rate of diffusion out as well as that due to active efflux from the cell. Our investigations at this time support the view that the rapid diffusional entry of fluoroquinolones rapidly results in an intracellular concentration capable of inhibiting DNA gyrase. Although studies are early it does not appear that the active efflux system plays a significant role in preventing an adequate intracellular concentration to inhibit gyrase (BRYAN et al. 1988).

Several workers have shown that resistance to fluoroquinolones may occur either through mutation affecting DNA gyrase or through a reduction of penetration of the compounds through the outer membrane. HIRAI et al. (1986a), HOOPER et al. (1986b), BEDARD et al. (1987) and HIRAI et al. (1987) have shown that resistance to various fluoroquinolones may arise as a result of either demonstrated or apparent changes in outer membrane permeability. Mutations resulting in loss of most or all of the F-porin in *Escherichia coli* are associated with reduced uptake of norfloxacin (HIRAI et al. 1986a; HOOPER et al. 1986b) or enoxacin (BEDARD et al. 1987). In *Pseudomonas aeruginosa* resistance to fluoroquinolones has been described associated with the acquisition of a new outer membrane protein of approximate molecular weight of 54000 daltons. The resistance phenotype was associated with a reduction of accumulation of norfloxacin (HIRAI et al. 1987). There is no evidence at the present time that mutations affecting the cytoplasmic membrane are associated with resistance to fluoroquinolones.

Most of the more recent quinolones are relatively hydrophilic compared to older quinolone antibiotics such as nalidixic acid. Studies by HIRAI et al. (1986b) have shown that most fluoroquinolones do not have a marked difference of activity when rough LPS derivatives are compared with their smooth parents. The activity of nalidixic acid was generally greater in mutants with rough LPS but these observations have not been seen for norfloxacin, enoxacin and ciprofloxacin.

In summary, it would appear that in *Escherichia coli* penetration of quinolones occurs principally through the F-porin and that smooth LPS is not a major barrier for the hydrophilic fluoroquinolones. Resistance results from a replacement of F-porin with C-porin in *E. coli* and may be seen in association with other more poorly defined outer membrane changes in *Pseudomonas aeruginosa*. In both gram-positive and gram-negative bacteria transport through the cytoplasmic membrane occurs by simple diffusion and resistance associated with change in this step of uptake has not been described.

Our own observations that *Pseudomonas aeruginosa* accumulates much lower quantities of ciprofloxacin and enoxacin than *E. coli* suggests that the somewhat greater activity of ciprofloxacin on *E. coli* is related to its better uptake in that organism (BEDARD and BRYAN, unpublished). Small changes in susceptibility of DNA gyrase between these organisms cannot yet be excluded. It is likely, however, again this difference in uptake would be manifest at the outer membrane level rather than at the cytoplasmic membrane.

2. Erythromycin

The present available evidence suggests that erythromycin is accumulated by a process of passive diffusion. Cellular association with erythromycin was measured using both time dependent kinetics uptake and equilibrium binding experiments (BARRE et al. 1986). A dissociation constant of 0.1 μM was determined, which is similar to that reflecting binding to bacterial ribosomes. No effect on accumulation by KCN or dinitrophenol was observed.

Maximal growth inhibition occurs with erythromycin A at about a pH of 8.5, which is very close to that of its p*Ka*. This is consistent with a process of diffusion suggesting the most active form is the non-protonated most lipophilic species.

LAMPSON et al. (1986) have described an unusual form of erythromycin resistance in *Staphylococcus aureus*. Resistance in plasmid-specified to only 14-member macrolides such as erythromycin but not to other macrolide-lincosamide-streptogramin antibiotics. Resistant derivatives accumulated less erythromycin but no inactivation or loss of binding affinity for ribosomes was detected. A 60K membrane protein was found in cells with the erythromycin plasmid. Thus, resistance my be due to altered permeability.

3. Clindamycin

It is not understood how clindamycin enters bacterial cells. Evidence has been advanced that clinidamycin utilizes a nucleoside transport system in polymorphonuclear leukocytes and alveolar macrophages. Resistance based on lack of transport to clindamycin has not been reported (STEINBERG and HAND 1984; HAND and KING-THOMPSON 1982).

4. Chloramphenicol

BURNS and SMITH (1987) have shown chloramphenicol is accumulated by *Haemophilus influenzae* by a process which has the characteristics of energy dependent transport and seems to be a saturable process. Chloramphenicol was concentrated within cells, its uptake was markedly decreased by 2,4-dinitrophenol and CCCP and inhibited by a fluorinated chloramphenicol analog SCH 24893. BURNS et al. (1985) propose that chloramphenicol is passively transported through the outer membrane which is supported by the presence of mutations defective in an outer membrane protein considered to be a porin in *Haemophilus influenzae*. There is also evidence that chloramphenicol utilizes the *Omp*F porin in *E. coli* (CHOPRA and ECCLES 1978). Following outer membrane diffusion it is proposed by Burns and Smith that entry across the cytoplasmic membrane occurs by the energy-dependent process characterized above. ABDEL-SAYED (1987) has also provided evidence for energy-dependent uptake of chloramphenicol in *E. coli* and *P. aeruginosa*.

BURNS et al. (1986) have recently cloned a portion of *Tn* 1696 from *P. aeruginosa* to *E. coli*. This is associated with reduced chloramphenicol uptake and the absence of 50K protein outer membrane protein. Some DNA homology was present with isolates of *Haemophilus influenzae* with reduced outer membrane permeability to chloramphenicol.

5. Others

A large additional list of antimicrobial agents exist which are not considered in this chapter. That is because they do not require a cytoplasmic transport process, for example, as *β*-lactams or very little is understood about them. Into the latter group such important agents as sulfonamides, trimethoprim, rifampicin and fusidic acid can be placed. It is likely agents like rifampicin and novobiocin which are hydrophobic compounds pass through the cytoplasmic membrane by means of diffusion. Polymyxin, a cationic compound, binds to both outer membrane and cytoplasmic membrane. It acts as a detergent to disorganize membranes and does not strictly speaking have a conventional transport system. Metronidazole uptake is associated with drug reduction and seems an essential step in its activity (RABIN and LOCKERBY 1984). It is not within the scope of this chapter to discuss ionophores which again do not themselves undergo transport but form transport channels with variable degrees of specificity.

References

Abdel-Sayed S (1987) Transport of chloramphenicol into sensitive strains of *Escherichia coli* and *Pseudomonas aeruginosa*. J Antimicrob Chemother 19:7–20

Acar JF, Goldstein FN, Lagrange F (1978) Human infections caused by thiamine or menadione-requiring *Staphylococcus aureus*. J Clin Microbiol 8:142–147

Adler LW, Rosen BP (1976) Properties of *Escherichia coli* mutants with alterations in Mg^{++}-adenosine triphosphatase. J Bacteriol 128:248–256

Anand J, Davis BD (1960) Damage by streptomycin to the cell membrane of *Escherichia coli*. Nature 185:22–23

Annear DI (1975) Unstable gentamicin resistance with linkage to colony size in *Pseudomonas aeruginosa*. Pathology 7:281–283

Anraku Y (1978) Active transport of amino acids. In: Rosen BP (ed) Bacterial transport. Dekker, New York, pp 171–220

Argast M, Beck CF (1985) Tetracycline uptake by susceptible *Escherichia coli* cells. Arch Microbiol 141:260–265

Atherton FR, Hall MJ, Hassal CH, Lambert RW, Lloyd WJ, Ringrose PS (1979) Phosphonopeptides as antibacterial agents: mechanism of action of alaphosphin. Antimicrob Agents Chemother 15:696–705

Atherton FR, Hall MJ, Hassal CH, Lambert RW, Lloyd WJ, Lord AV, Ringrose PS, Westmacott D (1983) Phosphonopeptides as substrates for peptide transport systems and peptidases of *Escherichia coli*. Antimicrob Agents Chemother 24:522–528

Avtalion RR, Ziegler-Schlomowitz R, Perl M, Wojdani A, Sompolinsky D (1971) Depressed resistance to tetracycline in *Staphylococcus aureus*. Microbios 3:165–180

Barre J, Furnet MP, Zini R, Defforge SL, Duval J, Tillment JP (1986) In vitro ^{3}H-erythromycin binding to *Staphylococcus aureus*. Biochem Pharmacol 35:1001–1004

Beck CF, Metzel R, Barbe J, Muller W (1982) A multifunctional gene (*tetR*) controls Tn*10*-encoded tetracycline resistance. J Bacteriol 150:633–642

Bedard J, Wong S, Bryan LE (1987) Accumulation of enoxacin by *Escherichia coli* and *Bacillus subtilis*. Antimicrob Agents Chemother 31:1348–1354

Braun V, Gunthner K, Hantke K, Zimmermann L (1983) Intracellular activation of albomycin in *Escherichia coli* and *Salmonella typhimurium*. J Bacteriol 156:308–315

Bryan LE, Kwan S (1981 b) Mechanisms of aminoglycoside resistance of anaerobic bacteria and facultative bacteria grown anaerobically. J Antimicrob Chemother [Suppl D] 8:1–8

Bryan LE, Kwan S (1983) Roles of ribosomal binding, membrane potential and electron transport in bacterial uptake of streptomycin and gentamicin. Antimicrob Agents Chemother 23:835–845

Bryan LE, van den Elzen HM (1975) Gentamicin accumulation by sensitive strain of *Escherichia coli* in *Pseudomonas aeruginosa*. J Antibiot (Tokyo) 28:696–703

Bryan LE, van den Elzen HM (1976) Streptomycin accumulation in susceptible and resistant strains of *Escherichia coli* in *Pseudomonas aeruginosa*. Antimicrob Agents Chemother 9:928–938

Bryan LE, van den Elzen HM (1977) Effects of membrane-energy mutations and cations on streptomycin and gentamicin accumulation by bacteria: a model for entry of streptomycin and gentamicin in susceptible and resistant bacteria. Antimicrob Agents Chemother 12:163–177
Bryan LE, Kowand SK, van den Elzen HM (1979) The basis of aminoglycoside antibiotic resistance in anaerobic bacteria: *Clostridium perfringens* and *Bacteroides fragilis*. Antimicrob Agents Chemother 15:7–13
Bryan LE, Nicas TI, Holloway BW, Crowther C (1980) Aminoglycoside-resistant mutation of *Pseudomonas aeruginosa* defective in cytochrome C_{553} and nitrate reductase. Antimicrob Agents Chemother 17:71–79
Bryan LE, O'Hara K, Wong S (1984) Lipopolysaccharide changes in permeability type aminoglycoside resistance in *Pseudomonas aeruginosa*. Antimicrob Agents Chemother 26:250–255
Bryan LE, Bedard J, Wong S, Chamberland S (1988) Quinolone antimicrobial agents: mechanism of action and resistance development. Clin Invest Med (in press)
Bryant RE (1984) Effect of the suppurative environment on antibiotic activity. In: Root RK, Sande MA (eds) New dimensions in antimicrobial therapy. Churchill Livingston, New York, pp 313–317
Burdett V (1986) Streptococcal tetracycline resistance mediated at the level of protein synthesis. J Bacteriol 165:564–569
Burdett V, Inamine J, Rajagopalam S (1982) Heterogeneity of tetracycline resistance for determinants in *Streptococcus*. J Bacteriol 149:995–1004
Burns JL, Smith AL (1987) Chloramphenicol accumulation by *Haemophilus influenzae*. Antimicrob Agents Chemother 31:686–690
Burns JL, Mendelman PN, Levy J, Stull TL, Smith AL (1985) A permeability barrier as a mechanism of chloramphenicol resistance in *Haemophilus influenzae*. Antimicrob Agents Chemother 27:46–54
Burns JL, Rubens CE, Mendelman PN, Smith AL (1986) Cloning and expression in *Escherichia coli* of a gene encoding non-enzymatic chloramphenicol resistance from *Pseudomonas aeruginosa*. Antimicrob Agents Chemother 29:445–450
Chopra I, Ball P (1982) Transport of antibiotics into bacteria. Adv Microb Physiol 23:184–240
Chopra I, Eccles NS (1978) Diffusion of tetracycline across the outer membrane of *Escherichia coli* K12 involvement of protein Ia. Biochim Biophys Res Commun 83:550–557
Cohen SP, Hooper DC, Wolfson JS, Souza KS, McMurry LM, Levy SB (1988) Endogenous active efflux of norfloxacin in susceptible *Escherichia coli*. Antimicrob Agents Chemother 32:1187–1191
Curiale MS, Levy S (1982) Two complementation groups mediate tetracycline resistance determined by Tn*10*. J Bacteriol 151:209–215
Damper TD, Epstein W (1981) Role of the membrane potential and bacterial resistance to aminoglycoside antibiotics. Antimicrob Agents Chemother 20:803–808
Davis BD, Chen L, Tai PC (1986) Misread protein creates membrane channels: an essential step in the bactericidal action of aminoglycosides. Proc Natl Acad Sci USA 83:6164–6168
Dette GA, Knothe H, Schonenbach B, Plage G (1983) Comparative study of fosomycin activity in Mueller-Hinton media and in tissues. J Antimicrob Chemother 11:517–524
Dickie P, Bryan LE, Pickard MA (1978) Effect of enzymatic adenylylation on dihydrostreptomycin accumulation in *Escherichia coli* carrying an R-factor: model explaining aminoglycoside resistance by inactivating mechanisms. Antimicrob Agents Chemother 14:569–580
Diver JM, Pidock LJV, Wyse R (1986) Investigations into the uptake of five fluoroquinolones by E. col. KL-16. (Abstr) 26th Interscience Conference on Antimicrobial Agents and Chemotherapy, New Orleans
Dockter ME, Magnuson JA (1974) Characterization of the active transport of chlorotetracycline in *Staphylococcus aureus* by a fluorescence technique. J Supramol Struct 2:32–44

Dosch DC, Salvasion FF, Epstein W (1984) Tetracycline resistant elements of pBR322 mediates potassium transport. J Bacteriol 160:1188–1190

Eisenberg ES, Mandel LJ, Kaback HR, Miller MH (1984) Quantitative association between electrical potential across the cytoplasmic membrane and early gentamicin uptake and killing in *Staphylococcus aureus*. J Bacteriol 157:863–867

Fayolle F, Privitera G, Sevald M (1980) Tetracycline transport in *Bacteroides fragilis*. Antimicrob Agents Chemother 18:502–505

Felle J, Porter JS, Slayman CL, Kaback HR (1980) Quantitative measurements of membrane potential in *Escherichia coli*. Biochemistry 19:3585–3590

Garcia-Riestra C, Perlin MH, Lerner SA (1985) Lack of accumulation of exogenous adenylyl dihydrostreptomycin by whole cells or spheroplasts of *Escherichia coli*. Antimicrob Agents Chemother 27:114–119

Gerber AU, Vatola AP, Brandel J, Craig WA (1982) Selection of aminoglycoside resistant variants of *Pseudomonas aeruginosa* in an in vivo model. J Infect Dis 146:691–697

Grappel SF, Giovenella AJ, Nisbet LJ (1985) Activity of a peptidyl prodrug alafosfalin against anaerobic bacteria. Antimicrob Agents Chemother 27:961–963

Hancock REW (1962) Uptake of ^{14}C-streptomycin by *Bacillus megaterium*. J Gen Microbiol 28:503–516

Hancock REW, Raffle VJ, Nicas TI (1981) Involvement of the outer membrane in gentamicin and streptomycin uptake and killing in *Pseudomonas aeruginosa*. Antimicrob Agents Chemother 19:777–785

Hand WL, King-Thompson NL (1982) Membrane transport of clindamycin and alveolar macrophages. Antimicrob Agents Chemother 21:241–247

Hartmann A, Fiedler H-P, Braun V (1979) Uptake and conversion of the antibiotic albomycin by *Escherichia coli* K12. Eur J Biochem 99:517–524

Hirai K, Aoyama H, Suzue S, Irikura T, Iyobe S, Mitsuhashi S (1986a) Isolation and characterization of norfloxacin-resistant mutants of *Escherichia coli* K12. Antimicrob Agents Chemother 30:248–253

Hirai K, Aoyama H, Iridura T, Iyobe S, Mitsuhashi S (1986b) Differences in susceptibility to quinolones of outer membrane mutants of *Salmonella typhimurium* and *Escherichia coli*. Antimicrob Agents Chemother 29:535–538

Hirai K, Suzue S, Irikura T, Iyobe S, Mitsuhashi S (1987) Mutations producing resistance to norfloxacin in *Pseudomonas aeruginosa*. Antimicrob Agents Chemother 31:582–586

Hillen W, Schollmeier K (1983) Nucleotide sequence of the Tn*10* encoded tetracycline resistance gene. Nucleic Acids Res 11:525–539

Hillen W, Clock G, Kaffenberger I, Wray LV, Reznikoff WS (1982) Purification of the TET repressor and TET operator from the transposon Tn*10* and characterization of their interaction. J Biol Chem 257:6605–6613

Hillen W, Gats C, Altschmide L, Scholmeier K, Meier I (1983) Control of expression of the *Rn*10-encoded tetracycline resistance genes. J Mol Biol 169:707–721

Holtje JV (1979) Induction of streptomycin uptake in resistant strains of *Escherichia coli*. Antimicrob Agents Chemother 15:177–181

Hooper DC, Wolfson JS, Souza KS, Schwartz MN (1986a) Binding of radiolabelled norfloxacin (NFX) to wildtype and mutant *Escherichia coli*. (Abstr) 26th Interscience conference on Antimicrobial Agents and Chemotherapy, New Orleans

Hooper DC, Wolfson JS, Souza KS, Tung C, McHugh GL, Swartz MN (1986b) Genetic and biochemical characterization of norfloxacin resistance in *Escherichia coli*. Antimicrob Agents Chemother 29:639–644

Hooper DC, Wolfson JS, Souza KS, Schwartz MN (1987) Effects of energy inhibitors on norfloxacin uptake by *Escherichia coli*. (Abstr) 27th Interscience Conference on Antimicrobial Agents and Chemotherapy, New York

Kadner RJ, Bassford PJ (1978) The role of the outer membrane in active transport. In: Rosen BP (ed) Bacterial transport. Dekker, New York, pp 413–462

Kahan FM, Kahan JS, Cassidy PJ, Kropp H (1974) The mechanism of action of fosfomycin (phosphonomycin). Ann NY Acad Sci 235:364–386

Kaneko M, Ayamaguchi A, Sawai T (1985) Energetics of tetracycline efflux system encoated by Tn*10* in *Escherichia coli*. FEBS Lett 193:194–198

Kogut M, Lightbown JW, Isaacson P (1965) Streptomycin action and anaerobiosis. J Gen Microbiol 39:155–164

Komatsu Y, Tanaka K (1972) A showdomycin-resistant mutant of *Escherichia coli* K12 with altered nucleoside transport character. Biochim Biophysics Acta 288:390–403

Komatsu Y, Tanaka K (1973) Deoxycytidine uptake by isolated membrane vesicles from *Escherichia coli* K12. Biochim Biophys Acta 311:496–506

Kono N, O'Hara K (1976) Mechanisms of streptomycin-resistance of highly streptomycin-resistant *Pseudomonas aeruginosa* strains. J Antibiot (Tokyo) 29:169–175

Kono N, O'Hara K (1977) Kanamycin-resistance mechanism of *Pseudomonas aeruginosa* governed by an R-plasmid independently of inactivating enzymes. J Antibiot (Tokyo) 30:688–690

Lampson BC, von David W, Parisi JT (1986) Novo mechanism for plasmid-mediated erythromycin resistance by pNE24 from *Staphylococcus epidermidis*. Antimicrob Agents Chemother 30:653–658

Leive L, Telesetsky S, Coleman WG, Carr D (1984) Tetracyclines of various hydrophobicities as a probe for permeability of *Escherichia coli* outer membrane. Antimicrob Agents Chemother 25:539–544

Levy SB (1984) Resistance to the tetracyclines. In: Bryan LE (ed) Antimicrobial drug resistance. Academic, Orlando, pp 191–240

Levy SB, McMurry L, Ognigman P, Saunders RM (1977) Plasmid-mediated tetracycline resistance in E. coli. In: Drews J, Hogenauer G (eds) R-factors: their properties and possible control. Springer, Berlin Heidelberg New York, pp 181–207 (Topics in infectious diseases, vol 2)

Lindley EV, Munscke GR, Magnuson JA (1984) Kinetic analysis of tetracycline accumulation by *Streptococcus faecalis*. J Bacteriol 158:334–336

Loh B, Grant C, Hancock REW (1984) Use of the fluorescent probe 1-*N*-phenylnaphthylamine to study the interactions of aminoglycoside antibiotics with the outer membrane of *Pseudomonas aeruginosa*. Antimicrob Agents Chemother 26:546–551

Mandel LJ, Eisenberg ES, Simkin NJ, Miller MH (1983) Effect of *N*, *N'*-dicyclohexylcarbodiimide and nigericin on *Staphylococcus aureus* susceptibility to gentamicin. Antimicrob Agents Chemother 24:440–442

Martin NL, Beveridge TJ (1986) Gentamicin interaction of *Pseudomonas aeruginosa* cell envelope. Antimicrob Agents Chemother 29:1079–1087

Mates SM, Eisenberg ES, Mandel LJ, Patel L, Kaback HR, Miller MH (1982) Membrane potential and gentamicin uptake in *Staphylococcus aureus*. Proc Natl Acad Sci USA 79:6693–6697

McEnroe AS, Taber HW (1984) Correlation between cytochrome aa_3 concentrations and streptomycin accumulation in *Bacillus subtilis*. Antimicrob Agents Chemother 26:507–512

McMurry LM, Levy S (1978) Two transport systems for tetracycline in sensitive *Escherichia coli*: critical role for an initial rapid uptake system in sensitive to energy inhibitors. Antimicrob Agents Chemother 14:201–209

McMurry LM, Cullinane JC, Petrucci RJ, Levy S (1981) Active uptake of tetracycline by membrane vesicles from susceptible *Escherichia coli*. Antimicrob Agents Chemother 20:307–313

McMurry LM, Cullinane JC, Levy S (1982) Transport of the lipophylic analog minocycline differs from that of tetracycline in susceptible and resistant *Escherichia coli* strains. Antimicrobial Agents Chemother 22:791–799

McMurry LM, Aronson DA, Levy SB (1983) Susceptible *Escherichia coli* cells can actively excrete tetracyclines. Antimicrob Agents Chemother 24:544–551

Miller MH, Edberg SC, Mandel LJ, Behar CF, Steigbeigel NH (1980) Gentamicin uptake in wild-type and aminoglycoside resistant small-colony mutants of *Staphylococcus aureus*. Antimicrob Agents Chemother 18:722–729

Muir ME, Hanwell DR, Wallace BJ (1981) Characterization of a respiratory mutant of *Escherichia coli* with reduced uptake of aminoglycoside antibiotics. Biochim Biophys Acta 638:234–241

Muir ME, Ballesteros M, Wallace BJ (1985) Respiration rate, growth rate and accumulation of streptomycin in *Escherichia coli*. J Gen Microbiol 131:2573–2579

Musher DM, Baughan RC, Templeton JB, Minuth JM (1977) Emergence of various forms of *Staphylococcus aureus* after exposure to gentamicin and infectivity of the variants in experimental animals. J Infect Dis 136:360–369

Musher DM, Baughan RC, Merrell GL (1979) Selection of small-colony variants of Enterobacteriaceae by in vitro exposure to aminoglycosides: pathogenicity for experimental animals. J Infect Dis 140:209–214

Nicas TI, Hancock REW (1980) Outer membrane protein H_1 of *P.* aeruginosa: involvement in adaptive and mutational resistance to EDTA, polymyxin B and gentamicin. J Bacteriol 143:872–878

Nichols WW, Young SN (1985) Respiration – dependent uptake of dihydrostreptomycin by *Escherichia coli.* Biochem J 228:505–512

Nikaido H, Vaara M (1985) Bacterial outer membrane permeability. Microbiol Rev 49:1–32

Nuesch J, Knusel F (1967) Sideromycins. In: Gottlieb D, Shaw PD (eds) Antibiotics I. Springer, Berlin Heidelberg New York, pp 499–541

Ohnuki T, Katoh T, Imanaka T, Aiba C (1985) Molecular cloning of tetracycline resistance genes from *Streptomyces rimosus.* in *Streptomyces griseus* and characterization of a cloned genes. J Bacteriol 161:1010–1016

Payne JW, Gilvarg C (1978) Transport of peptides in bacteria. In: Rosen BP (ed) Bacterial transport. Dekker, New York, pp 325–384

Pelletier LL, Richardson MR, Fiest N (1979) Virulent gentamicin-induced small-colony variants of *Staphylococcus aureus.* J Lab Clin Med 94:324–334

Postle K, Nguyen DT, Bertrand KP (1984) Nucleotide sequence of the repressor gene of the Tn*10* tetracycline resistance determinant. Nucleic Acids Res 12:4849–4863

Rabin HR, Lockerby DL (1984) Resistance to nitrofurans and nitroimidazoles. In: Bryan LE (ed) Antimicrobial drug resistance. Academic, Orlando, pp 317–344

Reynard AM, Nellis LF, Beck M (1971) Uptake of ^{3}H-tetracycline by resistant and sensitive *Escherichia coli.* Appl Microbiol 21:71–75

Rosen BP, Kashket ER (1978) Energetics of active transport. In: Rosen BP (ed) Bacterial transport. Dekker, New York, pp 559–620

Samra Z, Krausz-Steinmetz J, Sompolinsky D (1977) Transport of tetracyclines through the bacterial-cell membrane assayed by fluorescence – study with susceptible and resistant strains of *Staphylococcus aureus* and *Escherichia coli.* Microbios 21:7–21

Smith MC, Chopra I (1983) Limitations of a fluorescence assay for studies on tetracycline transport into *Escherichia coli.* Antimicrob Agents Chemother 23:175–178

Smith MC, Chopra I (1984) Energetics of tetracycline transport into *Escherichia coli.* Antimicrob Agents Chemother 25:446–449

Spagna VA, Fass RJ, Prior RB, Slama PG (1978) Report of a case of bacterial sepsis caused by a naturally occurring variant from of *Staphylococcus aureus.* J Infect Dis 138:277–278

Steinberg TH, Hand WL (1984) Effects of phagocytosis on antibiotic and leucocyte uptake by human polymorphonuclear leucocytes. J Infect Dis 149:397–403

Thomson TB, Crider BP, Eagon RG (1985) The kinetics of dihydrostreptomycin uptake in *Pseudomonas putida* membrane vesicles: absence of inhibition by cations. J Antimicrob Chemother 16:157–163

Tsuruoka T, Miyata A, Manada Y (1978) Two kinds of mutants defective in multiple carbohydrate utilization isolated from in vitro fosfomycin-resistant strains of *Escherichia coli* K12. J Antibiot (Tokyo) 31:192–201

Vastola AP, Altschaefl J, Harford S (1980) 5-epi-sisomicin and 5-epi-gentamicin B: substrates for aminoglycoside-modified enzymes that retain activity against aminoglycoside-resistant bacteria. Antimicrob Agents Chemother 17:798–802

Wargel RJ, Shadur CA, Neuhaus FC (1971) Mechanism of D-glycoserine action: transport mutants for D-alanine, D-cycloserine and glycine. J Bacteriol 105:1028–1035

Wray LV Jr, Jorgensen RA, Reznikoff WS (1981) Identification of the tetracycline resistance promoter and repressor in transposon Tn*10.* J Bacteriol 147:297–304

Yang HL, Zubay G, Levy S (1976) Synthesis of an R-plasmid protein associated with tetracycline resistance is negatively regulated. Proc Natl Acad Sci USA 73:1509–1512

CHAPTER 3

Susceptibility and Resistance of *Plasmodium falciparum* to Chloroquine *

D. J. KROGSTAD, P. H. SCHLESINGER, and I. Y. GLUZMAN

A. Introduction

Four species of malaria parasites infect humans: *Plasmodium falciparum, Plasmodium vivax, Plasmodium ovale* and *Plasmodium malariae*. Of these, only *P. falciparum* poses a significant risk of death in the non-immune patient because of its ability to invade red cells of any age and thus to produce overwhelming parasitemias $\geqq 10^6$ per µl (FIELD 1949; NEVA 1977). The other species produce less morbidity and mortality because they are able to invade only young (*P. vivax* or *P. ovale*) or old (*P. malariae*) red cells, respectively (NEVA 1977).

I. Magnitude of Malaria as a Medical Problem and the Importance of Antimalarials

Recent data suggest that there are more than 2 million deaths from malaria (most of which are among children less than 5 in Africa) and approximately 200–300 million cases each year (WYLER 1983). The incidence and mortality of malaria dwarf those of most other infectious diseases.

Antimalarials have been used since before the time of Hippocrates (JONES 1909), and were essential in settling the United States. However, antimalarial treatment has traditionally been empirical. The mechanisms of chloroquine action and resistance have been unknown although chloroquine has been the most widely used antimalarial for more than 40 years. This lack of knowledge is increasingly important because of the rising prevalence of chloroquine resistance. Many *P. falciparum* isolates from South America, Southeast Asia and Africa are now chloroquine-resistant (CENTERS FOR DISEASE CONTROL 1985, 1986, 1987; MILLER et al. 1986). In contrast, all *P. vivax, P. ovale* and *P. malariae* strains remain chloroquine-susceptible (CENTERS FOR DISEASE CONTROL 1985).

II. Potential Interventions – Vaccines Vs. Drugs

Current attempts to combat malaria include efforts to develop a malaria vaccine and better antimalarials. The effort to develop a malaria vaccine has been based primarily on the use of recombinant DNA technology to clone and identify the

---

* These investigations received the financial support of the UNDP/World Bank/WHO Special Programme for Research and Training in Tropical Diseases. They were also supported in part by grant AI 18911 from the National Institute of Allergy and Infectious Diseases and grant HL 26300 from the National Heart Lung and Blood Institute.

immunodominant epitopes of the parasite (ENEA et al. 1984). The consensus of most investigators is that an effective malaria vaccine will need to contain at least two and possibly three antigens – sporozoite, merozoite and gametocyte – in order to interfere with: initial infection of the liver by mosquito *sporozoites*, asexual replication in the bloodstream by *merozoites*, and transmission to the mosquito by *gametocytes*. Of these 3 parasite stages, the work on sporozoite antigens is most advanced. However, the fact that the initial sporozoite vaccine preparations have been less immunogenic than expected (BALLOU et al. 1987) suggests that an effective vaccine will not be available in the short-term future. Although the rising prevalence of chloroquine resistance has stimulated the effort to develop a malaria vaccine, a malaria vaccine is not expected to obviate the need for antimalarials. In fact, both approaches will likely be employed together in the future (MILLER et al. 1986).

III. The Effect of Parasite Stage

The understanding and development of better antimalarials is dependent on parasite stage because only asexual erythrocytic parasites produce clinical illness. Neither persistent exoerythrocytic hepatic parasites (hypnozoites) nor sexual parasites (gametocytes) produce recognizable clinical symptomatology. Therefore the antimalarials that produce rapid clinical improvement are those that inhibit the replication of asexual erythrocytic parasites. Different antimalarials are needed for treatment of the different parasite stages (Table 1).

Table 1. Stage dependence of antimalarial drugs

	Pharmacologic
Sporozoite	
Hypnozoite	Primaquine
Merozoite	
Asexual erythrocytic stages	Chloroquine
(ring, trophozoite, schizont)	Quinine
	Mefloquine
Gametocyte	Primaquine

IV. Drugs Active Against Asexual Erythrocytic Parasites

The most widely used agents active against asexual erythrocytic parasites are chloroquine, quinine, quinidine and mefloquine. Other important drugs include inhibitors of protein synthesis (such as tetracycline, which is used most frequently in combination with other agents) and antifolates (pyrimethamine and sulfonamides). In this chapter, we examine the action of chloroquine and other quinoline antimalarials, and the mechanism of chloroquine resistance.

B. Mechanism of Chloroquine Action

I. Previous Theories of Chloroquine Action

Previously, two theories have dominated thinking about the mechanism of chloroquine action against *P. falciparum*. However, in our opinion, neither theory satisfactorily explains the antiplasmodial activity of chloroquine. (1) *Intercalation of chloroquine into DNA* – Although chloroquine binds to DNA and other polyanions (Allison et al. 1965; Ciak and Hahn 1966; Parker and Irvin 1952), the extracellular chloroquine concentrations necessary to inhibit DNA synthesis by this mechanism (0.5–2 m*M*) (Cohen and Yielding 1965; O'Brien et al. 1966) are several orders of magnitude greater than those which inhibit the growth of chloroquine-susceptible plasmodia in vitro (1–20 n*M*) (Desjardins et al. 1979; Geary and Jensen 1983; Gluzman et al. 1987). In addition, chloroquine inhibits nucleic acid synthesis in virtually all prokaryotic and eukaryotic cells, in contrast to the exquisite specificity of chloroquine action against plasmodia in vivo. (2) *Binding of chloroquine to ferriprotoporphyrin IX (FP)* – Unlike mammalian cells, the malaria parasite is unable to break down the porphyrin ring of hemoglobin. Thus the parasite food vacuole (secondary lysosome) retains FP as the nondegradable residuum of hemoglobin internalized from its host red cell. Chloroquine has been shown to bind to FP with high affinity, and both FP and the chloroquine-FP complex can lyse the red cell and the parasite (Fitch 1983; Fitch et al. 1982; Orjih et al. 1981). However, it is not yet clear how the parasite normally protects itself from the potentially lytic action of FP (if biologically significant concentrations of free FP are present in the parasite vesicle). Although there may be specific FP-binding proteins in the vesicle, no such proteins have yet been identified. It is also not clear whether there are any differences between the FP or the FP-binding proteins of susceptible and resistant parasites which could contribute to chloroquine resistance.

II. Chloroquine and Acid Vesicles

Because neither intercalation into DNA nor binding to FP appears to explain the susceptibility of plasmodia to nanomolar concentrations of chloroquine or the specificity of chloroquine action, we have been interested in the possibility that chloroquine might act against the acid vesicle system of the parasite (Krogstad and Schlesinger 1987a, b). Chloroquine and other weak bases raise vesicle pH and interfere with acid vesicle function in mammalian cells. Acid intracellular vesicles have been shown to carry out a much more diverse range of functions than was suspected previously when lysosomes were envisioned simply as containers for the acidic degradation of internalized macromolecules (de Duve 1963; de Duve and Wattiaux 1966). It is now clear that the integrity of the acid vesicle system is essential for receptor-mediated endocytosis (of diverse ligands such as insulin, transferrin, low-density lipoprotein and growth factors), receptor recycling, membrane movement, secretion of basal lamina proteins, antigen processing, intracellular killing of toxoplasma and legionella, the intracellular targeting of lysosomal enzymes, and the cytoplasmic entry and action of several enveloped viruses and toxins (CAPLAN et al. 1987; DEAN et al. 1984; FORGAC et al. 1983; GOLDSTEIN et al. 1979; GONZALEZ-NORIEGA et al. 1980; HELENIUS and MARSH 1982; HORWITZ and MAXFIELD 1984; LEPPLA et al. 1980; SIBLEY et al. 1985; STONE et al. 1983; TIETZE et al. 1980; TYCKO and MAXFIELD 1983; WILLINGHAM and PASTAN 1980; ZIEGLER and UNANUE 1982). Taken together, these studies suggest that the ability of chloroquine to raise the pH of acid intracellular vesicles may play a major role in its antimalarial action.

III. Chloroquine as a Weak Base

More than a decade ago, Homewood and her collaborators suggested that chloroquine might raise the pH of the parasite's food vacuole as a weak base and thus inhibit the degradation of hemoglobin – resulting in the death of the parasite (HOMEWOOD et al. 1972). At the time it was proposed, this hypothesis was criticized because it did not explain the antiplasmodial activity of chloroquine at the low nanomolar extracellular chloroquine concentrations which are affective in vivo and in vitro. Because it was not possible to measure intravesicular pH in the parasite or the effect of chloroquine on intravesicular pH, it was not possible to test Homewood's hypothesis at that time.

IV. The Effect of Weak Bases on Lysosomal (Intravesicular) pH

De Duve and his colleagues first suggested a mechanism to explain the ability of weak bases to inhibit lysosomal proteolysis (DE DUVE 1963; DE DUVE and WATTIAUX 1966; DE DUVE et al. 1974). He proposed that weak bases (compounds with p*K*s from 7 to 11) inhibited the hydrolytic activity of lysosomes because of their "lysosomotropic" properties, which resulted from three facts:

1. Weak bases are membrane-permeable (cross plasma and vesicle membranes readily) in their unprotonated (uncharged) form.
2. Weak bases are impermeable (or much less permeable) in their protonated (charged) form.
3. Eukaryotic cells contain acid intracellular compartments which accumulate the protonated (charged) form of weak bases.

V. Concentration of Weak Bases Within Acid Vesicles

Because the unprotonated (neutral) form of a weak base crosses membranes freely, its concentration is the same in the different subcellular compartments (including acid intracellular vesicles), the cytoplasm, and the extracellular medium. In contrast, because the protonated (charged) form of a weak base is less permeable, its concentration typically varies in the different subcellular compartments according to their pH.

When the intravesicular pH is two units (100-fold) lower than extracellular (medium) pH, as is usually the case in acid intracellular vesicles, a monoprotic weak base is concentrated 100-fold inside the vesicle (Fig. 1, ROOS and BORON 1981). This process has two important consequences: (1) *Weak bases raise in-*

travesicular pH – Because weak bases enter the vesicle in their membrane-permeant unprotonated (uncharged) form, they consume protons from the interior of the vesicle as they are protonated and thus raise intravesicular pH. (As vesicle pH rises, the driving force for the concentration of additional weak base within the vesicle decreases.) (2) *Weak bases produce osmotic swelling of acid vesicles* – The total weak base concentration inside the vesicle can produce substantial osmotic swelling. Because protonation within the vesicle reduces the intravesicular concentration of the unprotonated (permeable) form of the weak base, additional unprotonated weak base continues to enter by diffusion – causing the vesicle to swell as free water enters to correct the transient osmotic dysequilibrium. Ultimately a steady state is reached in which the pH gradient, osmotic forces, proton pumping into the vesicle, and permeability of the protonated and unprotonated forms of the weak base are balanced against one another and the vesicle achieves a stable pH.

VI. Effects of Mono- and Diprotic Weak Bases on Vesicle pH

The accumulation of a weak base in an acid vesicle is a consequence of the p*K*(s) of the weak base and the difference in pH between the inside and the outside of the vesicle. This relationship can be described quantitatively using the Henderson-Hasselbalch equation (Roos and Boron 1981). In mammalian cells this relationship predicts correctly the observed increase in lysosomal pH as intravesicular protons are consumed by entry of the unprotonated weak base into a compartment with a pH lower than its p*K* (Krogstad and Schlesinger 1986). For monoprotic weak bases such as NH_4Cl, the relationship between the intravesicular consumption of protons and the concentration of the weak base has a simple 1 : 1 stoichiometry when the p*K* of the weak base is substantially greater than intravesicular pH. If the p*K* of the weak base approximates the pH of the vesicle, the con-

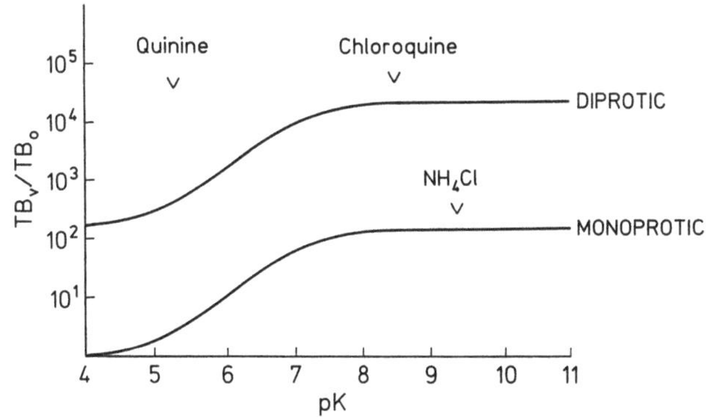

Fig. 1. The relative concentration of a monoprotic weak base within an acid vesicle (TB_v/TB_o) decreases to 1 as the dissociation constant (p*K*) of that weak base decreases. The medium pH is assumed to be 7.2 and the intravesicular pH 5.0. For diprotic weak bases, the more alkaline p*K* was set at 10.2 in performing these calculations. Note that the more acid lower p*K* of quinine (5.1) results in significantly less concentration of quinine within the vesicle – in comparison with chloroquine, which has a lower p*K* of 8.3

centration of the weak base within the vesicle is reduced in proportion to the fraction of the total intravesicular weak base which is unprotonated (Fig. 1).

For diprotic weak bases, one must include a second protonation in all the equations although the basic concept is unchanged. In practical terms, this means that a diprotic weak base is concentrated within the vesicle in proportion to the square of the proton gradient across the vesicle membrane – assuming that both p*K*s are substantially greater than intravesicular pH. As shown in Fig. 1, the intravesicular concentration of a diprotic weak base decreases to that of a monoprotic weak base as its p*K*s are reduced. As with monoprotic weak bases, the concentration of a diprotic weak base is reduced as intravesicular pH approaches the p*K*s of the weak base – i.e., as mono- or unprotonated forms of the diprotic weak base become a larger fraction of the total intravesicular weak base concentrations. Because chloroquine is a diprotic weak base (with p*K*s substantially greater than vesicle pH at 8.3 and 10.2), it is concentrated to a greater degree than a simple monoprotic weak base in an acid intracellular compartment. Thus chloroquine raises lysosomal pH in mammalian cells at lower external concentrations ($0.5–1 \times 10^{-6}$ *M*) than a simple monoprotic weak base such as NH_4Cl ($0.5–1 \times 10^{-3}$ *M*).

VII. The "Non-weak Base" Effect

Because the antimalarials employed most commonly (chloroquine, quinine and mefloquine) are diprotic weak bases, they should theoretically raise the pH of the parasite's acid vesicles at extracellular concentrations $\geqq 1$ μ*M*. However, a number of laboratories have demonstrated that susceptible strains of *P. falciparum* have an IC_{50} of 1–10 n*M* for chloroquine (DESJARDINS et al. 1979; GEARY and JENSEN 1983; GLUZMAN et al. 1987; KROGSTAD et al. 1985). Because these concentrations are 10^3 lower than the concentrations of chloroquine which raise pH in mammalian lysosomes, chloroquine cannot be acting only as a weak base in *P. falciparum*.

Despite this apparent discrepancy, several lines of evidence suggest that the food vacuole (the secondary lysosome of the parasite) is the site of chloroquine's antiplasmodial action. Autoradiographic studies with ^{3}H-chloroquine (AIKAWA 1972) indicate that chloroquine is concentrated in the parasite food vacuole. Furthermore, the parasite food vacuole, like the mammalian lysosome, receives material taken up from the host red cell cytoplasm by endocytosis, has an acid pH, acidifies by a mechanism which employs MgATP and alkalinizes in response to the addition of NH_4Cl (KROGSTAD et al. 1985; YAYON et al. 1984, 1985). Nevertheless, chloroquine raises the pH of parasite vesicles and inhibits parasite growth at extracellular chloroquine concentrations significantly lower than those which raise lysosomal pH in mammalian cells (1–10 n*M* for susceptible parasites and 100–300 n*M* for resistant parasites vs. 1–10 μ*M* for mammalian cells). Three conclusions follow from these observations:

1. The acid intracellular vesicles of the malaria parasite are similar to mammalian lysosomes in their ability to acidify with MgATP and in the response of their pH to weak bases.

2. The acid vesicles of the malaria parasite are unusually sensitive to the effects of chloroquine on vesicle pH.
3. The effects of chloroquine on acid vesicle pH are consistent with the ability of those same chloroquine concentrations to inhibit parasite growth.

The first of these conclusions lead to the prediction that any weak base should have antiplasmodial activity at concentrations that raise the internal pH of the parasites' vesicles.

1. Weak Bases Are Antimalarials

Therefore, we tested a diverse series of weak bases for antiplasmodial activity. Ammonium chloride, propylamine, benzylamine, cadaverine, and tributylamine each inhibit parasite growth at concentrations which increase the pH of the parasite's vesicles (KROGSTAD et al. 1986). Furthermore none of these compounds has significantly different activity against chloroquine-susceptible vs. -resistant parasites. These results are consistent with the hypothesis that raising intravesicular pH plays a major role in antimalarial action. They suggest also that there is no fundamental difference between chloroquine-susceptible and -resistant *P. falciparum* in their ability to maintain an acid intravesicular pH. This hypothesis was tested quantitatively by determining the total buffering capacity of acid vesicles in both chloroquine-susceptible and -resistant *P. falciparum*. The ability of a vesicle to resist alkalinization by a weak base is reflected in the total buffering capacity of the vesicle (KROGSTAD and SCHLESINGER 1986):

$$\text{Buffering capacity} = \frac{\text{Base equivalents required}}{\text{Change in vesicle pH}}$$

With a simple monoprotic weak base such as NH_4Cl, the buffering capacity of chloroquine-susceptible *P. falciparum*, chloroquine-resistant *P. falciparum* and mammalian cells is the same within experimental error (100–300 m*M* base required to raise intravesicular pH 1 pH unit) (KROGSTAD and SCHLESINGER 1986). This result demonstrates that there is no substantial difference in the baseline acidification of the parasite vesicle which can account for the greater ability of chloroquine to raise intravesicular pH in the parasite.

However, when vesicle buffering capacity is determined with chloroquine, there are striking differences which correlate with susceptibility to chloroquine. The calculated vesicle buffering capacity of resistant parasites is 500- to 800-fold less than that of mammalian cells. The calculated vesicle buffering capacity of susceptible parasites is 100-fold less than that of resistant parasites (KROGSTAD and SCHLESINGER 1986). These observations lead to 2 predictions about the mechanism of chloroquine action. Either chloroquine must alter the acid vesicles of the susceptible parasite so that they are unable to maintain an acid pH, or it must be concentrated to a much greater degree within the vesicles of susceptible parasites than in resistant parasites or mammalian cells.

VIII. Chloroquine Accumulation by *Plasmodium falciparum*

Beginning with the observations of Fitch (FITCH 1970, 1973) a number of investigators have demonstrated that susceptible *P. falciparum* accumulate more chloroquine than resistant parasites (GLUZMAN et al. 1987; KROGSTAD et al. 1985). We have shown also that raising intravesicular pH with NH_4Cl prevents (or reverses) chloroquine accumulation by both susceptible and resistant parasites. These observations indicate that the concentration of chloroquine by both susceptible and resistant parasite strains requires a low pH in the parasite's acid vesicles.

To compare the accumulation of chloroquine by mammalian cells, resistant and susceptible parasites, we calculated the concentration of chloroquine in the respective vesicle compartments after correcting for the number of vesicles per cell and vesicle size (KROGSTAD and SCHLESINGER, unpublished observations). This calculation indicates that the concentration of ^{3}H-chloroquine within the vesicles of susceptible parasites is 300- to 700-fold greater than within the vesicles of mammalian cells and 20- to 30-fold greater than within the vesicles of resistant parasites (Fig. 2). These results suggest that the greater effect of chloroquine on vesicle pH in susceptible parasites can be accounted for by their greater intravesicular accumulation of chloroquine. Because this result cannot be accounted for by the physicochemical factors which typically govern the concentration of weak bases within acid compartments (the p*K*s of the weak base and the ΔpH between the vesicle and the extracellular medium) (ROOS and BORON 1981), it has been called the "*non-weak base*" effect of chloroquine. However, two important and unanswered questions remain about this hypothesis of chloroquine action:

1. How do the vesicles of susceptible *P. falciparum* accumulate enough chloroquine to raise intravesicular pH at external chloroquine concentrations which do not affect intravesicular pH in mammalian lysosomes?
2. How does raising the pH of the parasite's acid vesicles inhibit parasite growth and ultimately kill the parasite?

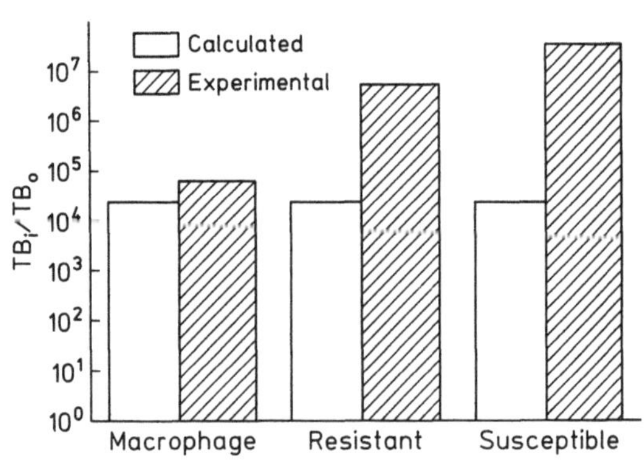

Fig. 2. The intravesicular accumulation of chloroquine by mammalian cells such as the macrophage is within 2- to 3-fold of that predicted by its properties as a weak base using the Henderson-Hasselbalch equation. In contrast, the intravesicular accumulation of chloroquine by *Plasmodium falciparum* is several orders of magnitude greater than that predicted by its properties as a diprotic weak base. Susceptible parasite vesicles accumulate approximately 40-fold more chloroquine than the vesicles of resistant parasites

At present, neither of these questions has a clear answer. In terms of the first question, the data presented above indicate that the vesicle of the susceptible parasite has a chloroquine-concentrating mechanism which is not present in mammalian cells. The nature of this concentrating mechanism is unknown. Factors which could contribute include differences between plasmodia and mammalian cells in permeability to the protonated or unprotonated forms of chloroquine, in membrane potential, or in chloroquine binding site(s) within the vesicle. In terms of the second question, recent studies of acid intracellular vesicles in eukaryotic cells suggest a number of potential mechanisms by which raising intravesicular pH might interfere with parasite growth (see below).

IX. Potential Biological Consequences of Raising Intravesicular pH

The role of acid vesicles in intracellular proteolysis (de Duve 1963; de Duve and Wattiaux 1966), receptor-mediated endocytosis (Stahl and Schwartz 1986), the intracellular targeting of lysosomal enzymes and the extracellular targeting of secreted proteins has been well described in mammalian cells (Caplan et al. 1987; Goldberg et al. 1984; Gonzalez-Noriega et al. 1980; Natowicz et al. 1979; Sly and Fischer 1982). However, mammalian cells survive for extended periods of time in the presence of weak bases (including chloroquine) which raise the pH of their acid intracellular vesicles and inhibit both receptor-mediated endocytosis and the intracellular targeting of newly synthesized lysosomal enzymes (Hasilik and von Figura 1984; Sly and Fischer 1982). Perhaps, as Homewood proposed (Homewood et al. 1972), the parasite may be more sensitive to inhibition and killing by chloroquine because it is critically dependent on the digestion of hemoglobin for essential amino acids and cannot obtain essential nutrients when antimalarials raise the pH of the parasite's food vacuole. Subcellular fractions of *P. falciparum* containing acid vesicles have been shown to degrade hemoglobin taken up by the intracellular form of the parasite prior to fractionation (Choi and Mego 1987). This proteolysis is stimulated by MgATP and is inhibited by weak bases such as NH_4Cl and chloroquine.

1. Other Potential Effects of Altering Vesicle pH

An alternative hypothesis would include the rise in intravesicular pH as the central event, but would also consider the multiple roles of acid intracellular vesicles (see above and Krogstad and Schlesinger 1987b). In mammalian cells, acid intracellular vesicles are essential for the intracellular transport of macromolecules and for the membrane movement necessary for differentiation (Bonner et al. 1986; Dean et al. 1984; Kent 1982; Lot and Bennett 1982). Both of these activities are disrupted by raising intravesicular pH in mammalian cells (Dean et al. 1984). During its intra-erythroyctic cycle, the malaria parasite undergoes extensive differentiation and development which must include the synthesis of several cellular organelles and extensive membranous reorganization. If the parasite employs receptor-mediated intracellular targeting of newly synthesized lysosomal enzymes similar to that of mammalian cells, that targeting will be disrupted by raising the pH of the parasite's acid intracellular vesicles. We know that the parasite has acid vesicles (KROGSTAD et al. 1985; YAYON et al. 1984, 1985) and proteases with acid pH optima (GYANG et al. 1982; VAN DER JAGT et al. 1984, 1986, 1987) so that the components of a lysosomal system are present. However, we do not yet know if they constitute a lysosomal system as found in mammalian cells, or if the biogenesis of this system follows the mammalian model. Disruption of the fundamental processes of intracellular targeting and membrane movement could produce the growth inhibition and parasite death that are observed in vitro with extracellular concentrations of chloroquine, quinine or mefloquine sufficient to raise parasite vesicle pH (KROGSTAD et al. 1985).

These observations suggest that the mechanism of chloroquine action is intimately related to the normal physiologic functions of the parasite's acid vesicles.

C. Mechanism of Chloroquine Resistance

Studies by many investigators, beginning with those of Fitch (FITCH 1970, 1973), have shown that chloroquine-resistant *P. falciparum* accumulate less chloroquine than susceptible parasites. However, the mechanism responsible for this difference in chloroquine accumulation has been unknown.

Furthermore, the genetic nature of chloroquine resistance has been unclear, because of the difficulty in performing genetic experiments with a haploid organism which requires cycling through its mosquito host in order to produce recombination. The available epidemiologic data are inconclusive. They suggest that chloroquine resistance in Africa may have been imported from Southeast Asia in the late 1970s. However, it is not clear whether there are any potential epidemiologic links between chloroquine resistance in Southeast Asia and the earlier resistance in South America. Thus, it is possible that most, or all, chloroquine resistance has been selected from one or a few genetic events in South America and/or Southeast Asia.

One could envision many potential mechanisms by which the parasite might have become resistant to clinically achievable concentrations of chloroquine. These include: (1) a defective concentrating mechanism so that the parasite vesicle would concentrate no more chloroquine than the vesicles of mammalian cells, (2) a permeability barrier which inhibited chloroquine accumulation (analogous to the altered penicillin-binding proteins observed in Enterobacteriaceae), (3) an enzyme(s) which modified the drug (analogous to β-lactamases or aminoglycoside-modifying enzymes) (NEU 1987), and (4) an altered target site (i.e., an acid vesicle system which functioned normally even when its pH was raised above 6.0).

Recent studies indicate that susceptible and resistant parasites initially accumulate chloroquine at the same rate (28–29 fmol per 10^6 parasitized red cells per minute) (KROGSTAD et al. 1987) and thus suggest that the chloroquine concentrating mechanism is intact in the resistant parasite. Examination of chloroquine which has been released from resistant parasites (using thin layer chromatography) reveals no evidence that it has been altered chemically (GLUZMAN et al.

1987). Studies with other weak bases such as NH_4Cl indicate that chloroquine-susceptible and -resistant parasites are both inhibited in vitro by concentrations of weak bases which raise intravesicular pH (KROGSTAD et al. 1986).

Although the studies described above did not define the mechanism of chloroquine resistance, recent studies demonstrate that resistant *P. falciparum* have a mechanism for releasing chloroquine (an efflux mechanism). This mechanism is either absent or greatly reduced in the susceptible parasite (KROGSTAD et al. 1987). The fact that the initial rates of chloroquine accumulation are the same in resistant and susceptible parasites suggests that this efflux mechanism causes the observed difference in steady-state chloroquine accumulation, and that it may be the only significant difference between resistant and susceptible parasites. Although there may be more than one mechanism of chloroquine resistance in *P. falciparum*, the rapid efflux phenotype has now been observed in isolates from Southeast Asia, South America and Africa. Thus this mechanism of resistance is present in each of the three continents with chloroquine-resistant *P. falciparum*.

These studies suggest also that the efflux of chloroquine from resistant *P. falciparum* may be dependent on intracellular calcium. Chloroquine efflux is inhibited by several calcium-channel blockers and by daunomycin (which may function as a calcium-channel blocker in some systems) (GIBBS 1985). The mechanism by which alterations in intracellular calcium might influence chloroquine efflux is not yet defined.

Alternatively, daunomycin, vinblastine and the calcium-channel blockers which inhibit chloroquine efflux may compete with chloroquine for a binding site similar to the P-glycoprotein of multidrug-resistant mammalian cancer cells. The efflux mechanism and the effects of calcium-channel blockers on chloroquine efflux in *P. falciparum* are strikingly similar to the phenomonon of multidrug resistance in mammalian cancer cells (CORNWELL et al. 1987; FOJO et al. 1985; SCOTTO et al. 1986). Those cells rapidly release anti-cancer drugs to which they are resistant (i.e., they have an efflux mechanism also). Calcium-channel blockers inhibit the efflux of anti-cancer drugs from these cells and thus increase their accumulation of, and susceptibility to, those anti-cancer agents.

This analogy is consistent with the effects of calcium-channel blockers and chloroquine against otherwise chloroquine-resistant *P. falciparum*. Studies by Martin et al. have shown that the combination of verapamil plus chloroquine in-

Table 2. Parallels between chloroquine resistance in *Plasmodium falciparum* and multidrug resistance in mammalian cancer cells

	P. falciparum	Mammalian cancer cells
Drug efflux from resistant cells	Enhanced efflux of chloroquine	Enhanced efflux of daunomycin and vinblastine
Effect of resistance phenotype on drug accumulation	Less accumulation of chloroquine	Less accumulation of daunomycin and vinblastine
Effect of calcium-channel blockers	Inhibition of efflux, resulting in greater accumulation of chloroquine	Inhibition of efflux, resulting in greater accumulation of daunomycin and vinblastine

hibits otherwise resistant *P. falciparum* in vitro (MARTIN et al. 1987). Taken together with the ability of calcium-channel blockers to inhibit chloroquine efflux, these results suggest that inhibition of chloroquine efflux produces the increased accumulation which enhances the effect of chloroquine against the resistant parasite. These results further suggest that the mechanism of chloroquine resistance in *P. falciparum* is similar (or identical) to that of multidrug resistance in mammalian cancer cells (Table 2).

D. Action of Mefloquine, Quinine, and Quinidine

I. Mechanism of Mefloquine Action

The effect of mefloquine on the acid vesicle system of *P. falciparum* has not been studied as carefully as that of chloroquine. However, it is a weak base with p*K*s similar to those of chloroquine and the data available indicate a similar mechanism of action. Against susceptible parasites, mefloquine has approximately the same activity as chloroquine (IC_{50}, 10 n*M*) (DESJARDINS et al. 1979; GEARY and JENSEN 1983; KROGSTAD et al. 1985). Nevertheless, the ability of mefloquine to raise parasite vesicle pH at such low concentrations indicates that, like chloroquine, it cannot be acting only as a weak base (KROGSTAD and SCHLESINGER 1986, 1987b). With mammalian cells, mefloquine increases lysosomal pH at concentrations consistent with its p*K*s (0.5–10 μ*M*) (KROGSTAD et al. 1985). As discussed above for chloroquine, this leads to the conclusion that the antiplasmodial action of mefloquine results from a specific interaction between the parasite vesicle and the drug. Although the mechanism of mefloquine action is less well characterized than that of chloroquine, it is clear that the parasite can become resistant independently to chloroquine, to mefloquine or to both drugs (DESJARDINS et al. 1979; GEARY and JENSEN 1983; KROGSTAD et al. 1985). These results suggest that resistance to either drug occurs by a mechanism that is independent of the "non-weak base" activity described above.

II. Quinine and Quinidine as Weak Bases

Quinine has been in clinical use longer than chloroquine and has been considered by some to be more effective. It is certainly more toxic. Quinine is a diprotic weak base which raises the pH of mammalian lysosomes and of parasite vesicles (KROGSTAD et al. 1985). Because the more acidic p*K* of quinine is 5.1 (vs. 8.3 for chloroquine – as shown in Fig. 1), quinine is concentrated in acid vesicles more like a monoprotic than a diprotic weak base at physiologic pH. This decreases the ability of quinine to raise vesicle as a weak base by 10- to 100-fold. Studies of vesicle buffering capacity have shown that quinine has much less (or no) "non-weak base" activity than chloroquine (KROGSTAD and SCHLESINGER 1986). Thus the data suggest that the antimalarial activity of quinine is due primarily to its properties as a weak base. Of interest but unexplored at the present time are observations which suggest that quinidine is more effective against *P. falciparum* than quinine (PHILLIPS et al. 1985; WHITE et al. 1981). Quinine and quinidine are stereochemical isomers and should have similar p*K*s and weak base properties. If quinidine has a greater ability to raise intravesicular pH in the parasite, the chemical isomerism between quinine and quinidine may be an important structural determinant of non-weak base activity. This would be consistent with our earlier hypothesis that non-weak base activity requires a specific interaction between the parasite vesicle and the drug in question.

III. Non-weak Base Activity and the Safety of Antimalarials

The recent observations of the non-weak base activity of chloroquine and the implication that mefloquine and quinidine display similar activity permits speculation concerning the effectiveness of antimalarials to inhibit parasite growth without producing side unwanted effects by increasing the pH of the acid vesicles of the host. Because of their activity at low extracellular concentrations (non-weak base properties), chloroquine and mefloquine raise vesicle pH in the parasite long before they affect vesicle pH in mammalian cells. This would explain the low incidence of side effects in the use of these drugs in humans. In contrast, quinine, which produces unwanted side effects much more frequently, raises vesicle pH in the parasite at concentrations similar to those at which it raises vesicle pH in mammalian cells. From this perspective, it is not surprising that quinine produces complications at concentrations which are effective clinically. This comparison emphasizes the importance of understanding the mechanism of chloroquine accumulation and its interaction with the parasite vesicle so that other safe and effective chemotherapeutic agents can be developed.

E. Summary of Basic Concepts and Prospects for the Future

I. The Acid Vesicle as a Pharmacologic Target Site

Recent studies indicate that the acid vesicle of the parasite is the major target of site of most of the antimalarials which have been employed successfully over the last 40 years. This observation indicates the importance of this organelle in the biology of the parasite. Recent studies indicate that the parasite has not substantially altered the pH or the functions of its acid vesicles in developing chloroquine resistance. This observation further strengthens the hypothesis that this organelle must remain functionally intact for parasite viability. A logical conclusion of these studies is that other agents which alter vesicle pH or other aspects of vesicle function should be considered in the development of future antimalarials.

II. Structure-Activity Relationships

Recent studies of chloroquine action and resistance suggest that these processes (the non-weak base activity associated with increased chloroquine accumulation by the susceptible parasite and the enhanced chloroquine efflux associated with the resistant parasite) result from specific interactions between the parasite and the drug. These interactions do not occur between chloroquine and other cell types, or between other weak bases and *P. falciparum*. Although these two processes appear to be unrelated, both depend on the chemical structure of the drug and not on more general properties such as p*K*s, which permit any weak base to be an antimalarial at concentrations high enough to raise vesicle pH. Therefore it should be possible to determine the conformational features of chloroquine in solution which confer non-weak base activity and those which permit rapid efflux from the resistant parasite. If these properties involve different structural features of the chloroquine molecule, it should be possible to develop compounds in which these features are altered in order to produce antimalarial (non-weak base) activity which circumvents the efflux mechanism of resistance.

III. Prospects for the Future

Because the efflux resistance mechanism is inhibited by calcium channel blockers, vinblastine and other compounds, it should be possible to develop drugs which inhibit the efflux mechanism without producing the severe side effects which have been seen when these compounds have been used with chloroquine to treat resistant *P. falciparum* infection in vivo. This strategy will be more likely to be successful if the ability of these compounds to reverse chloroquine resistance does not directly involve alterations of intracellular calcium. Success with either of these approaches will require considerable effort to define the biochemical mechanisms responsible for non-weak base activity and chloroquine efflux and to identify the parasite macromolecules responsible for these activities.

References

Aikawa M (1972) High-resolution autoradiography of malarial parasites treated with ^{3}H-chloroquine. Am J Pathol 67:277–284

Allison J, O'Brien RL, Hahn F (1965) DNA: reaction with chloroquine. Science 149:1111–1113

Ballou WR, Hoffmann SL, Sherwood JA, Hollingdale MR, Neva FA, Hockmeyer WT, Gordon DM, Schneider I, Wirtz RA, Young JF (1987) Safety and efficacy of a recombinant DNA *Plasmodium falciparum* sporozoite vaccine. Lancet I:1277–1281

Bonner JT, Suthers HB, Odell GM (1986) Ammonia orients cell masses and speeds up aggregating cells of slime moulds. Nature 323:630–632

Caplan MJ, Stow JL, Newman AP, Madri J, Anderson HC, Farquhar MG, Palade GE, Jamieson JD (1987) Dependence on pH of polarized sorting of secreted proteins. Nature 329:632–635

Centers for Disease Control (1985) Revised recommendations for preventing malaria in travelers to areas with chloroquine-resistant *Plasmodium falciparum*. Morbid Mortal Wkly Rep 34:185–195

Centers for Disease Control (1986) Need for malaria prophylaxis by travelers to areas with chloroquine-resistant *Plasmodium falciparum*. Morbid Mortal Wkly Rep 35:21–27

Centers for Disease Control (1987) Chloroquine-resistant *Plasmodium falciparum* in West Africa. Morbid Mortal Wkly Rep 36:13–14

Choi I, Mego JL (1987) Intravacuolar degradation of ^{125}I-labelled hemoglobin in *Plasmodium falciparum* digestive vacuoles. Fed Proc 46:4776

Ciak J, Hahn F (1966) Chloroquine: mode of action. Science 151:347–349

Cohen SN, Yielding KL (1965) Inhibition of DNA and RNA polymerase reactions by chloroquine. Proc Natl Acad Sci USA 54:521–527

Cornwell MM, Pastan IH, Gottesman MM (1987) Increased vinblastine binding to membrane vesicles from multidrug-resistant KB cells. J Biol Chem 261:7921–7928

Dean RT, Jessup W, Roberts CR (1984) Effects of exogenous amines on mammalian cells, with particular reference to membrane flow. Biochem J 217:27–40

De Duve C (1963) General properties of lysosomes: the lysosome concept. In: de Rueck AVS, Cameron MP (eds) Ciba foundation symposium on lysosomes. Little Brown, Boston, pp 1–31

De Duve C, Wattiaux R (1966) Functions of lysosomes. Annu Rev Physiol 28:435–492

De Duve C, de Barsy T, Poole B, Trouet A, Tulkens P, van Hoof F (1974) Lysosomotropic agents. Biochem Pharmacol 24:2495–2531

Desjardins RE, Canfield CJ, Haynes JD, Chulay JD (1979) Quantitative assessment of antimalarial activity in vitro by a semiautomated microdilution technique. Antimicrob Agents Chemother 16:710–718

Enea V, Ellis J, Zavala F, Aarnot DE, Asavanich A, Msuda A, Quakyi I, Nussenzweig RS (1984) DNA cloning of the *Plasmodium falciparum* circumsporozoite gene: amino acid sequence of repetitive epitope. Science 225:628–630

Field JW (1949) Blood examination and prognosis in acute falciparum malaria. Trans R Soc Trop Med Hyg 43:33–56

Fitch CD (1970) *Plasmodium falciparum* in owl monkeys: drug resistance and chloroquine-binding capacity. Science 169:289–290

Fitch CD (1973) Chloroquine-resistant *Plasmodium falciparum*: difference in the handling of ^{14}C-amodiaquin and ^{14}C-chloroquine. Antimicrob Agents Chemother 3:545–548

Fitch CD (1983) Mode of action of antimalarial drugs. Ciba Found Symp 94:222–232

Fitch CD, Chevli R, Banyal HS, Phillips GW Jr, Pfaller MA, Krogstad DJ (1982) Lysis of *Plasmodium falciparum* by ferriprotoporphyrin IX and a chloroquine-ferriprotoporphyrin IX complex. Antimicrob Agents Chemother 21:819–822

Fojo A, Akiyama S-I, Gottesman MM, Pastan IH (1985) Reduced drug accumulation in multiply drug-resistant human KB carcinoma cell lines. Cancer Res 45:3002–3007

Forgac M, Cantley L, Wiedenmann B, Altstiel L, Branton D (1983) Clathrin-coated vesicles contain an ATP-dependent proton pump. Proc Natl Acad Sci USA 80:1300–1303

Geary TG, Jensen JB (1983) Lack of cross-resistance to 4-aminoquinolines in chloroquine-resistant *Plasmodium falciparum* in vitro. J Parasitol 69:97–105

Gibbs CL (1985) Acute energetic effects of daunomycin on heart muscle. J Cardiovasc Pharmacol 7:556–561

Gluzman IY, Schlesinger PH, Krogstad DJ (1987) Inoculum effect with chloroquine and *Plasmodium falciparum*. Antimicrob Agents Chemother 31:32–36

Goldberg DE, Gabel C, Kornfeld S (1984) Processing of lysosomal enzyme oligosaccharide units. In: Dingle JT, Dean RT, Sly WS (eds) Lysosomes in biology and pathology, vol 7. Elsevier, Amsterdam, pp 45–62

Goldstein JL, Anderson RGW, Brown MS (1979) Coated pits, coated vesicles, and receptor-mediated endocytosis. Nature 279:679–685

Gonzalez-Noriega A, Grubb JH, Talkad V, Sly WS (1980) Chloroquine inhibits lysosomal enzyme pinocytosis and enhances lysosomal enzyme secretion by impairing receptor recycling. J Cell Biol 85:839–852

Gyang FN, Poole B, Trager W (1982) Peptidases from *Plasmodium falciparum* cultured in vitro. Mol Biochem Parasitol 5:263–273

Hasilik A, von Figura K (1984) Processing of lysosomal enzymes in fibroblasts. In: Dingle JT, Dean RT, Sly WS (eds) Lysosomes in biology and pathology, vol 7. Elsevier, Amsterdam, pp 3–16

Helenius A, Marsh M (1982) Encosytosis of enveloped animal viruses. Ciba Found Symp 92:59–76

Homewood CA, Warhurst DC, Peters W, Baggaley WC (1972) Lysosomes, pH and the antimalarial action of chloroquine. Nature 235:50–52

Horwitz MA, Maxfield FR (1984) *Legionella pneumophila* inhibits acidification of its phagosome in human monocytes. J Cell Biol 99:1936–1943

Jones WHS (1909) Malaria and Greek history. University Press, Manchester

Kent C (1982) Inhibition of myoblast fusion by lysosomotropic amines. Dev Biol 90:91–98

Krogstad DJ, Schlesinger PH (1986) A perspective on antimalarial action: effects of weak bases on *Plasmodium falciparum*. Biochem Pharmacol 35:547–552

Krogstad DJ, Schlesinger PH (1987a) The basis of antimalarial action: non-weak base effects of chloroquine on vesicle pH. Am J Trop Med Hyg 36:213–220

Krogstad DJ, Schlesinger PH (1987b) Acid vesicle function, intracellular pathogens, and the action of chloroquine against *Plasmodium falciparum*. N Engl J Med 317:542–549

Krogstad DJ, Schlesinger PH, Gluzman IY (1985) Antimalarials increase vesicle pH in *Plasmodium falciparum*. J Cell Biol 101:2302–2309

Krogstad DJ, Schlesinger PH, Gluzman IY, Koziol CM (1986) Weak bases are antimalarials. Clin Res 34:523A

Krogstad DJ, Gluzman IY, Kyle DE, Oduola AMJ, Martin SK, Milhous WK, Schlesinger PH (1987) Efflux of chloroquine from *Plasmodium falciparum*: mechanism of chloroquine resistance. Science 238:1283–1285

Leppla SH, Dorland RB, Middlebrook JL (1980) Inhibition of diphtheria toxin degradation and cytotoxic action by chloroquine. J Biol Chem 255:2247–2250

Lot TY, Bennett T (1982) The effects of chronic chloroquine administration in growing chicks. Med Biol 60:210–216

Martin SK, Oduola AMJ, Milhous WK (1987) Reversal of chloroquine resistance in *Plasmodium falciparum* by verapamil. Science 235:899–901

Miller LH, Howard RJ, Carter R, Good MF, Nussenzweig V, Nussenzweig RS (1986) Research toward malaria vaccines. Science 234:1349–1356

Natowicz MR, Chi MM-Y, Lowry OH, Sly WS (1979) Enzymatic identification of mannose-6-phosphate on the recognition marker for receptor-mediated pinocytosis of β-glucuronidase by human fibroblasts. Proc Natl Acad Sci USA 76:4322–4326

Neu HC (1987) The biochemical basis of antimicrobial and bacterial resistance. Bull NY Acad Sci 63:295–317

Neva FA (1977) Looking back for a view of the future: observations on immunity to induced malaria. Am J Trop Med Hyg [Suppl] 26:211–215

O'Brien RL, Olenick JG, Hahn FE (1966) Reactions of quinine, chloroquine and quinacrine with DNA and their effects on the DNA and RNA polymerase reactions. Proc Natl Acad Sci USA 55:1511–1517

Orjih AU, Banyal HS, Chevli R, Fitch CD (1981) Hemin lysis malaria parasites. Science 213:667–669

Parker FS, Irvin JL (1952) The interaction of chloroquine with nucleic acids and nucleoproteins. J Biol Chem 199:897–909

Phillips RE, Warrell DA, White NJ, Looareesuwan S, Karbwang J (1985) Intravenous quinidine for the treatment of severe falciparum malaria: clinical and pharmacokinetic studies. N Engl J Med 312:1273–1278

Roos A, Boron WF (1981) Intracellular pH. Physiol Rev 51:296–434

Scotto KW, Biedler JL, Melera PW (1986) Amplification and expression of genes associated with multidrug resistance in mammalian cells. Science 232:751–755

Sibley LD, Weidner E, Krahenbuhl JL (1985) Phagosome acidification blocked by intracellular *Toxoplasma gondii*. Nature 315:416–419

Sly WS, Fischer HD (1982) The phosphomannosyl recognition system for intracellular and intercellular transport of lysosomal enzymes. J Cell Biochem 18:67–85

Stahl PD, Schwartz AL (1986) Receptor-mediated endocytosis. J Clin Invest 77:657–662

Stone DK, Xie X-S, Racker E (1983) An ATP-driven proton pump in clathrin-coated vesicles. J Biol Chem 258:4059–4062

Tietze C, Schlesinger PH, Stahl PD (1980) Chloroquine and ammonium ion inhibit receptor-mediated endocytosis of mannose-glycoconjugates by macrophages: apparent inhibition of receptor recycling. Biochem Biophys Res Commun 93:1–8

Tycko B, Maxfield FR (1983) Rapid acidification of endocytic vesicles containing α_2-macroglobulin. Cell 28:643–651

Van der Jagt DL, Baack BR, Hunsaker LA (1984) Purification and characterization of an aminopeptidase from *Plasmodium falciparum*. Mol Biochem Parasitol 10:45–54

Van der Jagt DL, Hunsaker LA, Campos NM (1986) Characterization of a hemoglobin-degrading, low molecular weight protease from *Plasmodium falciparum*. Mol Biochem Parasitol 18:389–400

Van der Jagt DL, Hunsaker LA, Campos NM (1987) Comparison of proteases from chloroquine-sensitive and chloroquine-resistant strains of *Plasmodium falciparum*. Biochem Pharmacol 36:3285–3292

White NJ, Looareesuwan S, Warrell DA, Chongsuphajaisiddhi T, Bunnag D, Harinasuta T (1981) Quinidine in falciparum malaria. Lancet 2:1069–1071

Willingham MC, Pastan IH (1980) The receptosome: an intermediate organelle of receptor mediated endocytosis in cultured fibroblasts. Cell 21:67–77

Wyler DJ (1983) Malaria – resurgence, resistance, and research. N Engl J Med 308:875–878, 934–940

Yayon A, Cabantchik ZI, Ginsburg H (1984) Identification of the acidic compartment of *Plasmodium falciparum*-infected human erythrocytes as the target of the antimalarial drug chloroquine. EMBO J 3:2695–2700

Yayon A, Cabantchik ZI, Ginsburg H (1985) Susceptibility of human malaria parasites to chloroquine is pH-dependent. Proc Natl Acad Sci USA 82:2784–2788

Ziegler HK, Unanue ER (1982) Decrease in macrophage antigen catabolism caused by ammonia and chloroquine is associated with inhibition of antigen presentation to T cells. Proc Natl Acad Sci USA 79:175–178

CHAPTER 4

Resistance to β-Lactam Antibiotics Mediated by Alterations of Penicillin-Binding Proteins

B. G. SPRATT

A. Introduction

Beta-lactam antibiotics interfere with the biosynthesis of the bacterial cell wall by acting as analogues of the acyl-D-alanyl-D-alanine moiety of the lipid-linked disaccharide-pentapeptide substrate of the enzymes that catalyse the synthesis of crosslinked peptidoglycan (WAXMAN and STROMINGER 1983). These enzymes can be detected and studied as penicillin-binding proteins (PBPs) as they are essentially irreversibly acylated by penicillin, and other β-lactam antibiotics, resulting in an inactive penicilloyl-enzyme that is analogous to the acyl-enzyme formed during the processing of their normal peptide substrate (SPRATT and PARDEE 1975; SPRATT 1983).

In most bacteria the higher molecular weight (MW) PBPs are believed to be bifunctional enzymes that catalyse both a penicillin-sensitive peptidoglycan transpeptidase reaction, and a penicillin-insensitive transglycosylase reaction (NAKAGAWA et al. 1984). Inactivation of these high MW PBPs is believed to cause the lethal effects of the β-lactam antibiotics, whereas the inactivation of the lower MW PBPs, which catalyse the D-alanine carboxypeptidase reaction, is not thought to be of major physiological consequence (SPRATT 1975, 1983).

Our most detailed knowledge of the physiological role of PBPs derives from intensive studies with *E. coli*. This bacterium contains seven well-characterised PBPs, with MWs between 40000 and 94000, which are located in the cytoplasmic membrane (SPRATT 1977). β-lactams that preferentially bind to PBP 1A plus PBP 1B result in cell lysis (YOUSIF et al. 1985), while those that preferentially bind to PBP 2 or PBP 3 cause the formation of spherical cells or of filamentous cells respectively (SPRATT 1975).

Killing of *E. coli* by β-lactam antibiotics can therefore occur by the inactivation of three distinct killing targets, and most β-lactams act in vivo by inactivating more than one of these targets. Studies of the PBPs of a wide variety of bacteria have been reported. The general conclusions reached in the study of the *E. coli* PBPs are mostly applicable to the PBPs of other organisms.

Comparisons of the sequences of high MW PBPs, low MW PBPs, and class A and class C β-lactamases have shown that these enzymes, which all interact with penicillin via an acyl-enzyme mechanism involving an active-site serine residue, may be distantly related since very slight similarities in sequence are observed (SPRATT 1983; BROOME-SMITH et al. 1985a; FRÈRE and JORIS 1985).

Recent studies on the three-dimensional structures of a low MW secreted PBP from *Streptomyces* R61, and several class A β-lactamases, have shown that these enzymes have a remarkable similarity in the organisation of their secondary structure elements and leave little doubt that all of these enzymes are evolutionarily related (KELLY et al. 1986; SAMRAOUI et al. 1986; DIDEBERG et al. 1987; HERZBERG and MOULT 1987). It now seems likely that high MW PBPs, low MW PBPs, and those β-lactamases that have a serine mechanism, form a superfamily of penicillin-recognising enzymes that share a common three-dimensional structure, although they are highly diverged in their primary sequences.

In low MW PBPs, and β-lactamases, penicillin acylates an active-site serine residue that is located close to the amino-terminus (FRÈRE and JORIS 1985). In high MW PBPs the acylated serine residue is located towards the middle of the sequence (KECK et al. 1985) and the penicillin-sensitive transpeptidase domain is located towards the carboxy-terminus (HEDGE and SPRATT 1984). The amino-terminal region, which has no counterpart in the low MW PBPs and β-lactamases, is believed to contain the transglycosylase domain, although the evidence for this assignment is weak in most cases (NAKAGAWA et al. 1984).

A more detailed discussion of the enzymology and physiological functions of PBPs can be found in several recent reviews (SPRATT 1983; WAXMAN and STROMINGER 1983; REYNOLDS 1985; FRÈRE and JORIS 1985; SPRATT and CROMIE 1988).

B. Mechanisms of Resistance to β-Lactam Antibiotics

Clinicians generally define the sensitivity or resistance of a bacterium to antibiotics by reference to the levels of the antibiotic that can be achieved in the relevant tissue. In the case of β-lactam antibiotics some bacterial species may be "naturally" sensitive (e.g. *Neisseria gonorrhoeae*), whereas others may be "intrinsically" resistant (e.g. *Pseudomonas aeruginosa*). In addition, particular isolates of a bacterial species may have a significantly increased level of resistance to β-lactam antibiotics compared to that of typical members of the species, and for the purposes of this chapter I will define these isolates as resistant, although it should be noted that by this definition a resistant isolate of a bacterial species may still be treatable with β-lactam antibiotics. For example, a strain of *N. gonorrhoeae* with a minimum inhibitory concentration (MIC) of 0.5 μg/ml for benzylpenicillin would clearly be resistant by the above definition, but may still be eliminated by penicillin therapy.

Resistance to β-lactam antibiotics can occur by at least three routes. By far the most widespread cause of resistance is the production of a β-lactamase which catalyses the hydrolysis of the antibiotic to a biologically inert product (see Chap. 5, 6).

In gram-negative bacteria resistance to β-lactam antibiotics can also result from a decrease in the rate of penetration of the antibiotic through the outer membrane to the PBPs in the cytoplasmic membrane (see Chap. 1). This mechanism of resistance cannot give high levels of resistance since there is a limit to the extent that the permeability of the outer membrane can be reduced without seriously impairing the growth of the bacteria by limiting the uptake of nutrients. Resistance to β-lactam antibiotics by decreasing the access of the antibiotic to the PBPs has not been reported in gram-positive bacteria which lack an outer membrane.

The third mechanism of resistance to β-lactam antibiotics is via alterations in the properties of the physiological targets of the antibiotics – the penicillin-binding proteins.

C. Classification of PBP Alterations in β-Lactam-Resistant Strains

Increased levels of resistance to β-lactam antibiotics that are mediated by alterations of PBPs was first demonstrated in the laboratory (SPRATT 1978) and has been found in clinical isolates of an increasing number of bacterial species (reviewed MALOUIN and BRYAN 1986). PBP alterations can be broadly classified into four classes.

I. Alterations in the Affinities of PBPs for β-Lactam Antibiotics

In many ways the production of PBPs that are resistant to inhibition by β-lactams would seem an obvious strategy for bacteria to employ to protect themselves from the antibiotics. In practice, resistance mediated by the production of PBPs with reduced affinity for β-lactam antibiotics appears to be relatively rare for two main reasons (SPRATT 1978).

Firstly, β-lactam antibiotics generally kill bacteria by inhibiting more than one PBP. Thus ampicillin at the concentrations that are achieved in vivo would kill *E. coli* by inhibiting PBPs 1A/1B, 2 and 3. The development of a more ampicillin-resistant form of one of these PBPs would therefore have little or no effect on the resistance of the bacteria to ampicillin as killing would still occur by the inactivation of the other unaltered PBPs. Substantial levels of resistance to ampicillin would require the reduction in the affinity of each of the physiologically important PBPs, and would therefore be extremely difficult to achieve.

The second theoretical limitation on the development of β-lactam-resistant PBPs arises from the belief that β-lactam antibiotics are structural analogues of the acyl-D-alanyl-D-alanine moiety of the pentapeptide side chain of the substrate of PBPs (WAXMAN and STROMINGER 1983). It may be that numerous amino acid substitutions in a physiologically important PBP would result in a large reduction in the affinity of the PBP for the antibiotic, but the great majority of these substitutions would also drastically reduce the affinity of the enzyme for its normal substrate such that the enzyme could not function effectively in peptidoglycan synthesis.

The number of amino acid substitutions that allow a PBP to reduce substantially its affinity for β-lactam antibiotics, without reducing its affinity for substrate, and which also do not disrupt the overall structure of the active centre, is likely to be very small (see Sect. D.1). Amino acid substitutions that produce a more penicillin-resistant PBP, but which result in even a slight reduction in the ability of the enzyme to sustain the normal rate of transpeptidation, may be selected against in vivo.

II. Alterations in the Amounts of PBPs

The production of larger amounts of PBPs could provide a mechanism of resistance to β-lactam antibiotics by increasing the concentration of the antibiotic that is required to reduce the activity of a PBP to a level that limits peptidoglycan synthesis. However, the level of resistance obtained by this mechanism is likely to be very low. As in the case of alterations in the affinities of PBPs, an overproduction of each of the physiologically important PBPs would be required to obtain substantial levels of resistance to most β-lactam antibiotics.

We have investigated whether increased levels of PBP 3 can provide *E. coli* with elevated levels of resistance to those β-lactams that kill over a substantial concentration range exclusively by the inactivation of this target (HEDGE and SPRATT, unpublished results). A 50-fold increase in the amount of PBP 3 resulted in no increase in the MIC for most PBP 3-directed β-lactam antibiotics (including cephalexin, cefoperazone, cefotaxime, cefamandole and mezlocillin), but produced an 8-fold increase in the level of resistance to aztreonam, and a 5-fold increase in resistance to ceftazidime. The reason for the increased resistance to the latter compounds is unknown.

Increased resistance by the production of elevated levels of normal penicillin-sensitive PBPs has not been rigorously demonstrated in clinical isolates of any bacteria. Alterations in the levels of a β-lactam-resistant PBP are involved in methicillin-resistant strains of *S. aureus*, and in enterococci, but these examples are rather different to that discussed above (see Sects. E.5 and E.6).

III. Resistance by Illegitimate Acquisition of a Resistant PBP

In this mechanism bacteria gain resistance by acquiring from another bacterium a new PBP that has a low affinity for β-lactam antibiotics. The resistant PBP can then take over the functions of all of the normal PBPs of the bacteria when the latter are inactivated in the presence of antibiotic. The acquisition is illegitimate in the sense that the incoming piece of DNA encoding the PBP has no homologue in the recipient bacterium, and its integration into the chromosome does not involve homologous recombination. The resistant organism therefore contains all of the normal PBPs plus the extra resistant PBP. A clear example of this process is found in methicillin-resistant strains of *S. aureus* (Sect. E.5).

IV. Resistance by Homologous Acquisition of a Resistant PBP

An alternative way of acquiring a more resistant PBP is to replace one of the normal PBPs with that from a related species by the uptake, and integration by homologous recombination, of a piece of DNA encoding the more resistant PBP. Within a group of closely related bacteria the affinity of a particular PBP for β-lactam antibiotics will vary amongst the members of the group as a result of slight differences in the amino acid sequences of their transpeptidase domains. A species with the most penicillin-sensitive PBPs amongst this group could therefore obtain a more resistant PBP by the replacement of the region encoding some, or all, of the transpeptidase domain with the corresponding region from a more resistant member of the group. Although mechanism exist to limit the uptake and integration of homologous sequences from closely related species, the strong selective pressures provided by antibiotic therapy should be sufficient for homologous acquisition to occur. Provided that the necessary circumstances prevail, the acquisition of a more penicillin-resistant PBP from a closely related organism may be a less rare event than the accumulation of amino acid substitutions that are required to evolve a resistant PBP from a sensitive one.

The production of a PBP with decreased affinity for β-lactams by evolution (Sect. C.1), or by homologous acquisition, can only be distinguished by comparing the nucleotide sequences of PBP genes from sensitive and resistant isolates. At present this has only been achieved in *N. gonorrhoeae* (Sect. E.1) and *Streptococcus pneumoniae* (DOWSON et al. 1988a; Sect. E.4) and in the former organism there is evidence that the development of a PBP with decreased affinity for penicillin may have occurred by homologous acquisition in some resistant strains.

A probable (non-PBP-mediated) example of the acquisition of increased penicillin resistance by the introduction and recombination of a piece of DNA from a related organism has already been documented in a clinical isolate of *E. coli*. In this example the extremely low level of expression of the chromosomal β-lactamase appears to have been increased by exchanging the promoter of the *E. coli ampC* gene with the stronger promoter from the *ampC* gene of *Shigella sonnei* (OLSSON et al. 1983).

D. Laboratory Studies on the Development of β-Lactam-Resistant PBPs in *E. coli*

I. Amino Acid Substitutions That Decrease the Affinity of PBP 3 for β-Lactam Antibiotics

The extent to which a PBP can decrease its affinity for β-lactam antibiotics has been studied using PBP 3 of *E. coli* (HEDGE and SPRATT 1985a). Several β-lactam antibiotics have a much higher affinity for PBP 3 compared to either PBP1A/1B or PBP 2, and therefore kill *E. coli* over a wide concentration range exclusively by the inhibition of cell division. Thus, cephalexin results in killing by the inactivation of PBP 3 from 6 μg/ml (the MIC) up to about 400 μg/ml, and it is only above these levels that inactivation of PBP 1A/1B occurs, and the killing mechanism switches from inhibition of cell division to rapid cell lysis. It should therefore be possible in this system to detect alterations of PBP 3 that provide up to an 80-fold increase in cephalexin resistance.

In a very extensive study, using three different mutagens, the maximum level of resistance to cephalexin that could be obtained in a single step by alterations of PBP 3 was only 10-fold. Only three different amino acid substitutions in PBP 3 resulted in ≧7-fold increase in resistance to cephalexin (Thr-308 to Pro; Val-344 to Gly and Asn-361 to Ser). Each of the amino acid substitutions gave cross-resistance to structurally related cephalosporins, but not to other cephalosporins, or to penicillins or monobactams and, as expected, all were within the carboxy-terminal region of PBP 3 that has been proposed to be the transpeptidase domain.

Amino acid substitutions that allow PBP 3 to discriminate markedly between the binding of a β-lactam and its normal structurally analogous substrate should define residues that are located within the active centre of the transpeptidase domain. It is clear that Thr-308 is within the active centre as Ser-307 is the active-site residue acylated by penicillin (KECK et al. 1985). Asn-361 is also believed to be at the active centre of PBP 3, as this residue is conserved in all high MW PBPs (and also in low MW PBPs), and probably corresponds to Asn-132 of class A β-lactamases, which is located at approximately the same distance to the carboxy-terminal side of the active-site serine and, from the crystal structure of the β-lactamase of *S. aureus*, has been tentatively assigned a role in the binding of the carbonyl oxygen of the peptide bond in the side chain of β-lactam antibiotics (HERZBERG and MOULT 1987). It is less clear whether Val-344 of PBP 3 is within the active centre as it is difficult to produce a satisfactory alignment of the sequences of high MW PBPs and β-lactamases in this region. Interestingly, an amino acid insertion has occurred at the corresponding position in the development of all three of the more penicillin-resistant forms of the homologous PBP 2 of *N. gonorrhoeae* that have been sequenced (Sect. E.1), and extensive amino acid substitutions have occurred in the corresponding region of PBP 2G from a penicillin-resistant South African strain of *S. pneumoniae* (DOWSON et al. 1988a; Sect. E.4). The alterations of the equivalent region in these three studies suggest that it forms a part of the penicillin-binding site in the three-dimensional structure of high MW PBPs (DOWSON et al. 1988a).

The selection for cephalexin-resistant mutants in our initial studies appears to have been a particularly fortunate one, as subsequent experiments in which mutants were selected (after mutagenesis with one of four different mutagens) that had a ≧6-fold increase in their level of resistance to several other PBP 3-specific β-lactams (including ceftazidime, cefamandole cefoperazone, mezlocillin, piperacillin, carbenicillin and ticarcillin) failed to produce any in which the resistance was due to alterations of PBP 3 (CROMIE et al., unpublished experiments).

Although these studies have only been carried out with one PBP from one bacterial species, it is likely that the conclusions can be generalized to the physiologically important PBPs of other bacteria. Apparently single amino acid substitutions in PBPs cannot produce large changes in their ability to discriminate between β-lactam antibiotics and the normal peptide substrate. The evolution of PBPs that have high levels of resistance to inactivation by β-lactam antibiotics is therefore likely to have occurred by a multistep process in which each successive amino acid substitution in the PBP produces a further small reduction in its affinity for the antibiotic, without significantly decreasing its stability, or altering its ability to process the normal peptide substrate.

II. Re-modelling of the Active Centre of PBP 3 to Obtain High Level Resistance to β-Lactam Antibiotics

We have carried out a laboratory study to investigate the ease with which PBP 3 of *E. coli* can re-model its active centre to produce a PBP that has high levels of resistance to inactivation by β-lactam antibiotics (HEDGE and SPRATT 1985b). In this study we showed that a form of PBP 3 that was highly resistant to cephalosporins could be obtained by four amino acid substitutions within the transpeptidase domain of PBP 3. The evolution of the resistant form of PBP 3 involved two steps that reduced the affinity of PBP 3 for cephalosporins, but also decreased its thermostability, alternating with two steps that had little effect on affinity, but resulted in a re-stabilization of the enzyme. Interestingly, the highly cephalosporin-resistant form of PBP 3 showed no increase in its resistance to penicillins or monobactams. Attempts to introduce penicillin resistance, as well as cephalosporin resistance, into this form of PBP 3 were unsuccessful; introduction of increased levels of penicillin resistance could only be achieved at the expense of most of the cephalosporin resistance (HEDGE and SPRATT, unpublished experiments).

The laboratory study of the development of a cephalosporin-resistant form of PBP 3 has shown one route by which this end can be achieved. Our aim was to show the minimum number of amino acid substitutions that were needed to produce a highly β-lactam-resistant enzyme, and it is clear that the same result could have been obtained in other ways, e.g. by the introduction of substantially more amino acid substitutions that each have only a very slight alteration in the properties of the enzyme. The latter path may be preferred in nature since large reductions in the affinity of PBP 3 for cephalosporins were usually associated with a significant decrease in the stability of the enzyme (HEDGE and SPRATT 1985a, b).

Examples of resistant clinical isolates that produce PBPs with decreased affinity for β-lactam antibiotics are found in several species and the most well documented examples are described in the following sections.

E. PBP Alterations in Clinical Isolates

I. *Neisseria gonorrhoea*

β-Lactamase producing strains of *N. gonorrhoeae* first appeared in 1976 and are now widely disseminated. In addition to these highly penicillin-resistant strains, there has been a gradual increase in the prevalence of gonococcal isolates that have a decreased sensitivity to penicillin G. In many hospitals a substantial proportion of non-β-lactamase producing gonococci have MICs of >0.1 μg/ml and isolates with MICs of >1 μg/ml are not uncommon. Gonoccocal isolates that have an increased level of resistance to penicillin, but which do not produce β-lactamase, are generally called chromosomally mediated resistant *N. gonorrhoeae* (CMRNG).

DOUGHERTY et al. (1980) and BARBOUR (1981) have established the importance of PBP alterations in CMRNG isolates. *N. gonorrhoeae* possesses three PBPs with apparent MWs of approximately 88000 (PBP 1), 60000 (PBP 2) and 45000 (PBP 3) (DOUGHERTY et al. 1980; BARBOUR 1981). The lethal effects of penicillin apparently result from the inactivation of either PBP 1 or PBP 2. Two lines of evidence suggest that PBP 2 is specifically involved in peptidoglycan synthesis for cell division. Firstly, β-lactam antibiotics that show their highest affinity for PBP 2 results in a block in cell division and the production of enlarged spherical cells at their lowest effective concentration (BARBOUR 1981). Secondly, the amino acid sequence of PBP 2 of *N. gonorrhoeae* is very similar to that of PBP 3 of *E. coli* (the cell division PBP of this organism), whereas it shows very little similarity to any of the other *E. coli* PBPs (SPRATT 1988). Inhibition of PBP 1 of *N. gonorrhoeae* probably results in rapid cell lysis and this PBP is presumably analogous to PBP 1A/1B of *E. coli* and involved in non-septal peptidoglycan synthesis.

The genetics of the development of CMRNG strains have been analysed extensively and at least four genes involved in penicillin resistance have been identified (CANNON and SPARLING 1984). DNA from a penicillin-resistant isolate can transform a sensitive strain only to a slightly higher level of resistance. The first level resistant mutant can then be transformed with DNA from the resistant strain to a slightly higher level of resistance, and further cycles of transformation result in the production of a strain that has the level of penicillin resistance of the CMRNG strain from which the DNA was obtained (CANNON and SPARLING 1984; DOUGHERTY 1986; FARUKI and SPARLING 1986).

Analysis of the PBPs of CMRNG strains have shown that those with MICs of benzylpenicillin of $\geqq 1$ µg/ml produce altered forms of PBP 1 and PBP 2 that have substantially decreased affinity for penicillin G (DOUGHERTY et al. 1980, DOUGHERTY 1986). The analysis of the PBPs of an isogenic series of transformants showing increasing levels of penicillin resistance has shown that the first step in penicillin resistance (due to mutations in *pen*A) is due to a reduction in the affinity of PBP 2 for penicillin, and that the next two steps, which result in increased resistance to a number of unrelated antibiotics (*mtr* and *pen*B mutations), do not involve alterations of PBPs and probably result from alterations of the outer membrane. The fourth step involves a reduction in the affinity of PBP 1 for penicillin (DOUGHERTY et al. 1980; DOUGHERTY 1986).

Although the genetic dissection suggests that there are only four steps in the development of penicillin-resistant gonococci, the actual chronology of the molecular events that resulted in resistance in vivo are almost certainly much more complex since, in transformation, all of the multiple mutations that have accumulated in a resistance gene are likely to be incorporated into the genome of the recipient in a single step.

The pathway to the development of a penicillin-resistant gonococcus would be expected to involve the introduction of one, or more, amino acid substitutions into PBP 2 to reduce its affinity to an extent that killing at the MIC is no longer due to the inactivation of this PBP. At this point further reduction in the affinity of PBP 2 provides no further resistance to penicillin as killing at the MIC now results from the inactivation of PBP 1. The continuing pathway in the development of resistance should then involve the introduction of amino acid substitutions into PBP 1 until its affinity has been reduced to such an extent that killing at the MIC is now no longer due to the inactivation of PBP 1, but results again from inactivation of PBP 2. Further reductions in the affinity of the already partially penicillin-resistant PBP 2 are then required to produce a further increase in the MIC of the organism. As amino acid substitutions in proteins frequently decrease either their thermal stability or their susceptibility to proteolysis, the remodelling of the active centre of a PBP is likely to require amino acid substitutions that re-stabilise the enzyme in addition to those that decrease its affinity for antibiotic (HEDGE and SPRATT 1985 b).

The process by which penicillin resistance is gradually built up by the alternating reduction in the affinity of the two physiologically important PBPs could, in theory, continue indefinitely to result in a totally penicillin-resistant gonococcus. In practice the development of non-β-lactamase producing penicillin-resistant gonococci also involves mutations in the *mtr* and *penB* gene which reduce the penetration of the antibiotic through the gonococcal outer membrane.

We have recently cloned the PBP 2 gene of *N. gonorrhoeae* by making a gene library of DNA fragments from a penicillin-resistant isolate and isolating recombinant plasmids that transform a penicillin-sensitive gonococcus to a low level of penicillin resistance. The nucleotide sequences of the PBP 2 genes from two independent penicillin-sensitive strains and of three CMRNG strains have been compared (Spratt 1988).

The PBP 2 genes of the two unrelated penicillin-sensitive strains were almost identical in sequence throughout their entire coding regions. The nucleotide sequence of the PBP 2 gene of CDC77-124615 (MIC of 2 μg/ml) differed at 14 positions from that of the penicillin-sensitive strains. Seven of the nucleotide changes were neutral (in the sense that they did not alter the amino acid sequence), whereas the other changes resulted in five amino acid alterations (including the insertion of an additional amino acid) between the penicillin-sensitive and penicillin-resistant forms of PBP 2. The sequence of the PBP2 gene of another CMRNG strain (CDC84-060384, MIC of 4 μg/ml, from the outbreak of CMRNG infections in Durham, North Carolina; Faruki et al. 1985) was identical to that of CDC77-124615 except at one position.

The clear homology between PBP 2 of *N. gonorrhoeae* and PBP 3 of *E. coli* allows the identification of Ser-310 of the former protein as the active-site residue that is acylated by penicillin and predicts that the penicillin-sensitive transpeptidase domain of the gonococcal PBP extends from about residue 260 to the carboxy-terminus. The amino acid substitutions that distinguish PBP 2 of the penicillin-resistant strains from PBP 2 of the penicillin-sensitive strains all occur between residues 346 and 551. The development of the penicillin-resistant PBP has therefore, as expected, resulted from alterations of residues exclusively within the transpeptidase domain.

The finding that the PBP 2 gene of two penicillin-resistant strains, which were isolated several years apart, are identical (except at one position), but differ at 14 positions from the PBP 2 gene of penicillin-sensitive isolates, argues for a common origin of these resistant strains. The most persuasive evidence for the clonal origin of CDC77-124615 and CDC84-060384 is the fact that all seven of the neutral nucleotide substitutions in the PBP 2 gene are identical, since these changes have not occurred in response to selection, but presumably reflect the genetic background in which resistance emerged. A clonal origin of many CMRNG strains has often been suspected since these strains share common properties including increased resistance to tetracycline and erythromycin, proline auxotrophy, and serotype (Faruki et al. 1985).

We have also sequenced the PBP 2 gene of a third CMRNG strain (CDC84-060418; MIC = 1 μg/ml) that was shown by Dougherty (1986) to produce an altered from of PBP 2 with very low affinity for penicillin. The PBP 2 gene of CDC84-060418 was remarkable as it differed from that of penicillin-sensitive strains by only a few nucleotide substitutions, and one codon insertion (the same changes found in the other CMRNG strains), in the region encoding residues 1–517 but then diverged very extensively throughout the rest of the coding region. It is difficult to escape the conclusion that the PBP 2 gene of CDC84-060418 is a hybrid gene in which the promoter-distal region, encoding the carboxy-terminal part of the transpeptidase domain, has been replaced by homologous acquisition of sequences from another (*Neisseria*?) species.

Oligonucleotide probes based on nucleotide sequences that differ between the PBP 2 genes of penicillin-sensitive and CMRNG strains have been used to classify the PBP 2 genes in a collection of about 50 CMRNG strains from British hospitals (DOWSON et al. 1988b). This study has shown that the majority of CMRNG strains possess the altered PBP 2 genes found in CDC77-124615 and CDC84-060384 whereas the remainder possess the more extensively altered PBP 2 gene found in CDC84-060418. Since these two classes of altered PBP 2 genes have diverged from a common origin it is likely that the PBP 2 genes in all (or at least the great majority) of CMRNG strains have a clonal origin.

II. *Neisseria meningitidis*

Isolates of *Neisseria meningitidis* have until recently been uniformally sensitive to penicillin. Several non-β-lactamase-producing isolates that have low levels of resistance to penicillin have been reported recently in Spain (SAEZ-NIETO et al. 1987). These strains are about 10-fold more resistant to penicillin than typical penicillin-sensitive isolates and appear to arise from a reduction in the affinity of a PBP with a MW of 59000 that is the meningococcal analogue of PBP 2 of the gonococcus (MENDELMAN et al. 1988).

It would not be surprising if the development of penicillin resistance in *N. meningitidis* followed essentially the same pathway as in *N. gonorrhoeae* although, fortunately, the process might be expected to be considerably slower as the selective pressures for the development of resistance are likely to be much less in the meningococcus. A close monitoring of the low-level penicillin-resistant strains is required to prevent the emergence of meningococcal strains that have higher levels of penicillin resistance.

III. *Haemophilus influenzae*

Ampicillin-resistant, β-lactamase-producing, strains of pathogenic *Haemophilus influenzae* type b were first reported in 1974 and are now the most important cause of β-lactam resistance in this organism. Non-β-lactamase-producing ampicillin-resistant (NBLP Ap^R) strains of *H. influenzae* have been reported with increasing frequency since 1980. These strains are relatively rare amongst type b *H. influenzae*, which are the cause of purulent meningitis, but are more common amongst non-typable isolates, which are largely found in the respiratory tract and are implicated in nosocomial and community-acquired pneumoniae, and in pulmonary infections associated with chronic bronchitis and cystic fibrosis (PHILPOT-HOWARD 1984).

NBLP strains with MICs of ampicillin as high as 16 μg/ml have been reported (compared to an MIC of 0.5 μg/ml for a typical penicillin-sensitive isolate). These strains also show cross-resistance to other penicillins and to cephalosporins (including third generation compounds) and to moxalactam (MENDELMAN et al. 1984; PARR and BRYAN 1984). Surprisingly, the MIC values show a marked inoculum effect which, in the case of β-lactam antibiotics, is usually an indication that the resistance is due to β-lactamase production. The cause of the incoculum effect in the NBLP Ap^R strains of *H. influenzae* is unknown.

The mechanism of resistance apparently involves the production of altered forms of PBPs 3a and 3b that have decreased affinity for β-lactams (PARR and BRYAN 1984; MENDELMAN et al. 1984; SERFASS et al. 1986). β-lactams that bind preferentially to PBPs 3a and 3b result in the inhibition of cell division and the formation of filamentous cells (PARR and BRYAN 1984). The PBPs 3 of *H. influenzae* have very similar MWs to PBP 3 of *E. coli*, and PBP 2 of *N. gonorrhoeae*, and it is likely that they are all functionally homologous PBPs that act as peptidoglycan transpeptidases at cell division.

Since the organism is naturally transformable it has been possible to transfer resistance from ampicillin-resistant strains into an ampicillin-sensitive laboratory strain and to establish that the transfer of resistance is associated with the appearance of the altered forms of PBP 3a and PBP 3b (PARR and BRYAN 1984).

It is not clear why the alteration of both PBP 3a and PBP 3b is transferred in a single step. One possibility is that PBP 3a and PBP 3b are differently modified or processed forms of a single PBP. Alternatively, PBP 3a and PBP 3b may be the products of two distinct, but closely linked, genes that are co-transformed on a single piece of DNA. A third explanation that has been suggested by MALOUIN et al. (1987) is that the alterations in these PBPs may be the result of an alteration of a gene product that interacts with the PBPs and somehow modifies their properties.

In some NBLP Ap^R strains the full extent of ampicillin resistance, and of cross resistance to other β-lactams, could be transferred to a penicillin-sensitive strain in a single step by transformation. In other strains the full level of ampicillin resistance could be transferred in a single step but the level of cross resistance to some, or all, of the other β-lactam antibiotics tested was significantly less than in the original clinical isolate (MENDELMAN et al. 1984). It is therefore likely that at least in some NBLP Ap^R strains there are other alterations besides those that effect PBP 3a and PBP 3b, e.g. alterations of permeability, or of other PBPs.

The ability in *H. influenzae* to transform the full level of ampicillin resistance into a sensitive strain in a single step appears to be in sharp contrast to the situation in pneumococci and gonococci where several rounds of transformation are required to convert a sensitive organism to the full level of resistance of a penicillin-resistant clinical isolate. However, it should be remembered that the difference between the MICs of sensitive and resistant isolates is only about 30-fold in *H. influenzae* whereas it is about 1000-fold in both pneumococci and gonococci. The development of non-β-lactamase-mediated ampicillin resistance in *H. influenzae* has not therefore progressed as far as it has in pneumococci and gonococci.

Recently, MALOUIN et al. (1987) have reported the cloning of the gene(s) involved in ampicillin resistance in an NBLP Ap^R type b *H. influenzae* isolate. A cosmid library of DNA fragments isolated from the Ap^R strain was constructed, and a cosmid was obtained that transformed an ampicillin-sensitive laboratory strain of *H. influenzae* to ampicillin resistance.

Surprisingly two contiguous, but non-overlapping, fragments of the chromosomal insert in the cosmid were each able to transform an ampicillin-sensitive *H. influenzae* to (almost) the full level of ampicillin resistance, and the transformants obtained using either fragment expressed the altered forms of both PBP 3a and PBP 3b. Possible explanations for these results can be suggested but none of them convincingly explain why transformants obtained with either of the contiguous DNA fragments, or with the entire cosmid (which contains both fragments), have gained essentially the same level of resistance to all three β-lactam antibiotics that were examined, or why each fragment is able to introduce the altered forms of both PBP 3a and PBP 3b.

Several polypeptides have been shown to be expressed in *E. coli* minicells from the region of the cosmid that encodes the resistance determinant(s) but none of these correspond in size to that of PBP 3a or PBP 3b of *H. influenzae* (MALOUIN et al. 1987). This result does not eliminate the possibility that one or both of these PBP genes are present on the cosmid, since PBP genes are very poorly expressed in their natural host, and may not be expressed at a detectable level in a heterologous expression system. Clearly further work is necessary to clarify whether the DNA fragment that has been cloned encodes PBP 3A and/or PBP 3B, or whether it encodes another product that indirectly alters the properties of these PBPs.

It is probably not a coincidence that NBLP Ap^R strains are mainly found among non-typable *H. influenzae* since these strains are usually involved in recurrent pulmonary infections in chronic bronchitis, or cystic fibrosis, where patients often receive repeated courses of β-lactam antibiotics. Unlike the latter situation, which provides the ideal selective conditions for the emergence of resistant mutants with altered PBPs, or altered outer membrane permeability, the type b strains are generally associated with an acute episode of meningitis where the conditions for the emergence of resistance are much less favourable. The availability of transformation as a means of genetic exchange in *H. influenzae* is likely to allow the spread of resistance determinants from non-typable strains to type b strains.

The increased levels of resistance of non-typable strains to a broad range of β-lactam antibiotics (including the β-lactamase stable third generation cephalosporins) has not been convincingly associated with clinical treatment failure in respiratory tract infections. Treatment failure is likely to become significant with these strains, however, if the level of resistance increases due to further alterations of PBPs or of outer membrane permeability. Of more serious concern is the potential spread of resistance amongst type b strains that cause meningitis, since the levels of β-lactams that can be achieved in the cerebrospinal fluid are unlikely to be sufficient to eliminate these strains.

IV. *Streptococcus pneumoniae*

Until the late 1960s pneumococci were universally sensitive to benzylpenicillin and had MICs in the range 0.008–0.03 μg/ml. Isolates with decreased sensitivity to penicillin were first reported by HANSMAN and BULLEN (1967) and similar isolates with MICs of 0.1–0.5 μg/ml were reported with increasing frequency from several countries throughout the 1970s. Although these strains are still relatively sensitive to penicillin they are a cause for concern as they may be associated with treatment failure particularly in pneumococcal meningitis where sufficient levels of penicillin cannot be achieved in the cerebrospinal fluid.

Strains of pneumococci with high levels of resistance to benzylpenicillin were first reported from South Africa and these strains, unlike most of the less resistant isolates that had previously been described, were also resistant to several other classes of antibiotics (JACOBS et al. 1978). Isolates of pneumococci with high levels of resistance to penicillin (MICs of 1–10 μg/ml) have subsequently been reported from numerous countries, and have recently been the cause of community-acquired infections, whereas they were previously associated with nosocomial infections (FELDMAN et al. 1985).

Penicillin resistance in pneumococci is entirely due to alterations of the PBPs (HAKENBECK et al. 1980; ZIGHELBOIM and TOMASZ 1980). There have been no reports of β-lactamases in pneumococci, and mutations that reduce the accessibility of penicillin to the PBPs have not been described in gram-positive bacteria. The absence of these latter mechanisms of resistance, and the extensive clinical exposure of the pneumococcus to penicillin, have provided the ideal scenario for the development of resistance mediated by PBP alterations. It is therefore not surprising that the most advanced example of the development of penicillin resistance mediated by PBP alterations is found in this organism.

Evidence that alterations of PBPs are the only possible mechanism of resistance to penicillin in pneumococci (and by inference in any gram-positive bacteria where β-lactamases are unknown) has been provided by laboratory studies. Resistance to penicillin in the laboratory occurs by a stepwise mechanism (SHOCKLEY and HOTCHKISS 1970). Mutants that have increased levels of resistance arise at a frequency of about 10^{-8}–10^{-9} but show only a 2–4 fold increase in MIC. Second level mutants with a further slight increase in resistance can be obtained at low frequency, and the selection procedure can be repeated to obtain mutants with increasing levels of resistance. Analysis of these laboratory mutants has shown that in all cases the development of resistance is associated with alterations in the affinity of PBPs (HANDWERGER and TOMASZ 1986a; LAIBLE and HAKENBECK 1987).

Penicillin-sensitive isolates of *S. pneumoniae* contain five PBPs – PBPs 1a and 1b (MW 98000 and 95000), PBPs 2a and 2b (MW 81000 and 79000), and PBP 3 (MW 43000) (HAKENBECK et al. 1980; ZIGHELBOIM and TOMASZ 1980; PERCHESON and BRYAN 1980). Recently an additional PBP 2x (MW about 85000) has been reported (HAKENBECK et al. 1986). Attempts to correlate the binding of β-lactam antibiotics to particular PBPs, with the killing of the organism, or with a morphological effect, have been largely inconclusive (WILLIAMSON et al. 1980; WILLIAMSON and TOMASZ 1985; HAKENBECK et al. 1987).

The alterations of PBPs in laboratory mutants (HANDWERGER and TOMASZ 1986a; LAIBLE and HAKENBECK 1987), or clinical isolates (HAKENBECK et al. 1980; PERCHESON and BRYAN 1980; ZIGHELBOIM and TOMASZ 1980), that have increased levels of resistance to β-lactams mostly involve PBPs 1a, 2x, 2a and 2b, and it is likely that these are the physiologically important PBPs of pneumococci. PBP 3, in common with low MW PBPs in other bacteria, catalyses the D-alanine carboxypeptidase reaction and probably is not involved in the killing mechanism of β-lactam antibiotics in pneumococci (HAKENBECK and KOHIYAMA 1982).

The alterations in the PBPs of penicillin-resistant clinical isolates of pneumococci have been described by Tomasz and colleagues (ZIGHELBOIM and TOMASZ 1980; HAKENBECK et al. 1980; HANDWERGER and TOMASZ 1986b) and by PERCHESON and BRYAN (1980). These studies are difficult to analyse in detail as electrophoretic conditions that allow the clear resolution of each of the pneumococcal PBPs have not been used; consequently PBPs 1a and 1b and PBPs 2x, 2a and 2b have often not been studied individually but have been treated as PBP groups 1 and 2.

Pneumococci that have low levels of resistance to penicillin (MICs of 0.05–0.2 μg/ml) possess modified forms of PBP group 1 and 2 that have decreased affinity for penicillin. In the more resistant isolates, and particularly in the highly resistant isolates from South Africa (MICs >1 μg/ml) there are more complex PBP alterations involving the apparent loss of PBPs, and the appearance of "novel" PBPs, as well as alterations in the affinity of some of the PBPs for penicillin.

The most detailed studies of the PBPs of highly resistant pneumococci have been carried out with the South African strain 8249 (MIC of 6 μg/ml (ZIGHELBOIM and TOMASZ 1980; HANDWERGER and TOMASZ 1986b). In this strain only PBPs 1b, 2a and 3 can be labelled with radioactive penicillin (PBP 1b was not observed in earlier studies of strain 8249 but has subsequently been reported to be present; HAKENBECK et al. 1986). Neither PBP 1a or PBP 2b have been detected in strain 8249 using radioactive penicillin but a "novel" PBP 1c (MW 92000) is found (ZIGHELBOIM and TOMASZ 1980; HANDWERGER and TOMASZ 1986b).

The situation has been clarified by recent studies which have shown that the "novel" PBP 1c of the resistant strain is almost certainly an altered form of PBP 1a, since antibody raised against the latter PBP cross reacts with PBP 1c (HAKENBECK et al. 1986). PBP 1c of strain 8249 has a very low affinity for penicillin compared to the homologous PBP 1a of the laboratory strain R6. Low affinity forms of PBP 1a of variable MW are also seen in other highly penicillin-resistant strains from South Africa and in similar strains from Papua New Guinea (HAKENBECK et al. 1986).

The apparent absence of PBP 2b in strain 8249 has been shown to be due to a drastic decrease in its affinity for penicillin such that it is not detected by the PBP assay, since the protein is detected in strain 8249 using anti-PBP 2b antibody, rather than penicillin-labelling (HAKENBECK et al. 1986). In addition to these changes, PBP 2a (and perhaps PBP 1b) of strain 8249 has a greatly reduced affinity for penicillin compared to that in a penicillin-sensitive isolate. Indeed, the only PBP of strain 8249 that is not significantly altered in its properties is PBP 3 (ZIGHELBOIM and TOMASZ 1980; HANDWERGER and TOMASZ 1986b). Very similar alterations have been found in the PBPs of other highly penicillin-resistant pneumococci.

All of the remarkable differences between the PBPs of highly penicillin-resistant pneumococci, and those of penicillin-sensitive strains, can now be accounted for solely in terms of alterations in the affinity of the proteins and there is no evidence in pneumococci for the loss of PBPs or the acquisition of novel PBPs (as has occurred in methicillin-resistant strains of *Staphylococcus aureus*).

Differences in the apparent MWs of the corresponding PBPs of the penicillin-sensitive laboratory strain R6 and strains with moderate or high levels of penicillin resistance have frequently been observed. Examples have been found of alterations in the apparent MW of PBP 3 in a resistant strain from Papua New Guinea, and of PBP 2a, and PBP 1a, in moderately and highly penicillin-resistant strains from North America and South Africa (ZIGHELBOIM and TOMASZ 1980; HAKENBECK et al. 1980, 1986). These changes could have resulted from small insertions or deletions (or indeed point mutations, since there are examples of amino acid substitutions that alter the mobility of proteins on SDS polyacrylamide gels) in the PBP genes during the series of mutational events that led to the reduction in the affinities of the PBPs. However, slight differences are found in the mobilities of the PBPs of independent isolates of penicillin-sensitive pneumococci (HAKENBECK, personal communication). The differences between the apparent MWs of the PBPs of penicillin-resistant isolates and those of the R6 strain may therefore be unrelated to the alterations in the affinities of the PBPs and may simply reflect the fact that resistant PBPs have evolved in strains that are genetically distant from the R6 strain.

The causal link between the presence of PBPs with very low affinity for penicillin, and the high level of penicillin resistance of strain 8249, has been established by using DNA of the latter strain to transform the penicillin-sensitive strain R6 to increasing levels of penicillin resistance (ZIGHELBOIM and TOMASZ 1980). As expected, transformation of penicillin resistance occurs in a stepwise manner, and the PBPs of transformants with increasing levels of resistance become gradually like those of the DNA donor strain.

The gradual appearance of PBPs with decreasing affinity, or altered electrophoretic mobility, in the series of transformants with increasing levels of penicillin resistance appears to show the sequence of genetic events that have occurred during the evolution of a highly penicillin-resistant pneumococcus from a penicillin-sensitive one. As discussed in Sect. E.1, with reference to the gonococcus, the genetic events that have occurred in the evolution of highly penicillin-resistant pneumococci are likely to be very much more complex than those suggested by the transformation experiments. The evolution of resistant strains has almost certainly occurred by the introduction of a large number of mutations that gradually, and alternately, reduce the affinity of each of the physiologically important PBPs. In the transformation experiments all of the multiple mutations in a PBP gene should be introduced into the recipient in a single step and the number of steps required to transform a sensitive strain to the level of resistance of the DNA donor should approximate to the number of different genes involved in resistance.

According to both ZIGHELBOIM and TOMASZ (1980) and HANDWERGER and TOMASZ (1986b), the properties of individual PBPs change gradually in the isogenic series of increasingly penicillin-resistant transformants from those characteristic of the penicillin-sensitive recipient strain to those characteristic of the penicillin-resistant strain. Although a stepwise reduction in the affinity of PBPs in transformants with increasing levels of penicillin resistance seems at first sight entirely reasonable, it is difficult to explain at a molecular level as all of the mutations that distinguish a PBP gene of strain 8249 from the corresponding PBP gene of the recipient should be introduced in a single step since transformation occurs by the uptake and integration by homologous recombination of pieces of DNA that are large in comparison with the size of a gene. It would therefore be expected that all of the mutations in, for example, the PBP 1a gene would be introduced en bloc at the transformation step in which the introduction of a more resistant PBP 1a is required to obtain the next level of penicillin resistance. Transformants with the lowest level of penicillin resistance, which have not yet received the mutations in the PBP 1a gene, should therefore produce PBP 1a with the characteristic affinity of strain R6, and all of those with higher levels of resistance, which have received the multiply mutated PBP 1a gene, should possess a protein with the characteristically low affinity, and altered MW, of strain 8249. This anomaly is unresolved.

We have recently cloned and sequenced the PBP 2b gene from three penicillin-sensitive pneumococci (MICs of 0.008 μg/ml) and from a penicillin-resistant South African strain (MIC of 4 μg/ml). The amino acid sequences of PBP 2b from the three penicillin-sensitive strains were identical, whereas that of the penicillin-resistant strain differed at 17 positions within the transpeptidase domain (DOWSON et al. 1988 a). It therefore appears that the re-modelling of the active centre of PBP 2b to produce the low affinity form found in the penicillin-resistant strain, which can virtually exclude penicillin from its active centre without preventing its ability to bind its structurally analogous substrate, has required the introduction of 17 amino acid substitutions. The most remarkable difference in the penicillin-resistant strain was the substitution of seven consecutive residues in a region that probably forms a part of the penicillin-binding site in the three-dimensional structure of high MW PBPs (see Sect. D.1).

V. *Staphylococcus aureus*

Initial successes in the treatment of staphylococcal infections with benzylpenicillin were threatened by the appearance and spread of β-lactamase-producing strains in the 1950s. The introduction in 1959 of methicillin, which is resistant to hydrolysis by the class A β-lactamase found in *S. aureus* strains, was rapidly followed by the isolation of methicillin-resistant (MRSA) strains. During the 1960s these strains were responsible for serious nosocomial infections in many European hospitals and since then have become widespread also in North American, Australian and Japanese hospitals. MRSA are currently a serious problem in many hospitals as these strains are often resistant to aminoglycosides, macrolides, chloramphenicol, and tetracycline in addition to being untreatable with any of the β-lactam antibiotics.

Most MRSA strains are heterogeneous in that only a small fraction of the population expresses resistance when cells are grown at 37 °C in the absence of β-lactam antibiotics. In some heterogeneous strains growth at 30 °C results in all of the bacteria expressing high levels of methicillin resistance (thermosensitive heterogeneous strains), whereas in other MRSA strains heterogeneity of expression is maintained at the lower temperature (HARTMAN and TOMASZ 1986).

Homogeneously resistant MRSA strains are also found in which all of the cells express resistance at 30 °C or 37 °C.

Methicillin resistance in *S. aureus* is particularly interesting as it provides the only example where resistance appears to have been obtained by the illegitimate acquisition of a β-lactam-resistant PBP from another bacterium. The first clear indication that MRSA strains have altered PBPs compared to normal strains was provided by BROWN and REYNOLDS (1980), who reported that a heterogeneous MRSA strain possessed the same PBP profile as a methicillin-sensitive strain under conditions where methicillin resistance was not expressed, but contained large amounts of a modified PBP 3, or a new PBP, with very low affinity for β-lactam antibiotics, under conditions where methicillin resistance was expressed. Constitutive expression of a modified low affinity form of PBP 3 was reported at about the same time in a homogeneous MRSA strain by HAYES et al. (1981).

Subsequent studies using electrophoretic conditions that give better resolution of the PBPs have established that MRSA strains possess the four normal PBPs characteristic of staphylococci but, in addition, possess an extra PBP (now called PBP 2′) with a MW of about 78 000 that has a very low affinity for β-lactam antibiotics (HARTMAN and TOMASZ 1984; CHAMBERS et al. 1985; REYNOLDS and FULLER 1986; ROSSI et al. 1985; UBUKATA et al. 1985; UTSUI and YOKOTA 1985). In most heterogenous MRSA strains PBP 2′ is induced by growth in the presence of β-lactam antibiotics, whereas in homogeneous strains PBP 2′ is expressed constitutively (ROSSI et al. 1985; UBUKATA et al. 1985; REYNOLDS and FULLER 1986). PBP 2′ is not closely related to the normal PBPs of *S. aureus* since monoclonal antibodies directed against PBP 2′ do not cross react with any of the PBPs of methicillin-sensitive strains (O'HARA and REYNOLDS, personal communication).

Genetic studies have suggested that the methicillin resistance determinant (now known to be the gene encoding PBP 2′) is chromosomal but is carried on a piece of DNA that is not present in methicillin-sensitive strains (STEWARD and ROSENBLUM 1980). Recently the complete PBP 2′ gene has been cloned by taking advantage of its close genetic linkage to an aminoglycoside resistance gene in some MRSA strains (MATSUHASHI et al. 1986). A recombinant plasmid containing a 23.5-kb insert of MRSA DNA was obtained which encoded tobramycin resistance and resulted in the appearance in *E. coli* of a novel PBP that was very slightly larger than PBP 2′ of the MRSA strain. The novel PBP expressed in *E. coli* had the expected low affinity for β-lactams and was established to be PBP 2′ by comparing its penicilloyl-labelled proteolytic fragments with those of authentic PBP 2′ from the MRSA strain.

Cloning of the methicillin resistance determinant has also been reported by BECK et al. (1986) and by MATTHEWS et al. (1987). Hybridization studies have shown conclusively that the PBP 2′ gene is part of a large (>24-kb) region that is present in all MRSA strains so far examined and is absent from methicillin-sensitive strains (BECK et al. 1986; MATSUHASHI et al. 1986; MATTHEWS et al. 1987).

In some MRSA strains methicillin resistance can be lost at high frequency by growth at elevated temperatures, or spontaneously on storage, and loss of resistance is accompanied by loss of the PBP 2′ gene. The appearance in MRSA strains of a novel piece of genetic material encoding PBP 2′, its close linkage to other drug resistance genes in some strains, and its genetic instability, suggests that the PBP 2′

gene may be part of a transposable element. The presence of insertion sequences close to the methicillin resistance determinant has been proposed to explain the observed hybridisation between part of the determinant and regions on *S. aureus* plasmids (BECK et al. 1986; MATTHEWS et al. 1987). Direct evidence for insertion sequences flanking the methicillin resistance determinant is however lacking.

The origin of the PBP 2′ gene of MRSA strains is currently unknown but it is very likely that the gene has arrived in *S. aureus* from another species. The cloned PBP 2′ gene can now be used as a probe to search for the bacterial species from which the gene was acquired. Recently the PBP 2′ gene has been sequenced and the derived amino acid sequence has some similarity to that of other high MW PBPs (SONG et al. 1987). However most of the available sequences of high MW PBPs are from gram-negative species and it is more likely that PBP 2′ of MRSA strains was acquired from a gram-positive bacterium. The more meaningful comparison of PBP 2′ with the high MW PBPs of gram-positive species must await the cloning and sequencing of further gram-positive PBP genes.

The finding that the PBP 2′ gene of MRSA strains is inducible in some heterogeneous strains by growth in the presence of β-lactam antibiotics suggests that the acquired PBP gene has become under the control of a penicillin-regulated promoter. Many MRSA strains also express penicillinase, although this contributes little to their level of resistance to β-lactamase-stable β-lactams. Several studies suggest a correlation between the presence of a penicillinase plasmid and the inducibility of PBP 2′ (ROSSI et al. 1985; UBUKATA et al. 1985). In some MRSA strains loss of the penicillinase plasmid results in a change in the regulation of expression of PBP 2′ from inducible to constitutive, suggesting that repression of the PBP 2′ gene is mediated in these strains by the plasmid-encoded penicillinase repressor (UBUKATA et al. 1985).

The heterogeneity of expression of methicillin resistance in most MRSA strains is related to the inducibility of PBP 2′ in these strains. The $1:10^4$–$1:10^5$ cells that survive the addition of methicillin are likely to be those cells in the population that have transiently escaped repression and are producing high levels of PBP 2′ at the time of antibiotic challenge. The majority of the cells in a population of a heterogeneous MRSA strain die following addition of methicillin since the induction of PBP 2′ is too slow to produce a sufficiently high level of PBP 2′ to produce a methicillin-resistant peptidoglycan synthesising machinery before cell lysis occurs.

In β-lactam-sensitive strains of *S. aureus* the lethal effects of β-lactams are believed to be mediated by the inactivation of one or more of the higher MW PBPs 1, 2 or 3. In MRSA strains PBP 2′ can apparently take over all of the functions of the normal PBPs since, in the presence of high concentrations of methicillin, all of the PBPs except PBP 2′ should be acylated by the antibiotic, and yet growth and division continues.

Very high levels of PBP 2′ are found in MRSA strains (BROWN and REYNOLDS 1980) and may be needed because the enzyme has low enzymatic activity, but, alternatively, a large molar excess of the resistant PBP over the normal methicillin-sensitive PBPs may be required to obtain methicillin-resistant peptidoglycan synthesis. In *E. coli* a mixture of cephalexin-resistant and cephalexin-sensitive PBP 3 has been shown to result in cephalexin resistance only if the resistant PBP is in a substantial molar excess (HEDGE and SPRATT 1985a). This phenomenon probably occurs because PBPs act in concert to synthesise the cell wall and the inhibition of cephalexin-sensitive PBP 3 molecules can block peptidoglycan synthesis by cephalexin-resistant PBP 3 molecules (BROOME-SMITH et al. 1985b). The need to prevent the inactivated normal PBPs of *S. aureus* from stalling peptidoglycan synthesis catalysed by PBP 2′ in the presence of methicillin may be solved by the ability to express very large amounts of the resistant PBP.

PBP 2′ may function less efficiently than the normal PBPs of *S. aureus*. In the absence of methicillin the repression of the PBP 2′ gene in heterogeneous strains may be advantageous as it would prevent PBP 2′ from interfering with peptidoglycan synthesised by the normal complement of PBPs.

The differences in the levels of methicillin resistance of MRSA strains under different growth conditions may also be explained by differences in the stability, or expression, of PBP 2′. Thus the loss of methicillin resistance at low pH correlates with a failure to detect PBP 2′ in cells grown under these conditions (HARTMAN and TOMASZ 1986). However, the properties of some heterogeneous MRSA strains are not readily explained simply on the basis of the presence of an inducible PBP with low affinity for β-lactams, and some other factor that modulates the expression, or activity, of PBP 2′ has been invoked (HARTMAN and TOMASZ 1986).

BERGER-BACHI (1983) has provided evidence for a second gene involved in methicillin resistance. Methicillin-sensitive isolates obtained by insertional inactivation using Tn551 resulted from transpositions at a site that was not linked to the methicillin resistance determinant (the PBP 2′ gene). Similar insertion mutations have been identified by KORNBLUM et al. (1986) and result in the conversion of a homogeneous MRSA strain to heterogeneous expression of resistance.

MRSA strains appear to have varied properties with respect both to the expression of resistance, and to the expression of the PBP 2′ gene. It seems likely from the hybridisation studies so far carried out that the PBP 2′ gene is identical, or very similar, in all MRSA strains. The differences in the properties of different MRSA strains may be due to different solutions to the problem of regulating the expression of the new gene, or its gene product, so that it can achieve methicillin-resistant peptidoglycan synthesis in the presence of the inactivated normal PBPs, and yet not interfere with the function of the latter PBPs in the absence of antibiotics. In some MRSA strains regulation of expression by linkage to the regulatory circuit of the penicillinase gene may have arisen (SONG et al. 1987), whereas in other strains regulation of activity may have been achieved by interaction with other factors.

Methicillin resistance in *S. epidermidis* is also due to the presence of a novel PBP with very low affinity for β-lactam antibiotics (UBUKATA et al. 1985). Interestingly this novel PBP seems to be very closely related to PBP 2′ as it crossreacts with monoclonal antibodies raised against the latter protein (O'HARA and REYNOLDS, personal communication).

Resistance of *S. aureus* to penicillin in the laboratory can only be obtained in small stepwise increments (DEMEREC 1945). As expected in a β-lactamase-non-producing strains of a gram-positive bacteria, the stepwise build-up of resistance is due to the accumulative effects of mutations that result in small decreases in the affinities of the physiologically important PBPs (TONIN and TOMASZ 1986). Clinical isolates of *S. aureus* that have increased levels of resistance to β-lactams mediated by reductions in the affinities of the physiologically important PBPs have not so far been reported, although they may well exist.

VI. Enterococci

A wide range of sensitivities to β-lactam antibiotics is found amongst streptococci. Typical isolates of some species, e.g. group A, B, C and G streptococci (and *S. pneumoniae*), are extremely sensitive to penicillin (MICs of <0.01 µg/ml) whereas many group D streptococci (enterococci), e.g. *S. faecium*, *S. durans* and *S. faecalis*, are rather resistant to penicillin (MICs >1 µg/ml).

FONTANA et al. (1983) and WILLIAMSON et al. (1985) have shown that the penicillin resistance, or penicillin sensitivity, of streptococcal species correlates with the presence, or absence, of a PBP (MW about 80,000) that has a very low affinity for penicillin. In the laboratory, mutants with increased levels of resistance to penicillin have been shown to arise from the synthesis of elevated levels of the low affinity PBP 5 (FONTANA et al. 1983). The natural variation in the level of penicillin resistance, and in the levels of PBP 5, amongst some species of streptococci may reflect the presence or absence of mutations that increase the production of the resistant PBP.

The presence of a PBP with very low affinity for β-lactam antibiotics, which can take over the functions of all of the other PBPs, is very reminiscent of the situation in methicillin resistant strains of *S. aureus*. In the latter case the resistant PBP 2′ is encoded by a region of DNA that has been acquired from another species and which shows some of the properties of a mobile genetic element. The region encoding PBP 5 of *S. faecium* also appears to show unusual properties as penicillin resistance and PBP 5 can be lost at high frequency using conditions that efficiently cure plasmids, e.g. with novobiocin (ELIOPOULOS et al. 1982) or ethidium bromide (WILLIAMSON et al. 1985). However the cloned PBP 2′ gene of *S. aureus* does not hybridise with DNA from two β-lactam-resistant strains of *S. faecalis* (SONG et al. 1987).

F. Concluding Remarks

Resistance to β-lactam antibiotics mediated by alterations of PBPs is now well documented in several bacterial species. In other bacteria resistance by this mechanism has been suggested (e.g. *Pseudomonas aeruginosa*; GODFREY et al. 1981) but the evidence is not yet convincing. The development of resistant PBPs has occurred in species that are not known to produce β-lactamases (or where β-lactamase producing strains have only recently appeared), or in species where β-lactamase has been effectively disarmed by the availability of a β-lactam antibiotic that is resistant to hydrolysis by the enzyme (e.g. methicillin in the case of β-lactamase producing isolates of *S. aureus*).

It is perhaps not a coincidence that the two most significant examples of resistance due to PBP alterations have occurred in gram-positive organisms (*S.*

aureus and *S. pneumoniae*) where other resistance mechanisms are not available (or are not significant as in the case of β-lactamase production in *S. aureus*).

The emergence of resistance appears to have occurred mainly in bacteria that are involved in chronic infections where patients receive long term antibiotic therapy (e.g. in bacteria causing recurrent respiratory tract infections or, in the case of the gonococcus where prophylactic use of penicillin may be used by individuals repeatedly exposed to infection by this organism).

In these situations the long term presence of fluctuating levels of penicillin, and the large numbers of bacteria present in the infected tissues, provide the ideal conditions for the emergence of resistance. In contrast, bacteria that exist in low concentrations in asymptomatic carriers, and which occasionally cause acute infections that are treated with a single high dose of penicillin, provide much less favourable conditions for the emergence of resistance.

The difference between the rate of development of resistance in closely related bacteria that cause chronic or acute infections is striking. Thus resistance is widespread in the gonococcus but almost absent in the meningococcus; widespread in non-typable *H. influenzae* that cause pulmonary infections, but rare in type b isolates that cause meningitis.

References

Barbour AG (1981) Properties of penicillin-binding proteins in *Neisseria gonorrhoeae*. Antimicrob Agents Chemother 19:316–322

Beck WD, Berger-Bachi B, Kayser FH (1986) Additional DNA in methicillin-resistant *Staphylococcus aureus* and molecular cloning of *mec*-specific DNA. J Bacteriol 165:373–378

Berger-Bachi B (1983) Insertional inactivation of staphylococcal methicillin resistance by Tn551. J Bacteriol 154:479–487

Broome-Smith JK, Edelman A, Yousif S, Spratt BG (1985a) The nucleotide sequences of the *ponA* and *ponB* genes encoding penicillin-binding proteins 1A and 1B of *Escherichia coli*. Eur J Biochem 147:437–446

Broome-Smith JK, Hedge PJ, Spratt BG (1985b) Production of thiol-penicillin-binding protein 3 of *Escherichia coli* using a two primer method of mutagenesis. EMBO J 4:231–235

Brown DFJ, Reynolds PE (1980) Intrinsic resistance to β-lactam antibiotics in *Staphylococcus aureus*. FEBS Lett 122:275–278

Cannon JG, Sparling PF (1984) The genetics of the gonococcus. Annu Rev Microbiol 38:111–133

Chambers HF, Hartman BJ, Tomasz A (1985) Increased amounts of a novel penicillin-binding protein in a strain of methicillin-resistant *Staphylococcus aureus* exposed to nafcillin. J Clin Invest 76:325–331

Demerec M (1945) Production of staphylococcus strains resistant to various levels of penicillin. Proc Nacl Acad Sci USA 31:16–24

Dideberg O, Charlier P, Wery J-P, Dehottay P, Dusart J, Erpicum T, Frere J-M, Ghuysen J-M (1987) The crystal structure of the β-lactamase of *Streptomyces albus* G at 0.3 nm resolution. Biochem J 245:911–913

Dougherty TJ (1986) Genetic analysis and penicillin-binding protein alterations in *Neisseria gonorrhoeae* with chromosomally mediated resistance. Antimicrob Agents Chemother 30:649–652

Dougherty TJ, Koller AE, Tomasz A (1980) Penicillin-binding proteins of penicillin-susceptible and intrinsically resistant *Neisseria gonorrhoeae*. Antimicrob Agents Chemother 18:730–737

Dowson CG, Hutchison A, Spratt BG (1988a) Remodelling the active centre of a penicillin-binding protein in a penicillin-resistant strain of *Streptococcus pneumoniae*. Molecular Microbiology (in press)
Dowson CG, Jephcott AE, Gough K, Spratt BG (1988b) Penicillin-binding protein 2 genes of non-β-lactamase producing, penicillin-resistant, strains of *Neisseria gonorrhoeae* Molecular Microbiology (in press)
Eliopoulos GM, Wennersten C, Moellering RC (1982) Resistance to beta-lactam antibiotics in *Streptococcus faecium*. Antimicrob Agents Chemother 22:295–301
Faruki H, Sparling PF (1986) Genetics of resistance in a non-β-lactamase-producing gonococcus with relatively high-level penicillin resistance. Antimicrob Agents Chemother 30:856–860
Faruki H, Kohmescher RN, McKinney WP, Sparling PF (1985) A community-based outbreak of infection with penicillin-resistant *Neisseria gonorrhoeae* not producing penicillinase (chromosomally mediated resistance). N Engl J Med 313:607–611
Feldman C, Kallenbach JM, Miller SD, Thorburn JR, Koornhof HJ (1985) Community-acquired pneumonia due to penicillin-resistant pneumococci. N Engl J Med 313:615–617
Fontana R, Cerini R, Longini P, Grossato A, Canepari P (1983) Identification of a streptococcal penicillin-binding protein that reacts very slowly with penicillin. J Bacteriol 155:1343–1350
Frère J-M, Joris B (1985) Penicillin-sensitive enzymes in peptidoglycan synthesis. CRC Crit Rev Microbiol 4:299–396
Godfrey AJ, Bryan LE, Rabin HR (1981) β-lactam resistant *Pseudomonas aeruginosa* with modified penicillin-binding proteins emerging during cystic fibrosis treatment. Antimicrob Agents Chemother 19:705–711
Hakenbeck R, Kohiyama M (1982) Purification of penicillin-binding protein 3 from *Streptococcus pneumoniae*. Eur J Biochem 127:231–236
Hakenbeck R, Tarpay M, Tomasz A (1980) Multiple changes of penicillin-binding proteins in penicillin-resistant clinical isolates of *Streptococcus pneumoniae*. Antimicrob Agents Chemother 17:364–371
Hakenbeck R, Ellerbrok H, Briese T, Handwerger S, Tomasz A (1986) Penicillin-binding proteins of penicillin-susceptible and resistant pneumococci: immunological relatedness of altered proteins and changes in peptides carrying the β-lactam binding site. Antimicrob Agents Chemother 30:553–558
Hakenbeck R, Tornette S, Adkinson NF (1987) Interaction of non-lytic β-lactams with penicillin-binding proteins in *Streptococcus pneumoniae*. J Gen Microbiol 133:755–760
Handwerger S, Tomasz A (1986a) Alterations in penicillin-binding proteins of clinical and laboratory isolates of pathogenic *Streptococcus pneumoniae* with low levels of penicillin resistance. J Infect Dis 153:83–89
Handwerger S, Tomasz A (1986b) Alterations in kinetic properties of penicillin-binding proteins of penicillin-resistant *Streptococcus pneumoniae*. Antimicrob Agents Chemother 30:57–63
Hansman D, Bullen MM (1967) A resistant pneumococcus. Lancet 2:264–265
Hartman BJ, Tomasz A (1984) Low-affinity penicillin-binding protein associated with beta-lactam resistance in *Staphylococcus aureus*. J Bacteriol 158:513–516
Hartman BJ, Tomasz A (1986) Expression of methicillin resistance in heterogeneous strains of *Staphylococcus aureus*. Antimicrob Agents Chemother 29:85–92
Hayes MV, Curtis NAC, Wyke A, Ward JB (1981) Decreased affinity of a penicillin-binding protein for β-lactam antibiotics in a clinical isolate of *Staphylococcus aureus* resistant to methicillin. FEMS Microbiol Lett 10:119–122
Hedge PJ, Spratt BG (1984) A gene fusion that localises the penicillin-binding domain of penicillin-binding protein 3 of *Escherichia coli*. FEBS Lett 176:179–184
Hedge PJ, Spratt BG (1985a) Amino acid substitutions that reduce the affinity of penicillin-binding protein 3 of *Escherichia coli*. Eur J Biochem 151:111–121
Hedge PJ, Spratt BG (1985b) Resistance to β-lactam antibiotics by re-modelling the active site of an *E. coli* penicillin-binding protein. Nature 318:478–480

Herzberg O, Moult J (1987) Bacterial resistance to β-lactam antibiotics: crystal structure of β-lactamase from *Staphylococcus aureus* PC1 at 2.5A resolution. Science 236:694–701
Jacobs MR, Koornhof HJ, Robins-Browne RM, Stevenson CM, Vermaak ZA, Freiman M, Killer GB, et al. (1978) Emergence of multiply resistant pneumococci. N Engl J Med 299:735–740
Keck W, Glauner B, Schwarz U, Broome-Smith JK, Spratt BG (1985) Sequences of the active-site peptides of three of the high-MW penicillin-binding proteins of *Escherichia coli* K12. Proc Natl Acad Sci USA 82:1999–2003
Kelly JA, Dideberg O, Charlier P, Wery JP, Libert M, Moews PC, Knox JR, et al. (1986) on the origin of bacterial resistance to penicillin: comparison of a β-lactamase and a penicillin target. Science 231:1429–1431
Kornblum J, Hartman BJ, Novick RP, Tomasz A (1986) Conversion of a homogeneously methicillin-resistant strain of *Staphylococcus aureus* to heterogeneous resistance by Tn551-mediated insertional inactivation. Eur J Clin Microbiol 5:714–718
Laible G, Hakenbeck R (1987) Penicillin-binding proteins in β-lactam-resistant laboratory mutants of *Streptococcus pneumoniae*. Mol Microbiol 1:355–363
Malouin F, Bryan LE (1986) Modification of penicillin-binding proteins as mechanisms of β-lactam resistance. Antimicrob Agents Chemother 30:1–5
Malouin F, Schryvers AB, Bryan LE (1987) Cloning and expression of genes reponsible for altered penicillin-binding proteins 3a and 3b in *Haemophilus influenzae*. Antimicrob Agents Chemother 31:286–291
Matthews PR, Reed KC, Stewart PR (1987) The cloning of chromosomal DNA associated with methicillin and other resistances in *Staphylococcus aureus*. J Gen Microbiol 133:1919–1929
Matsuhashi M, Song MD, Ishino F, Wachi M, Doi M, Inoue M, Ubukata K, et al. (1986) Molecular cloning of the gene of a penicillin-binding protein supposed to cause high resistance to β-lactam antibiotics in *Staphylococcus aureus*. J Bacteriol 167:975–980
Mendelman PM, Chaffin DO, Stull TL, Rubens CE, Mack KD, Smith AL (1984) Characterization of non-beta-lactamase-mediated ampicillin resistance in *Haemophilus influenzae*. Antimicrob Agents Chemother 26:235–244
Mendelman PM, Campos J, Chaffin DO, Serfass DA, Smith AL, Saez-Nieto JA (1988) Relative penicillin G resistance in *Neisseria meningitidis* and reduced affinity of penicillin-binding protein. Antimicrob Agents Chemother 32:706–709
Nakagawa J, Tamaki S, Tomioka S, Matsuhashi M (1984) Functional biosynthesis of cell wall peptidoglycan by polymorphic bifunctional polypeptides. J Biol Chem 259:13937–13946
Olsson O, Bergstrom S, Lindberg FP, Normark S (1983) *ampC* β-lactamase hyperproduction in *Escherichia coli*: natural ampicillin resistance generated by horizontal chromosomal DNA transfer from *Shigella*. Proc Natl Acad Sci USA 80:7556–7560
Parr TR, Bryan LE (1984) Mechanism of resistance of an ampicillin-resistant, beta-lactamase-negative clinical isolate of *Haemophilus influenzae* type b to beta-lactam antibiotics. Antimicrob Agents Chemother 25:747–753
Percheson PB, Bryan LE (1980) Penicillin-binding components of penicillin-susceptible and -resistant strains of *Streptococcus pneumoniae*. Antimicrob Agents Chemother 12:390–396
Philpot-Howard J (1984) Antibiotic resistance and *Haemophilus influenzae*. J Antimicrob Chemother 13:199–208
Reynolds PE (1985) Inhibitors of bacterial cell wall synthesis. Symp Soc Gen Microbiol 38:13–40
Reynolds PE, Fuller C (1986) Methicillin-resistant strains of *Staphylococcus aureus*: presence of identical additional penicillin-binding protein in all strains examined. FEMS Microbiol Lett 33:251–254
Rossi L, Tonin E, Cheng YR, Fontana R (1985) Regulation of penicillin-binding protein activity: description of a methicillin-inducible penicillin-binding protein in *Staphylococcus aureus*. Antimicrob Agents Chemother 27:828–831

Saez-Nieto JA, Fontanals D, de Jalon G, de Artola VM, Pena P, Morera MA, Verdaguer R, et al. (1987) Isolation of *Neisseria meningitidis* strains with increase of penicillin minimal inhibitory concentrations. Epidemiol Infect 99:463–469

Samraoui B, Sutton BJ, Todd RJ, Artymiuk PJ, Waley SG, Phillips DC (1986) Tertiary structure similarity between a class A β-lactamase and a penicillin-sensitive D-alanyl carboxypeptidase-transpeptidase. Nature 320:378–380

Serfass DA, Mendelman PM, Chaffin DO, Needham CA (1986) Ampicillin resistance and penicillin-binding proteins of *Haemophilus influenzae*. J Gen Microbiol 132:2855–2861

Shockley TE, Hotchkiss RD (1970) Stepwise introduction of transformable penicillin resistance in pneumococcus. Genetics 64:397–408

Song MD, Maesaki S, Wachi M, Takahashi T, Doi M, Ishino F, Maeda Y, et al. (1987) Primary structure and origin of the gene of the β-lactam-inducible penicillin-binding protein that is responsible for methicillin resistance in strains of *Staphylococcus aureus*. FEMS Microbiol Lett 221:167–171

Spratt BG (1975) Distinct penicillin binding proteins involved in the division, elongation, and shape of *Escherichia coli*. Proc Natl Acad Sci USA 72:2999–3003

Spratt BG (1977) Properties of the penicillin-binding proteins of *Escherichia coli*. Eur J Biochem 72:341–352

Spratt BG (1978) *Escherichia coli* resistance to β-lactam antibiotics through a decrease in the affinity of a target for lethality. Nature 274:713–715

Spratt BG (1983) Penicillin-binding proteins and the future of β-lactam antibiotics. J Gen Microbiol 129:1247–1260

Spratt BG (1988) Hybrid penicillin-binding proteins in penicillin-resistant isolates of *Neisseria gonorrhoeae*. Nature 332:173–176

Spratt BG, Cromie KD (1988) Penicillin-binding proteins of gram-negative bacteria. Rev Infect Dis 10:699–711

Spratt BG, Pardee AB (1975) Penicillin-binding proteins and cell shape in *E. coli*. Nature 254:516–517

Stewart GC, Rosenblum ED (1980) Genetic behaviour of the methicillin resistance determinant in *Staphylococcus aureus*. J Bacteriol 144:1200–1202

Tonin E, Tomasz A (1986) β-lactam-specific resistant mutants of *Staphylococcus aureus*. Antimicrob Agents Chemother 30:577–583

Ubukata K, Yamashita N, Konno M (1985) Occurrence of a β-lactam-inducible penicillin-binding protein in methicillin-resistant staphylococci. Antimicrob Agents Chemother 27:851–857

Utsui Y, Yokota T (1985) Role of an altered penicillin-binding protein in methicillin- and cephem-resistant *Staphylococcus aureus*. Antimicrob Agents Chemother 28:397–403

Waxman DJ, Strominger JL (1983) Penicillin-binding proteins and the mechanism of action of β-lactam antibiotics. Annu Rev Biochem 52:825–869

Williamson R, Tomasz A (1985) Inhibition of cell wall synthesis and acylation of the penicillin-binding proteins during prolonged exposure of growing *Staphylococcus pneumoniae* to benzylpenicillin. Eur J Biochem 151:475–483

Williamson R, Hakenbeck R, Tomasz A (1980) In vivo interaction of β-lactam antibiotics with the penicillin-binding proteins of *Streptococcus pneumoniae*. Antimicrob Agents Chemother 18:629–637

Williamson R, Le Bouguenec C, Gutman L, Horaud T (1985) One or two low affinity penicillin-binding proteins may be responsible for the range of susceptibility of *Enterococcus faecium* to benzylpenicillin. J Gen Microbiol 131:1933–1940

Yousif SY, Broome-Smith JK, Spratt BG (1985) Lysis of *Escherichia coli* by β-lactam antibiotics: deletion analysis of the role of penicillin-binding proteins 1A and 1B. J Gen Microbiol 131:2839–2845

Zighelboim S, Tomasz A (1980) Penicillin-binding proteins of multiply antibiotic-resistant South African strains of *Streptococcus pneumoniae*. Antimicrob Agents Chemother 17:434–442

CHAPTER 5

Plasmid-Determined Beta-Lactamases

A. A. MEDEIROS

A. Introduction

The resistance of bacterial isolates to beta-lactam antibiotics is due principally to the production of beta-lactamases. Some beta-lactamases are determined by genes on the bacterial chromosome and others by genes on plasmids that can transfer from one species to another (DATTA and KONTOMICHALOU 1965). Moreover, twelve plasmid-determined beta-lactamases are known so far to be encoded by transposons (Table 1), genetic elements that can transfer from one plasmid to another and to and from plasmids and the bacterial chromosome (HEDGES and JACOB 1974).

The plasmid-determined beta-lactamases account for most of the beta-lactam resistance encountered in the most frequently isolated bacterial pathogens. They are an enormously diverse group of proteins that have manifested an ability to evolve rapidly into new structures capable of resisting newer beta-lactam anti-

Table 1. Beta-lactamase transposons

Transposon	Beta-lactamase	Phenotype	Size (kb)	Reference
Tn*3*	TEM-1	Ap	5	KOPECKO et al. (1976)
Tn*4*	TEM-1	ApSmSpSu	24	KOPECKO et al. (1976)
Tn*AB*	TEM-1	ApSm	14.3	HEDGES et al. (1977)
Tn*1699*	TEM-1	ApGmKm	9.3	RUBENS et al. (1979)
Tn*1700*	TEM-1	ApGmKmTm	9.3	RUBENS et al. (1979)
Tn*1*	TEM-2	Ap	5	HEDGES and JACOB (1974)
– [a]	SHV-1	Ap	14.3	NUGENT and HEDGES (1979)
Tn*1412*	LCR-1	ApGmKmSmSpSuTm	19	LEVESQUE and JACOBY (1988)
Tn*2603*	OXA-1	ApSmSpSuHg	20	YAMAMOTO et al. (1981)
Tn*2410*	OXA-2	ApSuHg	18.5	KRATZ et al. (1983)
Tn*1411*	OXA-3	ApCmGmKmSmSuTm	15	LEVESQUE and JACOBY (1988)
Tn*1409*	OXA-4	ApCmSmSpSuTp	14.6	LEVESQUE and JACOBY (1988)
Tn*1406*	OXA-5	ApGmKmSuTmHg	17.2	LEVESQUE and JACOBY (1988)
Tn*1401*	PSE-1	ApSmSpSuHg	12	MEDEIROS et al. (1982)
Tn*1403*	PSE-1	ApCmSmSp	18	MEDEIROS et al. (1982)
Tn*1404*	PSE-2	ApGmKmSmSpSuTm	9.6	PHILIPPON et al. (1983)
Tn*2521*	PSE-4	ApSmSpSu	6.8	SINCLAIR and HOLLOWAY (1982)
Tn*1405*	PSE-4	ApSmSpSu	8	LEVESQUE and JACOBY (1988)
Tn*1408*	CARB-3	ApCmSmSpSu	25.2	LEVESQUE and JACOBY (1988)

[a] Tn number not assigned.

biotics as they come into clinical use. Previous reviews have dealth with the molecular characteristics (COULSON 1985) and distribution of beta-lactamases and their R factors (MEDEIROS 1984; MEDEIROS and JACOBY 1986). This review will focus on newly discovered plasmid-determined beta-lactamases and on new information relating to the evolution and spread of these enzymes.

B. General Properties of Beta-Lactamases

Our understanding of beta-lactamases has been greatly elucidated by studies of the amino acid sequence of these proteins (AMBLER 1980; BERGSTROM et al. 1982; JAURIN and GRUNDSTROM 1981). Three classes have been defined. Class A beta-lactamases have a serine residue at the active site. They are proteins of molecular weight (MW) about 28000, exemplified by the "penicillinases" of *Staphylococcus aureus* PC1, *Bacillus licheniformis* 749/C, and the TEM-1 beta-lactamase. Class B beta-lactamases are metalloenzymes of MW ca. 23000, such as the cephalosporinase of *B. cereus*, rare among clinical isolates. Class C enzymes are the chromosomally determined cephalosporinases of *E. coli*. They share extensive sequence homology with *Shigella* and less with *Klebsiella*, *Salmonella*, *Serratia* and *Pseudomonas*.

The class A enzymes show genetic homology with L-alanine carboxypeptidase, a target site of penicillin action in *Bacillus* sp. This observation led to a hypothesis that the target sites of penicillin action, the penicillin-binding proteins (PBPs), share a common evolutionary origin with beta-lactamases (WAXMAN et al. 1979, 1982; YOCUM et al. 1979). This hypothesis has been supported by recent studies demonstrating that the tertiary structure, the three dimensional configuration, of the beta-lactamase of *B. licheniformis* is strikingly similar to the penicillin-binding protein of *Streptomyces* R6 despite limited sequence homology (KELLY et al. 1986; SAMRAOUI et al. 1986).

Beta-lactamases and PBPs also have similar functional characteristics. It is well known that many beta-lactamases are induced by exposure to beta-lactam antibiotics. Recent studies have shown that PBPs, notably the low affinity PBP found in methicillin-resistant *S. aureus*, are also inducible (CHAMBERS et al. 1985; UBUKATA et al. 1985). Indeed, the regulation of PBPs that determine methicillin resistance in *S. aureus* may be linked to regulation of staphylococcal beta-lactamase (BOYCE and MEDEIROS 1987). Similarly, the regulatory gene *bla*R1, required for induction of beta-lactamase in *B. licheniformis*, encodes a potential PBP (KOBAYASHI et al. 1987). Some penicillin-binding proteins act as weak beta-lactamases in that they are able to hydrolyze beta-lactam antibiotics at a slow rate (AMARAL et al. 1986). However, the converse is not true in that no direct function in cell wall metabolism has yet been identified for any beta-lactamase. Another shared characteristic is that mutations that result in modified affinity for cephalosporins occur in genes that determine both PBPs and beta-lactamases (HEDGE and SPRATT 1985; KLIEBE et al. 1985). As with beta-lactamases the genes that determine PBPs may be plasmid borne and may confer resistance to cephalosporins when transferred into a host strain where they replicate in high copy number (HEDGE and SPRATT 1985). Lastly, as suggested by ABRAHAM and CHAIN (1940), the ubiquity of beta-lactamases, in penicillin susceptible as well as penicillin resistant bacteria, further supports the hypothesis that these two proteins share a common origin and may share complementary functions as yet undiscovered.

C. Classification of Beta-Lactamases

Bacteria produce a great variety of beta-lactamases. This diversity has led to several classification schemes. The relative rates at which different beta-lactam antibiotics were hydrolyzed, i.e. the substrate profile, provided the basis for the earliest of the classification schemes (SAWAI et al. 1968; JACK and RICHMOND 1970). Inhibition of beta-lactamase by various compounds and reaction to antisera provided additional distinction.

A major advance in the classification of beta-lactamases occurred when MATTHEW et al. (1975) showed that specific beta-lactamases could be identified by flat-bed isoelectric focusing in polyacrylamide gel. Bands corresponding to specific beta-lactamases were identified by developing the gel with an overlay of nitrocefin, a chromogenic cephalosporin that changes color with hydrolysis. Specific beta-lactamases often showed patterns consisting of a main and several accessory bands which were reproducible and characteristic of that enzyme. An unknown beta-lactamase could be readily identified in a crude well extract by comparing its isoelectric point and banding pattern with reference enzymes run on the same gel. A matrix of highly purified agarose has also been used for isoelectric focusing of beta-lactamases, permitting shorter focusing time (VECOLI et al. 1983). Beta-lactamases may be further characterized in situ on polyacrylamide gels by overlaying the gel with an inhibitor prior to applying the nitrocefin overlay (SANDERS et al. 1986). Using concentrated cell extracts MATTHEW detected discrete beta-lactamase bands in virtually all gram-negative bacteria studied.

Matthew (MATTHEW 1979; MATTHEW et al. 1979) described 11 types of plasmid-determined beta-lactamases in gram-negative bacilli, all of which are produced constitutively, and grouped them into three broad classes: (a) those that hydrolyze benzylpenicillin and cephaloridine at similar rates (broad spectrum enzymes); (b) those that hydrolyze oxacillin and related penicillins rapidly (oxacillinases); and (c) those that break down carbenicillin readily (carbenicillinases). All of these enzymes possess a unique isoelectric point and most have a characteristic banding pattern on flat-bed isoelectric focusing. The patterns consist usually of a single major band and several satellite bands that develop late after overlay of nitrocefin onto the polyacrylamide gel. The number of plasmid-determined beta-lactamases now known is over 30 (Table 2). Figure 1 shows the band patterns of 29 plasmid-determined beta-lactamases in polyacrylamide gel approximately 20 min after the overlay of nitrocefin. The satellite bands of several are evident and in some instances bands representing weaker chromosomally determined beta-lactamases of the host strain are also seen.

Table 2. Properties of plasmid-determined beta-lactamases

Beta-lactamase	pI[a]	Relative rate of hydrolyses (penicillin G=100)								Inhibition by				Mol. wt. (×10³)	Reference
		Ampicillin	Carbenicillin	Oxacillin	Methicillin	Cloxacillin	Cephaloridine	Cephalothin	Cefamandole	Cloxacillin	pCMB[b]	NaCl	Clavulanic acid		
Broad spectrum															
HMS-1	5.2	253	14	<2	<2	<2	183	3		+	+	–		21.0	MATTHEW et al. (1979)
TEM-1	5.4	72	12	4	1	<0.2	60	13	20	+	–	–	+	22.0	MATTHEW et al. (1979) MEDEIROS et al. (1985)
TLE-1	5.55	67	13	4	5	6	52	15	24	+		–	+	19.8	MEDEIROS et al. (1985)
TEM-2	5.6	107	10	5	0	0	74	20		+	–	–	+	23.5	MATTHEW et al. (1969)
LCR-1	5.85 (6.5)	145	4		20	3	55	24		+	–		+	44.0	SIMPSON et al. (1983)
NPS-1	6.5	223	18	40	<0,1		3			–	–			25.0	LIVERMORE and JONES (1986a)
LXA-1	6.7														YANG et al. (1985)
OHIO-1	7.0	140	11	<0.5	<0.5	<0.5	79	8	15	+		–	+	22.0	SHLAES et al. (1986)
SHV-1	7.6	212	8	0	<2	<2	56	8		+	+/–	–		21.0	MATTHEW et al. (1979)
SHV-2	7.6	145		0			32	8		+	+/–		+		KLIEBE et al. (1985)
ROB-1	8.1	107	19			<0.2	37	4.5		+		–	+		MEDEIROS et al. (1986)
OXA-type															
Unnamed (GN11499)	6.9	357	43			271	71	57			+/–		+	41.5	SATO et al. (1983)
OXA-3	7.1	178	10	336	29	350	44	10		–	–	+		41.2	MATTHEW (1979)
OXA-1	7.4	419	65	271	342	119	112	43		–	+/–	+	–	23.3	MATTHEW (1979) PHILIPPON et al. (1986a)

OXA-4	7.45	325	57	188	357	121	110	20		–		+	–	23.0	MEDEIROS et al. (1985)
OXA-5	7.62	188	40	210	109	258	89	175	35	–		+	–	27.0	MEDEIROS et al. (1985)
OXA-7	7.65	545	48	702	424	494	136	51	47	–		+	–	25.3	MEDEIROS et al. (1985)
OXA-6	7.68	596	46	1048	585	301	149	24	82	+		–	–	40.0	MEDEIROS et al. (1985)
OXA-2	7.7	236	27	581	31	157	108	61	32	–	–	+	–	43.9	MEDEIROS et al. (1985)
CARB type															
CARB-4	4.3	130	79	1	2	<1	15	2		–	+	–	+	22.0	PHILIPPON et al. (1986b)
SAR-1	4.9	63	122		0	0	21		53	+	–		+	33.7	REID and AMYES (1986)
PSE-4 (CARB-1)	5.3	88	150	8	16	<2	40	4		–	–			32.0	MATTHEW (1979)
BRO-1	5.6	103	78		131	5	23	24	31						ELIASSON and KAMME (1985)
PSE-1 (Carb-2)	5.7	84	100	9	1.1	0	27	0	10	–	+			28.5	MATTHEW and SYKES (1977)
CARB-3	5.75	100	147	12.5	0.6	0.5	44	0.5						31.0	LABIA et al. (1981)
AER-1	5.9	38	98	0.9	0.3	0	26	77	18					22.0	HEDGES et al. (1985)
Unnamed (N-3)	6.0 (5.73)	113	113			<2	12	<2						24.0	TAKAHASHI et al. (1983)
PSE-2	6.1	173	87	273	286	902	50	11		–	+	+		12.4	PHILIPPON et al. (1983)
PSE-3	6.9	101	253			3	10				–			12.0	MATTHEW (1979)
Unnamed (N-29)	6.9 (6.83)	124	128			<2	6	<2						22.0	TAKAHASHI et al. (1983)
ampC type															
CEP-1	8.0													37.5	BOBROWSKI et al. (1976)
CEP-2	8.1		48				108	114	73					36.2	LEVESQUE et al. (1982); LEVESQUE and ROY (1982)

[a] Isoelectric point; values in parentheses are those obtained in our laboratory.
[b] *p*-Chloromercurobenzoate.

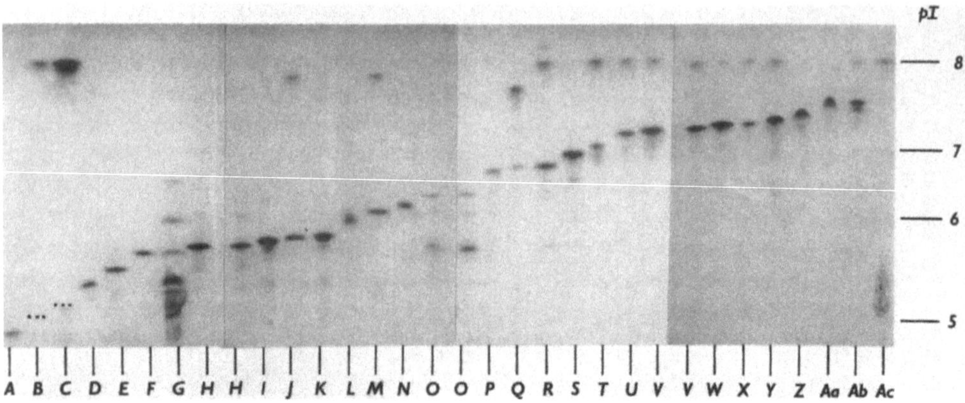

Fig. 1. Composite of isoelectric focusing gels showing the band patterns of 29 beta-lactamases determined by plasmids or transposons: (*A*) CARB-4, (*B*) SAR-1 (a band did not visualize on this gel, the reported pI is indicated by the *dotted line*), (*C*) HMS-1 (the position of the faint band of HMS-1 is indicated by the *dotted line*), (*D*) PSE-4, (*E*) TEM-1, (*F*) TLE-1, (*G*) BRO-1, (*H*) TEM-2, (*I*) PSE-1, (*J*) beta-lactamase specified by *P. mirabilis* N-3, (*K*) CARB-3, (*L*) LCR-1, (*M*) AER-1, (*N*) PSE-2, (*O*) NPS-1, (*P*) LXA-1, (*Q*) PSE-3, (*R*) beta-lactamase specified by *P. mirabilis* N-29, (*S*) OHIO-1, (*T*) OXA-3, (*U*) OXA-1, (*V*) OXA-4, (*W*) SHV-1, (*X*) SHV-2, (*Y*) OXA-5, (*Z*) OXA-7, (*Aa*) OXA-6, (*Ab*) OXA-2, (*Ac*) ROB-1. The producing strain was *E. coli* for all beta-lactamases, except CARB-4, PSE-4, CARB-3, LCR-1, PSE-2, NPS-1, PSE-3, OXA-6, which were produced by *P. aeruginosa*, and BRO-1 and ROB-1, which were produced by *B. catarrhalis* and *H. influenzae* respectively. An additional band representing the chromosomally encoded beta-lactamase of *E. coli* is seen in *lanes B, C, I, J, M, R, T, U, V, W, X, Y, Ab,* and that of *P. aeruginosa* in *lane Q*. A satellite band (pI c.6.2) as dense as the main band (pI 5.6), a pattern typical of BRO-1, is seen in *lane G* and an accumulation of activity at the anodic loading site, typical of ROB-1, is seen in *lane Ac*

D. Properties of Plasmid-Determined Beta-Lactamases

I. Broad-Spectrum Beta-Lactamases

The properties of the plasmid-determined beta-lactamases are summarized in Table 2. The broad-spectrum penicillinases (TEM-1, TEM-2, SHV-1 and HMS-1) all have nearly equal activity against benzylpenicillin and cephaloridine. The oxacillinases, on the other hand, hydrolyze oxacillin rapidly as exemplified by OXA-1, OXA-2 and OXA-3. The PSE enzymes have high activity against carbenicillin. Two of them, PSE-2 and BRO-1, resemble the oxacillinases in having a high relative activity against oxacillin as well. Three of these beta-lactamases (OXA-1, PSE-1 and PSE-2) hydrolyze cefotaxime at a significant rate (SIMPSON et al. 1982).

Cloxacillin inhibits the broad spectrum enzymes but does not inhibit the other classes. Sodium chloride inhibits the oxacillinases but does not inhibit the broad-spectrum beta-lactamases. Inhibition by *p*. chloromercuribenzoate is more variable (Table 2). The OXA-2 and OXA-3 beta-lactamases are known to be dimers with molecular weights of 44 600 and 41 200, respectively (DALE and SMITH 1976), whereas the molecular weight of the other beta-lactamases ranges between 12 000 and 32 000.

A survey of several hundred clinical isolates of ampicillin resistant *E. coli* revealed a novel TEM-like enzyme (MEDEIROS et al. 1980). *E. coli* 7604 was one of 70 Brazilian strains studied. It produced 2 beta-lactamases: TEM-1, and another enzyme, named TLE-1, with a substrate profile and molecular weight similar to TEM-1 but with a different isoelectric point. The strain contained two plasmids, each of which determined a different beta-lactamase (MEDEIROS et al. 1985).

Another novel TEM-like beta-lactamase was found in *Haemophilus influenzae* ROB, a type b strain isolated from a child with meningitis (RUBIN et al. 1981). This strain produced a beta-lactamase which resembled TEM-1 but hydrolyzed carbenicillin at a slightly higher rate and cephaloridine at a lower rate relative to benzylpenicillin. Extracts of the *Haemophilus* isolate demonstrated an enzyme band at pI 8.1 and an unusual accumulation of activity remaining at the anodic loading site on the gel. This observation suggested that the enzyme was membrane-bound, or possibly a lipoprotein. An additional strain of *H. influenzae* producing ROB-1 beta-lactamase was detected in a survey of 50 ampicillin-resistant clinical isolates from the United States (MEDEIROS et al. 1986).

SIMPSON et al. (1983) identified a third TEM-like beta-lactamase in a carbenicillin-resistant *Pseudomonas aeruginosa* burn isolate. Isoelectric focusing showed a single band nearly equidistant between those of PSE-1 and PSE-2, clearly distinguishing the LCR-1 beta-lactamase from TEM-1. The LCR-1 enzyme was similar in substrate profile to TEM-1 but had a slightly higher activity against methicillin.

A fourth broad spectrum beta-lactamase was first identified in an environmental isolate of *Enterobacter cloacae* from a hospital in Cleveland, Ohio (SHLAES 1986). A subsequent survey revealed OHIO-1 in clinical isolates from hospitals in Columbus and Cleveland, Ohio. Thirty-one clinical isolates of ten species of Enterobacteriaceae that produce OHIO-1 have since been found, all from Ohio (KRON et al. 1987). The OHIO-1 beta-lactamase has an isoelectric point of 7.0 and a substrate profile similar to that of TEM-1 but differs in susceptibility to inhibitors.

LIVERMORE and JONES (1986) discovered a novel broad spectrum plasmid-determined beta-lactamase, designated NPS-1, in two isolates of *P. aeruginosa* highly resistant to carbenicillin. The beta-lactamase had a pI of 6.5, distinct from previously described plasmid-mediated beta-lactamases, and had activity against both penicillins and cephalosporins. V_{max} rates for oxacillin and carbenicillin were less than 50% of the V_{max} for benzyl penicillin. The rate of hydrolysis of oxacillin relative to penicillin, however, was higher for NPS-1 than for other broad spectrum plasmid-mediated beta-lactamases. Cefsulodin caused a reversible reduction in the activity of NPS-1, suggesting that cefsulodin may alter the catalytic activity of the beta-lactamase by inducing a change in its conformation. The enzyme was encoded by a plasmid of molecular weight 41×10^6 that transferred readily to other *P. aeruginosa* strains but not to *E. coli* K12.

A beta-lactamase, designated LXA-1, that has an isoelectric point of 6.7 was found in isolates of *Klebsiella oxytoca*, *K. pneumoniae*, *E. cloacae*, and *Citrobacter freundii* (YANG et al. 1985). The beta-lactamase had predominantly penicillinase activity with an unusually low affinity for benzyl penicillin ($Km = 400$ μm) for a plasmid-mediated beta-lactamase. The production of LXA-1 along with TEM-1 and other resistances was determined by an 84 megadalton plasmid that was transferable by conjugation to *E. coli*. Production of the LXA-1 beta-lactamase alone resulted in very low levels of beta-lactam resistance in host strains.

II. Oxacillin-Hydrolyzing Beta-Lactamases

Four novel OXA-like beta-lactamases have been found; two among the *E. coli* isolates from Brazil, and two in *P. aeruginosa* (MEDEIROS et al. 1985; PHILIPPON et al. 1986a). An additional oxacillinase has been found in a strain of *B. fragilis* isolated in Japan and shown to be transferable by mating (SATO et al. 1983). All five of these OXA-like beta-lactamases have distinct isoelectric points ranging from 6.9 to 7.68. The OXA-6 enzyme and the beta-lactamase from *B. fragilis* have molecular weights of 40000 and 41500 respectively, whereas the molecular weights of the other OXA-like enzymes range between 23000 and 25000.

III. Carbenicillin-Hydrolyzing Beta-Lactamases

Four novel beta-lactamases have been detected that hydrolyze carbenicillin preferentially and that are determined by plasmids, transposons, or transposon-like elements. LABIA et al. (1981) studied a strain of *P. aeruginosa* that produced an enzyme termed CARB-3 with substrate profile similar to PSE-1 and PSE-4 but with a higher molecular weight and an isoelectric point of 5.75.

TAKAHASHI et al. (1983) have described two novel carbenicillin hydrolyzing beta-lactamases in *Proteus mirabilis* strains N-3 and N-29 that are plasmid-mediated. These enzymes, which have not yet been named, have substrate profiles and molecular weights similar to PSE-1 and PSE-4 but have distinct isoelectric points at 6.0 and 6.9. However, when focused in adjacent lanes in our laboratory the enzymes of *P. mirabilis* N-3, CARB-3, and PSE-1 have very similar pI values, ranging no more than half a pH unit overall (Table 2), indicating only minor differences between the charge properties of these enzymes. Similarly, the enzyme of strain N-29 has a pI value slightly higher than that of PSE-3 (A. A. MEDEIROS 1987).

Another carbenicillin-hydrolyzing beta-lactamase designated AER-1 has been found in *Aeromonas hydrophila*. The parent strain produced several beta-lactamase bands on isoelectric focusing but only a single enzyme with isoelectric point of 5.9 was transferred to *E. coli* by mating when a conjugative plasmid was introduced into the *Aeromonas* host (HEDGES et al. 1985).

A beta-lactamase with an unusually low isoelectric point of 4.3 was found in a strain of *P. aeruginosa* from France. The enzyme, designated CARB-4, hydrolyzed carbenicillin with a substrate profile similar to other carbenicillin hydrolyzing beta-lactamases found in *P. aeruginosa*. The enzyme conferred resistance to cefsulodin despite the lack of demonstrable hydrolytic activity (PHILIPPON et al. 1986b).

Another beta-lactamase with an unusally low pI value (circa 4.3) was isolated from two strains of *Vibrio cholerae* biotype El tor isolated in Tanzania. The beta-lactamase, named SAR-1, was a 33700 dalton protein (REID and AMYES 1986).

On flat-bed isoelectric focusing the enzyme had a similar pI to CARB-4 but had satellite bands discrete from those of CARB-4. Although the substrate profile of the SAR-1 beta lactamase was similar to PSE-1 and CARB-4, its inhibition profile was more like that of TEM-1.

A beta-lactamase transferable within the genus *Branhamella* and also from *Moraxella nonliquefaciens* to *B. catarrhalis* has been described by ELIASSON and KAMME (1985). The enzyme hydrolyzes carbenicillin and ampicillin at similar rates. Although the enzyme is classified among the CARB-type beta-lactamases, it hydrolyzes methicillin at a relatively rapid rate, similar to the PSE-2 beta-lactamase. BRO-1 appears to be more readily inhibited by cloxacillin and clavulanic acid than is TEM-1. Beta-lactamase positive transconjugant strains of *B. catarrhalis* acquire inoculum dependent resistance in both ampicillin and cefaclor. Although other beta-lactamases are produced by *B. catarrhalis*, BRO-1 appears to be the most common beta-lactamase found in strains from various regions.

IV. Amp C Type Beta-Lactamases

There have been two reports of plasmid-determined beta-lactamases with predominantly cephalosporinase activity. BOBROWSKI et al. (1976) described a plasmid originating in *P. mirabilis* that appeared to produce a beta-lactamase identical in enzymological and immunological properties to the chromosomal enzyme of *E. coli* K-12. LEVESQUE et al. (1982) and LEVESQUE and ROY (1982) have described a cephalosporinase determined by a plasmid from *Achromobacter*. This enzyme, which has been termed CEP-2 to indicate a relationship to the *Proteus* cephalosporinase or CEP-1, differed from CEP-1 in ability to hydrolyze carbenicillin and resistance to cloxacillin inhibition.

V. Staphylococcal Beta-Lactamases

Among the gram-positive bacteria staphylococci are the major pathogens which produce beta-lactamase. Four types (A–D) of closely related staphylococcal beta-lactamases have been distinguished by serological and enzymological criteria (RICHMOND 1965; ROSDAHL 1973). These enzymes have a molecular weight of 28 000 and preferentially hydrolyze penicillins. With the exception of type D, all types are inducible and are excreted extracellularly (DYKE 1979). Staphylococcal beta-lactamases share extensive sequence homology with beta-lactamases found in *Bacillus* species (DYKE 1979; AMBLER 1980). The beta-lactamases of both *B. cereus* and *S. aureus* have been found to be thioether lipoproteins (NIELSEN and LAMPEN 1982). The genes determining staphylococcal beta-lactamases are usually carried on small plasmids which can be transferred from cell to cell via transduction with bacteriophage. Larger plasmids carrying a beta-lactamase gene and resistance to other antibiotics have been described recently (MCDONNELL et al. 1983; GOERING and RUFF 1983). These genes can transfer by conjugation not only between strains of *S. aureus* but also between *S. aureus* and *S. epidermidis* (MCDONNELL et al. 1983; GOERING and Ruff 1983).

VI. Streptococcal Beta-Lactamases

In an extensive survey of the beta-lactamases produced by various clinical pathogens, MATTHEW and HARRIS (1976) found two strains of streptococci, one of *S. uberis*, and one of *S. faecalis*, which produced beta-lactamase. MURRAY and MEDERSKI-SAMORAJ described two ampicillin-resistant strains of *S. faecalis* that produce a plasmid-determined beta-lactamase encoded on different plasmids (MURRAY and MEDERSKI-SAMORAJ 1983; MURRAY et al. 1986b). Cloned staphylococcal penicillinase genes hybridized under stringent conditions with plasmid DNA from the *S. faecalis* strain, suggesting that the beta-lactamase is of staphylococcal origin (MURRAY et al. 1986a).

E. Relatedness of Plasmid-Determined Beta-Lactamases

I. Immunological Cross-Reactivity

Immunological cross-reaction using polyclonal antisera is observed within but not between these classes of beta-lactamase (Table 2). Antisera to TEM-1 cross-reacts with TEM-2 and TLE-1 and also partially inactivates SHV-1 but does not inactivate HMS-1, the OXA or PSE type bea-lactamases (SYKES and MATTHEW 1979; PAUL et al. 1981, 1985).

Antiserum to PSE-2 does not react with any of the other plasmid-determined beta-lactamases. However, antiserum prepared against CARB-3 cross-reacts with PSE-1 and PSE-4. Similarly, antiserum against the beta-lactamase of *P. mirabilis* N-29 cross-reacts with PSE-1, PSE-4, and with the enzyme from *P. mirabilis* N-3 but not with PSE-2, PSE-3, or TEM-2 (TAKAHASHI et al. 1983). These data indicate that there is a close immunological relationship between the beta-lactamases from *P. mirabilis* strains N-3, N-29, and the PSE-1, PSE-4, and CARB-3 beta-lactamases.

Antisera to OXA-1 reacts with OXA-4 but not with the other oxacillin-hydrolyzing enzymes (PAUL et al. 1985). Conversely, anti-OXA-4 serum reacts with OXA-1 (PHILIPPON et al. 1986a). HOLLAND and DALE (1985) found that antibodies to OXA-2 beta-lactamase inhibited OXA-3 but PAUL et al. (1985) found that anti-OXA-2 serum did not cross react with OXA-3 nor with any of 14 other plasmid-determined beta-lactamases tested. These data suggest that there is considerable homology between the OXA-1 and OXA-4 beta-lactamases. The relationship between the OXA-2 and OXA-3 beta-lactamases is less clear. Lack of immunological cross reactivity should not be taken as evidence of an absence of homology, however, since the beta-lactamases of *B. licheniformis* and *S. aureus* do not cross react (POLLOCK 1964) yet share regions of homology in their primary amino acid structures (AMBLER 1980).

MORIN et al. (1987) studied the cross reactivity of 16 monoclonal antibodies to the TEM-1 beta-lactamase against 20 other plasmid-determined beta-lactamases. The 16 monoclonal antibodies reacted with TEM-2 and TLE-1 and, to a lesser extent, SHV-1. Different levels of cross reactivity were also observed with OXA-3, OXA-7, OXA-1, OXA-6, and AER-1. The study suggests that biochemically distinct plasmid-mediated beta-lactamases share common epitopes. The extensive cross reactivity of these monoclonal antibodies limits the use of anti-TEM-1 monoclonal antibodies as a tool for the identification of a given plasmid-mediated beta-lactamase.

II. DNA Hybridization

The use of probes for DNA hybridization has further clarified the relationships between the diverse plasmid-determined beta-lactamases (Table 3). COOKSY et al. (1985) utilizing a 1000 base-pair TEM-1 probe showed cross-hybridization with the TEM-2 and OXA-2 beta-lactamases. Smaller probes of intragenic fragments of the TEM-1 gene have shown cross reactivity only with TEM-2 or TLE-1 beta-lactamases. OUELETTE et al. (1987b) constructed oligonucleotide probes of TEM-1 and TEM-2 that hybridized only with their respective beta-lactamase, making it possible to discriminate between genes (TEM-1 and TEM-2) that encode proteins that differ by a single amino acid substitution (AMBLER and SCOTT 1978; BARTHELEMY et al. 1985).

An intragenic probe for the OXA-1 beta-lactamase reacted only with OXA-4 (LEVESQUE et al. 1987). OUELLETTE and ROY (1986), on the other hand, found

Table 3. Cross hybridization between DNA probes and other beta-lactamase genes

Beta-lactamase probe	Size (bases)	Cross-hybridization	Reference
TEM-1	1000	TEM-2, OXA-2	COOKSEY et al. (1985)
	424	TEM-2, TLE-1	LEVESQUE et al. (1987)
	420	TEM-2, TLE-1	HUOVINEN et al. (1988b)
	700	(Not OHIO-1)	SHLAES et al. (1986)
	15	TEM-2	BOISSINOT et al. (1987)
	656	TEM-2	QUELLETE et al. (1987b)
	Oligo	(Not TEM-2)	QUELLETE et al. (1987b)
TEM-2	Oligo	(Not TEM-1)	QUELLETE et al. (1987b)
OHIO-1	2000	None	SHLAES et al. (1986)
SHV-1	780	SHV-2	HUOVINEN et al. (1988b)
ROB-1	250	None	LEVESQUE et al. (1987)
OXA-1	315	OXA-4	LEVESQUE et al. (1987)
	310	OXA-4	HUOVINEN et al. (1988b)
		(OXA-2)[a]	QUELLETE and ROY (1986)
	15	None	QUELLETE and ROY (1986)
OXA-2	510	(OXA-3)[a]	HUOVINEN et al. (1988b)
	12	OXA-3	BOISSINOT et al. (1987)
	15	None	BOISSINOT et al. (1987)
	18	None	BOISSINOT et al. (1987)
	45	None	BOISSINOT et al. (1987)
PSE-1	1300	PSE-4, CARB-3	LEVESQUE et al. (1987)
	1300	PSE-4, CARB-3	HUOVINEN et al. (1988b)
PSE-2	460	OXA-6 (OXA-5)[a]	HUOVINEN et al. (1988b)
PSE-4	180	PSE-1, CARB-3	HUOVINEN et al. (1988b)

[a] Beta-lactamases in parentheses hybridized weakly.

slight cross-reactivity between an OXA-1 probe and the OXA-2 gene but an oligo-nucleotide probe of OXA-1 failed to cross hybridize with other beta-lactamases. BOISSINOT et al. (1987) constructed four OXA-1 oligo-nucleotide probes, three of which reacted only with the respective OXA-1 beta-lactamase but one cross hybridized with OXA-3.

A PSE-1 probe reacted with PSE-4 and CARB-3 beta-lactamase genes, and a ROB-1 probe showed no cross hybridization (LEVESQUE et al. 1987; HUOVINEN et al. 1988 b). A PSE-1 probe hybridized with the OXA-6 gene under stringent conditions and weakly with OXA-5 (HUOVINEN et al. 1988b). A 2 kilobase probe of OHIO-1 did not hybridize with other TEM type or OXA type beta-lactamases (SHLAES et al. 1986). In sum, these studies suggest a high degree of genetic relatedness between the following beta-lactamases: TEM-1, TEM-2, and TLE-1; SHV-1 and SHV-2; OXA-1 and OXA-4; OXA-2 and OXA-3; PSE-1, PSE-4 and CARB-3; PSE-2 and OXA-6.

JOUVENOT et al. (1987) compared the sensitivity of isoelectric focusing and a TEM-1 probe in detecting the TEM-1 beta-lactamase in several hundred clinical isolates. Among those isolates that were positive either by isoelectric focusing or probe, 158 were positive by both methods, 16 were positive by probe but failed to demonstrate the TEM-1 beta-lactamase on isoelectric focusing and eight isolates were positive by isoelectric focusing but negative by probe. The false negative isolates (by probe) produced mainly cephalosporinases, presumably chromosomally determined. There was no explanation for the 16 isolates that were positive by probe but negative by isoelectric focusing. It was suggested that there may be "silent" TEM genes that are not phenotypically expressed.

HUOVINEN et al. (1988 b) compared isoelectric focusing with colony hybridization using DNA probes for TEM-1, SHV-1, OXA-1, OXA-2, PSE-1, PSE-2, and PSE-4 in 122 clinical isolates. Allowing for the cross-hybridizations noted above, only six strains gave false positive reactions. Thus, colony hybridization may prove useful as a screening method for detection of plasmid-mediated beta-lactamases.

III. Amino Acid and Nucleotide Sequencing

The nucleotide sequence of five plasmid-mediated beta-lactamases is known, i.e. TEM-1 (SUTCLIFFE 1978), TEM-2 (CHEN and CLOWES 1987), OXA-1 (OUELLETTE et al. 1987 a), OXA-2 (DALE et al. 1985), and PSE-2 (HUOVINEN et al. 1988 a). The OXA-1 and OXA-2 enzymes share greater than 48% homology but show no significant homology with the TEM enzymes nor with other class A or class C beta-lactamases except at the region adjacent to the active site. No homology exists between the OXA and class B beta-lactamases. OUELLETTE et al. (1987 a) thus propose that OXA-1 and OXA-2 be designated as class D beta-lactamases.

HUOVINEN et al. (1988 a) determined the sequence of the PSE-2 beta-lactamase, an enzyme that hydrolyzes both carbenicillin and oxacillin. PSE-2 shows a high degree of homology with the OXA-2 beta-lactamase but no homology with TEM-1 except near the active site serine. Although the oxacillin-hydrolyzing beta-lactamases, OXA-1, OXA-2, and PSE-2, share common sequences, they, nevertheless, differ considerably in their behavior towards various substrates and inhibitors.

A high degree of nucleotide sequence homology exists also between the plasmid-determined beta-lactamase, TEM-1, and the chromosomally encoded beta-lactamase of *K. pneumoniae LEN* (ARAKAWA et al. 1986). This beta-lactamase has a pI value of 7.1 (A. A. MEDEIROS, unpublished results) and is probably the same as the chromosomal beta-lactamase of *K. pneumoniae* 1103, an enzyme with kinetic properties nearly identical to TEM-1 (PITTON et al. 1978; LABIA et al. 1979). The SHV-1 beta-lactamase which is encoded by both chromosomal and plasmid determinants in *K. pneumoniae* (NUGENT and HEDGES 1979) also has extensive amino acid sequence homology with TEM-1 and the *K. pneumoniae* LEN beta-lactamase, suggesting that these enzymes have a common genetic origin (BARTHELEMY et al. 1987). These data support the hypothesis first proposed in the late 1960s by NAOMI DATTA (personal communication) that the TEM-1 beta-lactamase evolved from the beta-lactamase of *K. pneumoniae*.

The nucleotide sequence of the structural gene for *S. aureus* beta-lactamase has also been determined (CHAN 1986; WANG and NOVICK 1987). Interestingly, despite a high degree of homology between the beta-lactamases of *S. aureus* and *B. licheniformis*, the nucleotide sequence shows very low homology. The crystal structure of beta-lactamase of *S. aureus* PC1, recently determined (HERZBERG and MOULT 1987), shows similarities with the tertiary structures of two other class A beta-lactamases (KELLY et al. 1986; SAMRAOUI 1986).

F. Spread of Plasmid-Determined Beta-Lactamases in Patient Flora

The existence of beta-lactamase genes on plasmids and transposons ensures that a beta-lactamase originally confined to one group of bacteria sooner or later may appear in other groups. Widespread use of antibiotics fosters selection of the resistant organisms which rise in prevalence locally, then spread worldwide. A prime example of this process occurred with the TEM-1 beta-lactamase common in enterobacteria. In 1974 strains of *H. influenzae* producing TEM-1 were first discovered in the United States. Rare at first, they have since reached a prevalence of 38 percent in some regions (THORNSBERRY and MCDOUGAL 1982). In 1976 strains of *N. gonorrhea* producing the plasmid determined TEM-1 beta-lactamase appeared in England and one year later in the United States (PERINE et al. 1977; PERCIVAL et al. 1976). At first most of the cases were importations from Africa and the Far East, but eventually major outbreaks due to endemic transmission occurred in metropolitan areas. The incidence in the United States rose from 328 cases in 1979 to 3424 cases reported in the first 9 months of 1982, while similar increases in incidence occurred in other countries (Centers for Disease Control 1982).

The distribution of plasmid-determined beta-lactamases, as determined by isoelectric focusing, is summarized in Table 4. The data are a composite of results previously reported by MATTHEW (1979) combined with our own results on several hundred clinical isolates and other reports (CULLMANN et al. 1984; JOUVENOT et al. 1983; KATSU et al. 1981; MEDEIROS and JACOBY 1986; PHILIPPON et al. 1984a; ROY et al. 1983, 1985; SIMPSON et al. 1980, 1986; THABAUT et al. 1985; TIRADO et

Table 4. Distribution in gram negative bacilli of plasmid-determined beta-lactamases. Species producing two or more types of beta-lactamase

	TEM-1	TEM-2	SHV-1	HMS-1	OXA-1	OXA-2	OXA-3	PSE-1	PSE-2	PSE-3	PSE-4	Novel	Total
Pseudomonas aeruginosa	+	+				+	+	+	+	+	+	LCR-1, OXA-4, OXA-5, OXA-6, NPS-1, CARB-3, CARB-4	15
Escherichia coli	+	+	+		+	+	+	+	+			TLE-1, OXA-4, OXA-7, OHIO-1	12
Klebsiella sp.	+	+	+	+	+		+		+	+		LXA-1, OHIO-1	10
Proteus mirabilis	+	+	+	+	+	+		+				Enzymes specified by strains N-3 and N-29	9
Salmonella sp.	+	+	+		+	+		+					6
Providencia sp.	+	+			+		+		+			OHIO-1	6
Enterobacter sp.	+	+			+				+			LXA-1, OHIO-1	5
Citrobacter sp.	+	+		+								LXA-1, OHIO-1	5
Proteus (indole +)	+	+	+						+				4
Morganella sp.	+		+		+							OHIO-1	4
Serratia sp.	+	+				+						OHIO-1	4
Shigella sp.	+	+						+					3
Hemophilus influenzae	+											ROB-1	2
Vibrio cholera	+											SAR-2	2

Table 5. Types of beta-lactamases in clinical isolates of ampicillin-resistant *E. coli* from different regions

Geographic origin	Number tested	Chromo-somal only	Beta-lactamase-type											References
			TEM-1	TEM-2	OXA-1	SHV-1	OXA-2	PSE-1	Other	TEM-1 and PSE-1	TEM-1 and SHV-1	TEM-1 and OXA-1	TEM-1 and other	
Africa														
Senegal[f]	97	NS	NS			29					6			Shaokat et al. (1987)
South Africa	47	16 (34)[a]	23 (49)		5 (11)							3		Medeiros and Jacoby (1986)
Asia														
Bangkok[f]	29	0	27 (93)							1		1		Medeiros and Jacoby (1986)
Indonesia[f]	11	0	9 (82)		1 (9)			1						Medeiros and Jacoby (1986)
Europe														
England[d]	110	18 (16)	73 (66)		17 (16)	1								Simpson et al. (1980)
Germany	84	13 (16)	62 (74)		8 (10)									R. Marre, personal communication
Italy	16	NS	11	4		1								Esposito et al. (1985)
Italy	30	NS	28 (93)	2 (7)										Pagani et al. (1982)
Paris	21	3 (14)	16 (76)				2							Medeiros and Jacoby (1986)
Spain	90	0	86 (96)		2 (2)							1	1[c]	Roy et al. (1983)
South America														
Brazil	98	0	71 (72)		10 (10)	6		2	3[b]	2		3	1[b]	Medeiros and Jacoby (1986)
USA														
Boston	34	6 (18)	27 (79)		1 (3)									Medeiros and Jacoby (1986)
Providence	50	6 (12)	41 (82)		2 (4)		1							Medeiros and Jacoby (1986)
Germany, Amman, and South America[e]	130	17 (13)	99 (76)	5 (4)	7 (5)					1		1		Simpson et al. (1986)
Total	847 (100)	79 (9)	652 (77)	11	53 (6)	37 (4)	3	3	3	4	6	10	2	

[a] Percentage of total in parentheses.
[b] TLE-1.
[c] An uncharacterized beta-lactamase of pI 5.2.
[d] Urinary isolates.
[e] Fecal samples of healthy volunteers.
[f] Fecal samples of patients.
NS, not specified.

al. 1986; WHITAKER et al. 1983; WILLIAMS et al. (1984). The largest number of different types of beta-lactamases were found in *P. aeruginosa* (16), *E. coli* (12), *Klebsiella* (10), *P. mirabilis* (9), *Salmonella* (6), and *Providencia* (6).

Table 5 shows the beta-lactamases found in surveys of isolates of ampicillin-resistant *E. coli* from different countries. Most were random samplings of clinical isolates, except those from Indonesia and Thailand (enteropathogenic strains), from England (urinary isolates) (SIMPSON et al. 1980) and from Germany, South America or America (fecal samples of healthy volunteers) (SIMPSON et al. 1986). Overall, 77% produced TEM-1 whereas 6 percent produced OXA-1. Nine percent produced only chromosomal beta-lactamase. Interestingly, the distribution of beta-lactamase types in fecal samples from healthy volunteers paralleled that found in the surveys of clinical isolates suggesting that these strains do, indeed, represent the "gene pool" from which infections arise (SIMPSON et al. 1986). The collections from Brazil and Senegal were extraordinary in that three novel beta-lactamases and PSE-1 were found in the former and nearly a third of the isolates in the latter produced SHV-1. Although certain overall patterns are apparent, these data indicate that the distribution of beta-lactamase types within a particular species is not homogeneous worldwide.

In other species, TEM-1 is not the most prevalent beta-lactamase. All of 16 ampicillin-resistant strains of *Proteus mirabilis* isolated in Germany produced TEM-2 (R. MARRE, personal communication). Similarly, CULLMANN et al. (1982) reported TEM-2 in 8 of 11 beta-lactamase producing isolates of *P. mirabilis* and 12 of 13 isolates of *P. rettgeri* from 7 hospitals in Germany. Surveys of the beta-lactamases produced by isolates of *P. aeruginosa* from Spain (TIRADO et al. 1986) and several regions of France (THABAUT et al. 1985; JOUVENOT et al. 1983) showed a predominance of PSE-1 (Table 6). Interestingly, the TEM-2 beta-lactamase was more frequent than TEM-1 in a survey of 530 French isolates (THABAUT et al. 1985) as it was in an earlier worldwide sample (MATTHEW 1979a). The distribution of beta-lactamase types differed greatly among isolates from the United Kingdom, PSE-4 being the most common beta-lactamase (WILLIAMS et al. 1984). However, the majority of the PSE-4 producing strains from the United Kingdom belonged to a single serotype of *P. aeruginosa* indicating probable dissemination of that subtype in that region (LIVERMORE et al. 1985).

There is evidence that beta-lactamase genes may circulate between animal and human isolates (Table 7). In a study of 113 human and 146 animal isolates of ampicillin-resistant salmonellae from the United States, 81% and 77% of human and animal isolates, respectively, produced TEM-1 (MEDEIROS et al. 1981; A. A. MEDEIROS and T. F. O'BRIEN, unpublished data). However, the second commonest beta-lactamase in both human and animal isolates was OXA-2, an uncommon type in *E. coli*. Moreover, most of the isolates producing OXA-2 belonged to a relatively rare serotype, i.e., *S. typhimurium*, var. Copenhagen. This unexpected association in both human and animal isolates suggested that they shared the same resistance determinants. Indeed, endonuclease digests of plasmids from animal and human isolates from different regions of the United States were often identical (O'BRIEN et al. 1982).

Another form of ampicillin resistance that may have an animal reservoir is the ROB-1 beta-lactamase that has been found in human isolates of *H. influenzae* in

Table 6. Types of plasmid-determined beta-lactamases in clinical isolates of carbenicillin-resistant *P. aeruginosa*

Geographic origin	Number	Beta-lactamase type													Reference
		TEM-1	TEM-2	OXA-1	OXA-2	OXA-3	PSE-1	PSE-2	PSE-3	PSE-4	CARB-4	TEM-1 and OXA-1	pI 6.5	pI 7.8 (?OXA.6)	
UK	40	3	0	9 (23)	0	0	1	2	1	18 (45)	0	1	2	3	WILLIAMS et al. (1984)
Spain	73	28 (38)[a]	1	0	0	0	37 (51)	0	0	7 (10)	0	0	0	0	TIRADO et al. (1986)
France	530	21 (4)	28 (5)	56 (11)	89 (17)	2	288 (54)	8	14 (3)	3	1	0	0	20 (4)	THABAUT et al. (1985)
France	45	0	0	0	0	0	36 (80)	0	0	9 (20)	0	0	0	0	JOUVENOT et al. (1983)
Total	688 (100)	52 (8)	29 (4)	65 (9)	89 (13)	2	362 (53)	10	15 (2)	37 (5)	1	1	2	23 (3)	

[a] Percentage of total in parentheses.

Table 7. Types of beta-lactamase in human and animal isolates of ampicillin-resistant *Salmonella* from different regions

Geographic origin	Number	Beta-lactamase type								Reference
		TEM-1	TEM-2	SHV-1	OXA-1	OXA-2	PSE-1	TEM-1 and OXA-1	TEM-1 and PSE-1	
USA	119[a]	91 (76)[f]	0	0	1	18[c] (15)	6 (5)	2	1	MEDEIROS et al. (1981) and unpublished data
	146[b]	112 (77)	0	0	2	32[c] (22)	0	0	0	
France	53[a]	49 (92)	2 (4)	0	2 (4)	0	0	0	0	PHILIPPON et al. (1984b)
Senegal	52[a]	4 (8)	10[d] (19)	38[e] (73)	0	0	0	0	0	PHILIPPON et al. (1984b)
Total	370 (100)	256 (69)	12 (3)	38 (10)	5	50 (14)	6	2	1	

[a] Human isolates.
[b] Animal isolates.
[c] Most isolates were *S. typhimurium*, var Copenhagen.
[d] All isolates were *S. ordonez*.
[e] All isolates were *S. poona*.
[f] Percentage of total in parentheses.

the USA (RUBIN et al. 1981; MEDEIROS et al. 1986) and France (JOLY et al. 1987). ROB-1 has been discovered also in ampicillin-resistant isolates of the porcine pathogen *Haemophilus pleuropneumoniae* and in an ampicillin-resistant strain of *Pasteurella multocida* of porcine origin (MEDEIROS et al. 1986). PHILIPPON et al. (1986c) have also identified a beta-lactamase of pI greater than 8.0 that is probably ROB-1 in an ampicillin-resistant bovine strain of *P. multocida*.

The prevalence of different beta-lactamases can be expected to vary in time and place when strains become epidemic. Ampicillin-resistant strains of *S. typhimurium*, *S. typhi*, and *S. wien* which caused large-scale epidemics of salmonellosis in Europe, Africa, and the Middle East were found to produce OXA-1 whereas *S. ordonnez* which was epidemic in Senegal produced the SHV-1 beta-lactamase (Table 7) (MEDEIROS 1984; PHILIPPON et al. 1984b). A recent study of *E. coli* isolated from fecal samples of nonhospitalized patients in Senegal showed that 30% produced the SHV-1 beta-lactamase, a prevalence much higher than that seen in *E. coli* from other regions (Table 7) (SHAOKAT et al. 1987). These data suggest that the SHV-1 determinant spread between species in Senegal and continues to disseminate in the flora of the general population there.

The OHIO-1 beta-lactamase provides another example of a beta-lactamase gene that appears to be endemic within a geographic region (SHLAES et al. 1986). Over a 5-year period this enzyme was isolated from over 30 gram-negative bacilli comprising various species of *Enterobacteriaceae* from two hospitals in Ohio, Columbus and Cleveland, Ohio. It has not yet been identified outside of Ohio. Although multiple plasmids carried the OHIO-1 gene, endonuclease digestion and Southern hybridization showed that the plasmids had a common genetic origin (KRON et al. 1987). Why the OHIO-1 gene disseminated within this discrete geographical region is unclear.

I. Emergence of Variant Beta-Lactamases Active Against Newer Beta-Lactams

The success of the pharmaceutical industry in developing new beta-lactams resistant to hydrolysis by beta-lactamases led to the introduction into clinical use of the so-called third-generation beta-lactam antibiotics around 1978 in Europe and 1981 in the USA. These antibiotics, exemplified by cefotaxime, were very resistant to hydrolysis by the known plasmid-determined beta-lactamases. Then, in 1983 in Germany, isolates of *K. pneumoniae*, *E. coli*, *E. cloacae*, *S. marcescens*, and *K. ozaenae* were discovered that produced a plasmid-determined beta-lactamase of pI 7.6 that hydrolyzed cefotaxime, conferring resistance to it as well as to several other newer cephalosporins (BAUERNFEIND et al. 1985; KNOTHE et al. 1983; SHAH and STILLE 1983). KLIEBE et al. (1985) showed that this new beta-lactamase, called SHV-2, derived from a natural mutation in the well-known SHV-1 beta-lactamase commonly found in *Klebsiella*. The mutation resulted in an enhanced affinity of the SHV-1 beta-lactamase for cefotaxime. Similar strains producing SHV-2 have been found in France, Chile and Greece (A. A. MEDEIROS, unpublished data). More recently cefotaxime-resistant strains of *K. pneumoniae* producing a novel plasmid-encoded, TEM-like, cefotaxime-hydrolyzing beta-lactamase, designated CTX-1, have been recovered from patients in several hospitals in Paris and Clermont-Ferrand (BRUN-BUISSON et al. 1987; SIROT et al. 1987b). Also, three novel plasmid-encoded beta-lactamases of pI values 5.42, 5.5 and 5.9 that hydrolyze ceftazidime and aztreonam have appeared in clinical isolates from France and Germany (BAUERNFEIND and HORL 1987; GUTTMANN et al. 1987; SIROT et al. 1987a; A. BAUERNFEIND and A. A. MEDEIROS, unpublished data). Based on DNA hybridization studies these new beta-lactamases appear to be derivatives of the TEM-2 beta-lactamase (GOUSSARD et al. 1987; GUTTMANN et al. 1987), an enzyme found more commonly in European isolates. Thus, in response to new selection pressures engendered by the frequent use of third-generation cephalosporins mutations have occurred among the well established plasmid-determined beta-lactamases, resulting in dissemination of novel transferable beta-lactamases with an expanded spectrum of activity.

G. Contribution of Plasmid-Determined Beta-Lactamases to Beta-Lactam Antibiotic Resistance

Several parameters contribute to the level of antibiotic resistance mediated by a particular beta-lactamase in a population of bacteria. The efficiency of the beta-lactamase in hydrolyzing an antibiotic depends both an its rate of hydrolysis (V_{max}), conveniently expressed as a ratio relative to benzylpenicillin or cephaloridine, and its affinity for the antibiotic (*Km*), a value often difficult to obtain with substrates which are hydrolyzed weakly (LIVERMORE et al. 1986b). Another variable is the amount of beta-lactamase produced by the bacterial cell. The TEM-1 beta-lactamase activity of clinical isolates of *E. coli* may vary 100-fold (SIMPSON et al. 1986; MARRE et al. 1984). MARRE et al. (1984) and LIVERMORE et al. (1986b) demonstrated that the amount of TEM-1 enzyme produced by *E. coli* isolates determines levels of susceptibility to piperacillin and mezlocillin. High level production of plasmid-determined beta-lactamases in *E. coli* C600 transconjugants was associated with enhanced resistance to cefamandole and to some third generation cephalosporins (JACOBY and SUTTON 1985).

Within the bacterial cell, beta-lactamases contribute to antibiotic resistance in several ways. The simplest model is that of penicillinase-producing staphylococci in which the bacteria, upon exposure to penicillin, begin to produce beta-lactamase which they excrete into the media. Two events then take place concurrently: (1) penicillin lyses bacteria, and (2) beta-lactamase hydrolyzes penicillin. If viable bacterial cells remain after the level of penicillin has fallen below the minimal inhibitory concentration, regrowth of bacteria occurs (SYKES and MATTHEW 1976).

The second model shows a similar kinetic effect. It is exemplified by gram-negative bacilli which (1) produce a beta-lactamase that remains trapped in the periplasmic space and which (2) have no barrier to antibiotic penetration. An example is *H. influnenzae* strains that produce the TEM-1 beta-lactamase (MEDEIROS and O'BRIEN 1975). In both this model and the first one discussed, a marked inoculum effect occurs in that the minimal inhibitory concentration for a large inoculum (10^6 organisms/ml) may be a thousand-fold greater than with a small inoculum (10^2 organisms/ml). The low level of resistance of single cells has made it possible for ampicillin to cure some infections caused by beta-lactamase producing strains *H. influenzae*, when the inoculum of infecting bacteria was low (MOXON et al. 1977; MURPHY and TODD 1979). Greater levels of resistance may occur in *H. influenzae* when promoter mutations occur that result in greater expression of beta-lactamase activity (CHEN and CLOWES 1987).

The third model is exemplified by resistance to ampicillin of *E. coli* strains which produce the TEM-1 beta-lactamase. Beta-lactam antibiotics enter these bacteria through protein (porin) channels in the outer membrane (NIKAIDO 1985). The cells produce a beta-lactamase which remains localized to the periplasmic space. In this model, the kinetics are more complicated. The enzyme is strategically situated between the barrier to antibiotic penetration (outer membrane) and the antibiotic targets (penicillin binding proteins on the cytoplasmic membrane). In this position the enzyme can sequentially destroy antibiotic molecules as they make their way through the barrier, analogous to a sharpshooter with abundant ammunition who aims at targets passing through a single entry point. As a consequence, high levels of resistance occur with single bacterial cells, unlike the previous example (SYKES and MATTHEW 1976; PERCIVAL et al. 1963; MEDEIROS et al. 1974). Changes in the permeability of the bacterial outer membrane may occur due to regulation of porin production or mutational loss of porins, and may widen the spectrum of beta-lactam resistance in strains producing plasmid-determined beta-lactamases. As an example, a TEM-1 producing isolate of *S. typhimurium* acquired resistance to cephalosporins during therapy due to mutational loss of its ompC porin. The resistant variant manifested resistance only in high osmolality media where omp F porin production was physiologically repressed, leaving the cell without either type of porin (MEDEIROS et al. 1987).

Acknowledgment. I thank George Jacoby for discussions and information, Elaine Papa and Clotilde O'Gara for technical support, and Cheryl Marrone for secretarial assistance. This work was supported by The Miriam Hospital Foundation.

References

Abraham EP, Chain E (1940) An enyzme from bacteria able to destroy penicillin. Nature 373:837

Amaral L, Lee Y, Schwarz U, Lorian V (1986) Penicillin-binding site on the *Escherichia coli* cell envelope. J Bacteriol 167:492–495

Ambler RP (1980) The structure of beta-lactamases. Philos Trans R Soc Lond 289:321–331

Ambler RP, Scott GK (1978) Partial amino acid sequence of penicillinase coded by *Escherichia coli* plasmid R6K. Proc Natl Acad Sci USA 75:3732–3736

Arakawa Y, Ohta M, Kido N, Fujii Y, Komatsu T, Kato N (1986) Close evolutionary relationship between the chromosomally encoded beta-lactamase gene of *Klebsiella pneumoniae* and the TEM beta-lactamase gene mediated by R plasmids. FEBS Lett 207:69–74

Barthelemy M, Peduzzi J, Labia R (1985) Distinction between the primary structures of TEM-1 and TEM-2 beta-lactamases. Ann Inst Pasteur Microbiol 136[A]:311–321

Barthelemy M, Peduzzi J, Labia R (1987) N-terminal amino acid sequence of PIT-2 beta-lactamase (SHV-1). J Antimicrob Chemother 19:839–852

Bauernfeind A, Horl G (1987) Novel R-factor borne beta-lactamase of *Escherichia coli* conferring resistance to cephalosporins. Infection 15:257–259

Bauernfeind A, Shah P, Petermuller C, Motz M (1985) Plasmid-determined resistance to third generation cephalosporins in enterobacteria. Chemioterapia 4:30–31
Bergstrom S, Olsson O, Normark S (1982) Common evolutionary origin of chromosomal beta-lactamase genes in enterobacteria. J Bacteriol 150:528–534
Bobrowski MM, Matthew M, Barth PT, Datta N, Grinter NJ, Jacob AE, Kontomichalou P, Dale JW, Smith JT (1976) Plasmid-determined beta-lactamase indistinguishable from the chromosomal beta-lactamase of *Escherichia coli*. J Bacteriol 125:149–157
Boissinot M, Mercier J, Levesque RC (1987) Development of natural and synthetic DNA probes for OXA-2 and TEM-1 beta-lactamases. Antimicrob Agents Chemother 31:728–734
Boyce JM, Medeiros AA (1987) Role of beta-lactamase in expression of resistance by methicillin-resistant *Staphylococcus aureus*. Antimicrob Agents Chemother 31:1426–1428
Brun-Buisson C, Legrand P, Philippon A, Montravers F, Ansquer M, Duval J (1987) Transferable enzymatic resistance to third-generation cephalosporins during nosocomial outbreak of multiresistant *Klebsiella pneumoniae*. Lancet II:302–306
Centers for Disease Control (1982) Global distribution of penicillinase-producing *Neisseria gonorrhoeae* (PPNG). Conn Med 42:223
Chambers HF, Hartman BJ, Tomasz A (1985) Increased amounts of a novel penicillin-binding protein in a strain of methicillin-resistant *Staphylococcus aureus* exposed to nafcillin. J Clin Invest 76:325–331
Chan PT (1986) Nucleotide sequence of the *Staphylococcus aureus* PC1 beta-lactamase gene. Nucleic Acids Res 14:5940
Chen S-T, Clowes RC (1987) Nucleotide sequence comparisons of plasmids pHD131, pJB1, pFA3, and pFA7 and beta-lactamase expression in *Escherichia coli*, *Haemophilus influenzae*, and *Neisseria gonorrhoeae*. J Bacteriol 169:3124–3130
Cooksey RC, Clark NC, Thornsberry C (1985) A gene probe for TEM type beta-lactamases. Antimicrob Agents Chemother 28:154–156
Coulson A (1985) Beta-lactamases: molecular studies. Biotechnol Genet Eng Rev 3:219–253
Cullmann W, Flensberg T, Opferkuch W, Stieglitz M, Wiedemann B (1982) Correlation of beta-lactamase production and resistance to beta-lactam antibiotics in Enterobacteriaceae. Zentralbl Bakteriol Mikrobiol Hyg 252:480–489
Cullmann W, Opferkuch W, Steiglitz M, Dick W (1984) Influence of spontaneous and inducible beta-lactamase production on the antimicrobial activity of recently developed beta-lactam compounds. Chemotherapy 30:175–181
Dale JW, Smith JT (1976) The dimeric nature of an R-factor mediated beta-lactamase. Biochem Biophys Res Commun 68:1000–1005
Dale JW, Goodwin D, Mossakowska D, Stephenson P, Wall S (1985) Sequence of the OXA-2 beta-lactamase: comparison with other penicillin-reactive enzymes. FEBS Lett 191:39–44
Datta N, Kontomichalou P (1965) Penicillinase synthesis controlled by infectious R-factors in Enterobacteriaceae. Nature 208:239–241
Dyke KGH (1979) Beta-lactamases of *Staphylococcus aureus*. In: Hamilton-Miller JMT, Smith JT (eds) Beta-lactamases. Academic Press, London, pp 291–310
Eliasson I, Kamme C (1985) Characterization of the plasmid-mediated beta-lactamase in *Branhamella catarrhalis*, with special reference to substrate affinity. J Antimicrob Chemother 15:139–149
Esposito S, Galante D, Barba D, Pennucci D, Limauro D (1985) Correlation of beta-lactamase stability and antibacterial activity of beta-lactams in beta-lactamase-producing bacteria and respective transconjugants. Chemioterapia 4:33–35
Goering RV, Ruff EA (1983) Comparative analysis of conjugative plasmids mediating gentamicin resistance in *Staphylococcus aureus*. Antimicrob Agents Chemother 24:450–452
Goussard S, Sougakoff W, Gerbaud G, Courvalin P (1987) CTX-1, a wide-substrate-range enzyme, is a derivative of a TEM beta-lactamase. Program and abstracts of the twenty-seventh interscience conference on antimicrobial agents and chemotherapy. American Society for Microbiology, New York, No 517

Guttmann L, Kitzes MD, Billot-Klein MD, Goldstein FW, Tran Van Nhieu, Collatz R (1987) New plasmid-mediated TEM-derived beta-lactamase hydrolyzing ceftazidime. Program and abstracts of the twenty-seventh interscience conference on antimicrobial agents and chemotherapy, American Society for Microbiology, New York, No 518

Hedge PJ, Spratt BG (1985) Resistance to beta-lactam antibiotics by re-modelling the active site of an *E. coli* penicillin-binding protein. Nature 318:478–480

Hedges RW, Jacob AE (1974) Transposition of ampicillin resistance from RP4 to other replicons. Mol Gen Genet 132:31–40

Hedges RW, Matthew M, Smith DI, Cresswell JM, Jacob AE (1977) Properties of a transposon conferring resistance to penicillins and streptomycin. Gene 1:241–253

Hedges RW, Medeiros AA, Cohenford M, Jacoby GA (1985) Genetic and biochemical properties of AER-1, a novel carbenicillin-hydrolyzing beta-lactamase from *Aeromonas hydrophila*. Antimicrob Agents Chemother 27:479–484

Herzberg O, Moult J (1987) Bacterial resistance to beta-lactam antibiotics: crystal structure of beta-lactamase from *Staphylococcus aureus* PC1 at 2.5. A resolution. Science 236:694–701

Holland S, Dale JW (1985) Immunological comparison between OXA-2 beta-lactamase and those mediated by other R plasmids. Antimicrob Agents Chemother 27:989–991

Huovinen P, Huovinen S, Jacoby GA (1988 a) The sequence of PSE-2 beta-lactamase. Antimicrob Agents Chemother 32:134–136

Huovinen S, Huovinen P, Jacoby GA (1988 b) Detection of plasmid-mediated beta-lactamases using DNA probes. Antimicrob Agents Chemother 32:175–179

Jack GW, Richmond MH (1970) A comparative study of eight distinct beta-lactamases synthesized by gram-negative bacteria. J Gen Microbiol 61:43–61

Jacoby GA, Sutton L (1985) Beta-lactamases and beta-lactam resistance in *Escherichia coli*. Antimicrobial Agents Chemother 28:703–705

Jaurin B, Grundstrom T (1981) Amp C cephalosporinase of *Escherichia coli* K-12 has a different evolutionary origin from that of beta-lactamases of the penicillinase type. Proc Natl Acad Sci USA 78:4897–4901

Joly B, Delmas C, Rich C, Prere MF, Livrelli V, Dabernat H (1987) Un nouveau mécanisme de résistance à l'ampicilline par production de beta-lactamase ROB-1 chez une souche d'*Haemophilus influenzae* isolée en France. Presse Méd 16:916–917

Jouvenot M, Bonin P, Michel-Briand Y (1983) Frequency of beta-lactamases that are markedly active against carbenicillin in the *Pseudomonas aeruginosa* strains isolated in a Medical School Hospital. J Antimicrob Chemother 12:451–458

Jouvenot M, Deschaseaux ML, Royez M, Mougin C, Cooksey RC, Michel-Briand Y, Adessi GL (1987) Molecular hybridization versus isoelectric focusing to determine TEM-type beta-lactamases in gram-negative bacteria. Antimicrob Agents Chemother 31:300–305

Katsu K, Inoue M, Mitsuhashi S (1981) Plasmid-mediated carbenicillin hydrolyzing beta-lactamases of *Proteus mirabilis*. J Antibiot 43:1504–1506

Kelly JA, Kideberg O, Charlier P, Wery JP, et al. (1986) On the origin of bacterial resistance to penicillin: comparison of a beta-lactamase and a penicillin target. Science 231:1413–1429

Kliebe C, Nies BA, Meyer JF, Tolxdorff-Neutzling RM, Wiedemann B (1985) Evolution of plasmid-coded resistance to broad-spectrum cephalosporins. Antimicrob Agents Chemother 28:302–307

Knothe H, Shah P, Krcmery V, Antal M, Mitsuhashi S (1983) Transferable resistance to cefotaxmine, cefoxitin, cefamandole and cefuroxime in clinical isolates of *Klebsiella pneumoniae* and *Serratia marcescens*. Infection 11:315–317

Kobayashi T, Fang Zhu Y, Nicholls NJ, Oliver Lampen J (1987) A second regulatory gene, *bla*R1, encoding a potential penicillin-binding protein required for induction of beta-lactamase in *Bacillus licheniformis*. J Bacteriol 169:3873–3878

Kopecko DJ, Brevet J, Cohen SN (1976) Involvement of multiple translocating DNA segments and recombinational hotspots in the structural evolution of bacterial plasmids. J Mol Biol 108:333–360

Kratz J, Schmidt F, Wiedemann B (1983) Transposition of a gene encoding OXA-2 beta-lactamase. J Gen Microbiol 129:2951–2957

Kron MA, Shlaes DM, Currie-McMumber C, Medeiros AA (1987) Molecular epidemiology of OHIO-1 beta-lactamase. Antimicrob Agents Chemother 31:2007–2009

Labia R, Fabre C, Masson J-M, Barthelemy M (1979) *Klebsiella pneumoniae* strains moderately resistant to ampicillin and carbenicillin: characterization of a new beta-lactamase. J Antimicrob Chemother 5:375–382

Labia R, Guionie M, Barthelemy M, Philippon A (1981) Properties of three carbenicillin-hydrolyzing beta-lactamases (CARB) from *Pseudomonas aeruginosa*: identification of a new enzyme. J Antimicrob Chemother 7:49–56

Levesque R, Roy PH (1982) Mapping of the plasmid (pLQ3) from *Achromobacter* and cloning of its cephalosporinase gene in *Escherichia coli*. Gene 18:69–75

Levesque R, Roy PH, Letarte R, Pechere JC (1982) A plasmid-mediated cephalosporinase from *Achromobacter* species. J Infect Dis 145:753–761

Levesque RC, Jacoby GA (1988) Molecular structure and interrelationships of multiresistance beta-lactamase transposons. Plasmid (in press)

Levesque RC, Medeiros AA, Jacoby GA (1987) Molecular cloning and DNA homology of plasmid-mediated beta-lactamase genes. MGG 206:252–258

Livermore DM, Jones CS (1986) Characterization of NPS-1, a novel plasmid-mediated beta-lactamase from two *Pseudomonas aeruginosa* isolates. Antimicrob Agents Chemother 29:99–103

Livermore DM, Pitt TL, Jones CS, Crees-Morris JA, Williams RJ (1985) PSE-4 beta-lactamase: a serotype-specific enzyme in *Pseudomonas aeruginosa*. J Med Microbiol 19:45–53

Livermore DM, Moosdeen F, Lindridge MA, Ko P, Williams JD (1986) Behaviour of TEM-1 beta-lactamase as a resistance mechanism to ampicillin, mezlocillin and azlocillin in *Escherichia coli*. J Antimicrob Chemother 17:139–146

Marre R, Borner K, Schulz E (1984) Different mechanisms of TEM-1 and OXA-1 mediated resistance to piperacillin in *E. coli*. Zentralbl Bakteriol Mikrobiol Hyg 58:287–295

Matthew M (1979) Plasmid-mediated beta-lactamase of gram-negative bacteria: properties and distribution. J Antimicrob Chemother 5:349–358

Matthew M, Harris AM (1976) Identification of beta-lactamases by analytical isoelectric focusing: correlation with bacterial taxonomy. J Gen Microbiol 94:55–67

Matthew M, Sykes RB (1977) Properties of the beta-lactamase specified by the *Pseudomonas* plasmid RPL11. J Bacteriol 132:341–345

Matthew M, Harris AM, Marshall MJ, Ross GW (1975) The use of analytical isoelectric focusing for detection and identification of beta-lactamases. J Gen Microbiol 88:169–178

Matthew M, Hedges RW, Smith JT (1979) Types of beta-lactamase determined by plasmids in gram-negative bacteria. J Bacteriol 138:657–662

McDonnell RW, Sweendy HM, Cohen S (1983) Conjugational transfer of gentamicin resistance plasmids intra- and interspecifically in *Staphylococcus aureus* and *Staphylococcus epidermidis*. Antimicrob Agents Chemother 23:151–160

Medeiros AA (1984) Beta-lactamases. Br Med Bull 40:18–27

Medeiros AA, Jacoby GA (1986) Beta-lactamase-mediated resistance. In: Queener SF, Webber JA, Queener SW (eds) Beta-lactam antibiotics for clinical use. Dekker, New York, pp 49–84

Medeiros AA, O'Brien TF (1975) Ampicillin-resistant *Haemophilus influenzae* type b possessing a TEM-type beta-lactamase but little permeability barrier to ampicillin. Lancet I:716

Medeiros AA, Kent RL, O'Brien TF (1974) Characterization and prevalence of the different mechanisms of resistance to beta-lactam antibiotics in clinical isolates of *Escherichia coli*. Antimicrob Agents Chemother 6:791–801

Medeiros AA, Ximenez J, Blickstein-Goldworm K, O'Brien TF, Acar J (1980) Beta-lactamases of ampicillin-resistant *Escherichia coli* from Brazil, France and the United States. In: Nelson JD, Grassi C (eds) Current chemotherapy and infectious diseases. American Society for Microbiology, Washington DC, pp 761–762

Medeiros AA, Gilleece ES, O'Brien TF (1981) Distribution of plasmid type beta-lactamases in ampicillin-resistant salmonellae from humans and animals in the United States. In: Levy S, Clowes R, Koenig E (eds) Molecular biology, pathogenicity, and ecology of bacterial plasmids. Plenum, New York, p 634

Medeiros AA, Hedges RW, Jacoby GA (1982) Spread of a "*Pseudomonas*-specific" beta-lactamase to plasmids of enterobacteria. J Bacteriol 149:700–707

Medeiros AA, Cohenford M, Jacoby GA (1985) Five novel plasmid-determined beta-lactamases. Antimicrob Agents Chemother 27:715–719

Medeiros AA, Levesque R, Jacoby GA (1986) An animal source for the ROB-1 beta-lactamase of *Haemophilus influenzae* type b. Antimicrob Agents Chemother 29:212–215

Medeiros AA, O'Brien TF, Rosenberg EY, Nikaido H (1987) Loss of OmpC in a strain of *Salmonella typhimurium* causes increased resistance to cephalosporins during therapy. J Infect Dis 156:751–757

Morin CJ, Patel PC, Levesque RC, Letarte R (1987) Monoclonal antibodies to TEM-1 plasmid-mediated beta-lactamase. Antimicrob Agents Chemother 31:1761–1767

Moxon ER, Medeiros AA, O'Brien TF (1977) Beta-lactamase effect on ampicillin treatment of *Haemophilus influenzae* b bacteremia and meningitis in infant rats. Antimicrob Agents Chemother 12:461–464

Murphy D, Todd J (1979) Treatment of ampicillin-resistant *Haemophilus influenzae* in soft tissue infections with high doses of ampicillin. J Pediatr 94:983–987

Murray BE, Mederski-Samoraj B (1983) Transferrable beta-lactamase. A new mechanism for in vitro penicillin resistance in *Streptococcus faecalis*. J Clin Invest 72:1168–1171

Murray BE, Mederski-Samoraj B, Foster SK, Brunton JL, Harford P (1986a) In vitro studies of plasmid-mediated penicillinase from *Streptococcus faecalis* suggest a staphylococcal origin. J Clin Invest 77:289–293

Murray BE, Church DA, Wanger A, Zscheck K, Levison ME, Ingerman MJ, Abrutyn E, Mederski-Samoraj B (1986b) Comparison of two beta-lactamase-producing strains of *Streptococcus faecalis*. Antimicrob Agents Chemother 30:861–864

Nielsen JBK, Lampen JO (1982) Glyceride-cysteine lipoproteins and secretion by gram-positive bacteria. J Bacteriol 152:315–322

Nikaido H (1985) Role of permeability barriers in resistance to beta-lactam antibiotics. Pharmacol Ther 27:197–231

Nugent ME, Hedges RW (1979) The nature of the genetic determinant for the SHV-1 beta-lactamase. Mol Gen Genet 175:239–243

O'Brien TF, Hopkins JD, Gilleece ES, Medeiros AA, Kent RL, Blackburn BO, Holmes MB, Reardon JP, Vergeront JM, Schell WL, Christenson E, Bissett ML, Morse EV (1982) Molecular epidemiology of antibiotic resistance in salmonella from animals and human beings in the United States. N Engl J Med 307:1–6

Ouellette M, Roy PH (1986) Analysis by using DNA probes of the OXA-1 beta-lactamase gene and its transposon. Antimicrob Agents Chemother 30:46–51

Ouellette M, Bissonnette L, Roy PH (1987a) Precise insertion of antibiotic resistance determinants into Tn21-like transposons: nucleotide sequence of the OXA-1 beta-lactamase gene. Proc Natl Acad Sci USA 84:7378–7382

Ouellette M, Rossi JJ, Bazin R, Roy PH (1987b) Oligonucleotide probes for the detection of TEM-1 and TEM-2 beta-lactamase genes and their transposons. Can J Microbiol 33:205–211

Pagani L, Perduca M, Romero E (1982) Prevalence and distribution of R plasmid-mediated beta-lactamases in *Enterobacteriaceae*. Microbiologica 5:179–184

Paul G, Philippon A, Barthelemy M, Labia R, Nevot P (1981) Immunological distinction between constitutive beta-lactamases of gram-negative rods with antisera TEM-1 and CARB-3. Program and abstracts of the 21st interscience conference on antimicrobial agents and chemotherapy. American Society for Microbiology, Chicago, No 681

Paul G, Philippon A, Nevot P (1985) Immunological identification of beta-lactamases: specificity of an immune serum anti-OXA-2. Chemioterapia 4:31–33

Percival A, Brumfitt W, de Louvois J (1963) The role of penicillinase in determining natural and acquired resistance of gram-negative bacteria to penicillins. J Gen Microbiol 32:77–89

Percival A, Rowlands J, Corkhill JE, Alergant CD, Arya OP, Rees E (1976) Penicillinase-producing gonococci in Liverpool. Lancet II:1379–1382
Perine PI, Schalla W, Siegel MS; Thornsberry C, Biddle J, Wong K-H, Thompson SE (1977) Evidence for two distinct types of penicillinase-producing *Neisseria gonorrhoeae*. Lancet II:993–995
Philippon AM, Paul GC, Jacoby GA (1983) Properties of PSE-2 beta-lactamase and genetic basis for its production in *Pseudomonas aeruginosa*. Antimicrob Agents Chemother 24:362–369
Philippon A, Thabaut A, Meyran M, Nevot P (1984a) Distribution des beta-lactamases constitutives chez *Pseudomonas aeruginosa*. Presse Méd 13:772–776
Philippon A, Fournier G, Cornel E, Paul G, LeMinor L, Nevot P (1984b) Les beta-lactamases des *Salmonella* résistantes à l'ampicilline. Ann Microbiol (Paris) 135:229–238
Philippon AM, Paul GC, Jacoby GA (1986a) New plasmid-mediated oxacillin-hydrolyzing beta-lactamase in *Pseudomonas aeruginosa*. J Antimicrob Chemother 17:415–422
Philippon AM, Paul GC, Thabaut AP, Jacoby GA (1986b) Properties of a novel carbenicillin-hydrolyzing beta-lactamase (CARB-4) specified by an IncP-2 plasmid from *Pseudomonas aeruginosa*. Antimicrob Agents Chemother 29:519–520
Philippon A, Joly B, Reynaud D, Paul G, Martel JL, Sirot D, Cluzel R, Nevot P (1986c) Characterization of a beta-lactamase from *Pasteurella multocida*. Ann Inst Pasteur Microbiol 137[A]:153–158
Pitton JS, Heitz M, Labia R (1978) Characterization of two new beta-lactamases from *Klebsiella* spp. Current Chemotherapy – 10th International Congress, pp 482–484
Pollock MR (1964) Stimulating and inhibiting antibodies for bacterial penicillinase. Immunology 7:707–723
Reid AJ, Amyes SGB (1986) Plasmid penicillin resistance in *Vibrio cholerae*: identification of new beta-lactamase SAR-1. Antimicrob Agents Chemother 30:245–247
Richmond MH (1965) Wild-type variants of exopenicillinase from *Staphylococcus aureus*. Biochem J 94:584–593
Rosdahl VT (1973) Naturally occurring constitutive beta-lactamase of novel serotype in *Staphylococcus aureus*. J Gen Microbiol 77:229–231
Roy C, Foz A, Segura C, Tirado M, Fuster C, Reig R (1983) Plasmid-determined beta-lactamases identified in a group of 204 ampicillin-resistant Enterobacteriaceae. J Antimicrob Chemother 12:507–510
Roy C, Segura C, Tirado M, Reig R, Hermida M, Teruel D, Foz A (1985) Frequency of plasmid-determined beta-lactamases in 680 consecutively isolated strains of *Enterobacteriaceae*. Eur J Clin Microbiol 4:146–147
Rubens CE, McNeill WF, Farrar WE Jr (1979) Evolution of multiple-antibiotic-resistance plasmids mediated by transposable plasmid deoxyribonucleic acid sequences. J Bacteriol 140:713–719
Rubin LG, Medeiros AA, Yolken RH, Moxon ER (1981) Ampicillin treatment failure of apparently beta-lactamase-negative *Haemophilus influenzae* type B meningitis due to novel beta-lactamase. Lancet II:1008–1010
Samraoui B, Sutton BJ, Todd RJ, Artymiuk PJ, et al. (1986) Tertiary structural similarity between a class A beta-lactamase and a penicillin-sensitive L-alanyl carboxypeptidase-transpeptidase. Nature 320:378–380
Sanders CC, Sanders WE Jr, Moland ES (1986) Characterization of beta-lactamases in situ on polyacrylamide gels. Antimicrob Agents Chemother 30:951–952
Sato K, Matsuura Y, Inoue M, Mitsuhashi S (1983) Properties of a new penicillinase type produced by *Bacteriodes fragilis*. Antimicrob Agents Chemother 22:579–584
Sawai T, Mitsuhashi S, Yamagishi S (1968) Comparison of beta-lactamases in gram-negative rod bacteria resistant to p-aminobenzylpenicillin. Jpn J Microbiol 12:423–434
Shah PM, Stille W (1983) *Escherichia coli* and *Klebsiella pneumoniae* strains more susceptible to cefoxitin than to third generation cephalosporins. J Antimicrob Chemother 11:597–601
Shaokat S, Ouellette M, Sirot D, Joly B, Cluzel R (1987) Spread of SHV-1 beta-lactamase in *Escherichia coli* isolated from fecal samples in Africa. Antimicrob Agents Chemother 31:943–945

Shlaes DM, Medeiros AA, Kron MA, Currie-McCumber C, Papa E, Vartian CV (1986) Novel plasmid-mediated beta-lactamase in members of the family *Enterobacteriaceae* from Ohio. Antimicrob Agents Chemother 30:220–224

Simpson IN, Harper PB, O'Callaghan CH (1980) Principal beta-lactamases responsible for resistance to beta-lactam antibiotics in urinary tract infections. Antimicrob Agents Chemother 17:929–936

Simpson IN, Plested SJ, Harper PB (1982) Investigation of the beta-lactamase stability of ceftazidime and eight other new cephalosporin antibiotics. J Antimicrob Chemother 9:357–368

Simpson IN, Plested SJ, Budin-Jones MJ, Lees J, Hedges RW, Jacoby GA (1983) Characterization of a novel plasmid-mediated beta-lactamase and its contribution to beta-lactam resistance in *Pseudomonas aeruginosa*. FEMS Microbiol Lett 19:23–27

Simpson IN, Knoth H, Plested SJ, HArper PB (1986) Qualitative and quantitative aspects of beta-lactamase production as mechanisms of beta-lactam resistance in a survey of clinical isolates from faecal samples. J Antimicrob Chemother 17:725–737

Sinclair MI, Holloway BW (1982) A chromosomally located transposon in *Pseudomonas aeruginosa*. J Bacteriol 151:569–579

Sirot J, Labia R, Thabaut A (1987a) *Klebsiella pneumoniae* strains more resistant to ceftazidime than to other third-generation cephalosporins. J Antimicrob Chemother 20:611–612

Sirot D, Sirot J, Labia R, et al. (1987b) Transferable resistance to third-generation cephalosporins in clinical isolates of *Klebsiella pneumoniae*: identification of CTX-1, a novel beta-lactamase. J Antimicrob Chemother 20:323–334

Sutcliffe JG (1978) Nucleotide sequence of the ampicillin resistance gene of *Escherichia coli* plasmid pBR322. Proc Natl Acad Sci USA 75:3737–3741

Sykes RB, Matthew M (1976) The beta-lactamases of gram-negative bacteria and their role in resistance to beta-lactam antibiotics. J Antimicrob Chemother 2:115–157

Sykes RB, Matthew M (1979) Detection, assay and immunology of beta-lactamases. In: Hamilton-Miller JMT, Smith JT (eds) Beta-lactamases. Academic Press, London, pp 17–49

Takahashi I, Tsukamoto K, Harada M, Sawai T (1983) Carbenicillin-hydrolyzing penicillinases of *Proteus mirabilis* and the PSE-type penicillinases of *Pseudomonas aeruginosa*. Microbiol Immunol 27:995–1004

Thabaut A, Philippon A, Meyran M (1985) Beta-lactamases of *Pseudomonas aeruginosa* and susceptibility against beta-lactam antibiotics. Chemioterapia IV:36–42

Thornsberry C, McDougal LK (1982) Ampicillin-resistant *Haemophilus influenzae*: incidence, mechanism, and detection. Postgrad Med 71:135–145

Tirado M, Roy C, Segura C, Reig R, Hermida M, Foz A (1986) Incidence of strains producing plasmid determined beta-lactamases among carbenicillin resistant *Pseudomonas aeruginosa*. J Antimicrob Chemother 18:453–458

Ubukata K, Yamashita N, Konno M (1985) Occurrence of a beta-lactam-inducible penicillin-binding protein in methicillin-resistant staphylococci. Antimicrob Agents Chemother 27:851–857

Vecoli C, Prevost FE, Ververis JJ, Medeiros AA, O'Leary GP Jr (1983) A comparison of polyacrylamide and agarose gel thin-layer isoelectric focusing for the characterization of beta-lactamase. Antimicrob Agents Chemother 24:186–189

Wang P-Z, Novick RP (1987) Nucleotide sequence and expression of the beta-lactamase gene from *Staphylococcus aureus* plasmid pI258 in *Escherichia coli*, *Bacillus subtilis*, and *Staphylococcus aureus*. J Bacteriol 169:1763–1766

Waxman DJ, Amanuma H, Strominger JL (1979) Mechanism of penicillin action: penicillin and substrate bind covalently to the same active site serine in two bacterial L-alanine carboxypeptidases. Proc Natl Acad Sci USA 76:2730–2734

Waxman DJ, Amanuma H, Strominger JL (1982) Amino acid sequence homologies between *Escherichia coli* penicillin-binding protein 5 and class A beta-lactamases. FEBS Lett 139:159–163

Whitaker S, Hajipieris P, Williams JD (1983) Distribution and type of beta-lactamase amongst 1000 gram-negative rod bacteria. Proc 13th Int Congr Chemother 89:10–11

Williams RJ, Livermore DM, Lindridge MA, Said AA, Williams JD (1984) Mechanisms of beta-lactam resistance in British isolates of *Pseudomonas aeruginosa*. J Med Microbiol 17:283–293

Yamamoto T, Tanaka M, Nohara C, Fukunaga Y, Yamagishi S (1981) Transposition of the oxacillin-hydrolyzing penicillinase gene. J Bacteriol 145:808–813

Yang YJ, Livermore DM, Jones CS (1985) LXA-1, a new plasmid determined beta-lactamase from enterobacteria. Abstr 2nd Eur Congr Clin Microbiol

Yocum RR, Waxman DJ, Rasmussen JR, Strominger JL (1979) Mechanism of penicillin action: penicillin and substrate bind covalently to the same active site serine in two bacterial L-alanine carboxypeptidases. Proc Natl Acad Sci USA 76:2730–2734

CHAPTER 6

The Chromosomal Beta-Lactamases

C. C. SANDERS

A. Introduction

Virtually all gram-negative bacteria studied to date produce a chromosomal beta-lactamase. Thus, it is not surprising that there is a great diversity among these enzymes in substrate profile, susceptibility to inhibitors, genetic control of expression and molecular makeup. Some enzymes have been studied extensively while others have been examined only superficially. Some appear to have great clinical relevance mediating resistance to a broad array of beta-lactam antibiotics. Others play little role in resistance or occur in organisms with little pathogenicity for humans. Many have been included in detailed general reviews on beta-lactamases (RICHMOND and SYKES 1973; SYKES and MATTHEW 1976; RICHMOND 1979; MITSUHASHI and INOUE 1981; HAMILTON-MILLER 1982; BUSH and SYKES 1984; MEDEIROS 1984) and others have been examined specifically in reviews concerning the inducible chromosomal enzymes (LIVERMORE 1987a; SANDERS 1987; SANDERS and SANDERS 1987). The genetic control mechanisms responsible for these enzymes have also been recently reviewed in this and other publications (LINDBERG and NORMARK 1986a; CHAMBERLAND, Chap. 7, this volume). Thus, the purpose of this chapter is to present a broad-based view of chromosomal beta-lactamases emphasizing the biochemical, physicochemical and molecular aspects as they are now known. The diverse nature of these enzymes will be presented and used in a multitiered classification system. Due to the very large number of different chromosomal enzymes known to exist and our uneven knowledge of them, this chapter will focus primarily on those enzymes of clinical importance that have been studied to the greatest extent. Thus, chromosomal beta-lactamases of gram-negative bacteria will be the major emphasis of this review.

B. General Characteristics

I. The Reaction Catalyzed

Regardless of the specific enzyme and substrate involved, the reaction catalyzed by all beta-lactamases is essentially the same.

$$\mathrm{ENZ} + \beta\mathrm{lac} \underset{1}{\rightleftarrows} \mathrm{ENZ} \cdot \beta\mathrm{lac} \underset{2}{\rightarrow} \mathrm{ENZ} - \beta\mathrm{lac} \underset{3}{\rightarrow} \mathrm{ENZ} + \mathrm{PROD}$$

In this reaction, ENZ represents the beta-lactamase, βlac represents the substrate drug and PROD represents the product of the reaction, i.e. inactivated drug. Two covalent bonds are broken and one is formed over the reaction sequence. In the first step a reversible, noncovalent enzyme/substrate intermediate, *ENZ·βlac*, is formed. In the second step, the beta-lactam bond is hydrolyzed and a new covalent bond between the enzyme and substrate is formed. Thus, there is an acyl-enzyme, *ENZ-βlac*, intermediate. The third step involves deacylation which regenerates active enzyme and hydrolyzed product. None of the substrate intermediates nor the product is biologically active. For most chromosomal beta-lactamases the rate limiting step is deacylation, step 3, while for most plasmid-mediated enzymes, step 2 is rate limiting (KNOTT-HUNZIKER et al. 1982b; EMANUEL et al. 1986). This difference became very important with the development of the newer so-called beta-lactamase stable cephalosporins and monobactams.

In vitro assays with many of the newer beta-lactam antibiotics indicated that these drugs were highly resistant to hydrolysis by chromosomal enzymes. Thus, it was very surprising to learn that high levels of certain chromosomal enzymes (primarily the cephalosporinases) found in various mutants conferred resistance to many of the newer drugs (SANDERS 1987). This resistance led to a series of hypotheses on how a beta-lactamase could mediate resistance to such poor substrate drugs. These included theories that, in the face of enzyme excess *in situ*, poor substrate drugs for which the chromosomal enzymes had high affinity would be "trapped" in inactive complexes either as *ENZ·βlac* (THEN and ANGEHRN 1982; GUTMANN and WILLIAMSON 1983; PHELPS et al. 1986; SANDERS and SANDERS 1986a) or as *ENZ-βlac* (MURAKAMI and YOSHIDA 1985; LIVERMORE 1987b). This would allow inactivated product to be slowly generated without having large concentrations of biologically active drug build up in the cell. Furthermore, the normally slow permeation of most beta-lactam drugs into the gram-negative cell readily augments the protection afforded by the enzyme so that slow hydrolysis (i.e. deacylation) of poor substrate drugs can be a very efficient mechanism of resistance (LIVERMORE 1985; VU and NIKAIDO 1985; NAYLER 1987; SANDERS 1987).

Thus it has become amply clear that resistance to poor substrate drugs can be mediated by a beta-lactamase as long as affinity for the drug is high and hydrolysis operates efficiently under the physiologic conditions present in the intact cell. Since in vitro assays with isolated beta-lactamases are usually not conducted under physiologic conditions, it is not surprising that in vitro hydrolysis (or lack thereof) of a substrate drug is often not an accurate predictor of a drug's activity against the intact bacterium.

II. Classification Schemes

A number of schemes have been proposed in an attempt to classify bacterial beta-lactamases (SYKES 1982). Some of these are based on kinetic and physicochemical characteristics of the enzymes (RICHMOND and SYKES 1973; SYKES and MATTHEW 1976; MITSUHASHI and INOUE 1981) while others are more molecular in their approach (AMBLER 1980; KNOTT-HUNZIKER et al. 1982b). Since each has attempted to classify all or most all beta-lactamases, it is not surprising that the chromosomal enzymes are generally poorly differentiated from each other in these schemes.

Table 1. Amino acid sequence around the active site serine of chromosomal beta-lactamases

Molecular class	Organism	Amino acid sequence	Reference
A	*Bacillus licheniformis* 749/C	Phe-Ala-**Phe**-**Ala**-Ser*-Thr-**Ile**-Lys	AMBLER (1980)
	Bacillus cereus 569/H(βI)	Phe-Ala-**Phe**-**Ala**-Ser-Thr-**Tyr**-Lys	AMBLER (1980)
	Klebsiella aerogenes 1082E	Phe-Ala-**Met**-**Asn**-Ser-Thr-**Ser**-Lys	EMANUEL et al. (1986)
	Klebsiella pneumoniae SC10436	Phe-Ala-**Met**-**Cys**-Ser-Thr-**Ser**-Lys	JORIS et al. (1987)
C	*Escherichia coli* K12	Thr-Leu-Phe-Glu-Leu-Gly-Ser-Val-Ser-Lys	KNOTT-HUNZIKER et al. (1982a)
	Citrobacter freundii OS60	Thr-Leu-Phe-Glu-Leu-Gly-Ser-Val-Ser-Lys	LINDBERG and NORMARK (1986b)
	Pseudomonas aeruginosa 1822S/H	Thr-Leu-Phe-Glu-**Ile**-Gly-Ser-Val-Ser-Lys	KNOTT-HUNZIKER et al. (1982a)
	Enterobacter cloacae P99	Thr-Leu-Phe-Glu-Leu-Gly-Ser-**Ile**-Ser-Lys	JORIS et al. (1984)
	Serratia marcescens SC8247	Thr-Leu-Phe-Glu-**Val**-Gly-Ser-**Leu**-Ser-Lys	JORIS et al. (1986)

* Active site serine at position 70

In the scheme of RICHMOND and SYKES (1973), the chromosomal beta-lactamases comprised three of five classes. Class I included the chromosomal cephalosporinases, most of which were inducible; class II included the extremely rare chromosomal penicillinases; and class IV included the constitutive chromosomal broad-spectrum enzymes. In the molecular classification of AMBLER (1980) as extended by KNOTT-HUNZIKER et al. (1982 b), all of the chromosomal cephalosporinases of gram-negative bacteria studied initially fell into class C. This class was comprised of enzymes with serine in their active site which shared a high degree of amino acid sequence homology among class members around the active site (Table 1). Among gram-positive bacteria, the chromosomal beta-lactamase of *Bacillus licheniformis* and *Bacillus cereus* (I) belonged to molecular class A – a second group of serine containing enzymes showing a high degree of homology around the active site (Table 1). Molecular class B had but a single representative, the chromosomal metalloenzyme of *Bacillus cereus* (II).

The chromosomal enzymes were separated into two groups by MITSUHASHI and INOUE (1981) based primarily upon substrate profile. These were the cephalosporinases (CSase) and the cefuroximases (CXase) both groups of which contained inducible and constitutively expressed enzymes. Many of the CSases and CXases have been referred to as "species specific" enzymes since antisera directed against one rarely show any cross-reactivity with another chromosomal enzyme even from strains within the same genus (FUJII-KURIYAMA et al. 1977; OHYA et al. 1980; HIRAI et al. 1981; MITSUHASHI and INOUE 1981; MURATA et al. 1981; TAJIMA et al. 1981; TODA et al. 1981; TAJIMA et al. 1982). The genetic relatedness of the chromosomal enzymes within the same species was also highlighted by the work of MATTHEW and HARRIS (1976), who showed a high correlation between the isoelectric point (pI) of such enzymes and bacterial taxonomy. Within the same species there was an extremely limited distribution of pIs while much greater diversity was observed between species or genera.

All in all, previous classification schemes have served to identify many important characteristics of chromosomal beta-lactamases. However, they by necessity have been too general to allow highly specific distinctions between the various chromosomal enzymes. The ever growing list of clinically important chromosomal beta-lactamases requires that these enzymes be examined in detail separately from their plasmid-mediated counterparts. To begin such an examination, it is easiest to divide the chromosomal enyzmes into four major groups: (1) cephalosporinases, (2) oxyiminocephalosporinases, (3) penicillinases, and (4) broad spectrum beta-lactamases. The first group comprises by far the most commonly encountered chromosomal enzymes.

C. Cephalosporinases

I. Inducible Cephalosporinases

Many different gram-negative bacteria produce inducible cephalosporinases (RICHMOND and SYKES 1973; SYKES and MATTHEW 1976; MITSUHASHI and INOUE 1981; SANDERS 1987). The most thoroughly studied are those produced by *Enterobacter cloacae*, *Citrobacter freundii*, *Serratia mercescens* and *Pseudomonas aerugi-*

nosa. The amino acid sequence around the active site serine has been determined for each of these enzymes which belong to molecular class C (KNOTT-HUNZIKER et al. 1982a; JORIS et al. 1984; JORIS et al. 1986; LINDBERG and NORMARK 1986b). These enzymes, although produced by widely divergent genera, show almost identical amino acid sequences around the active site serine (Table 1). Inducible cephalosporinases similar to these are also produced by other species of *Enterobacter* and *Serratia* (SYKES and MATTHEW 1976) *Morganella morganii* (FUJII-KURIYAMA et al. 1977; MITSUHASHI and INOUE 1981; TODA et al. 1981) *Proteus (Providencia) rettgeri* (MATSUURA et al. 1980; OHYA et al. 1980; LABIA 1982), *Proteus inconstans* (*Providencia stuartii*, OHYA et al. 1980) and *Chromobacterium violaceum* (FARRAR and O'DELL 1976a).

1. General Characteristics

Although inducible cephalosporinases are produced by different genera of bacteria, they share many general characteristics. As the name implies, they hydrolyze the cephalosporins five to fifty times as rapidly as benzylpenicillin (SYKES and MATTHEW 1976). Although they do not rapidly hydrolyze the newer cephalosporins, cephamycins, monobactams or carbenicillin, they nonetheless mediate resistance to these drugs once mutation leading to high intracellular enzyme levels has occurred (SANDERS 1987; see Sect. B.I above). The inducible cephalosporinases are inhibited by cloxacillin, iodine, Hg^{2+} but not parachloromercuribenzoate (pCMB), clavulanic acid or sulbactam (RICHMOND and SYKES 1973; SYKES and MATTHEW 1976; MINAMI et al. 1980a; TAJIMA et al. 1980; MURATA et al. 1981; TAJIMA et al. 1981). They generally have alkaline pIs and molecular weights between 25000 and 40000 (RICHMOND and SYKES 1973; SYKES and MATTHEW 1976; MITSUHASHI and INOUE 1981).

2. Induction/Derepression

The molecular mechanism responsible for the induction of chromosomal cephalosporinases has not been delineated. Compounds capable of inducing these enzymes include both non-specific (metabolic) and specific beta-lactam inducers (SANDERS 1987). Only the latter will be considered here. After exposure to beta-lactam inducers, enzyme levels rise very rapidly and reach their peak in 1–2 hours (NORDSTRÖM and SYKES 1974; MINAMI et al. 1980a; MITSUHASHI and INOUE 1981; GOOTZ and SANDERS 1983; MINAMI et al. 1983; OKONOGI et al. 1985). Levels remain elevated as long as the inducer persists in the environment with its beta-lactam ring intact. Physical removal or enzymatic hydrolysis of the beta-lactam inducer is followed by a rapid decline to basal (uninduced) enzyme levels. In *Enterobacter cloacae*, induction is not subject to catabolite repression by glucose and is unaffected by exogenous cyclic AMP (GOOTZ and SANDERS 1983). Cells in lag or mid logarithmic phase respond to inducers while stationary phase cells do not (MITSUHASHI and INOUE 1981; ARONOFF and SHALES 1987). Induction can be prevented by inhibitors of protein or RNA synthesis (NORDSTRÖM and SYKES 1974; GOOTZ and SANDERS 1983), suggesting that new protein must be synthesized for induction to occur. In certain wild type and mutant strains induction shows thermosensitivity (SAWAI et al. 1977; GOOTZ et al. 1982; CURTIS et al. 1987). Genetic studies indicate that at least two regulatory genes *ampR* and *ampD* are required for induction to occur (LINDBERG and NORMARK 1986a; LIVERMORE 1987a). The precise role of the proteins encoded by these genes in the induction process is unknown but they appear to exert both positive (activator) and negative (repressor) effects (LINDBERG and NORMARK 1986a; CURTIS et al. 1987). From the data gathered to date, it appears that induction of chromosomal cephalosporinases by beta-lactam compounds results from a direct effect of the drugs themselves interacting with the *ampR* and/or *ampD* loci or their products.

The ability of different beta-lactams to function as inducers of chromosomal cephalosporinases is highly variable and has been the subject of numerous investigations (GARBER and FRIEDMAN 1970; MINAMI et al. 1980c; MITSUHASHI and INOUE 1981; GOOTZ and SANDERS 1983; MINAMI et al. 1983; OKONOGI et al. 1985; MOOSDEEN et al. 1986; SANDERS and SANDERS 1986b; ARONOFF and SHLAES 1987) and has been reviewed recently (SANDERS 1987). Certain beta-lactams are excellent inducers regardless of the organism examined or the concentration of inducer. These include the cephamycins like cefoxitin and cefmetazole, imipenem, ampicillin, 6-amino-penicillanic acid and benzylpenicillin. Other compounds are highly variable inducers. Some induce only when tested at very high, superinhibitory concentrations while others appear almost species or strain specific in their inducer activity. Most of the cephalosporins, monobactams, ureidopenicillins and beta-lactamase inhibitors like clavulanic acid fall into these latter two categories. Thus, only through direct testing can the inducer potential of a beta-lactam for any strain be properly assessed. One such test devised by CURTIS et al. (1986) involves the determination of minimal inhibitory concentrations (MICs) for beta-lactams against a wild type strain possessing an inducible enzyme and two mutants obtained from it. One mutant produces only basal levels of enzyme equivalent to the wild type but is not inducible. The second mutant is stably derepressed for enzyme production, expressing enzyme at levels equivalent to the wild type following induction. If a beta-lactam is a poor inducer, MICs for the wild type and basal mutant will be similar since the beta-lactam will not elevate enzyme levels in the former. However, if a beta-lactam is an efficient inducer, MICs for the wild type will be similar to the derepressed mutant and higher than the MIC for the basal mutant. Such a result reflects the elevated enzyme levels in the wild type due to the inducer activity of the drug. Using this assay system CURTIS et al. (1986) showed the aminothiazolyl-oxime beta-lactams, ureidopenicillins and cefoperazone were generally poor inducers; cefazolin, cefamandole and cefuroxime were variable inducers; and the cephamycins were generally good inducers.

Induction is but one way in which levels of chromosomal cephalosporinases can become elevated. The second involves mutation of the wild type to the stably derepressed state. Such a mutation occurs at a frequency of 10^{-6} to 10^{-9} (FINDELL and SHERRIS 1976; GOOTZ et al. 1982; DEL ROSARIO VALENCIA et al. 1984; GOOTZ et al. 1984; CURTIS et al. 1986; GATES et al. 1986; SHANNON and PHILLIPS 1986; BUSCHER et al. 1987; CULLMANN et al. 1987). For Enterobacteriaceae, a single mutation usually leads to complete derepression (i.e. constitutive expression) while in *Pseudomonas aeruginosa* two mutations are required (GATES et al. 1986).

Once mutation to the stably derepressed state occurs, resistance to multiple beta-lactam antibiotics is expressed (SYKES and MATTHEW 1976; SAWAI et al. 1981; GOOTZ et al. 1982; SANDERS et al. 1982; BRYAN et al. 1984; DEL ROSARIO VALENCIA et al. 1984; GOOTZ et al. 1984; CURTIS et al. 1986; ENG et al. 1986; SANDERS and SANDERS 1986b; SHANNON and PHILLIPS 1986; ASHBY et al. 1987; BÜSCHER et al. 1987; LIVERMORE and YANG 1987). These include not only the older penicillins and cephalosporins, which are good substrates for the enzymes, but also the newer cephalosporins, cephamycins and monobactams, which are relatively poor substrates. Among the beta-lactams, only amdinocillin, imipenem and related compounds are not resisted. The mechanism by which this multiple beta-lactam resistance occurs in the presence of very high enzyme levels resultant from derepression has been discussed in Sect. B.I.

Mutation to the stably derepressed state is of great clinical importance (SANDERS and SANDERS 1987). It has been responsible for the emergence of multiple beta-lactam resistance during therapy with the newer cephalosporins, monobactams, and some penicillins. When this occurs, patients often relapse or fail therapy completely. Retreatment of such patients is complicated since therapeutic alternatives almost always involve non-beta-lactam agents and drug combinations. Among patients at risk (i.e. those infected with an organism possessing an inducible beta-lactamase) emergence of resistance and therapeutic failures occur in 10% to 50% of patients treated with one of the newer cephalosporins (SANDERS and SANDERS 1987).

The production of very large quantities of chromosomal cephalosporinase after mutation to the stably derepressed state has one notable positive attribute. It allows the easy recovery of large amounts of enzyme for biochemical and physicochemical studies. Thus, most of the specific characteristics of chromosomal cephalosporinases have been obtained in studies utilizing enzymes recovered from stably derepressed mutants.

3. The Enzymes

The chromosomal cephalosporinase of *Enterobacter cloacae* is one of the most widely studied beta-lactamase of gram-negative bacteria. This is perhaps due to the fact that the P99 enzyme reported by FLEMING et al. (1963), in what was probably a derepressed mutant of *Enterobacter cloacae*, was the first cephalosporinase ever described. HENNESSEY (1967) was the first to describe the normally inducible expression of the enzyme in this species. Over the last twenty years, the chromosomal cephalosporinases from various strains of *Enterobacter cloacae* have been purified and their biochemical and physicochemical properties described (HENNESSEY and RICHMOND 1968; MARSHALL et al. 1972; ROSS and BOULTON 1973; MINAMI et al. 1980a; BUSH et al. 1982; LABIA 1982; SAWAI et al. 1982; SEEBERG et al. 1983; OKONOGI et al. 1985). From comparisons of pIs, there appear to be two and possibly three subgroups of enzymes (SEEBERG et al. 1983). Most enzymes studied to date possess pIs of 7.8 (subgroup B) or 8.8 (subgroup A). A few have pIs of 8.3–8.4 (subgroup C). Enzymes from strains P99 and 214 are examples of subgroup B (FLEMING et al. 1963; HENNESSEY 1967), those from strains 208 and 1194E are examples of subgroup A (SEEBERG et al. 1983; GUERIN et al. 1986), and

Table 2. Properties of various chromosomal cephalosporinases produced by specific strains of bacteria[a]

Strain	Relative rate of hydrolysis[b]										K_i (μ*M*)		MWt (k)	pI	Class[c]	Reference[d]
	CFL	CF	CXM	CTX	CFX	MOX	AZT	IMI	PEN	CLOX	CLOX	CLAV				
Cephalosporinases																
Enterobacter cloacae GN7471	100	190	<1	<1	<1	<1			10		0.02	>100	44	8.4	I/C	MINAMI et al. (1980a)
Pseudomonas aeruginosa GN10362	100	450	<1	<1	<1	<1			30		0.006	>100	37	8.7	I/C	MURATA et al. (1981)
Citrobacter freundii GN7391	100	130	<1	<1	<1	<1			5		0.006	>100	37	8.6	I/C	TAJIMA et al. (1980)
Serratia marcescens GN10857	100	90	<1	<1	<1	<1			5		0.001	>100	38	8.9	I/C	MITSUHASHI and INOUE (1981)
Escherichia coli GN5482	100	270	<1	<1	<1	<1			60		0.007	>100	39	8.7	I/C	MINAMI et al. (1980b)
Oxyiminocephalosporinases																
Proteus vulgaris GN7919	100	180	1140	80	<1	<1	20	<1	20		1.3	1.1	30	8.8	I	MITSUHASHI and INOUE (1981)
Pseudomonas capacia GN11164	100	320	240	170	<1	<1	20	<1	160		3.4	1.7	24	9.3	I	HIRAI et al. (1980)
Bacteroides fragilis GN11477	100	50	40	20	<1	<1	4	<1	5		0.4	0.2	32	5.2	I	SATO et al. (1983)
Penicillinase																
Alkaligenes faecalis GN14061[e]	<1	<1	<1	<1	<1		<1	<1	100	70	–	>100	29	5.9		FUJII et al. (1985a)
Broad spectrum enzymes																
a) Metalloenzymes																
Pseudomonas maltophilia GN12873	100		500	20		1	<1	400	1670		–	>100	32	6.9	E?	SAINO et al. (1982)
Flavobacterium odoratum GN14053	100	690	2750	1100	80	80	<1	1060	210		–	>100	26	5.8		SATO et al. (1985)
Legionella gormanii ATCC 33297	100	160	90	50	10	90	<1	5	7	20	–	>100	25	10.5		FUJII et al. (1986)
Bacteroides fragilis G 237	100	110	70	80	50	260	<1	470	260	320	–	>100	26	4.8		YOTSUJI et al. (1983)
b) *Klebsiella enzymes*																
Klebsiella oxytoca GN10650	100	120	20	5	<1	1	10		200	20	–	0.5	27	5.3		INOUE et al. (1983)
Klebsiella pneumoniae SC10436	100	50	20	5	<1	1	60	<1	280	30		0.2[f]	27	6.5	IV/A	BUSH et al. (1982); BUSH (unpublished results)

[a] Strains were selected on the basis of the largest amount of data available

[b] Hydrolysis of cephaloridine placed at 100. All other rates are relative to cephaloridine. A value of <1 indicates that no hydrolysis was observed under the conditions of the test. Drug names: cephaloridine (CFL), cephalothin (CF), cefuroxime (CXM), cefotaxime (CTX), cefoxitin (CFX), moxalactam (MOX), aztreonam (AZT), imipenem (IMI), penicillin G (PEN), cloxacillin (CLOX), clavulanic acid (CLAV)

[c] RICHMOND and SYKES class indicated by Roman numeral, molecular class indicated by letter

[d] Original reference describing the strain. Some data are also from other references listed in the text

[e] For relative rate of hydrolysis, hydrolysis of penicillin G is 100

[f] I

that from strain GN7471 is an example of subgroup C (MINAMI et al. 1980a). Observed molecular weights for purified enzymes have ranged from 35000 to 44000. The biochemical and physical characteristics of the GN7471 enzyme are listed in Table 2 as an example of the *Enterobacter cloacae* cephalosporinase. Among the *Enterobacter cloacae* cephalosporinases, the P99 enzyme has been most extensively studied. Its amino acid composition, N-terminal sequence and active site sequence have been determined (HENNESSEY and RICHMOND 1968; JORIS et al. 1984; JORIS et al. 1985). X-ray crystallography of the P99 enzyme (CHARLIER et al. 1983) shows orthorhombic mmm Laue symmetry and space group $P2_12_12$ with unit cell dimensions $a = 77.4$ Å, $b = 69.4$ Å and $c = 63.6$ Å. There is one molecule of molecular weight 39000 in the asymmetric unit.

The chromosomal cephalosporinase of *Pseudomonas aeruginosa* is often called the Sabath/Abraham enzyme after the investigators who first described it (SABATH and ABRAHAM 1964; SABATH et al. 1965). The biochemical and physical properties of this enzyme have been examined by a number of investigators (SABATH et al. 1965; FLETT et al. 1976; LABIA et al. 1976b; FURTH 1979; MURATA et al. 1981; BERKS et al. 1982). Results from studies with strain GN10362 are listed in Table 2. As with *Enterobacter cloacae*, the enzymes in *Pseudomonas aeruginosa* show a limited discrete range of pIs. MATTHEW and HARRIS (1976) listed four pIs of 8.15, 7.95, 7.5 and 7.2 representing 8%, 65%, 24% and 2% respectively of 49 strains studied. In a more recent study (GATES and SANDERS, unpublished data) four distinct pIs of 9.6, 9.2, 8.7 and 8.4 representing 11%, 37%, 22% and 10% respectively of 70 strains studied were also noted. Although the pIs varied approximately 1.2 units between the two studies (which was probably due to methodologic differences) there does appear to be four distinct subgroups of cephalosporinases from *Pseudomonas aeruginosa* based upon pI alone. Interestingly, enzymes with multiple discrete pIs can also be observed in a single strain following mutation to the stably derepressed state (GATES et al. 1986). It is possible that these different pIs represent minor amino acid sequence variations in the structural genes or slight differences in post-translational processing. Nevertheless, the similarities in the discrete pIs observed among many strains and within the same strain is surprising.

Among the other inducible cephalosporinases, various properties of the enzymes produced by *Citrobacter freundii* (SYKES and MATTHEW 1976; TAJIMA et al. 1980; MITSUHASHI and INOUE 1981; SAWAI et al. 1982; LINDBERG and NORMARK 1986b) and *Serratia marcescens* (FARRAR and O'DELL 1976b; SYKES and MATTHEW 1976; MITSUHASHI and INOUE 1981; TAJIMA et al. 1981; SAWAI et al. 1982; JORIS et al. 1986) have been described. This includes the amino acid composition and sequence around the active site. Examples of enzymes from each of these organisms are shown in Table 2.

II. Constitutive Cephalosporinase

Among the Enterobacteriaceae that do not produce an inducible cephalosporinase, virtually every species studied to date possesses a cephalosporinase that is expressed constitutively at a very low level (MATTHEW and HARRIS 1976; BERGSTRÖM et al. 1982). The enzyme produced by *Escherichia coli* is the most extensively studied and will be considered here as the prototype for this type of cephalosporinase.

Although the expression of the *Escherichia coli* enzyme is quite different from those discussed previously, all of the chromosomal cephalosporinases have a common evolutionary origin. This has been demonstrated in hybridization studies with a probe prepared from *ampC*, the structural gene for the *Escherichia coli* enzyme (BERGSTRÖM et al. 1982). The *Escherichia coli* enzyme, however, is normally not involved in clinically significant resistance to beta-lactam antibiotics since it is usually expressed at a very low level. Nevertheless, mutations causing the production of elevated enzyme levels have been described and these can lead to multiple beta-lactam resistance similar to that seen in derepressed mutants of *Enterobacter cloacae* (KABINS et al. 1966; BERGSTRÖM and NORMARK 1979; TAKAHASHI et al. 1980; CHABBERT and JAFFÉ 1982; LABIA et al. 1986; LINDBERG and NORMARK 1986a). Since the kinetic properties of the *Escherichia coli* enzyme are very similar to those of the inducible cephalosporinases (Table 2), resistance to both good and poor substrates is probably mediated by the same mechanisms as described above. However, the mutations leading to elevated enzyme levels in *Escherichia coli* are very different due to the lack of a complex control system in this organism (LINDBERG and NORMARK 1986a).

The biochemical and physicochemical properties of the *Escherichia coli* cephalosporinase have been extensively studied. The substrate profile is very similar to that of the inducible cephalosporinases with cephalothin hydrolyzed more rapidly than penicillin G. The newer cephalosporins, cephamycins and monobactams are hydrolyzed very poorly if at all under standard assay conditions (LABIA et al. 1976a; SYKES and MATTHEW 1976; MINAMI et al. 1980b; TAKAHASHI et al. 1980; MITSUHASHI and INOUE 1981; SAWAI et al. 1982). The *Escherichia coli* enzyme is sensitive to inhibition by cloxacillin, iodine and Hg^{2+}, but not by pCMB clavulanic acid or sulbactam. Alkaline pIs between 8.7 and 9.3 have been reported while molecular weights vary from 32000 to 39000. The kinetic and physicochemical properties of the cephalosporinase from strain GN5482 are listed in Table 2. For *Escherichia coli* K12, the amino acid sequence around the active site is identical to that for *Citrobacter freundii* OS60 (KNOTT-HUNZIKER et al. 1982a, Table 1). The entire 1536 nucleotide sequence of the *ampC* gene of strain K12 has also been determined and found to code for a protein of 377 amino acids of which the first 19 form a signal peptide (JAURIN and GRUNDSTRÖM 1981). The molecular weight of the mature enzyme is 39600 and its entire amino acid sequence has been deduced from its nucleotide sequence (JAURIN and GRUNDSTRÖM 1981).

D. Oxyiminocephalosporinases

I. Inducible Oxyiminocephalosporinases

These enzymes are found in *Proteus vulgaris* (HIRAI et al. 1981; LABIA et al. 1981; MATSUBARA et al. 1981; MITSUHASHI and INOUE 1981; TAJIMA et al. 1982; MINAMI et al. 1983; MITSUHASHI 1985; OKONOGI et al. 1986) and its indole-negative counterpart *Proteus penneri* (GRACE et al. 1986; GRACE et al. 1987), *Pseudomonas ce-*

pacia (HIRAI et al. 1980; HIRAI et al. 1981; MITSUHASHI and INOUE 1981; MITSUHASHI 1985), *Pseudomonas maltophilia* (L-2 enzyme, SAINO et al. 1982; SAINO et al. 1984) and *Pseudomonas pseudomallei* (LIVERMORE et al. 1987). They have been referred to in the past as cefuroximases (MITSUHASHI and INOUE 1981) and belong to Richmond and Sykes class I enzymes (RICHMOND and SYKES 1973; SYKES and MATTHEW 1976). Although the amino acid composition of the enzyme from *Proteus vulgaris* 1427 has been ascertained (TAJIMA et al. 1982), the sequence around the active site has not been determined for any of the oxyiminocephalosporinases. Thus, the molecular class to which they belong is unknown.

The oxyiminocephalosporinases have the same substrate profile as the cephalosporinases but they also hydrolyze aztreonam and the oxyiminocephalosporins like cefuroxime and cefotaxime quite readily. They do not hydrolyze the cephamycins, moxalactam, or imipenem. The inhibitor profile of the oxyiminocephalosporinases is quite different from that of the cephalosporinases. The oxyiminocephalosporinases are less susceptible to inhibition by cloxacillin but are more susceptible to inhibition by clavulanic acid, sulbactam and pCMB (HIRAI et al. 1980; MATSUBARA et al. 1981; MITSUHASHI and INOUE 1981; TAJIMA et al. 1982; SAINO et al. 1984; MITSUHASHI 1985; GRACE et al. 1987; LIVERMORE et al. 1987). They are also inhibited by iodine and Hg^{2+}. The molecular weight of oxyiminocephalosporinases tends to be lower than those of cephalosporinases, ranging from 24000 to 30000 (HIRAI et al. 1980; MATSUBARA et al. 1981; TAJIMA et al. 1982; SAINO et al. 1984; MITSUHASHI 1985; GRACE et al. 1986; LIVERMORE et al. 1987). Like the cephalosporinases, the inducible oxyiminocephalosporinases generally have alkaline pIs (MITSUHASHI 1985). The properties of two inducible oxyiminocephalosporinases are shown in Table 2.

Induction of the oxyiminocephalosporinases, although less well studied, proceeds similarly to that described previously for the cephalosporinases. Specific induction by beta-lactam compounds has been examined in *Proteus vulgaris* (MITSUHASHI and INOUE 1981; MINAMI et al. 1983; OKONOGI et al. 1986). Results have been fairly similar to those obtained in tests with organisms possessing inducible cephalosporinases; i.e. cephamycins, imipenem, 6-aminopenicillanic acid, benzylpenicillin, and ampicillin are good inducers. However, cefmenoxime at high concentrations is also a good inducer for *Proteus vulgaris* (IKEDA et al. 1987). This results in a paradoxical effect of no growth in low concentrations but good growth in high concentrations during MIC determinations due to the induction of enzyme under the latter but not former conditions. Elevated enzyme levels can also occur via mutation to the stably derepressed state which leads to multiple beta-lactam resistance similar to that observed with the cephalosporinases (SAWAI et al. 1981; CHIESA et al. 1986). However, since the enzymes are sensitive to inhibition by clavulanic acid, resistance mediated by them can be counteracted by the inclusion of this beta-lactamase inhibitor.

II. Constitutive Oxyiminocephalosporinases

Certain members of the *Bacteroides fragilis* group produce the most well characterized constitutive oxyiminocephalosporinases (NORD 1986). These include *Bacteroides fragilis*, *Bacteroides thetaiotaomicron* and *Bacteroides vulgatus* (ANDER-

SON and SYKES 1973; DELBENE and FARRAR 1973; OLSSON et al. 1976; LEUNG and WILLIAMS 1978; PECHÈRE et al. 1980; SATO et al. 1980; MISUHASHI and Inoue 1981; Timewell et al. 1981; SIMPSON et al. 1982; SATO et al. 1983; MITSUHASHI 1985; ELEY and GREENWOOD 1986).

The substrate profiles of these enzymes are similar to those of the inducible oxyiminocephalosporinases; however, they do not hydrolyze cefotaxime or penicillin as readily as other oxyiminocephalosporinases (MITSUHASHI and INOUE 1981; SATO et al. 1983; MITSUHASHI 1985). Inhibitor profiles are similar as they are susceptible to inhibition by pCMB, clavulanic acid, sulbactam, iodine and Hg^{2+}. They are less susceptible to inhibition by cloxacillin than the cephalosporinases (OLSSON et al. 1976; SATO et al. 1980; MITSUHASHI and INOUE 1981; SIMPSON et al. 1982; SATO et al. 1983; MITSUHASHI 1985; NORD 1986). The molecular weight of these enzymes range from 29000 to 31000 and pIs are in the acidic range of 4.6–5.4 (SIMPSON et al. 1982; NORD 1986). They have been previously classified as Richmond and Sykes class I enzymes (SYKES and MATTHEW 1976). Antisera made against the oxyiminocephalosporinase of any one of these three species within the *Bacteroides fragilis* group cross-react with enzymes of the other two species (SATO et al. 1983).

The enzyme is produced primarily during the logarithmic phase of growth and unlike many other gram-negative enzymes is released to a large extent into the surrounding medium (OLSSON et al. 1976; PECHÈRE et al. 1980; SATO et al. 1983). These enzymes are responsible for much of the beta-lactam resistance commonly observed in the *Bacteroides fragilis* group. An example of the oxyiminocephalosporinase of *Bacteroides fragilis* is shown in Table 2.

E. Penicillinases

Eleven years ago, SYKES and MATTHEW (1976) noted that only four strains of gram-negative bacteria had ever been reported to produce chromosomally mediated penicillinase. These had been designated class II enzymes by RICHMOND and SYKES (1973). However, SYKES and MATTHEW (1976) noted that three of the four were perhaps on plasmids since failure to transfer the resistance did not rule out a plasmid location. Only the Dalgleish enzyme from *Pseudomonas aeruginosa* and an inducible penicillinase from *Pseudomonas thomasii* were considered to be true examples of chromosomal penicillinases (SYKES and MATTHEW 1976). However, since that review was written, the Dalgleish enzyme has been shown to be on a plasmid specifying what is now referred to as the PSE-4 beta-lactamase (MATTHEW 1979). Thus, penicillinases that are unequivocally specified by chromosomal genes are indeed very rare.

To date, very few enzymes have been described that are likely candidates for chromosomal penicillinases. One has been described in *Alkaligenes faecalis* (FUJII et al. 1985). Although a chromosomal location has not been proven for this enzyme, its inducible nature suggests a chromosomal location. This inducible penicillinase has been purified from *Alkaligenes faecalis* GN14061. It has a molecular weight of 29000 and pI of 5.9. It hydrolyzes the penicillins including cloxacillin but does not hydrolyze any cephalosporin, aztreonam or imipenem

(Table 2). It is not inhibited by clavulanic acid or sulbactam but is inhibited by iodine and Hg^{2+}. The role played by this enzyme in the resistance of *Alkaligenes faecalis* to beta-lactam drugs is unknown. Its substrate profile is not predictive of susceptibility or resistance to various beta-lactam drugs (FUJII et al. 1985).

F. Broad-Spectrum Beta-Lactamases

I. Metalloenzymes

The first chromosomally specified metalloenzyme ever described was the type II enzyme of *Bacillus cereus* (KUWABARA and ABRAHAM 1967), which belongs to molecular class B (AMBLER 1980). In 1982 a second metalloenzyme, designated L-1, was described in a strain of *Pseudomonas maltophilia* (SAINO et al. 1982). This zinc-requiring enzyme is inducible, exists as a tetramer of 123000 molecular weight comprised of four 31600 subunits (SAINO et al. 1982; BICKNELL et al. 1985). The L-1 enzyme has a very broad substrate profile hydrolyzing the penicillins including cloxacillin, the cephalosporins and imipenem (Table 2). It does not hydrolyze aztreonam or moxalactam appreciably (SAINO et al. 1982; MITSUHASHI 1985). Its activity is inhibited by EDTA, iodine and Hg^{2+} but not by clavulamic acid or pCMB. The N-terminal amino acid sequence of the L-1 enzyme of *Pseudomonas maltophilia* has been determined and shows no similarity to that of beta-lactamase II from *Bacillus cereus* (BICKNELL et al. 1985). It also differs from beta-lactamase II in metal content, thiol content and activity, substrate profile and many other properties (BICKNELL et al. 1985). Thus, this L-1 enzyme may well belong to a new molecular class (E?). It does appear to be responsible for much of the beta-lactam resistance in *Pseudomonas maltophilia* especially resistance to imipenem (SAINO et al. 1982).

Several other imipenem-hydrolyzing enzymes have been described which may also be chromosomal metalloenzymes. These include beta-lactamases produced by *Flavobacterium odoratum* (SATO et al. 1985; MITSUHASHI 1985), *Legionella gormanii* (MITSUHASHI 1985; FUJII et al. 1986) and *Bacteroides fragilis* (YOTSUJI et al. 1983; MITSUHASHI 1985; CUCHURAL et al. 1986). Each of these enzymes have been shown either to require zinc or to be sensitive to inhibition by EDTA. They are very broad spectrum enzymes hydrolyzing virtually every major group of beta-lactam except aztreonam (Table 2). They are generally not sensitive to inhibition by clavulanic acid but are inhibited by iodine, Hg^{2+} and pCMB. The multiple beta-lactam resistance of the producer organisms is thought to be due, in large part, to the production of these enzymes. Proof of their chromosomal location and strict requirement for a metal cofactor await further study.

II. Enzymes from *Klebsiella*

A number of broad spectrum enzymes have been isolated from species of *Klebsiella* which are responsible for resistance to various beta-lactam antibiotics in this genus. These include strains of *Klebsiella aerogenes* (HAMILTON-MILLER 1963; MARSHALL et al. 1972; ROSS and BOULTON 1973; MATTHEW and HARRIS 1976;

SYKES and MATTHEW 1976; EMANUEL et al. 1986), *Klebsiella pneumoniae* (SAWAI et al. 1973; SYKES and MATTHEW 1976; BUSH et al. 1982; SYKES et al. 1982; JORIS et al. 1987) and *Klebsiella oxytoca* (HART and PERCIVAL 1982; INOUE et al. 1983; MITSUHASHI 1985; LABIA et al. 1986).

The similarities among these enzymes is not surprising since *Klebsiella aerogenes* is not a separate species but a biogroup of *Klebsiella pneumoniae* and *Klebsiella oxytoca* varies from *Klebsiella pneumoniae* only in its ability to produce indole (BRENNER 1984). Thus, all three "species" are very closely related. In fact, *Klebsiella aerogenes* 1082E, one of the most thoroughly examined strains, is indole positive (MATTHEW and HARRIS 1976) as is *Klebsiella pneumoniae* SC10436 (K. BUSH, personal communication). Thus, it would probably be more appropriate today to refer to these strains as *Klebsiella oxytoca*.

The chromosomal beta-lactamases produced by *Klebsiella* have been designated by Richmond and Sykes as class IV enzymes (RICHMOND and SYKES 1973; SYKES and MATTHEW 1976) and are often referred to as K1 enzymes (BUSH et al. 1982; SYKES et al. 1982; EMANUEL et al. 1986; JORIS et al. 1987). The amino acid sequence around the active site has been determined for the enzymes produced by *Klebsiella aerogenes* 1082E (EMANUEL et al. 1986) and *Klebsiella pneumoniae* SC10436 (JORIS et al. 1987). The two sequences are very similar to each other and most resemble that of enzymes belonging to molecular class A (Table 1). Like class A enzymes, hydrolysis of the beta-lactam bond is the rate limiting step in the reaction sequence (EMANUEL et al. 1986).

The broad spectrum beta-lactamases of *Klebsiella* spp. show a slight preference toward penicillins with rates of hydrolysis for penicillin G greater than that for cephaloridine or cephalothin (HAMILTON-MILLER 1963; MARSHALL et al. 1972; ROSS and BOULTON 1973; SAWAI et al. 1973; INOUE et al. 1983; MITSUHASHI 1985; EMANUEL et al. 1986). However, many of the enzymes also hydrolyze cloxacillin, the oxyiminocephalosporins, and aztreonam (MARSHALL et al. 1972; MATTHEW and HARRIS 1976; SYKES and MATTHEW 1976; BUSH et al. 1982; HART and PERCIVAL 1982; INOUE et al. 1983; MITSUHASHI 1985; LABIA et al. 1986). They generally do not hydrolyze the cephamycins, ceftazidime, moxalactam or imipenem. These broad spectrum enzymes are generally not susceptible to inhibition by cloxacillin or EDTA but are inhibited by pCMB, Hg^{2+}, iodine and clavulanic acid (SYKES and MATTHEW 1976; HART and PERCIVAL 1982; MITSUHASHI 1985; EMANUEL et al. 1986). Their pIs are generally in the acidic range (4.9–6.8) but values between 7.2 and 7.7 have also been reported (SAWAI et al. 1973; MATTHEW and HARRIS 1976; SYKES and MATTHEW 1976; HART and PERCIVAL 1982; MITSUHASHI 1985; LABIA et al. 1986). Molecular weights between 23000 and 27000 have been obtained for the *Klebsiella* enzymes (ROSS and BOULTON 1973; SYKES and MATTHEW 1976; INOUE et al. 1983; EMANUEL et al. 1986; JORIS et al. 1987). Examples of enzymes from two strains of indole positive *Klebsiella* are shown in Table 2.

Table 3. Classification scheme for chromosomal beta-lactamases

Bush[a] class	Desciption	Molecular class	Substrate profile[b]									Inhibitor profile					
			PEN	OXA	CARB	CEPH	CXM	CTX	MOX	AZT	IMI	CLOX	CLAV	pCMB	I	Hg^{2+}	EDTA
1	Cephalosporinases	C	+	−	−	+++	−	−	−	−	−	+	−	−	+	+	−
2a	Penicillinases		++	+	+	+/−	−	−	−	−	−	−	−	−	+	+	−
2b	Broad spectrum enzymes	A	+++	+	+	++	+	+	−	+	−	−	+	+	+	+	−
2e	Oxyiminocephalosporinases		+	−	−	++	++	++	−	+	−	+/−	+	+	+	+	−
3	Metalloenzymes	A, E?	+++	+++	+++	++	+	+	++	−	+++	−	−	+	+	+	+

[a] Bush (1988)
[b] Number of pluses (+) indicates substrate preferences
Abbreviations: PEN, penicillin; OXA, oxacillin; CARB, carbenicillin; CEPH, cephalothin; CXM, cefuroxime; CTX, cefotaxime; MOX, moxalactam; AZT, aztreonam; IMI, imipenem; CLOX, cloxacillin; CLAV, clavulanic acid; I, iodine; Hg^{2+}, mercurials

G. Subclassification Scheme for Chromosomal Beta-Lactamases

Recently, Bush proposed a new classification scheme for bacterial beta-lactamases (BUSH 1988). This scheme incorporates both biochemical and molecular aspects and divides the enzymes into three classes. Class 1 includes the chromosomal cephalosporinases (molecular class C). Class 2 includes the penicillinases (2a), broad spectrum beta-lactamases (2b), cloxacillinases (2c), carbenicillinases (2d) and oxyiminocephalosporinases (2e). Those relatively few class 2 enzymes for which the active site sequence is known belong to molecular class A. Class 3 includes the metalloenzymes (molecular class B and E). Using this classification scheme, the chromosomal beta-lactamases can be characterized in more detail by substrate and inhibitor profiles summarized from the data presented in this review (Table 3). This scheme should serve to differentiate the chromosomal enzymes that have been described to date. It should also provide the foundation for classifying any additional enzymes that may be described in the future as well as accomodate new information on previously described enzymes as it becomes available.

References

Ambler RP (1980) The structure of β-lactamases. Philos Trans R Soc Lond [Biol] 289:321–331

Anderson JD, Sykes RB (1973) Characterization of a β-lactamase obtained from a strain of *Bacteroides fragilis* resistant to β-lactam antibiotics. J Med Microbiol 6:201–206

Aronoff SC, Shales DM (1987) Factors that influence the evolution of β-lactam resistance in β-lactamase inducible strains of *Enterobacter cloacae* and *Pseudomonas aeruginosa.* J Infect Dis 155:936–941

Ashby J, Kirkpatrick B, Piddock LJV, Wise R (1987) The effect of imipenem on strains of Enterobacteriaceae expressing Richmond and Sykes class I β-lactamases. J Antimicrob Chemother 20:15–22

Bergström S, Normark S (1979) β-lactam resistance in clinical isolates of *Escherichia coli* caused by elevated production of *ampC*-mediated chromosomal β-lactamase. Antimicrob Agents Chemother 16:427–433

Bergström S, Olsson O, Normark S (1982) Common evolutionary origin of chromosomal β-lactamase genes in Enterobacteria. J Bacteriol 150:528–534

Berks M, Redhead K, Abraham EP (1982) Isolation and properties of an inducible and a constitutive β-lactamase from *Pseudomonas aeruginosa.* J Gen Microbiol 128:155–159

Bicknell R, Emanuel EL, Gagnon J, Waley SG (1985) The production and molecular properties of the zinc β-lactamase of *Pseudomonas maltophilia.* Biochem J 229:791–797

Brenner DJ (1984) Enterobacteriaceae. In: Krieg NR (ed) Bergey's manual of systematic bacteriology, vol 1. Williams and Wilkins, Baltimore, p 408

Bryan LE, Kwan S, Godfrey AJ (1984) Resistance of *Pseudomonas aeruginosa* mutants with altered control of chromosomal β-lactamase to piperacillin, ceftazidime, and cefsulodin. Antimicrob Agents Chemother 25:382–384

Büscher K-H, Cullmann W, Dick W, Stieglitz M (1987) Selection frequency of resistant variants by various β-lactam antibiotics in clinical *Enterobacter cloacae* isolates. Chemotherapy 33:40–51

Bush K (1988) Recent developments in β-latamase research and their implications for the future. Rev Infect Dis 10:681–690

Bush K, Sykes RB (1984) Interaction of β-lactam antibiotics with β-lactamases as a cause for resistance. In: Bryan LE (ed) Antimicrobial drug resistance. Academic, New York, p 1

Bush K, Freudenberger JS, Sykes RB (1982) Interaction of azthreonam and related monobactams with β-lactamases from gram-negative bacteria. Antimicrob Agents Chemother 22:414–420
Chabbert Y, Jaffé A (1982) Sch 29482: activity against susceptible and β-lactam resistant variants of Enterobacteriaceae. J Antimicrob Chemother 9 [Suppl C]:203–212
Charlier P, Dideberg O, Frère J-M, Moews PC, Knox JR (1983) Crystallographic data for the β-lactamase from *Enterobacter cloacae* P 99. J Mol Biol 171:237–238
Chiesa C, Labrozzi PH, Aronoff SC (1986) Decreased baseline β-lactamase production and inducibility associated with increased piperacillin susceptibility of *Pseudomonas cepacia* isolated from children with cystic fibrosis. Pediatr Res 20:1174–1177
Cuchural GJ Jr, Malamy MH, Tally FP (1986) β-lactamase-mediated imipenem resistance in *Bacteroides fragilis*. Antimicrob Agents Chemother 30:645–648
Cullmann W, Büscher KH, Dick W (1987) Selection and properties of *Pseudomonas aeruginosa* variants resistant to beta-lactam antibiotics. Eur J Clin Microbiol 6:467–473
Curtis NAC, Eisenstadt RL, Rudd C, White AJ (1986) Inducible Type I β-lactamases of gram-negative bacteria and resistance to β-lactam antibiotics. J Antimicrob Chemother 17:51–61
Curtis NAC, East SJ, Cornford RJ, Walker LA (1987) Properties of spontaneous *Enterobacter cloacae* mutants with temperature-conditional derepression of Type I β-lactamase synthesis. J Antimicrob Chemother 19:417–428
DelBene VE, Farrar WE Jr (1973) Cephalosporinase activity in *Bacteroides fragilis*. Antimicrob Agents Chemother 3:369–372
delRosario Valencia AM, Vuye A, Pijck J (1984) Selection of resistant mutants of *Citrobacter freundii* by second and third generation cephalosporins and imipenem. Infection 12:402–404
Egger R, Lebek G (1986) The development of chromosomally coded beta-lactamase production by *Escherichia coli* after in vitro selection with ampicillin, cefoxitin and ceftriaxzone. Chemotherapy 32:515–520
Eley A, Greenwood D (1986) Characterization of β-lactamases in clinical isolates of *Bacteroides*. J Antimicrob Chemother 18:325–333
Emanuel EL, Gagnon J, Waley SG (1986) Structural and kinetic studies on β-lactamase K1 from *Klebsiella aerogenes*. Biochem J 234:343–347
Eng RHK, Smith SM, Cherubin CE (1986) In vitro emergence of β-lactam-resistant variants of *Pseudomonas aeruginosa*. J Antimicrob Chemother 17:717–723
Farrar WE Jr, O'Dell NM (1976a) β-lactamase activity in *Chromobacterium violaceum*. J Infect Dis 134:290–293
Farrar WE Jr, O'Dell NM (1976b) β-lactamases and resistance to penicillins and cephalosporins in *Serratia marcescens*. J Infect Dis 134:245–251
Findell CM, Sherris JC (1976) Susceptibility of *Enterobacter* to cefamandole: evidence for a high mutation rate to resistance. Antimicrob Agents Chemother 9:970–974
Fleming PC, Goldner M, Glass DG (1963) Observations on nature, distribution and significance of cephalosporinase. Lancet 1:1399
Flett F, Curtis NAC, Richmond MH (1976) Mutant of *Pseudomonas aeruginosa* 18S that synthesizes type Id β-lactamase constitutively. J Bacteriol 127:1585–1586
Fujii T, Sato K, Inoue M, Mitsuhashi S (1985) Purification and properties of inducible penicillin β-lactamase isolated from *Alkaligenes faecalis*. Antimicrob Agents Chemother 27:608–611
Fujii T, Sato K, Mujata K, Inoue M, Mitsuhashi S (1986) Biochemical properties of β-lactamase produced by *Legionella gormanii*. Antimicrob Agents Chemother 29:925–926
Fujii-Kuriyama Y, Yamamoto M, Sugawara S (1977) Purification and properties of beta-lactamase from *Proteus morganii*. J Bacteriol 131:726–734
Furth A (1979) The β-lactamases of *Pseudomonas aeruginosa*. In: Hamilton-Miller JMT (ed) β-lactamases. Academic, New York, p 403
Garber N, Friedman J (1970) β-lactamase and the resistance of *Pseudomonas aeruginosa* to various penicillins and cephalosporins. J Gen Microbiol 64:343–352
Gates ML, Sanders CC, Goering RV, Sanders WE Jr (1986) Evidence for multiple forms of type I chromosomal β-lactamase in *Pseudomonas aeruginosa*. Antimicrob Agents Chemother 30:453–457

Gootz TD, Sanders CC (1983) Characterization of β-lactamase induction in *Enterobacter cloacae*. Antimicrob Agents Chemother 23:91–97
Gootz TD, Sanders CC, Goering RV (1982) Resistance to cefamandole: derepression of β-lactamases by cefoxitin and mutation in *Enterobacter cloacae*. J Infect Dis 146:34–42
Gootz TD, Jackson DB, Sherris JC (1984) Development of resistance to cephalosporins in clinical strains of *Citrobacter* spp. Antimicrob Agents Chemother 25:591–595
Grace ME, Gregory FJ, Fu KP (1986) Purification and properties of a β-lactamase from *Proteus penneri*. J Antibiot [Tokyo] 39:938–942
Grace ME, Fu KP, Gregory FJ, Hung PP (1987) Interaction of clavulanic acid, sulbactam, and cephamycin antibiotics with β-lactamases. Drugs Exp Clin Res 13:145–148
Guerin S, Paradis F, Guay R (1986) Cloning and characterization of chromosomally encoded cephalosporinase gene of *Enterobacter cloacae*. Can J Microbiol 32:301–309
Gutmann L, Williamson R (1983) A model system to demonstrate that β-lactamase-associated antibiotic trapping could be a potential means of resistance. J Infect Dis 148:316–321
Hamilton-Miller JMT (1963) Penicillinase from *Klebsiella aerogenes*. A comparison with penicillinases from gram-positive species. Biochem J 87:209–214
Hamilton-Miller JMT (1982) β-lactamases and their clinical significance. J Antimicrob Chemother 9 [Suppl B]:11–19
Hart CA, Percival A (1982) Resistance to cephalosporins among gentamicin-resistant klebsiellae. J Antimicrob Chemother 9:275–286
Hennessey TD (1967) Inducible β-lactamase in *Enterobacter*. J Gen Microbiol 49:277–285
Hennessey TD, Richmond MH (1968) The purification and some properties of a β-lactamase (cephalosporinase) synthesized by *Enterobacter cloacae*. Biochem J 109:469–473
Hirai K, Iyobe S, Inoue M, Mitsuhashi S (1980) Purification and properties of a new β-lactamase from *Pseudomonas cepacia*. Antimicrob Agents Chemother 17:355–358
Hirai K, Sato K, Matsubara N, Katsumata R, Inoue M, Mitsuhashi S (1981) Immunological properties of beta-lactamases that hydrolyze cefuroxime and cefotaxime. Antimicrob Agents Chemother 20:262–264
Ikeda Y, Nishino T, Tanino T (1987) Paradoxical antibacterial activity of cefmenoxime against *Proteus vulgaris*. Antimicrob Agents Chemother 31:865–869
Inoue M, Haller I, Mitsuhashi S (1983) Purification and properties of chromosomally mediated beta-lactamases from *Klebsiella oxytoca*. In: Spitzy KH, Karrer K (eds) Proceedings of the 13th International Congress of Chemotherapy 51:21–24
Jaurin B, Grundström T (1981) *amp C* cephalosporinase of *Escherichia coli* K-12 has a different evolutionary origin from that of β-lactamases of the penicillinase type. Proc Natl Acad Sci USA 78:4897–4901
Joris B, Dusart J, Frère J-M, VanBeeumen J, Emanuel EL, Petursson S, Gagnon J, Waley SG (1984) The active site of the P99 β-lactamase from *Enterobacter cloacae*. Biochem J 223:271–274
Joris B, DeMeester F, Galleni M, Reckinger G, Coyette J, Frère J-M (1985) The β-lactamase of *Enterobacter cloacae* P99. Chemical properties, N-terminal sequence and interaction with 6 β-halogenopenicillanates. Biochem J 228:241–248
Joris B, DeMeester F, Galleni M, Masson S, Dusart J, Frère J-M, VanBeeumen J, Bush K, Sykes R (1986) Properties of a class C β-lactamase from *Serratia marcescens*. Biochem J 239:581–586
Joris B, DeMeester F, Galleni M, Frère J-M, VanBeeumen J (1987) The K1 β-lactamase of *Klebsiella pneumoniae*. Biochem J 243:561–567
Kabins SA, Sweeney HM, Cohen S (1966) Resistance to cephalothin in vivo associated with increased cephalosporinase production. Ann Intern Med 65:1271–1277
Knott-Hunziker V, Petursson S, Jayatilake GS, Waley SG, Jaurin B, Grundström T (1982a) The chromosomal β-lactamases of *Pseudomonas aeruginosa* and *Escherichia coli*. Biochem J 201:621–627
Knott-Hunziker V, Petursson S, Waley SG, Jaurin B, Grundström T (1982b) The acyl-enzyme mechanism of β-lactamase action. The evidence for class C β-lactamases. Biochem J 207:315–322

Kuwabara S, Abraham EP (1967) Some properties of two extracellular β-lactamases from *Bacillus cereus* 569/H. Biochem J 103:27C–30C

Labia R (1982) Moxalactam: an oxa-β-lactam antibiotic that inactivates β-lactamases. Rev Infect Dis 4 [Suppl]:S529–S535

Labia R, Brunet G, Guionie M, Philippon A, Heitz M, Pitton J-S (1976a) Céphalosporinases constitutives de *Escherichia coli*. Ann Inst Pasteur Microbiol 127[B]:453–461

Labia R, Fabre C, Guionie M (1976b) Étude cinétique d'une nouvelle céphalosporinase de *Pseudomonas aeruginosa*. Biochimie 58:913–915

Labia R, Berguin-Billecog R, Guionie M (1981) Behaviour of ceftazidime towards β-lactamases. J Antimicrob Chemother 8 [Suppl B]:141–146

Labia R, Morand A, Guionie M, Heitz M, Pitton J-S (1986) Bêtalactamases de *Klebsiella oxytoca*: étude de leur action sur les céphalosporines de troisième génération. Pathol Biol [Paris] 34:611–615

Leung T, Williams JD (1978) β-lactamases of subspecies of *Bacteroides fragilis*. J Antimicrob Chemother 4:47–54

Lindberg F, Normark S (1986a) Contribution of chromosomal β-lactamases to β-lactam resistance in enterobacteria. Rev Infect Dis 8 [Suppl]:S292–S304

Lindberg F, Normark S (1986b) Sequence of the *Citrobacter freundii* OS60 chromosomal *amp C* β-lactamase gene. Eur J Biochem 156:441–445

Livermore DM (1985) Do β-lactamases "trap" cephalosporins? J Antimicrob Chemother 15:511–514

Livermore DM (1987a) Clinical significance of beta-lactamase induction and stable derepression in gram-negative rods. Eur J Clin Microbiol 6:439–445

Livermore DM (1987b) "Covalent trapping" and latimoxef resistance in β-lactamase-derepressed *Peudomonas aeruginosa*. J Antimicrob Chemother 20:7–13

Livermore DM, Yang Y-J (1987) β-lactamase lability and inducer power of newer β-lactam antibiotics in relation to their activity against β-lactamase-inducibility mutants of *Pseudomonas aeruginosa*. J Infect Dis 155:775–782

Livermore DM, Chau PY, Wong AIW, Leung PK (1987) β-lactamase of *Pseudomonas pseudomallei* and its contribution to antibiotic resistance. J Antimicrob Chemother 20:313–321

Marshall MJ, Ross GW, Chanter KV, Harris AM (1972) Comparison of the substrate specificities of the β-lactamases from *Klebsiella aerogenes* 1082E and *Enterobacter cloacae* P99. Appl Microbiol 23:765–769

Matsubara N, Yotsuji A, Kumano K, Inoue M, Mitsuhashi S (1981) Purification and some properties of a cephalosporinase from *Proteus vulgaris*. Antimicrob Agents Chemother 19:185–187

Matsuura M, Nakazawa H, Inoue M, Mitsuhashi S (1980) Purification and biochemical properties of β-lactamase produced by *Proteus rettgeri*. Antimicrob Agents Chemother 18:687–690

Matthew M (1979) Plasmid-mediated β-lactamases of gram-negative bacteria: properties and distribution. J Antimicrob Chemother 5:349–358

Matthew M, Harris AM (1976) Identification of β-lactamases by analytical isoelectric focusing: correlation with bacterial taxonomy. J Gen Microbiol 94:55–67

Medeiros AA (1984) Beta-lactamases. Br Med Bull 40:18–27

Minami S, Inoue S, Mitsuhashi S (1980a) Purification and properties of a cephalosporinase from *Enterobacter cloacae*. Antimicrob Agents Chemother 18:853–857

Minami S, Inoue M, Mitsuhashi S (1980b) Purification and properties of cephalosporinase in *Escherichia coli*. Antimicrob Agents Chemother 18:77–80

Minami S, Yotsuji A, Inoue M, Mitsuhashi S (1980c) Induction of β-lactamase by various β-lactam antibiotics in *Enterobacter cloacae*. Antimicrob Agents Chemother 18:382–385

Minami S, Matsubara N, Yotsuji A, Araki H, Watanabe Y, Yasuda T, Saikawa I, Mitsuhashi S (1983) Induction of cephalosporinase production by various penicillins in Enterobacteriaceae. J Antibiot [Tokyo] 36:1387–1395

Mitsuhashi S (1985) Resistance to β-lactam antibiotics in bacteria. In: Ishigami J (ed) Recent advances in chemotherapy. Antimicrobial section 1. University of Tokyo Press, Tokyo, p 3

Mitsuhashi S, Inoue M (1981) Mechanisms of resistance to β-lactam antibiotics. In: Mitsuhashi S (ed) Beta-lactam antibiotics. Springer, Berlin Heidelberg New York, p 41
Moosdeen F, Keeble J, Williams JD (1986) Induction/inhibition of chromosomal β-lactamases by β-lactamase inhibitors. Rev Infect Dis 8 [Suppl]:S562–S568
Murakami K, Yoshida T (1985) Covalent binding of moxalactam to cephalosporinase of *Citrobacter freundii*. Antimicrob Agents Chemother 27:727–732
Murata T, Minami S, Yasuda K, Iyobe S, Inoue M, Mitsuhashi S (1981) Purification and properties of cephalosporinase from *Pseudomonas aeruginosa*. J Antibiot [Tokyo] 34:1164–1170
Nayler JHC (1987) Resistance to β-lactams in gram-negative bacteria: relative contributions of β-lactamase and permeability limitations. J Antimicrob Chemother 19:713–732
Nord CE (1986) Mechanisms of β-lactam resistance in anaerobic bacteria. Rev Infect Dis 8 [Suppl 5]:S543–S548
Nordström K, Sykes RB (1974) Induction kinetics of β-lactamase biosynthesis in *Pseudomonas aeruginosa*. Antimicrob Agents Chemother 6:734–740
Ohya S, Fujii-Kuriyama Y, Yamamoto M, Sugawara S (1980) Purification and properties of β-lactamases from *Proteus rettgeri* and *Proteus inconstans*. Microbiol Immunol 24:815–824
Okonogi K, Sugiura A, Kuno M, Higashide E, Kondo M, Imada A (1985) Effect of β-lactamase induction on susceptibility to cephalosporins in *Enterobacter cloacae* and *Serratia marcescens*. J Antimicrob Chemother 16:31–42
Okonogi K, Kuno M, Higashide E (1986) Induction of β-lactamase in *Proteus vulgaris*. J Gen Microbiol 132:143–150
Olsson B, Nord CE, Wadström, T (1976) Formation of beta-lactamase in *Bacteroides fragilis*: cell-bound and extracellular activity. Antimicrob Agents Chemother 9:727–735
Pechère JC, Guay R, Dubois J, Letarte R (1980) Hydrolysis of cefotaxime by a beta-lactamase from *Bacteroides fragilis*. Antimicrob Agents Chemother 17:1001–1003
Phelps DJ, Carlton DD, Farrell CA, Kessler RE (1986) Affinity of cephalosporins for β-lactamase as a factor in antibacterial efficacy. Antimicrob Agents Chemother 29:845–848
Richmond MH (1979) β-lactam antibiotics and β-lactamases: two sides of a continuing story. Rev Infect Dis 1:30–36
Richmond MH, Sykes RB (1973) The β-lactamases of gram-negative bacteria and their possible physiological role. Adv Microb Physiol 9:31–88
Ross GW, Boulton MG (1973) Purification of β-lactamases on QAE-sephadex. Biochim Biophys Acta 309:430–439
Sabath LD, Abraham EP (1964) Synergistic action of penicillins and cephalosporins against *Pseudomonas pyocyanea*. Nature 204:1066–1069
Sabath LD, Jago M, Abraham EP (1965) Cephalosporinase and penicillinase activities of a beta-lactamase from *Pseudomonas pyocyanea*. Biochem J 96:739–752
Saino Y, Kobayashi F, Inoue M, Mitsuhashi S (1982) Purification and properties of inducible penicillin β-lactamase isolated from *Pseudomonas maltophilia*. Antimicrob Agents Chemother 22:564–570
Saino Y, Inoue M, Mitsuhashi S (1984) Purification and properties of an inducible cephalosporinase from *Pseudomonas maltophilia* GN12873. Antimicrob Agents Chemother 25:362–365
Sanders CC (1987) Chromosomal cephalosporinases responsible for multiple resistance to newer β-lactam antibiotics. Ann Rev Microbiol 41:573–593
Sanders CC, Sanders WE Jr (1986a) Trapping and hydrolysis are not mutually exclusive mechanisms for β-lactamase-mediated resistance. J Antimicrob Chemother 17:121–122
Sanders CC, Sanders WE Jr (1986b) Type I β-lactamases of gram-negative bacteria: interactions with β-lactam antibiotics. J Infect Dis 154:792–800
Sanders CC, Sanders WE Jr (1987) Clinical importance of inducible beta-lactamases in gram-negative bacteria. Eur J Clin Microbiol 6:435–437
Sanders CC, Moellering RC Jr, Martin RR, Perkins RL, Strike DG, Gootz TD, Sanders WE Jr (1982) Resistance to cefamandole: a collaborative study of emerging clinical problems. J Infect Dis 145:118–125

Sato K, Inoue M, Mitsuhashi S (1980) Activity of β-lactamase produced by *Bacteroides fragilis* against newly introduced cephalosporins. Antimicrob Agents Chemother 17:736–737
Sato K, Matsuura Y, Mujata K, Inoue M, Mitsuhashi S (1983) Characterization of cephalosporinases from *Bacteroides fragilis*, *Bacteroides thetaiotaomicron* and *Bacteroides vulgatus*. J Antibiot [Tokyo] 36:76–85
Sato K, Fujii T, Okamoto R, Inoue M, Mitsuhashi S (1985) Biochemical properties of β-lactamase produced by *Flavobacterium odoratum*. Antimicrob Agents Chemother 27:612–614
Sawai T, Yamagishi S, Mitsuhashi S (1973) Penicillinases of *Klebsiella pneumoniae* and their phylogenetic relationship to penicillinases mediated by R factors. J Bacteriol 115:1045–1054
Sawai T, Nakajima S, Morohoshi T, Yamagishi S (1977) Thermolabile repression of cephalosporinase synthesis in *Citrobacter freundii*. Microbiol Immunol 21:631–638
Sawai T, Yoshida T, Tsukamoto K, Yamagishi S (1981) A set of bacterial strains for evaluation of β-lactamase-stability of β-lactam antibiotics. J Antibiot [Tokyo] 34:1418–1326
Sawai T, Kanno M, Tsukamoto K (1982) Characterization of eight β-lactamases of gram-negative bacteria. J Bacteriol 152:567–571
Seeberg AH, Tolxdorff-Neutzling RM, Wiedemann B (1983) Chromosomal β-lactamases of *Enterobacter cloacoe* are responsible for resistance to third-generation cephalosporins. Antimicrob Agents Chemother 23:918–925
Shannon K, Phillips I (1986) The effects on β-lactam susceptibility of phenotypic induction and genotypic derepression of β-lactamase synthesis. J Antimicrob Chemother 18 [Suppl E]:15–22
Simpson IN, Page CD, Harper PB (1982) The contribution of β-lactamases to β-lactam resistance in *Bacteroides fragilis*. J Antimicrob Chemother 9:29–45
Sykes RB (1982) The classification and terminology of enzymes that hydrolyze β-lactam antibiotics. J Infect Dis 145:762–765
Sykes RB, Matthew M (1976) The β-lactamases of gram-negative bacteria and their role in resistance to β-lactam antibiotics. J Antimicrob Chemother 2:115–157
Sykes RB, Bonner DP, Bush K, Georgopapadakou NH (1982) Azthreonam (SQ 26,776), a synthetic monobactam specifically active against aerobic gram-negative bacteria. Antimicrob Agents Chemother 21:85–92
Tajima M, Takenouchi Y, Sugawara S, Inoue M, Mitsuhashi S (1980) Purification and properties of chromosomally mediated β-lactamase from *Citrobacter freundii* GN7391. J Gen Microbiol 121:449–456
Tajima M, Masuyoshi S, Inoue M, Takenouchi Y, Sugawara S, Mitsuhashi S (1981) Purification and properties of β-lactamases from *Serratia marcescens*. J Gen Microbiol 126:179–184
Tajima M, Takenouchi Y, Ohya S, Sugawara S (1982) Purification and properties of β-lactamase from *Proteus vulgaris*. Microbiol Immunol 26:531–534
Takahashi I, Sawai T, Ando T, Yamagishi S (1980) Cefoxitin resistance by a chromosomal cephalosporinase in *Escherichia coli*. J Antibiot [Tokyo] 33:1037–1042
Then RL, Angehrn P (1982) Trapping of non-hydrolyzable cephalosporins by cephalosporinases in *Enterobacter cloacae* and *Pseudomonas aeruginosa* as a possible resistance mechanism. Antimicrob Agents Chemother 21:711–717
Timewell R, Taylor E, Phillips I (1981) The β-lactamases of *Bacteroides* species. J Antimicrob Chemother 7:137–146
Toda M, Inoue M, Mitsuhashi S (1981) Properties of cephalosporinase from *Proteus morganii*. J Antibiot [Tokyo] 34:1469–1475
Vu H, Nikaido H (1985) Role of β-lactam hydrolysis in the mechanism of resistance of a β-lactamase constitutive *Enterobacter cloacae* strain to expanded spectrum β-lactams. Antimicrob Agents Chemother 27:393–398
Yotsuji A, Minami S, Inoue M, Mitsuhashi S (1983) Properties of novel β-lactamase produced by *Bacteroides fragilis*. Antimicrob Agents Chemother 24:925–929

CHAPTER 7

Beta-Lactamases: Genetic Control

S. CHAMBERLAND

A. Introduction

Beta-lactamases have been recognized as the major determinant of beta-lactam resistance in gram-positive and gram-negative bacteria. Beta-lactamases were discovered as early as 1940, when an extract of a strain of *E. coli* was shown to inactivate a solution of benzylpenicillin (ABRAHAM et al. 1940). A few years later the importance of beta-lactamases was demonstrated in gram-positive bacteria when *S. aureus* producing such an enzyme was shown to be responsible for clinical resistance to penicillin (SEGALOVE 1947).

After the introduction of semi-synthetic penicillins and cephalosporins, the attention was shifted onto the beta-lactamases of gram-negative bacteria. These organisms were shown to produce many types of beta-lactamases capable of destroying the new beta-lactams and, therefore, rapidly became an important clinical problem (MEDEIROS 1984).

In this chapter, the mechanisms by which beta-lactamase expression is controlled will be discussed. The regulation of beta-lactamase (*bla*) operons has been studied for many years. Bacterial gene expression is controlled at the trancription and/or at the translation level, and the regulation of the *bla* operons is not different. However, the *bla* operon is a complex system of regulation and, at this point in time, only partial understanding of its structure and control has been achieved.

B. Classification of Beta-Lactamases

Beta-lactamases form a family of heterogeneous enzymes which catalyse the hydrolysis of the amide bond in the beta-lactam ring of penicillins and related molecules, leading to the inactivation of those antibacterial agents.

Because a wide variety of beta-lactamases have been identified, attempts have been made to design comprehensive classification schemes.

The first classification to be recognized and extensively used was elaborated by RICHMOND and SYKES (1973). The beta-lactamases were classified by the following criteria: substrate and inhibitor profiles, genetic locus (plasmid or chromosomally mediated) and the nature of enzyme expression (constitutive or inducible). Five classes of beta-lactamases were defined. The chromosomally mediated beta-lactamase of *Escherichia coli* was a class IV enzyme, while the inducible and still chromosomally determined beta-lactamases of *Enterobacter cloacae* and *Pseudomonas aeruginosa* were classified together as type I enzymes. The major limitations of this classification include the heterogeneity among enzymes in the same class, the difficulty to classify an enzyme if the genetic locus implicated has not been localized, and the difficulty in determining inhibitor profiles under certain conditions (MEDEIROS 1984).

An improved classification scheme is now available. Based on molecular analysis of the enzymes, such as determination of isoelectric point, amino acid and nucleotide sequences, and kinetic parameters, three evolutionary distinct classes of enzyme have been defined (AMBLER 1980; BERGSTROM et al. 1982).

Class A is composed of highly homologous enzymes having a molecular weight of 29000 daltons. They are referred to as "serine" enzymes because a serine residue in the active site region of the molecule is responsible for the interaction with the substrate. They also show preferential hydrolysis of penicillins. This group includes the plasmid-mediated TEM-1 beta-lactamase widely distributed among gram-negative bacteria, as well as enzymes of gram-positive bacteria such as *Staphylococcus aureus* and *Bacillus licheniformis*. The amino acid sequence around the active site of the class A enzymes shows extensive homology with the penicillin binding site of the D-alanine carboxypeptidase of two *Bacillus* species, supporting the hypothesis that beta-lactamases may have derived from penicillin-binding proteins involved in peptidoglycan synthesis (YOCUM et al. 1979, WAXMAN et al. 1982).

The class B enzymes are metalloenzymes that require metal cofactor (Zn^{2+}) for activity. The beta-lactamase II of *Bacillus cereus* (ABRAHAM and WALEY 1979), as well as an enzyme elaborated by *Bacteroides fragilis*, fall into this category (CUCHURAL et al. 1986). The regulation of these enzymes has not yet been investigated and therefore will not be discussed in this chapter.

The chromosomally mediated beta-lactamases of *E. coli* K12, *Shigella*, *Klebsiella*, *Salmonella*, *Serratia*, *Enterobacter*, *Citrobacter* and *Pseudomonas* species form the class C enzymes. Using a ^{32}P-labelled DNA probe made from the beta-lactamase structural *amp*C gene of *E. coli*, BERGSTROM et al. (1982) showed extensive sequence homologies with *Shigella* sp. and could detect a homologous sequence in every species mentioned previously. Partial amino acid sequence determination around the active site of the chromosomal beta-lactamase from *Pseudomonas aeruginosa* revealed extensive homologies with the *E. coli* enzyme (KNOTT-HUNZIKER et al. 1982). The class C enzymes have a molecular weight of about 39000 daltons and, like the class A beta-lactamases, are serine enzymes. However, there is no sequence homology between these two classes of enzymes.

The class C enzyme can still be divided into two groups. All beta-lactamases of this group are chromosomally mediated, but some organisms like *E. coli* and *Shigella* sp. express the enzyme at a low constitutive level, while others like *Enterobacter cloacae* and *Pseudomonas aeruginosa* have an inducible enzyme.

C. Regulation of Class A Enzymes

The regulation of class A beta-lactamase expression has been extensively studied in gram-positive bacteria. The enzymes elaborated by *B. licheniformis* and *S. aureus* are secreted in the surrounding environment and are therefore known as exocellular beta-lactamases. However, a fraction of the elaborated enzyme is membrane-bound and is thought to be the precursor of the free beta-lactamase. Class A beta-lactamases are inducible enzymes thought to be under repressor control. Induction by enzyme substrates, the beta-lactams, would cause the release of the putative repressor from the operator gene and allow transcription of the beta-lactamase structural gene. Studies on *B. licheniformis* and *S. aureus* beta-lactamase operons have led to the elaboration of comprehensive models of regulation in which some regulatory genetic elements have been identified.

I. *Bacillus licheniformis*

1. Enzyme Properties

Two types of class A enzymes have been identified in *B. licheniformis*. The first type is an exoenzyme of 29000 daltons. It is a single polypeptide chain of 265 amino acids as sequenced by AMBLER and MEADWAY (1969). The second type of beta-lactamase is a membrane-bound enzyme. It is larger than the exo-beta-lactamase and strongly hydrophobic. YAMAMOTO and LAMPEN (1976) have shown that both enzymes possess the same C-terminal sequence although the membrane-bound form has a leader sequence of 25 amino acid residues attached at the N-terminal of the original exoenzyme sequence. Upon cloning of the structural gene, it was shown that the leader peptide contains 34 amino acid residues with a hydrophilic N-terminal region and a hydrophobic core region (KROYER and CHANG 1981). This peptide extension is thought to provide the anchor for the membrane-bound beta-lactamase and is also a secretion signal peptide (NEUGEBAUER et al. 1981). The specific proteolytic cleavage of this peptide generates the exo-beta-lactamase (AIYAPPA et al. 1977).

2. Kinetics of Induction

Penicillin is a potent inducer of *B. licheniformis* beta-lactamase. Radiolabelled penicillin irreversibly binds to the cells and is not released during induction (DAVIES 1969). There is, however, a time lag of about 1 h between the binding of the inducer and maximum expression of beta-lactamase, indicating that the inducer does not directly inactivate the repressor of the *bla* operon. It was proposed that the beta-lactam interacts with some specific target on the cell membrane. Such interaction would modify the level of a second effector in the cytoplasm, which would directly act on a repressor and regulate the transcription of the beta-lactamase gene (COLLINS 1979).

3. Genetic

The genetic determinants encoding class A beta-lactamase in *B. licheniformis* are chromosomally specified. Transformation analysis showed that at least three regulatory genes control the expression of the structural gene, *bla*P, in this species. *bla*I is the gene encoding the repressor and is closely linked to *bla*P. *bla*I$^-$ mutants produce large amounts of enzyme constitutively. Complementation analysis of mero- and heteropolyploids also indicates that *bla*I codes for the repressor (IMA-

NAKA et al. 1981). Two more regulatory genes have been identified, R1 and R2 genes. The former is 50% linked to *bla*P, while R2 is unlinked to the structural gene. $R1^-$ mutants produce normal basal level of enzyme, but cannot be induced at the parental level. $R2^-$ mutants are noninducible and produce less beta-lactamase than the parent strain (COLLINS 1979).

Transcriptional analysis of the beta-lactamase operon of *B. licheniformis* has recently been done (MCLAUGHLIN et al. 1982; SALERNO and LAMPEN 1986). The mRNA half-life was 2 min. It was shown that without inducer the level of beta-lactamase mRNA was low. Upon induction, the mRNA level reached a peak at 1 h and declined slowly during several hours. As mentioned before, this correlates with the rate of beta-lactamase synthesis observed upon induction, indicating that regulation of the beta-lactamase occurs at the transcriptional level. Moreover, three *bla*P mRNAs of 1.2, 2.9 and 3.4 kb were identified. The 1.2 kb mRNA represents 97% of the *bla*P mRNA population. It ends at an efficient terminator located at 60 bases 3′ to *bla*P, indicating that *bla*P and *bla*I genes are not transcribed on a polycistronic mRNA. The isolation of the longer *bla*P mRNA species (2.9 and 3.4 kb) indicates potential locations of genetically linked regulatory elements of beta-lactamase synthesis.

Since the nature of the repressor protein and the nature of the R1 and R2 gene products have not been established, it is still premature to conclude on the regulation of beta-lactamase expression in *B. licheniformis*. Two models of such regulation have been proposed by COLLINS (1979). Both models agree that the beta-lactam inducer acts on a specific target at the cytoplasmic membrane. In the first model, this interaction stimulates a second unidentified effector in the cytoplasm, which in turn binds and specifically inactivates the repressor. The second model is based on the fact that beta-lactams inhibit the synthesis of peptidoglycan. Accumulation of peptidoglycan precursors would act on the regulatory system(s) controlling cell wall synthesis, as well as on the *bla* operon, and inactivation of the repressor would take place. In this last model, only the repressor is specific to the *bla* operon.

II. *Staphylococcus aureus*

1. Enzyme Properties

Staphylococcus aureus produces four serologically different beta-lactamases, classified as types A to D. Types A, B, and C are inducible enzymes, while type D enzymes are expressed constitutively (ROSDAHL 1973). Like *B. licheniformis* beta-lactamases, staphylococcal beta-lactamases are exoenzymes as well as membrane-bound enzymes. The membrane-bound enzymes are also thought to be precursors of the exo-beta-lactamases (DYKE 1979). Upon amino acid sequencing, it was determined that the type A pre-beta-lactamase (32000 daltons) carries a signal peptide of 24 amino acid residues. This signal peptide would be cleaved during secretion, leading to an exocellular beta-lactamase of 28800 daltons. This polypeptide chain of 257 amino acids does not contain any cysteine or tryptophan residue (MCLAUGHLIN et al. 1981).

2. Kinetics of Induction

Staphylococcal beta-lactamases are induced by a wide variety of penicillins and cephalosporins. There is a time lag of about 10 min between the moment the inducer is added to the culture medium and the moment beta-lactamase production is increased.

Nonspecific induction has also been reported. As previously mentioned, the beta-lactamase does not contain any tryptophan, but incorporation of a tryptophan analog into the bacterial protein leads to beta-lactamase induction. It was proposed that a repressor protein was inactivated by incorporation of the analog (IMSANDE 1973).

3. Genetic

a) Location

Staphylococcal beta-lactamases are generally plasmid-specified enzymes; however, the beta-lactamase genes can also be found on the bacterial chromosome.

Plasmids encoding *S. aureus* beta-lactamases can be divided into five groups: alpha, beta, gamma, delta, and unrelated plasmids. Studies on the structure of these plasmids and the increasing rate of isolation of *S. aureus* with chromosomally specified beta-lactamases led to the hypothesis that beta-lactamase genes are carried on transposable elements. Several beta-lactamase transposons have now been characterized (LYON and SKURRAY 1987).

b) Regulation

At least two regulatory genes, *bla*I and *bla*R2, have been identified in *S. aureus*. The *bla*I gene specifies the repressor protein and is closely linked to the structural gene *bla*Z. Using heterodiploid construction, it was shown that the repressor is a tetramer of four similar subunits (IMSANDE 1978). The *bla*R2 gene is not linked to *bla*Z and is always located on the chromosome and regulates chromosomal as well as plasmid-specified beta-lactamase expression. *bla*R2$^-$ mutants produce a large amount of enzyme constitutively; *bla*R2 is thought to specify an inactive antirepressor protein. In the presence of inducer, the antirepressor would be activated and would interact with the repressor protein leading to derepression of the *bla* operon (IMSANDE 1978).

D. Regulation of Class C Enzymes

The regulation of the chromosomally mediated class C enzymes elaborated by Enterobacteria, such as *E. coli*, *E. cloacae*, and *C. freundii*, has been extensively studied in the past few years and comprehensive reviews of the topic are now available (LINDBERG and NORMARK 1986b; LINDBERG et al. 1986; NORMARK et al. 1986).

The following section will summarize the current knowledge on the regulation of class C enzyme expression and will provide new information about the expression of this enzyme in *Pseudomonas aeruginosa*.

I. Constitutive: *Escherichia coli*

1. Enzyme Properties

The class C chromosomally mediated beta-lactamase of *E. coli* is encoded by the *ampC* gene (BURMAN et al. 1973). This gene codes for a pre-beta-lactamase of 377 amino acids, of which the first 19 residues form a signal peptide. This signal peptide has been shown to be necessary for proteolytic processing leading to the mature enzyme and is necessary for the secretion of the beta-lactamase into the periplasmic space. Therefore, amino acid substitutions in that peptide or deletion of the *amp*C region encoding the signal peptide result in a reduced expression of active beta-lactamase (KADONAGA et al. 1984; KADONAGA et al. 1985). The mature enzyme has a molecular weight of 39 600 daltons (JAURIN et al. 1981). This enzyme preferentially hydrolyses cephalosporins and therefore is termed cephalosporinase. As mentioned above, this enzyme is expressed at a low constitutive level that cannot contribute to beta-lactam resistance. In fact, the mutational inactivation of the *ampC* gene of *E. coli* resistant to 2 μg of ampicillin per ml does not decrease this minimal resistance (BURMAN et al. 1973). However, following mutational events, the beta-lactamase can be expressed at high constitutive levels and becomes a primary determinant of beta-lactam resistance in laboratory-derived mutants, as well as in clinical isolates (BERGSTROM and NORMARK 1979; JACOBY and SUTTON 1985). The mechanism of such a phenomenon and its implication in bacterial resistance will be discussed in a following section.

2. Genetic

The first genetic loci responsible for beta-lactamase expression in *E. coli* were identified some 20 years ago. By studying *E. coli* ampicillin-resistant mutants (MIC of 10 μg/ml) producing more beta-lactamase than the wild type parent, the locus *amp*A was designated as a regulatory region governing beta-lactamase expression (ERICKSSON-GRENNBERG et al. 1965; ERICKSSON-GRENNBERG et al. 1968; LINDSTROM et al. 1970). A stepwise increase in resistance was also identified. The first level of resistance (ampicillin MIC: 10 μg/ml) was provided by a mutation in the *amp*A locus, while a second step mutation increasing resistance up to 50 μg ampicillin per ml was explained by a double mutation affecting the *amp*A and *amp*B loci. The *amp*B gene was reported to be distant from the *amp*A locus (ERICKSSON-GRENNBERG et al. 1968; NORDSTROM et al. 1968). A few years later the structural gene, *amp*C, was identified by the analysis of low-beta-lactamase producing mutants of *E. coli*, and was shown to map very close to the *amp*A locus previously described (BURMAN et al. 1973). In fact, after the cloning and sequencing of this DNA region, it was shown that *amp*A was a regulatory region included in the *amp*C locus (GRUNDSTROM et al. 1980; JAURIN et al. 1981). Today the genetic locus of the *E. coli* beta-lactamase is known as *amp*C and is mapped at 94 min on *E. coli* K12 chromosome (BACHMANN 1983).

The *amp*C gene of wild type *E. coli* K12 is poorly expressed. The beta-lactamase represents less than 0.01% of the total protein. The level of expression is not affected by the addition of beta-lactams, indicating that the enzyme is constitutively expressed (LINDBERG and NORMARK 1986b). JAURIN et al. (1981) showed that the poor expression of the *amp*C gene is due to an inefficient promoter and to the presence of an attenuator structure situated between the promoter and the structural gene and responsible for early termination of transcription.

The expression of the chromosomally mediated beta-lactamase was shown to be influenced by the growth rate of *E. coli*, being higher in rich media, and was thought to be due to greater transcriptional readthrough beyond the attenuator. It was postulated that the leader RNA possesses a potential ribosome binding site and may form a translation inhibition complex. The formation of such a complex would protect a RNA region necessary for the formation of the termination stem and loop structure and therefore inhibits their formation, allowing the RNA polymerase to transcribe the structural beta-lactamase region. Since the number of ribosomes increases proportionally to the growth rate, if binding of ribosomes to the *amp* leader RNA is proportional to the cellular concentration of ribosomes, the previous hypothesis would explain why at a higher growth rate there is less premature termination of transcription and greater *amp*C expression.

Operons are generally regarded as well-defined functional units that do not interact with adjacent operons on the same chromosome. However, the fumarate reductase (*frd*) operon and the *amp*C operon have been shown to overlap. Overlapping genes are defined as a single nucleotide sequence coding for more than one polypeptide. This was first observed in phages and was thought to allow packaging of a maximum amount of genetic information. However, it is now known that overlapping genes are present in mitochondrial DNA, insertion elements and bacterial genomes. Such gene arrangements are thought to be involved in regulation of expression.

The *frd* operon is composed of four genes encoding the subunits of the membrane-found fumarate reductase. Fumarate reductase is only produced in anaerobiosis, where it is essential for growth on non-fermentable substrates and when fumarate is the terminal electron acceptor (COLE et al. 1982). Upon DNA sequencing it was found that the *amp*C promoter was located within the *frd*D gene in such a way that the 10 carboxyterminal amino acids of the *frd*D protein were encoded by the *amp*C promoter sequence. The transcriptional terminator for the *frd* operon is situated in the leader region of the *amp*C operon and acts as an attenuator for the *amp*C operon (GRUNDSTROM and JAURIN 1982; NORMARK et al. 1983).

3. Mechanisms Increasing Beta-Lactamase Gene Expression

As previously mentioned, resistant *E. coli* hyperproducing chromosomal beta-lactamase can be readily isolated in the laboratory and is also encountered in clinical samples.

The hyperproduction of the beta-lactamase can be achieved in many ways. Beta-lactamase synthesis can be increased by amplification of the *amp*C gene. DNA repetitions carrying the *amp*C gene were identified in hyperproducing mutants of *E. coli*. As many as 10 identical repeats organized in tandem could be generated by a normal mutation frequency (EDLUND et al. 1979; NORMARK et al. 1977). Mutations in the promoter and attenuator region described previously can lead to an increased rate of transcription of the *amp*C gene. For instance, a single base-pair insertion in the *amp*C promoter resulted in a significant increase in the frequency of transcriptional initiation (JAURIN et al. 1981). However, since the promoter sequence in shared by the *frdD* gene of the *frd* operon, mutations affecting positively the *ampC* promoter might have a negative effect on the *fdr*D gene expression. Therefore, a low number of mutations are allowed in the promoter region and this explains a mutation frequency of about 10^{-10}. Mutations in the attenuator site are more frequent (10^{-8}). These mutations increase beta-lactamase production to confer resistance to beta-lactams that are good substrates. However, resistance to beta-lactamase-stable beta-lactams has been observed and is thought to be due to the combined effort of two mutations affecting both the promoter and the attenuator, leading to a higher expression of the *amp*C gene. Such combined mutations are encountered at a very low frequency (10^{-18}) (LINDBERG and NORMARK 1986b).

II. Inducible

Probably all species of gram-negative bacteria elaborate a chromosomally mediated class C enzyme and among them, some elaborate an inducible enzyme.

Induction refers to the ability of bacteria to synthesize the beta-lactamase or to increase the rate of production of this enzyme, only when its substrates, the beta-lactams, are present. Induction of the *bla* operon significantly increases the level of beta-lactam resistance. But as we have seen in *E. coli*, organisms expressing class C enzyme can also mutate and overproduce this enzyme in a constitutive fashion. The mutation events leading to derepression occur at high frequency (10^{-7}). Such mutants are produced in the laboratory but have also been observed in clinical isolates. The new beta-lactamase-stable cephalosporins are particularly effective in selecting derepressed mutants. Moreover, a high level of class C beta-lactamase mediates resistance to substrate and nonsubstrate beta-lactams and therefore becomes a major clinical problem. Therapeutic failures due to the selection of mutants with derepressed beta-lactamase expression are well documented (SANDERS and SANDERS 1986; CURTIS et al. 1986; WIEDEMANN 1986).

1. *Citrobacter freundii*

The *C. freundii amp*C gene encodes for a 380 amino-acid-long precursor (pre-beta-lactamase) with a 19-residue signal peptide. The mature beta-lactamase has a molecular weight of 39781 daltons (LINDBERG and NORMARK 1986a). In *C. freundii*, the *bla* and *frd* operons are sitting beside each other on the chromosome but do not overlap as in the case of *E. coli*. They are separated by about 1100 base pairs determining the inducible property of the enzyme. This gene has been termed *amp*R and encodes a 31000 dalton polypeptide. It was shown that, in the absence of inducer, the *amp*R protein represses *amp*C expression. However, in the presence of beta-lactam, the *amp*R was necessary for induction and therefore it was concluded that this gene has a positive effect on *amp*C expression in the presence of inducer (BERGSTROM et al. 1983; LINDBERG et al. 1985; YAMAMOTO et al. 1983). The mutation leading to overproduction of beta-lactamase is not located in the *amp*R-*amp*C region. The high mutation frequency observed (10^{-7}) indicates the destruction of a repressor gene, not by specific alteration but by several possible changes. It has been hypothesized that this repressor, instead of being a conventional repressor protein, would be a low-molecular-weight metabolite, possibly an intermediate in peptidoglycan synthesis (LINDBERG and NORMARK 1986b).

More recently, LINDBERG et al. (1987) reported that the expression of the *C. freundii ampC* gene and its regulatory elements cloned in *E. coli* could also be modulated by an *E. coli* chromosomal determinant. When *C. freundii bla* operon is cloned in *E. coli*, its expression is inducible. A chromosomal mutation mapped between *nad*C and *aro*P at 2.4 min on the *E. coli* chromosome leads to semiconstitutive overproduction of *C. freundii* beta-lactamase. This gene was called *ampD*. The wild type *amp*D gene trans-complemented the *amp*D mutant, indicating a diffusible gene product. Since the inactivation of *amp*D gene resulted in induction of beta-lactamase expression, it was concluded that the *amp*D product is inactivated during this process. Finally, since *amp*D is present in *E. coli* which does not express an inducible beta-lactamase, *amp*D may not be a specific regulatory element of the *bla* operon.

2. *Enterobacter cloacae*

a) Enzyme Properties

In 1967, HENNESSY showed that *Enterobacter cloacae* could be induced to produce a beta-lactamase, if exposed to benzylpenicillin. This enzyme showed preferential hydrolysis of cephalosporins and was therefore termed cephalosporinase. The purification of this enzyme from *E. cloacae* strains of different origins identified two forms of class C serine enzyme in this bacterial species. The first enzyme described (A) was shown to have a molecular weight of 44000 daltons, a pI of 8.4, an optimal pH of 8.5 and optimal temperature of 40 °C (MINAMI et al. 1980). The second enzyme (B) isolated from *E. cloacae* P99 has a molecular weight of 39000 daltons, a pI of 7.8 but the same pH and temperature optima described for the form A. The two enzyme types are not produced by the same organism (JORIS et al. 1984; JORIS et al. 1985; SEEBERG et al. 1983).

b) Induction Specificity and Derepression

Like all inducible class C enzymes, the production of *E. cloacae* beta-lactamase was shown to be induced in the presence of beta-lactams and rapidly repressed as the concentration of inducer decreases in the culture medium. All beta-lactams tested so far, including the enzyme-stable cephalosporins such as cefoxitin, were proved to be powerful inducers. Once the beta-lactamase production was induced, the enzyme mediated high level resistance to most beta-lactams. Further experiments showed that the degree of induction of the beta-lactamase was directly related to the stability of the inducer to degradation by the enzyme (LAMPE et al. 1982; GOOTZ and SANDERS 1983; SEEBERG et al. 1983; OKONOGI et al. 1985).

The production of this beta-lactamase can also be induced by compounds not related to the beta-lactam antibiotics. This induction is therefore considered nonspecific. Bicyclic molecules such as folic acid, thiamine, tryptophan or haemin proved to be good inducers. Complex media such as trypticase soy broth, serum, pleural fluid and cerebrospinal fluid also showed induction potency. This last finding indicates that beta-lactamase induction can easily take place in vivo and be a considerable factor in development of resistance to beta-lactams (CULLMAN et al. 1983; CULLMAN et al. 1984).

Catabolite repression often controls the expression of inducible systems in gram-negative bacteria. However, it was demonstrated that glucose or exogeneous cAMP in the culture medium does not affect beta-lactamase specific or nonspecific induction, indicating that the organization of this inducible system is somehow different (GOOTZ and SANDERS 1983; CULLMAN et al. 1984).

Mutants of *E. cloacae* overproducing a constitutive beta-lactamase can be isolated under selective pressure (passage on cefamandole or other cephalosporins). Interestingly, these mutants can still be induced by specific or nonspecific inducers, even with compounds that have been proven to have no effect on the parent strain (CULLMAN and DICK 1985).

Finally, clindamycin, a protein synthesis inhibitor, was shown to selectively prevent derepression of the beta-lactamase in some strains of *Enterobacter cloacae*. Other protein synthesis inhibitors, such as chloramphenicol, have shown preferential inhibitory effect of inducible enzymes compared to constitutively expressed enzymes. However, clindamycin did not affect all inducible enzymes since beta-galactosidase derepression was not inhibited. This specific inhibitory effect of clindamycin on the *E. cloacae* beta-lactamase system still remains unclear (SANDERS et al. 1983 a; SANDERS et al. 1983 b).

c) Genetic

Cloning of the DNA region encoding the inducible cephalosporinase of *E. cloacae* has been achieved. The DNA fragment cloned codes for seven polypeptides. Among them, a 42000-dalton protein and a 39500-dalton protein represent the pre-beta-lactamase and the beta-lactamase respectively. The beta-lactamase precursor contains a 20-residue-long signal peptide. When the regulatory region was deleted, the cephalosporinase was expressed at low level and could not be induced by beta-lactams (GUERIN et al. 1985 b).

Further nucleotide sequence analysis of the cloned DNA region gave some insight in the regulation of the production of this beta-lactamase. The promoter includes a −35 (TTAAGAC) region and a −10 (TATAAC) region which is immediately followed by the consensus sequence determining the ribosome attachment site. An initiation codon immediately follows this sequence. Four sets of dyad symmetries are located downstream of the initiation codon, three of which lay within the structural cephalosporinase gene. This arrangement is immediately followed by the terminator region and a presumed antitermination signal.

Transcriptional analysis showed that several mRNA species were synthesized. One corresponded to the pre-beta-lactamase while three others would be translated in truncated beta-lactamase proteins of molecular weights ranging from 40700 to 24700 daltons. These proteins were found to be active beta-lactamases with conserved active site. These truncated proteins might explain the observation of satellite bands on isoelectric focusing of *E. cloacae* beta-lactamase. Finally, one mRNA species corresponded to a readthrough over the cephalosporinase gene terminator. The gene that follows immediately the beta-lactamase gene has been shown to encode a 44000-dalton protein. The role of this protein is still unknown (GUERIN et al. 1985a).

Recent findings indicate that the *amp*R region of *E. cloacae* is highly similar to the *amp*R gene of *C. freundii* previously described. This regulatory region is 800 base pairs long and the gene product has a size of 31 000 daltons. The *amp*R function can be transcomplemented between the two species indicating a very similar regulation of *bla* operon. Finally, complementation experiments also suggest direct interaction of the *amp*R gene product with the *amp*C gene (LINDBERG and NORMARK 1987; NICOLAS et al. 1987).

3. *Pseudomonas aeruginosa*

a) Enzyme Properties

All *Pseudomonas aeruginosa* strains possess a chromosomally mediated inducible beta-lactamase (LIVERMORE 1982). It was first shown that this enzyme could be induced by high concentrations of benzylpenicillin or cephalosporin C and that it contributed to the high level of resistance to these beta-lactams (SABATH et al. 1965).

Attempts made to purify and characterize this beta-lactamase showed slight variations between enzymes of different strains. The enzyme, purified by MCPHAIL and FURTH (1973) from *P. aeruginosa* NCTC 8203, had an apparent molecular weight of 42000 daltons, as determined by SDS-PAGE and gel filtration. The maximum activity was reached at pH 8.0, and the enzyme was stable between 4 °C and 27 °C but labile at 40 °C. The beta-lactamase had a pI of 8.1 but up to 10 very minor satellite bands were observed upon isoelectric focusing analysis. Comparison of this enzyme with the beta-lactamase constitutively expressed of another *P. aeruginosa* strain showed no major differences (BERKS et al. 1982). However, MURATA et al. (1981) isolated an enzyme with an apparent molecular weight of 34000 daltons, as determined by SDS-PAGE and gel filtration. The optimal pH and optimal temperature of the purified enzyme were 8.0 and 40 °C, respectively. This beta-lactamase had a pI of 8.7. However, no significant differences were observed in the substrate profile of these enzymes, both preferentially hydrolysed cephalosporins.

b) Induction Specificity and Derepression

Class C beta-lactamase expression is minimal in *P. aeruginosa* and its synthesis is greatly enhanced in the presence of penicillins or cephalosporins, but the penicillins, at low concentrations, are not powerful inducers (JACOBS et al. 1984). Once induced, the enzyme constitutes a defense against most beta-lactams, including the "nonhydrolysable" cephalosporins (LIVERMORE 1983; JACOBS et al. 1984).

Like the *E. cloacae* enzyme previously described, the *P. aeruginosa* enzyme is not only induced in the presence of beta-lactams. Nonspecific inducers such as aromatic amino acids and histidine have been identified. Complex culture media also have an induction potential (DALHOFF and CULLMAN 1984).

Derepressed mutants, producing constitutively a high level of beta-lactamase, have also been isolated in laboratory and from patients. The derepression is stable and associated with high level resistance to cephalosporins. Selection of derepressed mutants in patients by antibiotherapy using the new beta-lactams has also led to therapeutic failure (BELL et al. 1985; KING et al. 1983; LIVERMORE 1985; NICHOLS and MAKI 1985). Therefore, induction and derepression seem to occur in vivo. DALHOFF and CULLMAN (1984) studied the in vivo induction of the beta-lactamase of *P. aeruginosa*, in a granuloma pouch model in rats. They showed that in animals treated with carbenicillin, ticarcillin, piperacillin, azlocillin and cefsulodin the *P. aeruginosa* beta-lactamase was rapidly induced, reaching a constant level approximately 8 h after infection. Interestingly, in nontreated animals the beta-lactamase was also induced to the same extent. They therefore concluded that nonspecific induction was produced by body fluids.

More recently, GATES et al. (1986) reported the isolation of laboratory mutants partially (mutational frequency 10^{-7}) and fully derepressed (mutational frequency 10^{-9}) for beta-lactamase production, by single passage in broth containing cefotaxime. It was shown that the beta-lactamases produced by these isolates were significantly different by their kinetic parameters, substrate profiles and pIs. The partially derepressed mutant was shown to synthesize a beta-lactamase with a pI of 8.4. However, two forms of beta-lactamase were identified by isoelectric focusing of the fully derepressed mutant crude extract. These two beta-lactamases, pI 8.4 and 7.5, could also be observed upon induction of the wild type parent strain of *P. aeruginosa*.

c) Genetics

The beta-lactamase gene of *P. aeruginosa* has not yet been cloned, and therefore analysis of the molecular structure of the gene, leading to the elucidation of the regulation mechanism that governs beta-lactamase expression in this bacterial species, cannot be done.

However, classical genetic techniques have been used to localize the beta-lactamase (*bla*) gene(s) on *P. aeruginosa* chromosome. MATSUMOTO and TERAWAKI (1981) produced a set of isogenic mutants by chemical mutagenesis. These mutants included beta-lactamase negative strains, some weak producers of beta-lactamase and some derepressed mutants with constitutive high level expression of the enzyme. By conjugation between constitutive and inducible strains, it became evident that three loci were implicated in the induction system. They were termed *bla*I, *bla*J and *bla*K. Mutants in these regions expressed the beta-lactamase constitutively. Mutants lacking beta-lactamase expression had mutations in the structural gene termed *bla*P. The *bla*I gene was mapped near *met*-9011 at 50–55 min, but was not cotransducible with this marker. The *bla*J, *bla*K and *bla*P genes were located between *str*A and *pro*A at 35–40 min on the PAO map. The *bla*J and *bla*P genes were cotransducible. MATSUMOTO and TERAWAKI (1981) concluded that since *bla*J was close to *bla*P, this gene could be the operator region of the structural gene. No functions were proposed for the *bla*I and *bla*K genes. More recently, one more locus (*bla*L) was mapped close to *bla*I (HOLLOWAY and MORGAN 1986). It is interesting to note that genes distant of the operator and structural regions do affect beta-lactamase expression in *P. aeruginosa*.

Further work is needed in order to determine if *amp*D and *amp*R functions described in Enterobacteria are also regulatory elements of the *bla* operon in *P. aeruginosa*.

E. Conclusion

The rigorous studies conducted on the regulation of class A and class C beta-lactamase expression have led to the establishment of some regulation models.

Studies on class A beta-lactamase expression have demonstrated that at least three regulatory elements control beta-lactamase expression in gram-positive bacteria (*bla*I, *bla*R1 and *bla*R2). Somehow the control of beta-lactamase expression could be coupled to some control elements of the cell wall synthesis system.

Studies conducted in *C. freundii* and *E. cloacae* have shown that the expression of the class C beta-lactamase structural gene (*amp*C) is regulated by two elements, the *amp*R and *amp*D gene products. The *amp*R gene would specify a repressor protein while the *amp*D gene would specify a sensor interacting directly with the beta-lactam inducer. This type of genetic organisation may be proven right for all gram-negative bacteria elaborating an inducible class C beta-lactamase.

References

Abraham EP, Chain EB (1940) An enzyme from bacteria able to destroy penicillin. Nature 146:837–845

Abraham EP, Waley SG (1979) Beta-lactamases from *Bacillus cereus*. In: Hamilton-Miller JMT, Smith JT (eds) Beta-lactamases. Academic, London, p 311

Ambler RP (1980) The structure of beta-lactamases. Philos Trans R Soc Lond [Biol] 289:321–331

Ambler RP, Meadway RJ (1969) Chemical structure of bacterial penicillinases. Nature 222:24–26

Aiyappa PS, Traficante LJ, Lampen JO (1977) Penicillinase-releasing protease of *Bacillus licheniformis*: purification and general properties. J Bacteriol 129:191–197

Bachmann BJ (1983) Linkage map of *Escherichia coli* K-12, Edition 7. Microbiol Rev 47:180–230

Bell SM, Pham JN, Langarone JYM (1985) Mutation of *Pseudomonas aeruginosa* to piperacillin resistance mediated by beta-lactamase production. J Antimicrob Chemother 15:665–670

Bergstrom S, Normark S (1979) Beta-lactam resistance in clinical isolates of *Escherichia coli* caused by elevated production of the *amp*C-mediated chromosomal beta-lactamase. Antimicrob Agents Chemother 16:427–433

Bergstrom S, Olsson O, Normark S (1982) Common evolutionary origin of chromosomal beta-lactamase genes in Enterobacteria. J Bacteriol 150:528–534

Bergstrom S, Lindberg FP, Olsson O, Normark S (1983) Comparison of the overlapping *frd* and *amp*C operons of *Escherichia coli* with the corresponding DNA sequences in other gram-negative bacteria. J Bacteriol 155:1277–1305

Berks M, Redhead K, Abraham EP (1982) Isolation and properties of an inducible and a constitutive beta-lactamase from *Pseudomonas aeruginosa*. J Gen Microbiol 128:155–159

Burman LG, Park JR, Lindstrom EB, Boman HG (1973) Resistance of *Escherichia coli* to penicillins: identification of the structural gene for the chromosomal penicillinase. J Bacteriol 116:123–130

Cole ST, Grundstrom T, Jaurin B, Robinson JJ, Weiner JH (1982) Location and nucleotide sequence of *frd*B, the gene coding for the iron-sulphur protein subunit of the fumarate reductase of *Escherichia coli*. Eur J Biochem 126:211–216

Collins JF (1979) The *Bacillus licheniformis* beta-lactamase system. In: Hamilton-Miller JMT, Smith JT (eds) Beta-lactamases. Academic, London, p 351

Cuchural GJ Jr, Malamy MH, Tally FP (1986) Beta-lactamase-mediated imipenem resistance in *Bacteroides fragilis*. Antimicrob Agents Chemother 30:645–648

Cullman W, Dick W (1985) Evidence for nonspecific induction of beta-lactamase in overproducing variants of *Enterobacter cloacae* and *Citrobacter freundii*. Eur J Clin Microbiol 4:34–40

Cullman W, Dick W, Dalhoff A (1983) Non-specific induction of beta-lactamase in *Enterobacter cloacae*. J Infect Dis 148:765

Cullman W, Dalhoff A, Dick W (1984) Nonspecific induction of beta-lactamase in *Enterobacter cloacae*. J Gen Microbiol 130:1781–1786

Curtis NAC, Eisenstadt RL, Rudd C, White AJ (1986) Inducible type I beta-lactamases of gram-negative bacteria and resistance to beta-lactam antibiotics. J Antimicrob Chemother 17:51–61

Dalhoff A, Cullman W (1984) Specificity of beta-lactamase induction in *Pseudomonas aeruginosa*. J Antimicrob Chemother 14:349–357

Davies JW (1969) Regulation of penicillinase synthesis in *Bacillus licheniformis*: binding of inducer to cells, and half-life of the messenger ribonucleic acid. Biochem J 115:44P

Dyke KGH (1979) Beta-lactamases of *Staphylococcus aureus*. In: Hamilton-Miller JMT, Smith JT (eds) Beta-lactamases. Academic, London, p 291

Edlund T, Grundstrom T, Normark S (1979) Isolation and characterization of DNA repetitions carrying the chromosomal beta-lactamase gene of *Escherichia coli* K-12. Mol Gen Genet 173:115–125

Eriksson-Grennberg KG (1968) Resistance of *Escherichia coli* to penicillins. II. An improved mapping of the *amp*A gene. Genet Res 12:147–156

Eriksson-Grennberg KG, Boman HG, Jansson JAT, Thoren S (1965) Resistance of *Escherichia coli* to penicillins. I. Genetic study of some ampicillin-resistant mutants. J Bacteriol 90:54–62

Gates ML, Sanders CC, Goering RV, Sanders EJR (1986) Evidence for multiple forms of type I chromosomal beta-lactamase in *Pseudomonas aeruginosa*. Antimicrob Agents Chemother 30:453–457

Gootz TD, Sanders CC (1983) Characterization of beta-lactamase induction in *Enterobacter cloacae*. Antimicrob Agents Chemother 23:91–97

Grundstrom T, Jaurin B (1982) Overlap between *amp*C and *frd* operons on the *Escherichia coli* chromosome. Proc Natl Acad Sci USA 79:1111–1115

Grundstrom T, Jaurin B, Edlund T, Normark S (1980) Physical mapping and expression of hybrid plasmids carrying chromosomal beta-lactamase genes of *Escherichia coli* K-12. J Bacteriol 143:1127–1134

Guerin S, Guay R, Letarte R, Levesque R (1985a) Multiple forms of *Enterobacter cloacae* cephalosporinase gene (*cpa*) products: role of regulatory sequences. Interscience Conference on Antimicrobial Agents and Chemotherapy, Minneapolis, 28 Sept 2 Oct, Abstract no 700

Guerin S, Paradis F, Guay R (1985b) Cloning and characterization of chromosomally encoded cephalosporinase gene of *Enterobacter cloacae*. Can J Microbiol 32:301–309

Hennessey TD (1967) Inducible beta-lactamase in *Enterobacter*. J Gen Microbiol 49:277–285

Holloway BW, Morgan AF (1986) Genome organization in *Pseudomonas*. Annu Rev Microbiol 40:79–105

Imanaka T, Tanaka T, Tsunekawa H, Aiba S (1981) Cloning of the genes for penicillinase, *pen*P and *pen*I of *Bacillus licheniformis* in some vector plasmids and their expression in *Escherichia coli*, *Bacillus subtilis*, and *Bacillus licheniformis*. J Bacteriol 147:776–786

Imsande J (1973) Repressor and antirepressor in the regulation of Staphylococcal penicillinase synthesis. Genetics 75:1–17

Imsande J (1978) Genetic regulation of penicillinase synthesis in gram-positive bacteria. Microbiol Rev 42:67–83
Jacobs JY, Livermore DM, Davey KWM (1984) *Pseudomonas aeruginosa* beta-lactamase as a defence against azlocillin, mezlocillin and piperacillin. J Antimicrob Chemother 14:221–229
Jacoby GA, Sutton L (1985) Beta-lactamases and beta-lactam resistance in *Escherichia coli*. Antimicrob Agents Chemother 28:703–705
Jaurin B, Grundstrom T, Edlund T, Normark S (1981) The *E. coli* beta-lactamase attenuator mediates growth rate-dependent regulation. Nature 290:221–225
Joris B, Dusart J, Frere J-M, Van Belumen J, Emanuel EL, Petursson S, Gagnon J, Waley SG (1984) The active site of the P99 beta-lactamase from *Enterobacter cloacae*. Biochem J 223:271–274
Joris G, DeMeester F, Galleni M, Reckinger G, Coyette J, Frere J-M (1985) The beta-lactamase of *Enterobacter cloacae* P99. Chemical properties, N-terminal sequence and interaction with 6 beta-halogenopenicillinates. Biochem J 228:241–248
Kadonaga JT, Gautier AE, Straus DR, Charles AD, Edge MD, Knowles JR (1984) The role of beta-lactamase signal sequence in the secretion of proteins by *Escherichia coli*. J Biol Chem 259:2149–2154
Kadonaga JT, Pluckthun A, Knowles JR (1985) Signal sequence mutants of beta-lactamase. J Biol Chem 260:16192–16199
King A, Shannon K, Eykyn S, Phillips I (1983) Reduced sensitivity to beta-lactam antibiotics arising during ceftazidime treatment of *Pseudomonas aeruginosa* infections. J Antimicrob Chemother 12:363–370
Knott-Hunziker V, Petursson S, Jayatilako GS, Waley SG, Jaurin B, Grundstrom T (1982) Active sites of beta-lactamases. The chromosomal beta-lactamases of *Pseudomonas aeruginosa* and *Escherichia coli*. Biochem J 201:621–627
Kroyer J, Chang S (1984) The promoter-proximal region of the *Bacillus licheniformis* penicillinase gene: nucleotide sequence and predicted leader peptide sequence. Gene 15:343–347
Lampe MF, Allan BJ, Minshew BH, Sherris JC (1982) Mutational enzymatic resistance of *Enterobacter* species to beta-lactam antibiotics. Antimicrob Agents Chemother 21:655–660
Lindberg F, Normark S (1986a) Sequence of the *Citrobacter freundii* 0560 chromosomal *amp*C beta-lactamase gene. Eur J Biochem 156:441–445
Lindberg F, Normark S (1986b) Contribution of chromosomal beta-lactamases to beta-lactam resistance in *Enterobacteria*. Rev Infect Dis [Suppl 8] 3:5292–5304
Lindberg F, Normark S (1987) Common mechanism of *amp*C beta-lactamase induction in *Enterobacteria*: regulation of the cloned *Enterobacter cloacae* P99 beta-lactamase gene. J Bacteriol 169:758–763
Lindberg F, Westman L, Normark S (1985) Regulatory components in *Citrobacter freundii* *amp*C beta-lactamase induction. Proc Natl Acad Sci USA 82:4620–4624
Lindberg F, Lindquist S, Normark S (1986) Induction of chromosomal beta-lactamase expression in enterobacteria. J Antimicrob Chemother [18 Suppl C]:43–50
Lindberg F, Lindquist S, Normark S (1987) Inactivation of the *amp*D gene causes semiconstitutive overproduction of the inducible *Citrobacter freundii* beta-lactamase. J Bacteriol 169:1923–1928
Lindstrom EB, Boman HG, Steele BB (1970) Resistance of *Escherichia coli* to penicillins VI. Purification and characterization of the chromosomally mediated penicillinase present in *amp*A-containing strains. J Bacteriol 101:218–231
Livermore DM (1982) Beta-lactamases of *Pseudomonas aeruginosa*. J Antimicrob Chemother 10:168–171
Livermore DM (1983) Kinetics and significance of the activity of the Sabath and Abrahams beta-lactamase of *Pseudomonas aeruginosa* against cefotaxime and cefsulodin. J Antimicrob Chemother 11:169–179
Livermore DM (1985) Do beta-lactamases "trap" cephalosporins? J Antimicrob Chemother 15:511–521

Lyon BR, Skurray R (1987) Antimicrobial resistance of *Staphylococcus aureus*: genetic basis. Microbiol Rev 51:88–134
Matsumoto H, Terawaki Y (1981) Chromosomal location of the genes participating in the formation of beta-lactamase in *Pseudomonas aeruginosa*. Symposium on Microbial Drug Resistance, Tokyo, p 207
McLaughlin JR, Murray CL, Rabinowitz JC (1981) Unique features in the ribosome binding site sequence of the gram-positive *Staphylococcus aureus* beta-lactamase gene. J Biol Chem 21:11283–11291
McLaughlin JR, Chang S-Y, Chang S (1982) Transcriptional analyses of the *Bacillus licheniformis penP* gene. Nucleic Acids Res 10:3905–3919
McPhail M, Furth AJ (1973) Purification and properties of an inducible beta-lactamase from *Pseudomonas aeruginosa* N.C.T.C. 8203. Biochem Soc Trans 1:1260–1263
Medeiros AA (1984) Beta-lactamases. Br Med Bull 40:18–27
Minami S, Inoue M, Mitsuhashi S (1980) Purification and properties of a cephalosporinase from *Enterobacter cloacae*. Antimicrob Agents Chemother 18:853–857
Murata T, Minami S, Yasuda K, Iyobe S, Inoue M, Mitsuhashi S (1981) Purification and properties of cephalosporinase from *Pseudomonas aeruginosa*. J Antibiot [Tokyo] 34:1164–1170
Neugebauer K, Sprengel R, Schaller H (1981) Penicillinase from *Bacillus licheniformis*: nucleotide sequence of the gene and implications for the biosynthesis of a secretory protein in a gram-positive bacterium. Nucleic Acids Res 9:2577–2588
Nichols L, Maki DG (1985) The emergence of resistance to beta-lactam antibiotics during treatment of *Pseudomonas aeruginosa* lower respiratory tract infections: is combination therapy the solution? Chemioterapia 4:102–109
Nicolas M-H, Honore N, Jarlier V, Philippon A, Cole ST (1987) Molecular genetic analysis of cephalosporinase production and its role in beta-lactam resistance in clinical isolates of *Enterobacter cloacae*. Antimicrob Agents Chemother 31:295–299
Nordstrom K, Eriksson-Grennberg KG, Bowman HG (1968) Resistance of *Escherichia coli* to penicillins. III *amp*B, a locus affecting episomally and chromosomally mediated resistance to ampicillin and chloramphenicol. Genet Res 12:157–168
Normark S, Edlund T, Grundstrom T, Bergstrom S, Wolf-Watz H (1977) *Escherichia coli* K-12 mutants hyperproducing chromosomal beta-lactamase by gene repetitions. J Bacteriol 132:912–922
Normark S, Bergstrom S, Edlund T, Grundstrom T, Jaurin B, Lindberg FP, Olsson O (1983) Overlapping genes. Annu Rev Genet 17:499–525
Normark S, Lindquist S, Lindberg F (1986) Chromosomal beta-lactam resistance in *Enterobacteria*. Scand J Infect Dis [Suppl] 49:38–45
Okonogi K, Suguira A, Kuno M, Higeshide E, Kondo M, Imada A (1985) Effect of beta-lactamase induction on susceptibility to cephalosporins in *Enterobacter cloacae* and *Serratia marcescens*. J Antimicrob Chemother 16:31–42
Richmond MH, Sykes RB (1973) The beta-lactamases of gram-negative bacteria and their possible physiological role. Adv Microb Physiol 9:31–38
Rosdahl VT (1973) Naturally occurring constitutive beta-lactamase of novel serotype in *Staphylococcus aureus*. J Gen Microbiol 77:229–231
Sabath LD, Jago M, Abraham EP (1965) Cephalosporinase and penicillinase activities of a beta-lactamase from *Pseudomonas pyocyanea*. Biochem J 96:739–752
Salerno AJ, Lampen JO (1986) Transcriptional analysis of beta-lactamase regulation in *Bacillus licheniformis*. J Bacteriol 166:769–778
Sanders CC, Sanders WE Jr (1986) Trapping and hydrolysis are not mutually exclusive mechanisms for beta-lactamase-mediated resistance. J Antimicrob Chemother 17:121–127
Sanders CC, Sanders WE Jr, Goering RV (1983a) Influence of clindamycin on derepression of beta-lactamases in *Enterobacter* spp. and *Pseudomonas aeruginosa*. Antimicrob Agents Chemother 24:48–53
Sanders CC, Sanders WE Jr, Goering RV (1983b) Effects of clindamycin on derepression of beta-lactamases in gram-negative bacteria. J Antimicrob Chemother 12 [Suppl C]:97–104

Seeberg AH, Tolxdorff-Neutzling RM, Wiedemann B (1983) Chromosomal beta-lactamases of *Enterobacter cloacae* are responsible for resistance to third-generation cephalosporins. Antimicrob Agents Chemother 23:918–925
Segalove M (1947) The effect of penicillin on growth and toxin production by enterotoxic Staphylococci. J Infect Dis 81:228–243
Waxman DJ, Amanuma H, Strominger JL (1982) Amino acid sequence homologies between *Escherichia coli* penicillin-binding protein 5 and class A beta-lactamase. FEBS Lett 139:159–163
Wiedemann B (1986) Selection of beta-lactamase producers during cephalosporin and penicillin therapy. Scand J Infect Dis [Suppl] 49:100–105
Yamamoto S, Lampen JO (1976) Membrane penicillinase of *Bacillus licheniformis* 749/C. Sequence and possible repeated tetrapeptide structure of the phospholipopeptide region. Proc Natl Acad Sci USA 73:1457–1461
Yamamoto T, Murayama SY, Sawai T (1983) Cloning and expression of the gene(s) for cephalosporinase production of *Citrobacter freundii*. Mol Gen Genet 190:85–91
Yocum RR, Waxman DJ, Rasmussen JR, Strominger JL (1979) Mechanism of penicillin action: penicillin and substrate bind covalently to the same active site serine in two bacterial L-alanine carboxypeptidases. Proc Natl Acad Sci USA 76:2730–2734

CHAPTER 8

Resistance to Quinolones and Fluoroquinolones

L. J. V. Piddock

A. Introduction

The quinolone class of oral antimicrobial agents has enjoyed rapid expansion and development over recent years and a revival in interest in the earlier agents nalidixic and oxolinic acid. The quinolone class (which includes 4-pyridone antibacterials) share the 4-quinolone nucleus and also a carboxylic acid substituent at position 3 (Fig. 1). During the last twenty-five years many compounds have

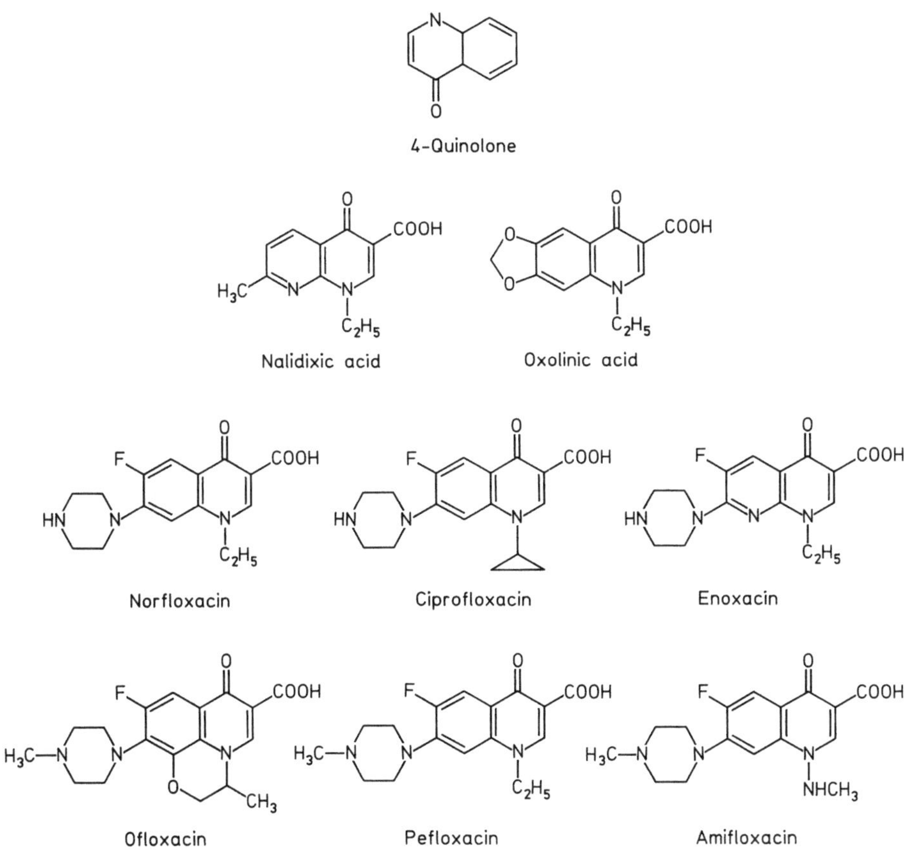

Fig. 1. The quinolone class of oral antimicrobial agents

been synthesised with additional substituents upon the basic nucleus and have been evaluated for use in antimicrobial chemotherapy. The early agents, nalidixic and oxolinic acid, were only active against gram-negative bacteria and the achievable serum concentrations were below the concentration needed to inhibit most pathogens. Consequently, these agents were limited to the treatment of urinary tract infections. In recent years many compounds have been synthesised with a fluorine substituent at position 6 of the quinolone nucleus (Fig. 1). This was found to enhance the antibacterial activity and enable adequate serum concentrations to be achieved (HOOPER and WOLFSON 1985). Other substituents in addition to the fluorine have been added to the nucleus with the aim of increasing the anti-gram positive bacterial activity. There are now approximately one dozen significant quinolone and fluoro-quinolone compounds (referred to as "quinolone" for the rest of the chapter) which are active against a broad spectrum of pathogens, including those causing systemic infections. The spectrum of activity for the agents in Fig. 1 has been recently reviewed (WOLFSON and HOOPER 1985) as has the pharmacology, clinical uses and toxicities in humans (HOOPER and WOLFSON 1985).

B. Mechanism of Action

I. DNA Gyrase

The majority of duplex DNA in vivo exists in a negatively supercoiled state. Supercoiling is very important as the double helix of DNA poses topological problems that the bacterial cell must overcome so that it may replicate and pass on its genetic information. The discovery that DNA existed in a circular form in bacterial cells and the problem of unravelling two strands of DNA by semiconservative replication indicated the necessity of a "swivel" in the circular DNA. The swivel composing of two intertwined single stranded rings permitting strand separation (CAIRNS 1963). In 1976, GELLERT et al. described an enzyme, DNA gyrase, that introduced negative supercoils into DNA. The study of the action of DNA gyrase (DNA topoisomerase II) has often utilised two compounds which had been shown to inhibit DNA replication, nalidixic acid and oxolinic acid. Studies upon DNA gyrase have resulted in the elucidation of the primary mechanism of action of nalidixic and oxolinic acids and hence quinolones.

In 1977 the *nal* A gene product was purified and shown to be the target of nalidixic acid (SUGINO et al. 1977). Comparison of the inhibition of purified DNA gyrase from *nal* A mutant cells and wild-type cells by nalidixic acid established a relationship between the *nal* A gene and DNA gyrase (SUGINO et al. 1977; GELLERT et al. 1977).

Purification of DNA gyrase from *Escherichia coli* and *Micrococcus luteus* has shown the enzyme to be composed of two sub-units, the A sub-unit and the B sub-unit (PEEBLES et al. 1978; GELLERT et al. 1978; LIU and WANG 1978; BROWN et al. 1979). Sub-unit A has been shown to be the target of nalidixic acid (PEEBLES et al. 1978). Purification of A and B sub-units and mixing under the appropriate conditions provides a reconstituted DNA gyrase. It has been shown that there is ten times more sub-unit A than sub-unit B in bacterial cells (HIGGINS et al. 1978). Sub-unit A comprises a dimer of two homogeneous protomers of 105000 daltons each; sub-unit B is a dimer of two homogeneous protomers each of 85 000 daltons (HIGGINS et al. 1978). Each protomer has an active site, and the reconstituted DNA gyrase comprises one dimer of A sub-units and one dimer of B sub-units, with a total molecular weight of 400 000.

The structural gene assignments of DNA gyrase *gyr* A and *gyr* B replaced the genetic terms *nal* A and *cou* in *E. coli* as the gene products of *gyr* A and *nal* A were shown to be identical, as were those of *cou* and *gyr* B (PEEBLES et al. 1978; HANSEN and VON MEYENBURG 1979; HIGGINS et al. 1978; MIZUUCHI et al. 1978; KREUZER and COZZARELLI 1979).

DNA gyrase negatively supercoils DNA, i.e. reduces the linking number of circular double stranded DNA and this reaction is ATP-dependent. The linking number is the number of times one strand of the double helix passes over the other if the molecule were constrained to lie in one plane. Since the linking number is changed, there must be a transient break of one or both strands of the DNA (BAUER 1978). DNA gyrase is a type II DNA topoisomerase; enzymes of this class in addition to supercoiling DNA have also been shown to catalyse the catenation/decatenation (interlinking/unlinking) and knotting and unknotting of circular DNA.

The current models of the mechanism of action of DNA gyrase all involve the movement of a portion of DNA through a double strand break, usually involving site-specific binding of DNA gyrase (LIU et al. 1980; BROWN and OZZARELLI 1979; WANG et al. 1981; MIZUUCHI et al. 1980; KREUZER and COZZARELLI 1980). Each model differs slightly in the precise geographical movements of DNA. Essentially DNA gyrase binds preferentially to specific sites on DNA and introduces local positive wrapping of the DNA. ATP is bound to the complex and the upper helix of DNA is transported through the lower necessitating a double stranded break in the DNA and a change in the conformation of DNA gyrase, thereby reducing the linking number by two. ATP is hydrolysed and the transported DNA portion prepares the system for another cycle of supercoiling (Fig. 2). There is evidence that there are 33 domains of supercoiling of the bacterial chromosome (CRUMPLIN and SMITH 1975). As can be seen supercoiling reduces the three-dimensional size of circular DNA thereby enabling the bacterial chromosome to fit within the bacterial cell! DNA gyrase and supercoiling correspondingly play a fundamental role in bacterial chromosome structure and function and it may be anticipated that inhibition of DNA gyrase is lethal to the bacterial cell.

Two biochemical assays have been developed for the measure of DNA gyrase activity. The first assay measures the conversion of relaxed plasmid DNA to its native supercoiled form using purified and reconstituted DNA gyrase (SUGINO and COZZARELLI 1980). The second assay utilises commercially available supercoiled plasmid DNA and examines the effect of inhibitor-DNA gyrase-DNA complex by measuring the production of linear DNA (DOMAGALA et al. 1986). From the first assay an I_{50} value corresponding to the concentration of inhibitor (in micrograms per millilitre) required to inhibit the supercoiling activity of DNA gyrase can be calculated. In the second assay a DNA gyrase cleavage value corresponding to the minimum concentration of inhibitor to produce linear DNA is obtained. It has been shown using these two assays that quinolones inhibit the supercoiling activity of DNA gyrase (SUGINO et al. 1977; GELLERT et al. 1977; YA-

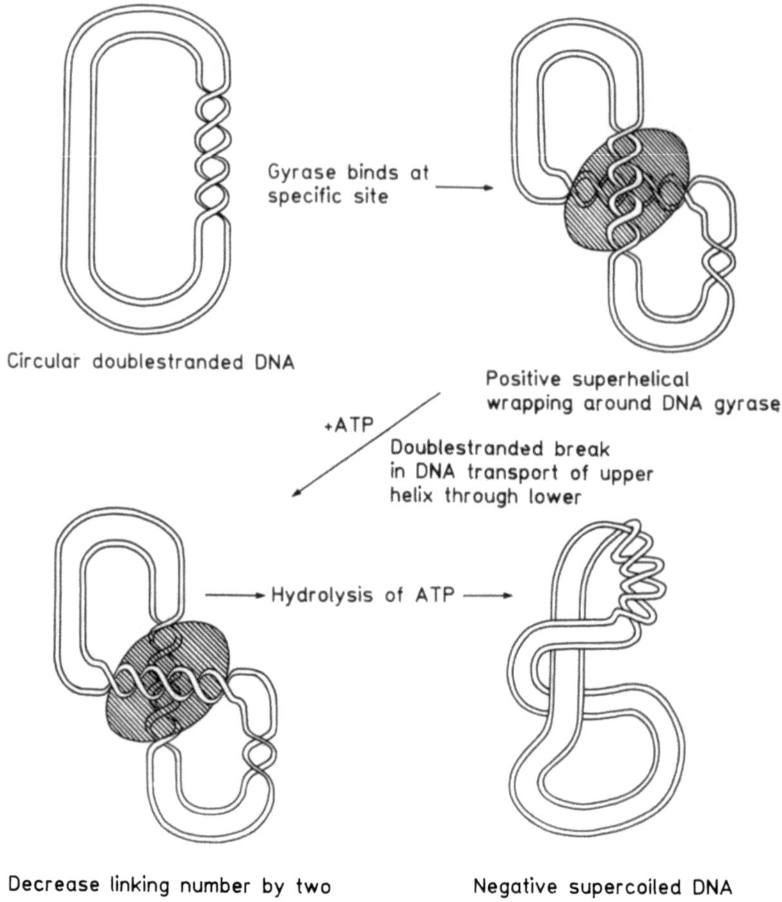

Fig. 2. Supercoiling of DNA. Adapted from GELLERT (1981)

MAGISHI et al. 1981; HOGBERG et al. 1984; DOMAGALA et al. 1986), and that this activity therefore resides at the A sub-unit. It is thought that nalidixic acid inhibits the nicking and resealing reaction catalysed by DNA gyrase, thereby preventing supercoiling (DRLICA et al. 1980), and more specifically the geographical location has been implicated as being at the DNA replication fork.

A number of reviews covering DNA gyrase activity have been published in recent years, and readers are directed to those for precise biochemical details of the activities of type II DNA topoisomerases (CHAMPOUX 1978; COZZARELLI 1980; GELLERT 1981; DRLICA 1984; WANG 1985).

II. SOS Response

Exposure of *E. coli* to agents or conditions that damage or interfere with DNA and its replication cause an increase in the expression of genes involved in DNA repair, collectively known as the SOS response. The expression of the SOS re-

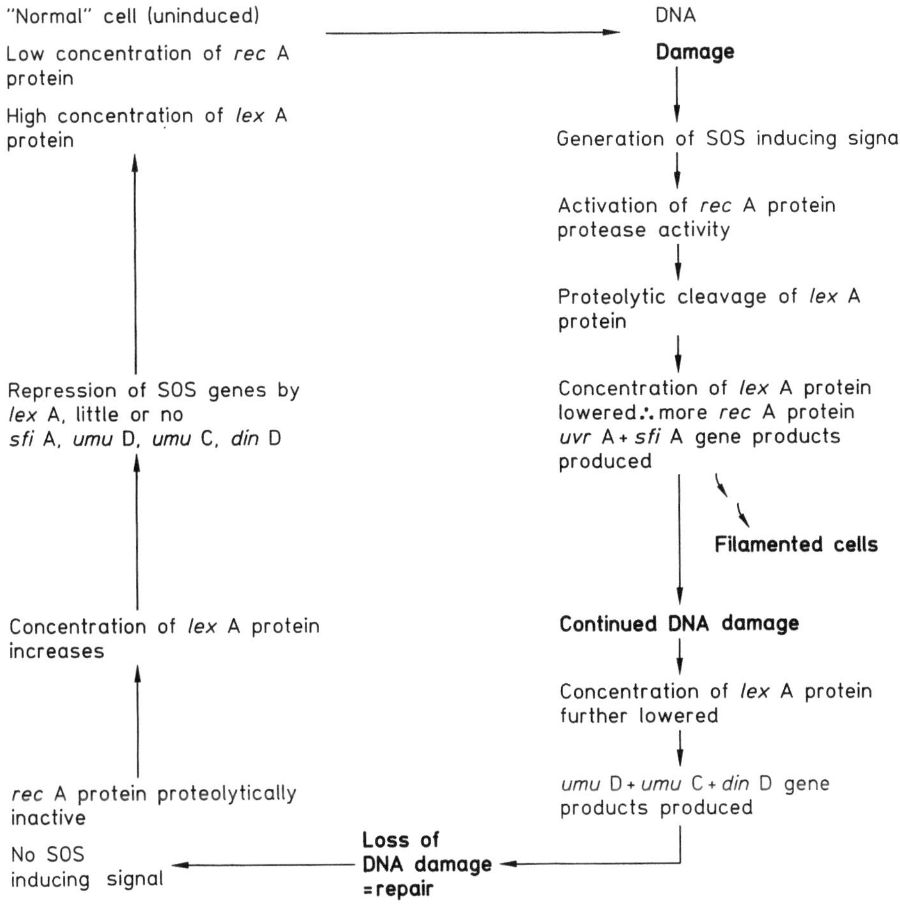

Fig. 3. The SOS regulatory system in *Escherichia coli*

sponse directly affects the mutagenic consequences of a variety of DNA-damaging treatments.

The present model of the physiology of the SOS responses has been described in detail in review articles (WITKIN 1976; LITTLE and MOUNT 1982; WALKER 1984). Essentially in an uninduced wild-type *E. coli* the *lex* A gene product acts as a repressor by binding to the operator sequences for many unlinked genes involved in the SOS response, including *rec* A and *lex* A itself (Fig. 3). (Some genes in this response have more than one operator sequence; in those cases the *lex* A gene product binds to all operator sites.) In the repressed wild-type state there is still considerable expression of *rec* A and *lex* A, such that there is sufficient Rec A protein produced to act in homologous recombination (KARU and BELK 1982; SALLES and PAOLETTI 1983). If there is damage to DNA or DNA replication is inhibited, an (unknown) inducing signal is generated. This signal reversibly activates the proteolytic activity of the Rec A protein which cleaves the *lex* A gene product (repressor). The concentration of Lex A therefore decreases, allowing several genes to be transcribed. As may be anticipated, the genes with weakly binding operator sites to Lex A are expressed primarily, but if the induction continues even genes with tightly bound operator sites are expressed. As a result of the pleiotropic expression of many genes, DNA is repaired and the inducing signal is therefore decreased, leading to repression of the activated genes by Lex A once again.

Many diverse physiological functions occur as part of the SOS response, including prophage induction, inhibition of cell division, induced radioresistance, and repair of double stranded DNA breaks to list a few (BROOKS and CLARK 1967; HERTMAN and LURIA 1967; COLE 1983; HUISMAN and D'ARI 1981). It is thought that nalidixic and oxolinic acids form a complex in which the A sub-units of DNA gyrase and the drug are bound to DNA acting as replication fork barriers thereby allowing the accumulation of gapped or single stranded DNA which has been proposed as the inducing signal (SALLES and DEFRAIS 1984). It has been shown that nalidixic acid and more recently new quinolones induce the SOS response (GUDAS and PARDEE 1976; PIDDOCK et al. 1988 a). Induction of the SOS response by quinolones may also be affected by factors other than inhibition of DNA gyrase and hence DNA synthesis, as greater induction of *rec* A is caused by higher concentrations of quinolones than lower even though both concentrations inhibit DNA synthesis to the same extent (GUDAS and PARDEE 1976; DIVER et al. 1987). The inducing signal for *rec* A expression requires wild-type *rec* B and *rec* C as *rec* BC mutants are non-inducible by quinolones (PIDDOCK et al. 1988 a). An increase in the concentration of quinolone gives an increase in the bactericidal activity up to an optimum concentration, the "most bactericidal concentration" (CRUMPLIN and SMITH 1975; RATCLIFFE and SMITH 1984); above this concentration the rate of bactericidal action is diminished. Maximum induction of *rec* A expression occurs at the "most bactericidal concentration;" above this concentration the quinolone inhibits protein synthesis hence inhibiting further SOS response (DIVER et al. 1987). Values greater than 90% inhibition of DNA synthesis, and presumably DNA gyrase activity, are achieved well below the most bactericidal concentration (DIVER et al. 1987).

One of the effects of SOS regulation is induction of the *sfi* A gene, whose product inhibits the *sfi* B (ftz) protein, which has been shown to be required for cell division (MANES et al. 1983). Most quinolones cause filamentation and presumably inhibit the production of the *sfi* B protein; recovery to wild-type cell division occurs when quinolone is removed and evidence indicates that this recovery requires competent lon proteins, which is thought to degrade the *sfi* A protein after DNA repair (DRLICA 1984). *lon* mutants exposed to nalidixic acid exhibit lethal filamentation (KANTOR and DEERING 1968). Continuous induction of the SOS response by quinolones prevents recovery from inhibition of cell division and is proposed to be one of the major mechanisms of cell death of these agents (PIDDOCK et al. 1988 a).

III. Other Properties of Quinolones

It has been shown that nalidixic acid and new quinolones eliminate plasmid DNA from bacterial cells at subinhibitory concentrations (BOUANCHAUD and CHAB-

BERT 1971; HAHN and CIAK 1976; TRAUB and KLEBER 1973; WEISSER and WEIDEMANN 1985). It is possible that this property may enhance the clinical attributes of these agents, as there would be firstly no plasmid-mediated mechanism of resistance; and secondly quinolones could be used in combination with other antimicrobial agents, e.g. aminoglycosides to treat infections that are caused by organisms harbouring plasmid-mediated mechanisms of resistance, e.g. to gentamicin and are "borderline" susceptible to quinolones (see Sect. D.I). In this case it is thought that the quinolone would aid elimination of the plasmid, rendering the infectious organism susceptible to gentamicin. It has also been shown that quinolones inhibit the transfer of plasmid DNA from bacterial cell to cell during conjugation (ANDERSON et al. 1973; BURMAN 1977; RENZINI et al. 1982; WEISSER and WEIDEMANN 1987). However, the concentrations of quinolone required to give >90% inhibition of conjugation were between one and six times the minimum inhibitory concentration (MIC), a concentration which also caused lethal effects to the donor and recipient (WEISSER and WEIDEMANN 1987). This would therefore cause doubt to be shed on the clinical importance of this property, and in addition clinical evidence that this occurs is to date anecdotal.

C. Mechanisms of Resistance

I. Properties of DNA Gyrase Mutants

As has been described on preceding pages, the primary mechanism of action or target of quinolones is the A sub-unit of DNA gyrase although the actual mechanism of bactericidal action may involve a cascade of cellular events. It therefore follows that the easiest mutants to select in the laboratory are those with altered DNA gyrase. The gene coding for the A sub-unit of DNA gyrase maps at 48 min (GELLERT et al. 1976) and a mutation at this gene causes high level resistance to the bacterial cell due to the production of a DNA gyrase, which is far less susceptible to nalidixic acid than the wild type. *gyr* A mutations have been well characterised in *E. coli* and exhibit cross-resistance between nalidixic acid and all quinolones (SMITH 1984). Strains expressing *gyr* A mutations do not exhibit cross-resistance to chemically unrelated antimicrobial agents (Table 1). Strains of *E. coli* containing *gyr* A mutations can be selected in the laboratory as spontaneous, single step events at a frequency of approximately 10^{-7}. Other Enterobacteriaceae produce spontaneous mutants at a similar frequency and with a similar phenotype to that expressed by an *E. coli gyr* A mutant [Table 3; PIDDOCK et al. manuscript submitted for publication (b)]. DNA gyrase has been shown to exist in all bacterial species examined to date (GELLERT 1981), and there is evidence that in *Pseudomonas aeruginosa*, *Haemophilus influenzae* and *Citrobacter freundii nal* A mutations similar to *gyr* A in *E. coli* also code for a DNA gyrase A sub-unit that is less susceptible to inhibition by nalidixic acid (RELLA and HAAS 1982; HIRAI et al. 1987; SETLOW et al. 1985; INOUE et al. 1987; AOYAMA et al. 1988). The *nal* A gene in *Ps. aeruginosa* maps between 51 and 52 min on the bacterial chromosome (HOLLOWAY and MORGAN 1986).

As can be seen, alteration of the A sub-unit of DNA gyrase from *E. coli* as a mechanism of resistance to nalidixic acid has been well characterised. By exa-

Table 1. Mutation causing decreased susceptibility to quinolones in *E. coli*

Genotype	Phenotype (MIC, μg ml⁻¹)							Locatio genetic (mins)
	Nal	Nor	Cip	Cefox	Tet	Chlor	Gent	
E. coli KL-16 wt	4	0.06	0.03	4	2	4	1	–
E. coli KL-16 *gyr A*	>128	0.5	0.5	4	> 2	4	0.5	48
nal B	16	0.06	0.03	–	–	–	0.5	88
nal-24	128	0.008	<0.008	–	–	–	0.5	83
nal-31	32	0.12	0.06	–	–	–	0.5	83
icd	> 8	–	–	–	–	–	–	25
cya	> 8	–	–	–	–	–	–	85
crp	> 8	–	–	–	–	–	–	74
nfx B	16	0.32	–	>32	16	32	–	20–22
nor B	12.5	0.20	0.10	25	–	12.5	1.56	34
nor C	0.78	0.20	0.05	6.25	–	3.13	1.56	8
nal D	(6)24	–	–	4	4	4	0.25	89.5

Nal, nalidixic acid; Nor, norfloxacin; Cip, ciprofloxacin; Cefox, cefoxitin; Tet, tetracycline; Chlor, chloramphenicol; Gent, gentamicin
Please see text for details of mutations

mining such mutants for susceptibility to new quinolones, a mechanism of resistance has been implied. Recently, two reports have documented a mechanism of resistance in *E. coli* to norfloxacin that maps at approximately 48 min on the genetic map and codes for a DNA gyrase A sub-unit that is less susceptible to norfloxacin inhibition than the enzyme from the parent wild-type strain (HOOPER et al. 1986; HIRAI et al. 1986); this mutation was deduced by both groups of workers to be an allele of *gyr* A, and designated *nfx* A and *nor* A respectively. There are also reports that a ciprofloxacin-resistant *E. coli* and *Enterobacter cloacae*, and an ofloxacin-resistant strain of *E. coli* derived in the laboratory, are also resistant due to a mutation at *gyr* A (HOOPER et al. 1987; YAMASHITA et al. 1986; SATO et al. 1986). Recently an *nfx* A mutation has been described for *Ps. aeruginosa* (HIRAI et al. 1987), and shown to be an allele of *nal* A which is thought to be the gene analagous to *gyr* A of *E. coli*. There is therefore growing evidence that *gyr* A mutations in *E. coli* (and probably other gram-negative bacteria) encode resistance to all quinolone compounds. The clinical relevance of this is discussed in Sect. D.

Two other DNA gyrase mutants of *E. coli* have also been isolated in the laboratory, *nal*-24, and *nal*-31, which occur at 83 min on the genetic map. The *nal*-24 (formerly *nal* D) confers resistance to nalidixic acid, pipemidic acid and a slight decrease in susceptibility to some new quinolones. The *nal*-31 (formerly *nal* C) confers resistance to nalidixic acid and hypersusceptibility to pipemidic acid and other quinolones possessing a piperazine substituent at carbon-7 on the quinolone nucleus (SMITH 1984). It is interesting to note that both of these mutations occur at the *gyr* B gene, but neither cause decreased susceptibility to novobiocin. The DNA gyrase of *nal*-31 and *nal*-24 express resistance or hypersusceptibility, correlating well with the antimicrobial activity of selected quinolones (YAMAGISHI et al. 1981). Neither mutation causes decreased susceptibility to chemically unrelated antimicrobial agents. Recently the nucleotide sequences of the *gyr* B gene, and that of the *nal*-31 and *nal*-24 mutants, has been determined (YAMAGISHI et al. 1986). Both *nal* mutations were shown to be due to a translation of nucleotides in the *gyr* B gene, and to reside in one of the two domains of the *gyr* B gene product, represented by *V*, thought to be the portion of the *gyr* B gene product that is necessary (when combined with A subunit) to reconstitute the DNA breakage-reunion activity of DNA gyrase. The other domain of the *gyr* B gene product contains the ATP binding site and is susceptible to the action of novobiocin. The *nal*-24 and *nal*-31 mutations cause changes in the overall electric charge of DNA gyrase; the *nal*-24 causes a decrease of minus charge and the *nal*-31 an increase in minus charge. This compares well with the data available for the electric charge associated with quinolones and that the *nal*-31 mutation confers hypersusceptibility to compounds that are positively charged. The data from the mechanism of resistance afforded by the *nal*-24 and *nal*-31 mutants demonstrate that electric charge is important in drug-DNA gyrase interactions. There is also some evidence that the *nal*-24 mutation confers decreased permeability to nalidixic acid (INOUYE et al. 1978).

II. Other Genetically Characterised Mutations Conferring Quinolone Resistance

It has been shown that in *E. coli* there are mutations in several genes that code for products unrelated to the apparent activity of DNA gyrase, and yet cause a decrease in susceptibility to nalidixic acid (MIC >8 μg ml^{-1}), such genes as *icd*, *cya*, *pur* B and *crp* (coding for enzyme 1 of the phosphoenol pyruvate-dependent-phosphotransferase system, adenyl cyclase, adenylosuccinase and CAMP-receptor protein respectively). Such mutants were selected in the laboratory using 8 μg ml^{-1} nalidixic acid and shown not to be mutations at *gyr* A or *gyr* B. The susceptibility of such mutants to new quinolones is unknown (KUMAR 1980).

A mutation in *E. coli* designated *nal* B has been described, mapping at 58 minutes on the chromosomal map, causing resistance to nalidixic acid (HANE and WOOD 1969). The mechanism of resistance afforded by the *nal* B mutant was purported to be a change in the permeability of nalidixic acid, although measurements of the uptake of nalidixic acid into the bacterial cell, and outer membrane protein profiles were not examined; however, EDTA treatment enhanced DNA synthesis inhibition, i.e. DNA gyrase inhibition, whereas similar treatment to a *gyr* A mutant was ineffective (BOURGINON et al. 1973). Another mutation causing decreased susceptibility in *E. coli* to nalidixic acid has also been described (HREBENDA et al. 1985), *nal* D. The gene coding for this mutation occurs between 89 and 89.5 minutes on the genetic map and is susceptible to 6 μg ml^{-1} nalidixic acid at 30 °C, but is resistant to nalidixic acid at 37 °C (MIC = 24 μg ml^{-1}). This mutant shows a decrease in the uptake of [^{3}H]nalidixic acid and [^{3}H]glycerol compared to the wild-type parent strain, but no change in the outer membrane protein profile or cross-resistance to chemically unrelated antimicrobial agents. It is hypothesized that this strain contains a mutation causing a phospholipid bilayer alteration. The susceptibility of this mutant to new quinolones was not described.

Two laboratories have recently described mechanisms of norfloxacin resistance which have been characterised in laboratory derived strains of *E. coli* K-12, *nfx* B and *nor* B. In both studies, a mechanism of resistance was determined at a genetic locus distant to *gyr* A (HOOPER et al. 1986; HIRAI et al. 1986 a). However, whilst each study describes mutants that have similar phenotypes (Table 1), each apparently maps at different locations (20–22 min and 34 min respectively). Both mutants were shown to be lacking OMP F and lower uptake of norfloxacin compared to the parent wild type. Both mutants demonstrated cross-resistance to cephalosporins, tetracycline and chlorampherícol, the activity of which has been shown to be affected by the absence of OMP F (JAFFE et al. 1982; PUGSLEY and SCHNAITMANN 1978; REEVE and DOHERTY 1968). The *nfx* B gene apparently occurs at or close to the structural gene for OMP F which maps at 22 min on the bacterial chromosome (HOOPER et al. 1986). The *nor* B gene occurs close to the *mar* A gene, which has been shown to encode multiple antibiotic resistance such as decreased susceptibility to tetracycline and chloramphenicol (GEORGE and LEVY 1983). Two recently described mutations, *cfx* B and *ofx* B, with similar phenotypes to *nor* B have also been shown to occur close to *mar* A (HOOPER et al. 1987). It is possible that *nor* B, *cfx* B and *ofx* B are alleles of *mar* A. Whilst the role of OMP F in causing decreased susceptibility to quinolones has been implicated, strains of *E. coli* expressing decreased production of OMP F do not always show a decrease in susceptibility to new quinolones (PIDDOCK and WISE 1986); however the differences in susceptibility for OMP F strains exhibited by HOOPER et al. (1986) and HIRAI et al. (1986 a) may not have been detected in the experimental procedure employed by PIDDOCK and WISE (1986).

HIRAI et al. also described a third *E. coli* mutant with decreased susceptibility to norfloxacin, *nor* C. This mutation mapped at 8 min on the genetic map and was shown to have altered expression of OMP F and a change in the lipopolysaccharide (LPS) structure of the outer membrane. The *nor* B and *nor* C mutants demonstrate the same decrease in uptake of norfloxacin (and the absence of OMP F) and yet the *nor* C mutant does not show the same decrease in susceptibility to cefoxitin and chloramphenicol. The *nor* C mutant is hypersusceptible to cloxacillin, novobiocin, sodium dodecyl sulphate and gentian violet and showed changes in the LPS. Alterations to the LPS have been shown previously to cause a change in susceptibility to penicillin and detergents (HIRUMA et al. 1984).

HIRAI et al. (1987) have recently transferred their studies of laboratory derived norfloxacin resistance to *Ps. aeruginosa* and described a *nfx* B gene that codes for a decrease in susceptibility to norfloxacin and hypersusceptibility to beta lactam and aminoglycoside antimicrobial agents (Table 2). The *nfx* B mutant exhibited a wild-type outer membrane profile with the addition of an extra band at 54000 daltons. The uptake of norfloxacin was shown to be decreased when compared with the wild-type parent strain. It can be seen that the *nfx* B mutant of *Ps. aeruginosa* is not similar to the *nfx* B mutant of *E. coli.* There has been a *nal* B gene described for *Ps. aeruginosa*, which maps at approximately 32 min on the genetic map, and encodes resistance to nalidixic acid and some β-lactams but not gentamicin, rifampicin or tetracycline (Table 2) (RELLA and HAAS 1982); however, uptake studies and outer membrane protein profiles were not examined. The *nal* B gene of *Ps. aeruginosa* may be similar to the *nor* B gene of *E. coli.*

Table 2. Mutations causing decreased susceptibility to quinolones in *Ps. aeruginosa*

Genotype	Phenotype (MIC, μg ml^{-1})								Location on genetic map (mins)
	Nal	Nor	Cip	Gent	Carb	Cefs	Tet	Chlor	
Ps. aeruginosa									
PA04009 (wt)	100	0.5	0.12	2	64	2	32	64	–
nal A	>1024	4	1	2	64	2	32	64	50–52
nal B	800	–	–	–	200	–	–	–	31–32
nfx B	200	6.25	0.78	0.39	12.5	0.78	25	50	4– 8

Nal, nalidixic acid; Nor, norfloxacin; Cip, ciprofloxacin; Gent, gentamicin; Carb, carbenicillin; Cefs, cefsulodin; Tet, tetracycline; Chlor, chloramphenicol
Please see text for details of mutations

III. Properties of Mutants Defective in Components of the SOS Response

To increase the probability of survival, bacteria have developed the ability to repair damaged DNA, the SOS response (see Sect. B.II). Mutants defective in various components of the SOS response have been examined for the ability to survive in the presence of nalidixic acid. As might be anticipated strains defective in *rec* A, *rec* F, *rec* B *rec* C, *rec* B, rec C *rec* F are hypersusceptible to nalidixic acid (McDaniel et al. 1978). It is now possible to select in the laboratory strains of *E. coli* that constitutively produce *rec* A protein (one of the major components of the SOS response); this may give the bacterial cell an advantage in repairing its DNA by providing a ready pool of *rec* A protein that only needs to be catalysed to proteolytic activity to initiate the SOS response. Preliminary data suggest that such mutants may be less susceptible to the action of quinolones (Piddock, unpublished observations).

IV. Properties of Strains of Gram-Negative Bacteria with Phenotypically Characterised Mechanisms of Resistance

There have been various studies of in vitro mutants of Enterobacteriaceae with decreased susceptibility to quinolones. Several groups have examined the ability of different species for the ability to produce spontaneous mutants with a phenotype similar to that of an *E. coli gyr* A mutant, that is high level resistance to nalidixic acid, cross resistance to other quinolones and no cross-resistance to chemically unrelated antimicrobial agents. It has been found that most Enterobacteriaceae examined will produce spontaneous quinolone resistant mutants, although the techniques employed by the various groups differ (Barry and Jones 1984; King et al. 1984; Tenney et al. 1983; Chin and Neu 1983; Piffaretti et al. 1983; Cullman et al. 1985). Dependent on the selecting concentration of quinolone, all Enterobacteriaceae except *Proteus* spp. will produce spontaneous mutants with a *gyr* A phenotype at a frequency of approximately 1 in 10^7 (Cullmann et al. 1985; Piddock et al. 1988 b). Previous reports have shown that some new quinolones do not select resistant variants; however, that has usually been because the selecting concentration of quinolone employed is above the MIC of a *gyr* A type mutant.

Several groups have selected mutants of *Enterobacteriaceae with decreased susceptibility to quinolones, and several unrelated antimicrobial agents. A multi-resistant phenotype in Klebsiella pneumoniae* was described in 1984 by Sanders and her co-workers, which was selected with decreased susceptibility to norfloxacin and also decreased susceptibility to β-lactams, chloramphenical and tetracycline (Table 3). This strain also had a decrease in certain outer membrane proteins, putatively identified as porin proteins. Using different strains but from the same species, *Olsson-Llilequist* et al. (1985) also showed the selection of norfloxacin-resistant strains of *K. pneumoniae* and *E. cloacae* with an altered outer membrane profile and a multi-resistant phenotype. GUTMANN et al. (1985) selected mutants with decreased susceptibility to nalidixic acid and which were shown to have a concomitant decrease in susceptibility to some β-lactams, chloramphenicol and trimethoprim. Outer membrane protein profiles demonstrated a decrease in certain outer membrane proteins, again putatively identified as porin proteins, and the uptake of radiolabelled chloramphenicol and glucose was also shown to be decreased. Both studies concluded that the mechanism of resistance to all agents was due to a decrease in the production of porin proteins.

To verify whether a multi-resistant Enterobacteriaceae phenotype selected using nalidixic acid or a newer quinolone is cross resistant to other agents, strains of *E. cloacae*, *K. pneumoniae* and *Citrobacter freundii* were examined (PIDDOCK et al. 1988b). The selected phenotype did not always agree with that published by Sanders and Gutmann (Table 3). Moreover, only the multi-resistant phenotype of only one strain of *E. cloacae* showed decreased susceptibility to trimethoprim, and not all multi-resistant phenotypes had a change in outer membrane protein profile. Strains with a change in outer membrane profile showed a concomitant decrease in the uptake of [^{14}C]pefloxacin. From these three studies it is apparent that there are pleiotropic mechanisms of resistance, although one would expect that a one-step spontaneous mutation causing a simultaneous change to the susceptibility of the bacteria to several agents would be due to a mutation at a single gene. Until chromosome maps of each of the individual strains are available it will be difficult to interpret the observed phenotypes and the exact role of outer membrane proteins in quinolone resistance.

V. Mechanisms of Resistance in Bacteria Selected In Vivo

It has been shown that between 1% and 2% of urinary isolates of gram-negative bacteria are clinically resistant to nalidixic acid and which exhibited laboratory cross-resistance to new quinolones (SLACK 1984; PIDDOCK et al. 1986). All nalidixic acid resistant isolates from the latter study exhibited a *gyr* A mutant phenotype (Table 3). One strain of *E. coli* from this study which was highly resistant to nalidixic acid (MIC = > 512 μg ml^{-1}) was shown to contain altered A subunits of DNA gyrase (WYKE and CULLEN, personal communication). There have been two descriptions of *E. coli* expressing high level resistance to norfloxacin (MIC = 100 μg ml^{-1}) which has been isolated from an upper urinary tract infection (SATO et al. 1987; AOYAMA et al. 1987). The DNA gyrase from the strain in the first re-

Table 3. Phenotypes of Enterobacteriaceae selected with decreased susceptibility to quinolones

Description	Species	Susceptibility (μg ml⁻¹)								OMP change	Decrease in quinolone uptake
		Nal	Nor	Cip	Cefox	Tet	Chlor	Gent	Tmp		
wt[a]	*E. cloacae*	8	0.12	0.015	256	>128	>128	0.25	0.15	–	
gyr A type[a]	*E. cloacae*	512	2	0.5	256	>128	>128	0.25	0.15	×	×
multi-R type[a]	*E. cloacae*	64	1	0.25	256	>128	>128	0.25	8	√	√
N[b]	*E. cloacae*	64	–	–	–	–	128	–	16	√	–
wt[a]	*S. marcescens*	8	0.25	0.06	16	8	8	0.5	0.5	–	–
gyr A type[a]	*S. marcescens*	256	4	0.5	16	8	8	0.5	1	×	×
multi-R type[a]	*S. marcescens*	16	1	0.25	64	16	64	0.5	1	√	×
N[b]		256	–	–	–	–	256	–	16	√	–
wt[a]	*K. pneumoniae*	8	0.5	0.06	16	>128	8	0.25	32	–	–
gyr A type[a]	*K. pneumoniae*	>512	4	0.5	16	>128	8	0.25	32	×	×
multi-R type[a]	*K. pneumoniae*	256	4	0.5	128	>128	128	0.5	32	√	×
N[b]	*K. pneumoniae*	64	–	–	–	–	128	–	8	√	–
NOR-6[c]	*K. pneumoniae*	64	2	0.5	256	32	> 32	–	–	√	–

[a] PIDDOCK et al. (1988b)
[b] GUTMANN et al. (1985)
[c] SANDERS et al. (1984)
Abbreviations as Tables 1 and 2. Please see text for details

port has been purified and the A subunits shown to be less susceptible to inhibition by norfloxacin and other new quinolones, resulting in supercoiling activity that was highly resistant to quinolone action, correlating well with the antibacterial activities of these drugs. Whilst the chromosomal location of the gene involved was not determined, the evidence would indicate that alterations to DNA gyrase causing a decrease in affinity for quinolones causes clinical resistance. It is of interest to note, however, that the change in susceptibility observed in this strain and in the strain obtained in the UK was far higher than that observed for laboratory derived *gyr* A mutations. The strain described in the second report also had a DNA gyrase less susceptible to quinolone inhibition, however this strain also lacked OMP F and, so, the authors concluded that both factors contributed to resistance.

It is likely that DNA gyrase alterations also cause a decrease in susceptibility to enoxacin (and other new quinolones), as strains of *Ps. aeruginosa* isolated after enoxacin therapy from the sputum of patients suffering from chronic obstructive airways disease show a similar phenotype to that observed for a strain expressing a *nal* A mutation (PIDDOCK et al. 1987 a). There was also one pair of isolates from this study where the post-enoxacin-therapy isolate showed a decrease in susceptibility to quinolones, and some β-lactams. Examination of this strain showed the absence of OMP F and a decrease in the uptake of [^{14}C]enoxacin (PIDDOCK et al. 1987 b). Genetic analysis indicated a *nal* B type mutation. It is interesting to note that clinical isolates of *Ps. aeruginosa* treated with polymyxin B nonapeptide had increased sensitivity to quinolones (KUBESCH et al. 1987).

Alterations in outer membrane protein profile have also been implicated to cause a decrease in susceptibility to ciprofloxacin in a strain of *Serratia marcescens* isolated from the sputum of a patient suffering from a fatal bacteraemia,

Table 4. In vivo development of resistance during quinolone treatment

Site of infection	Organism(s)	Therapy	Reference
Gastrointestinal tract	*Shigella dysenteriae*	Nalidixic acid	PANHOTRA and DESAI (
Gastrointestinal tract	*Shigella dysenteriae*	Nalidixic acid	PANHOTRA et al. (1985)
Lungs	*Ps- aeruginosa*	Ciprofloxacin	ROBERTS et al. (1985)
Wound	*Ps. aeruginosa*	Ciprofloxacin	CROOK et al. (1985)
Lungs	*Staph. aureus*	Ciprofloxacin	HUMPHREYS and MULV (1985)
Lung, blood	*Kleb. pneumoniae*	Ciprofloxacin	CHAPMAN et al. (1985)
Blood	*E. cloacae*	Ciprofloxacin	CHAPMAN et al. (1985)
Bone	*Ps. aeruginosa*	Ciprofloxacin	CHAPMAN et al. (1985)
Chest	*Ps. aeruginosa*	Ciprofloxacin	CHAPMAN et al. (1985)
Blood	Staphylococci	Ciprofloxacin	SMITH et al. (1985)
Genitals	*Neisserie gonorrhoeae*	Enoxacin	WAGENVOORT et al. (19
Blood	*Ps. aeruginosa*	Ciprofloxacin	AZADIAN et al. (1986)
Lungs	*Ps. aeruginosa*	Enoxacin	PIDDOCK et al. (1987)
Urine	*Kleb. pneumoniae*	Enoxacin	WISE et al. (1987)
Gastric mucosa	*Campylobacter pyloridis*	Ofloxacin	GLUPCZYNSKI et al. (1
Blood	*Corynebacterium jeikeium* (group JK)	Ciprofloxacin	MURPHY and FERGUSO (1987)

although the patient was treated with ticarcillin and tobramycin (SANDERS and WATANAKUNAKORN 1986).

There have been several reports of quinolone resistant strains emerging during therapy with new quinolones (Table 4); however no biochemical or genetic analysis has been made. Susceptibility determination for all strains except the *Klebsiella pneumoniae* demonstrates only a decrease in susceptibility to quinolones, implicating a DNA gyrase alteration (PIDDOCK, unpublished observations). The *K. pneumoniae* demonstrate cross-resistance to β-lactams but no apparent change in the outer membrane protein profile (PIDDOCK, unpublished observations). There has been one report of plasmid mediated resistance to nalidexic acid in *Shigella dysenteriae*, but the mechanism of resistance encoded on the plasmid was not characterized. Cross resistance to new quinolones was not demonstrated (MUNSHI et al. 1987).

VI. Inherent Resistance

In the preceding sections (Sects. I–V) the mechanisms of resistance described are for *E. coli* or other gram-negative bacteria. It has long been realised that nalidixic acid displays little or no useful antibacterial activity against gram-positive bacteria; however, with the development of newer more active quinolones the gram-positive activity has been improved (WOLFSON and HOOPER 1985). It can be seen however that whilst the susceptibility of most gram-positive bacteria is within the therapeutically achievable concentrations of many new quinolones (please see Sect. D) the susceptibility of such species as *Staphylococcus aureus* and *Streptococcus pneumoniae* is far less than that of the Enterobacteriaceae, and resistant mutants can be selected easily in experimental infections (KAATZ et al. 1981). It is thought that this lower susceptibility is due to a DNA gyrase that is inherently less susceptible to the action of quinolones (N. Georgopapadakou, personal communication). Descriptions of the DNA gyrase of medically important gram-positive species has yet to be published; however, data are available for the enzyme from *Micrococcus luteus* and *Bacillus subtilis* (LIU and WANG 1978; SUGINO and BOTT 1980). A mutation at *gyr* A in *B. subtilis* causing decreased susceptibility to nalidixic acid (MIC > 300 μg ml^{-1}) has been mapped between *pur* A and *cys* A on the chromosomal map (VAZQUEZ-RAMOS and MANDELSTRAM 1981). Two mutations conferring decreased susceptibility to oxolinic acid were also described, *oxr*-1 and *oxr*-2; however, they were not thought to be alleles of *gyr* A as they did not map at the same location. The *gyr* A mutation conferred a larger decrease in susceptibility than *oxr*-1 and *oxr*-2, and DNA synthesis was not inhibited by oxolinic acid (unlike *oxr*-1 and *oxr*-2); the authors therefore suggested *oxr*-1 and *oxr*-2 may code for a mutation affecting the uptake of nalidixic acid and oxolinic acids.

D. Clinical Implications of Resistance Mechanisms

I. Pharmacokinetics

Bacterial resistance to an antimicrobial agent is one of the major causes of therapeutic failure. The identification of not only resistance to an agent but the mechanism of that resistance are important to the clinician in deciding whether to continue the same therapy (a common statement by medical microbiologists is that the patient recovered in spite of the bacteria being resistant) or what other antimicrobial therapy options are left available. Therapeutic failures due to resistance to an antimicrobial agent in the clinical setting can be due to one or a combination of several factors; firstly the pathogen may be inherently resistant to the antimicrobial agent used, secondly the dose administered of the chosen antimicrobial agent may be too low and finally the patient displays unusual pharmacokinetic parameters allowing a higher than expected concentration of the agent to be excreted so that an insufficient concentration reaches the site of infection. The result of the second two situations is that a subpopulation of bacteria with decreased susceptibility to the antimicrobial agent, perhaps due to a spontaneous mutation, is allowed to proliferate allowing the emergence of a resistant population. Alternatively, superinfection by a species whose growth was inhibited by the original pathogen may now emerge. In vitro studies of the mechanisms of resistance prevalent in spontaneous mutants indicate the possible types of resistance that can occur to an antimicrobial agent in vivo.

There have been essentially two classes of quinolone resistance described to date, mutations affecting DNA gyrase and mutations affecting OMP F production and/or permeability (Sect. C). The susceptibility of an example of each class for five species of Enterobacteriaceae is shown in Table 5. By comparison with the maximum achievable concentrations (C_{max}) in selected body fluids in healthy human volunteers (Table 6) certain conclusions as to the clinical relevance of characterised mechanisms of resistance can be made. For ciprofloxacin, ofloxacin and pefloxacin a sufficient concentration can be achieved in the serum and urine to inhibit even the "high level" resistance exhibited by a laboratory derived *gyr* A mutant, and it might be anticipated that in a patient displaying "normal" pharmacokinetics that bacterial resistance would not occur. However, a strain of

Table 5. Susceptibility of selected laboratory mutants to a range of quinolones

Strain	Susceptibility (μg ml^{-1})								
	Nal	Nor	Cip	Enox	Ami	Per	Ofl	Ro	S-3
E. coli gyr A	>256	1	0.25	0.5	4	2	1	2	4
E. coli multi-R	16	0.25	0.03	0.5	0.5	0.5	0.12	0.5	2
E. cloacae gyr A	>256	2	0.5	2	4	2	1	2	4
E. cloacae multi-R	64	1	0.25	1	4	2	1	1	4
S. marcescens gyr A	>256	1	0.5	4	4	1	1	2	4
S. marcescens multi-R	16	1	0.25	1	1	1	1	0.5	2
K. pneumoniae gyr A	>256	2	0.5	2	4	2	1	2	4
K. pneumoniae multi-R	64	0.5	0.5	1	1	1	0.5	0.5	2
C. freundii gyr A	>256	2	0.25	4	4	2	1	2	4
C. freundii multi-R	64	1	0.12	2	1	2	1	1	4

All data from PIDDOCK et al. (1988b)
Nal, nalidixic acid; Nor, norfloxacin; Cip, ciprofloxacin; Enox, enoxacin; Ami, amifloxacin; Per, perfloxacin; Ofl, ofloxacin; Ro, Ro 236240; S-30, S-25930

Table 6. Pharmacology of quinolones in humans

Drug	Dose (mg)	Route	Serum C_{max} (μg ml^{-1})	Urine C_{max} (μg ml^{-1})	Sputum (μg ml^{-1})
Nalidixic acid	1000	p.o.	–	50–500[b]	–
Ciprofloxacin	500	p.o.	1.9–2.9[a]	–	0.8–1.5[b]
	200		–	255[b]	–
Norfloxacin	400	p.o.	1.5[a]	98–114[a]	–
Enoxacin	600	p.o.	3.7[a]	288[a]	3.7[b]
Ofloxacin	600	p.o.	11[a]	–	–
	200	p.o.	–	216[b]	4.6[b]
Pefloxacin	400	p.o.	3.8[a]	–	–

[a] Data from Hooper and Wolfson (1985)
[b] Data from Wise (personal communication)

E. coli selected in vivo and shown to have quinolone resistance due to a DNA gyrase with decreased susceptibility to quinolones (Sato et al. 1987) has an MIC to ciprofloxacin and ofloxacin above the clinically achievable concentrations in serum and sputum. It is possible that the patient from this study had abnormal pharmacokinetics allowing the organisms to bathe in a low level of quinolone, providing ideal conditions for the selection of resistant variants.

Comparison of the susceptibility of the *gyr*-A phenotype (not genetically characterised) displayed by strains of Enterobacteriaceae other than *E. coli* suggest that certain species can become outside the therapeutic spectrum of norfloxacin and enoxacin if the infection were in the blood. Such mutants would not be inhibited by the achievable concentrations of enoxacin and ciprofloxacin in sputum, either. It may be prudent to suggest that if a strain of such a species is resistant to >64 μg ml^{-1} nalidixic acid then it will probably be clinically resistant to norfloxacin, enoxacin and ciprofloxacin at certain sites. If one allows greater than four-fold multiple of the MIC as the minimum required clinically achievable concentration (as argued by many clinicians) then the majority of the new quinolones would not retain their therapeutic spectrum against *gyr*-A type mutation in species such as *K. pneumoniae* infecting the lungs or blood.

It is of interest to note that the species of bacteria (e.g. *Staph. aureus, Ps. aeruginosa*) that are dominating the collection of resistant variants isolated to date (Table 4) are species that are less susceptible to most quinolones than the majority of species examined (Enterobacteriaceae, Neissericeae) in in vitro antimicrobial agents screening programmes. They are also the species infecting sites such as the lungs where in certain patient populations, e.g. cystic fibrotics, the achievable concentrations in the sputum may be far lower than those in a normal human volunteer. The selection of patients from which the resistant variants were isolated often also had underlying defects in their host defences which might enhance the selection of strains with decreased susceptibility to quinolones.

It may be that a quinolone will be combined with another antimicrobial agent for serious infections which would be active against any variants expressing a *gyr*-A type mutation; perhaps what is more worrying is a mechanism of resistance that causes decreased susceptibility to several chemically unrelated agents, such as the multiresistant phenotype (abbreviated to multi-R) observed in certain Enterobacterioaceae (which is similar to the *E. coli nfx* B, *nor* B, etc.). If the susceptibility of such strains is examined it is possible that the achievable concentrations of ciprofloxacin, norfloxacin and enoxacin in sputum, serum, sputum and serum respectively would be insufficient.

A current body of opinion is that as quinolones such as ofloxacin and ciprofloxacin achieve concentrations in body fluids such as serum that are up to one hundred fold excess of the inhibitory concentration of many bacterial species that the selection of resistant organisms and hence therapy failure is extremely unlikely. Coupled with the apparent information that the susceptibility of strains of *E. coli* expressing *gyr* A mutations is still within the spectrum of quinolone activity the likelihood of resistant variants emerging is very remote. However, evidence is appearing that what may be the case for laboratory strains of *E. coli* certainly is not the case for other species. The strains from Table 4 all expressed a larger decrease in susceptibility to all quinolones than one might anticipate from laboratory studies (PIDDOCK and DIVER, unpublished observations). It is worrying that for this class of antimicrobial agents that laboratory derived resistant variants may not be emulating their in vivo isolated counterparts; this is perhaps a facet of quinolone activity that differs from other chemical classes of antimicrobial agent.

The actual numbers of nalidixic acid-resistant variants that are cross resistant to quinolones occurring to date is still low (PIDDOCK et al. 1986) and the available statistics of the occurrence of clinical resistance to new quinolones confirm this. As quinolones are used to treat a wider range of infections in a larger number of patients, isolates of certain species expressing resistance to certain agents at certain sites will probably increase. From the evidence to date the species will include *Ps. aeruginosa*, *Staph. aureus*, *K. pneumoniae* and *Ent. cloacae* infecting the lungs or blood, and the actual mechanism(s) of that resistance have yet to be confirmed.

II. Pathogenicity

It has been suggested that strains of *E. coli* isolated in the laboratory expressing decreased susceptibility to quinolones are at a physiological disadvantage compared to a wild-type sensitive strain (CRUMPLIN 1985; RAVIZZOLA et al. 1987). Such strains have new nutritional requirements and do not exhibit the same growth kinetics as the parent strain from which they were derived. It is possible that the strains isolated in this study exhibit the mutations described by HELLING and KUKORA (1971) and KUMAR (1980) such as *pur* B as well as *gyr* A type mutations. Other workers in the field have not noted any physiological differences between wild-type strains and characterised mutants which would almost certainly have been observed, if present, during chromosomal mapping experiments. Strains expressing altered porin production often have a longer doubling time than the wild type, and although this has not been recorded for the *E. coli nfx* B, *nor* B or *nor* C mutants it might be expected. The post-enoxacin therapy quinolone resistant *Ps. aeruginosa* had a doubling time that was 8 minutes longer than the apparent isogenic original sensitive isolate, but this slower growth rate obviously did not have a deleterious effect on the survival of the resistant variant (PIDDOCK et al. 1987 b). To prove or disprove the theory that quinolone resistant variants are at a physiological disadvantage, and are therefore less likely to cause infection, i.e. be pathogenic, animal studies need to be performed. The occurrence of quinolone resistant variants causing infections in clinical practice perhaps indicates that such studies are unnecessary.

E. Summary and Conclusions

Quinolones have been shown to exert their bactericidal action via inhibition of the A subunits of DNA gyrase. Resistance to quinolones has been characterised in *E. coli* and shown to be caused either by a mutation at *gyr* A conferring DNA gyrase A subunits with decreased affinity for quinolones or by a determinant conferring decreased susceptibility to quinolones, β-lactams, chloramphenicol and tetracycline. The involvement of OMP F and decreased uptake of these agents has been identified as the mechanism of this resistance. Genetic studies have not been performed for other Enterobacteriaceae, but phenotypic characterisation suggests that two similar categories also exist. The mechanisms of quinolone resistance exhibited by clinical isolates is to date primarily the *gyr* A type. The frequency of occurrence of quinolone resistant variants is at present low; however, with an increase in usage, it may be predicted that the incidence will rise.

Acknowledgements. I thank J. T. Smith, A. Wyke, and N. Georgopapadakou for preprints and/or discussions of their unpublished work. I also thank R. Wise for helpful discussions of human pharmacokinetics and J. Diver and D. Griggs for technical assistance for certain studies described in this chapter. Lastly, I thank Central Clerical Services at Birmingham University for typing this manuscript.

References

Anderson JD, Ingram LC, Richmond MH, Weidemann B (1973) Studies on the nature of plasmids arising from conjugation in the human gastro-intestinal tract. J Med Microbiol 6:475–486

Aoyama H, Sato K, Kato T, Hirai K, Mitsuhashi S (1987) Norfloxacin resistance in a clinical isolate of *Escherichia coli.* Antimicrob Agents Chemother 31:1640–1641

Aoyama H, Sato K, Fujii T, Fujimaka K, Inoue M, Mitsuhashi S (1988) Purification of *Citrobacter freundii* DNA gyrase and inhibition by quinolones. Antimicrob Agents Chemother 32:104–109

Azadian BS, Bendig JW, Samson DM (1986) Emergence of ciprofloxacin resistant *Pseudomonas aeruginosa* after combined therapy with ciprofloxacin and amikacin. J Antimicrob Chemother 18:771

Barry AL, Jones RN (1984) Cross-resistance among cinoxacin, ciprofloxacin, DJ-6783, enoxacin, nalidixic-acid, norfloxacin and oxolinic acid after in vitro selection of resistant populations. Antimicrob Agents Chemother 25:775–777

Bauer WR (1978) Structure and reactions of closed duplex DNA. Annu Rev Biophys Bioeng 7:287–313

Bounchchaud DH, Chabbert YA (1971) Practical effectiveness of agents curing R-factors and plasmids. Ann NY Acad Sci 182:305–311

Bourginon GJ, Levitt M, Sternglanz R (1973) Studies on the mechanism of action of nalidixic acid. Antimicrob Agents Chemother 4:479

Brooks K, Clark AJ (1967) Behaviour of lambda bacteriophage in a recombination deficient strain of *Escherichia coli*. J Virol 1:283–293

Brown PO, Cozzarelli NR (1979) A sign inversion mechanism for enzymatic supercoiling of DNA. Science 206:1081–1083

Brown PO, Reebles CI, Cozzarelli NR (1979) A topoisomerase from *Escherichia coli* related to DNA gyrase. Proc Natl Acad Sci USA 76:6110

Burman L (1977) R-plasmid transfer and its response to nalidixic acid. J Bacteriol 131:76–81

Cairns J (1963) The chromosome of *Escherichia coli*. Cold Spring Harbour. Symp Quant Biol 28:43–45

Champoux JJ (1978) Mechanism of the reaction catalysed by the DNA untwisting enzyme: attachment of the enzyme to 3′-terminus of the nicked DNA. J Mol Biol 118:441–446

Chapman ST, Speller DC, Reeves DS (1985) Resistance to ciprofloxacin. Lancet 2(8445):39

Chin N-X, Neu H (1983) In vitro activity of enoxacin, a quinolone carboxylic acid, compared with those of norfloxacin, new β-lactams, aminoglycosides, and trimethoprim. Antimicrob Agents Chemother 24:754–763

Cole ST (1983) Characterisation of the promoter for the Lex A regulated *sul* A gene of *Escherichia coli*. Mol Gen Genet 189:400–404

Cozzarelli NR (1980) DNA gyrase and the supercoiling of DNA. Science 207:953–960

Crook SM, Selkon JB, McLardy-Smith PD (1985) Clinical resistance to long-term oral ciprofloxacin. Lancet 1(8440):1275

Crumplin GC (1985) Development and consequences of resistance to antimicrobial agents acting upon DNA gyrase. Annual Conference of the American Society of Microbiology

Crumplin GC, Smith JT (1975) Nalidixic acid: an antibacterial paradox. Antimicrob Agents Chemother 8:251–261

Cullman W, Stieglitz M, Baars B, Opferkuch W (1985) Comparative evaluation of recently developed quinolone compounds – with a note on the frequency of resistant mutants. Chemotherapy 31:19–28

Diver JM, Piddock LJV, Wise R (1987) Investigations into the mechanism of cell death of *E. coli* K12 after exposure to quinolone antibacterials. 15th International Congress of Chemotherapy, Istanbul

Domagala JM, Hanna LD, Heifetz CL, Hutt MP, Mich TF, Sanchez JP, Solomon M (1986) New structure-activity relationships of the quinolone antibacterials using the target enzyme. The development and application of a DNA gyrase assay. J Med Chem 29:394–404

Drlica K (1984) Biology of bacterial deoxyribonucleic acid topoisomerases. Microbiol Rev 48:273–289

Drlica K, Engle EC, Manes SH (1980) DNA gyrase on the bacterial chromosome: possibility of two levels of action. Proc Natl Acad Sci USA 77:6879–6883

Gellert M (1981) DNA topoisomerases. Annu Rev Biochem 50:879–910

Gellert M, Mizuuchi K, O'Dea MH, Nash HA (1976) DNA gyrase: an enzyme that introduces superhelical turns into DNA. Proc Natl Acad Sci USA 73:3872–3876

Gellert M, Mizuuchi K, O'Dea MH, Itoh T, Tomizawa J (1977) Nalidixic acid resistance: a second genetic character involved in DNA gyrase activity. Proc Natl Acad Sci USA 74:4767

Gellert M, Mizuuchi K, O'Dea MH, Ohmori H, Tomizawa J (1978) DNA gyrase and DNA supercoiling. Cold Spring Harbour Symp Quant Biol 43:35

George A, Levy SB (1983) Gene in the major cotransduction map of the *Escherichia coli* K-12 linkage map required for the expression of chromosomal resistance to tetracycline and other antibiotics. J Bact 155:531–540

Glupczynski Y, Labbe M, Burette A, Delmee M, Avesari V, Bruck C (1987) Treatment failure of ofloxacin in *Campylobacter pylori* infection. Lancet 1(8541):1096

Gudas LJ, Pardee AB (1976) DNA synthesis inhibition and the induction of protein X in *Escherichia coli*. J Mol Biol 101:459–477

Gutmann L, Williamson R, Moreau N, Kitzis MD, Collatz E, Acar JF, Goldstein FW (1985) Cross-resistance to nalidixic acid, trimethoprim and chloramphericol associated with alterations in outer membrane proteins of *Klebsiella*, *Enterobacter* and *Serratia*. J Infect Dis 151:501–507

Hahn FE, Ciak J (1976) Elimination of resistance determinants from R-factor R1 by intercalative compounds. Antimicrob Agents Chemother 9:77–80

Hane MW, Wood TH (1969) *Escherichia coli* K-12 mutants resistant to nalidixic acid: genetic mapping and dominance studies. J Bacteriol 99:238–241

Hansen FG, von Meyenberg K (1979) Characterisation of the *dna*A, *gyr* B and other genes in the *dna* A region of the *Escherichia coli* chromosome on specialised transducing phages lambda tna. Mol Gen Genet 175:135

Helling RB, Kukora JS (1971) Nalidixic acid-resistant mutants of *Escherichia coli* deficient in isocitrate dehydrogenase. J Bacteriol 105:1224–1226

Hertman I, Luria SE (1967) Transduction studies on the role of *rec*-gene in ultraviolet induction of prophage lambda. J Mol Biol 23:117–133

Higgins NP, Peebles CL, Sugino A, Cozzarelli NR (1978) Purification of subunits of *Escherichia coli* DNA gyrase and reconstitution of enzymatic activity. Proc Natl Acad Sci USA 75:1773–1777

Hirai K, Aoyama H, Irikura T, Iyobe S, Mitsuhashi S (1986a) Differences in susceptibilities to quinolones of outer membrane mutants of *Salmonella typhimuruiri* and *Escherichia coli*. Antimicrob Agents Chemother 29:535–538

Hirai K, Aoyama H, Suzue S, Irikura T, Iyobe S, Mitsuhashi S (1986b) Isolation and characterisation of norfloxacin-resistant mutants of *Escherichia coli* K-12. Antimicrob Agents Chemother 30:248–253

Hirai K, Suzue S, Irikura T, Iyobe S, Mitsuhashi S (1987) Mutations producing resistance to norfloxacin in *Pseudomonas aeruginosa*. Antimicrob Agents Chemother 31:582–586

Hiruma R, Yamaguchi A, Sawai T (1984) The effect of LPS on lipid bilayer permeability of β-lactam antibiotics. FEBS Lett 170:268

Hogberg T, Khanna I, Drake SD, Mitscher LA, Shen LL (1984) Structure activity relationships among DNA gyrase inhibitions. Synthesis and evaluation of 1,2-dihydro-4-dimethyl-1-oxo-2-napthalene carboxylic acids as 1 carba bioesters of oxolinic acid. J Med Chem 27:306–310

Holloway BW, Morgan AP (1986) Genone organisation in Pseudomonas. Annu Ref Microbiol 40:79–105

Hooper D, Wolfson J (1985) The fluoroquinolones: pharmacology, clinical uses, and toxicities in humans. Antimicrob Agents Chemother 28:716–721

Hooper D, Wolfson J, Souza KS, Tung C, McHugh G, Swartz M (1986) Genetic and biochemical characterisation of norfloxacin resistance in *Escherichia coli*. Antimicrob Agents Chemother 29:639–644

Hooper D, Wolfson J, Ng E, Swartz M (1987) Mechanisms of action of and resistance to ciprofloxacin. Am J Med 82(4A):12–20

Hrebenda J, Heleszko H, Brzostek K, Bielecki H (1985) Mutation affecting resistance of *Escherichia coli* K12 to nalidixic acid. J Gen Microbiol 131:2285–2292

Huisman O, d'Ari R (1981) An inducible DNA replication-cell division coupling mechanism in *E. coli*. Nature 290:797–799

Humphreys H, Mulvihill E (1985) Ciprofloxacin-resistant *Staphylococcus aureus*. Lancet 2(8451):383

Inoue Y, Sato K, Fujii T, Kirai K, Inoue M, Shizuko I, Mitsuhashi S (1987) Some properties of subunits of DNA gyrase from *Pseudomonas aeruginosa* PA01 and its nalidixic acid-resistant mutant. J Bacteriol 169:2322–2325

Inouye S, Ohne T, Yamagishi J, Nakamura S, Shimuzu M (1978) Mode of incomplete cross-resistance among pipemidic, piromidic and nalidixic acids. Antimicrob Agents Chemother 14:240–245

Jaffe A, Chabbert YA, Sernonin Q (1982) Role of porin proteins OMP F and OMP C in the permeation of β-lactams. Antimicrob Agents Chemother 22:942–948

Kaatz GW, Barriere SL, Schaberg DR, Fekety R (1987) The emergence of resistance to ciprofloxacin during treatment of experimental *Staphylococcus aureus* endocarditis. J Antimicrob Chemother 20:753–758
Kantor GJ, Deering RA (1968) Effect of nalidixic acid and hydroxy urea on division ability of *Escherichia coli* fil$^+$ and *lon*-strains. J Bacteriol 95:520–530
Karu AE, Belk ED (1982) Induction of *E. coli rec* A protein via *rec* BC and alternate pathways: quantitation by enzyme-linked immunosorbent assay (ELISA). Mol Gen Genet 185:275–282
King A, Shannon K, Phillips I (1984) The in vitro activity of ciprofloxacin compared with that of norfloxacin and nalidixic acid. J Antimicrob Chemother 13:325–331
Kreuzer KN, Cozzarelli NR (1979) *Escherichia coli* mutants thermosensitive for deoxyribonucleic acid gyrase subunit A: effects on deoxyribonucleic acid replication, transcription and bacteriophage growth. J Bacteriol 140:424–435
Kreuzer KN, Cozzarelli NR (1980) Formation and resolution of DNA catenates by DNA gyrase. Cell 20:245–254
Kubesch P, Wehsling M, Tummler B (1987) Membrane permeability of *Pseudomonas aeruginosa* to 4-quinolones. Zentralbl Bakteriol Mikrobiol Hyg (A) 265:197–202
Kumar S (1980) Types of spontaneous nalidixic acid resistant mutants of *Escherichia coli.* Indian J Exp Biol 18:341–343
Little JW, Mount DW (1982) The SOS regulatory system of *Escherichia coli.* Cell 29:11–22
Liu LF, Wang JC (1978) *Micrococcus luteus* DNA gyrase: active components and a model for its supercoiling of DNA. Proc Natl Acad Sci USA 75:2098
Liu LF, Liu C-C, Alberts BM (1980) Type II DNA topoisomerases: enzymes that can unknot a topologically knotted DNA molecule via a reversible double-strand break. Cell 19:697–708
Manes SH, Pruss GJ, Drlica K (1983) Inhibition of RNA synthesis by oxolinic acid is unrelated to average DNA supercoiling. J Bacteriol 155:420–423
McDaniel LS, Rogers LH, Hill WE (1978) Survival of recombination-deficient mutants of *Escherichia coli* during incubation with nalidixic acid. J Bacteriol 134:1195–1198
Mizuuchi K, Gellert M, Nash HA (1978) Involvement of supertwisted DNA in integrative recombination of bacteriophage lambda. J Mol Biol 212:375–392
Mizuuchi K, Fischer LM, O'Dea M, Gellert M (1980) DNA gyrase B action involves the introduction of transient double stranded breaks into DNA. Proc Natl Acad Sci USA 77:1847–1851
Munshi MH, Haider K, Rahaman M, Sack D, Ahmed Z, Morshed M (1987) Plasmid-mediated resistance to nalidixic acid in *Shigella dysenteriae* type I. Lancet 2:419–421
Murphy PG, Ferguson WP (1987) *Corynebacterium jeikeium* (group JK) resistance to ciprofloxacin emerging during therapy. J Antimicrob Chemother 20:922–923
Olsson-Llilequist B, Gezelius L, Svensson SB (1985) Selection of multiple antibiotic resistance by norfloxacin and nalidixic acid in *Klebsiella* and *Enterobacter*: correlation with outer membrane protein profiles. 25th ICAAC, Minneapolis
Panhotra BR, Desai B (1983) Resistant *Shigella dysenteriae*. Lancet 2(8364):1420
Panhotra BR, Desai B, Sharma PL (1985) Nalidixic-acid-resistant *Shigella dysenteriae* I. Lancet 1(8431):763
Peebles CL, Higgins NP, Krenzer KN, Morrison A, Brown PO, Sugino A, Cozzarelli NR (1978) Structure and activities of *Escherichia coli* DNA gyrase. Cold Spring Harbour Symp Quant Biol 43:41–52
Piddock LJV, Wise R (1986) The effect of altered porin expression in *Escherichia coli* upon susceptibility to 4-quinolones. J Antimicrob Chemother 18:547–552
Piddock LJV, Wise R (1987) Induction of the SOS response by 4-quinolones. FEMS Microbiol Letts 41:289–294
Piddock LJV, Diver JM, Wise R (1986) Cross-resistance of nalidixic acid resistant enterobacteriaceae to new quinolones and other antimicrobials. Eur J Clin Microbiol 5:411–415
Piddock LJV, Wijnands WJA, van Klingeran B, Wise R (1987a) Characterisation of the mechanism of decreased susceptibility to enoxacin in a strain of *Pseudomonas aerugi-*

nosa isolated from a patient after enoxacin therapy. 5th International congress of chemotherapy, Istanbul
Piddock LJV, Wijnands WJA, Wise R (1987 b) Quinolone ureidopenicillin cross resistance. Lancet 17:907
Piddock LJV, Diver JM, Wise R (1988 a) Correlation of the biochemical responses with the bactericidal action of quinolone antimicrobial agents in *E. coli* K-12 (submitted)
Piddock LJV, Griggs D, Wise R (1988 b) The selection and phenotypic characterisation of the mechanism of resistance of selected Enterobacteriaceae to quinolones. Proceedings of the 2nd symposium of new quinolones, Geneva
Piffaretti JC, Demarta A, Leidi-Bulla L, Peduzzi R (1983) In vitro emergence of *Escherichia coli* and *Pseudomonas aeruginosa* strains resistant to norfloxacin and nalidixic acid. Antimicrob Agents Chemother 23:641–648
Pugsley A, Schnaitman CC (1978) Outer membrane proteins of *Escherichia coli* VII. Evidence that bacteriophage-directed protein 2 functions as a pore. J Bact 133:1181–1189
Ratcliffe NT, Smith JT (1985) Norfloxacin has a bactericidal mechanism of action unrelated to that of other 4-quinolones. J Pharm Pharmacol 37:92P
Ravizzola G, Pirali F, Paolucci A, Terlenghi L, Peroni L, Columbi A, Turano A (1987) Reduced virulence in ciprofloxacin-resistant variants of *Pseudomonas aeruginosa* strains. J Antimicrob Chemother 20:825–829
Reeve EC, Doherty P (1968) Linkage relationships of two genes causing partial resistance to chloramphenicol in *Escherichia coli* K-12. Genet Res II:303–309
Rella M, Haas D (1982) Resistance of *Pseudomonas aeruginosa* PAO to nalidixic acid and low levels of *β*-lactam antibiotics: mapping of chromosomal genes. Antimicrob Agents Chemother 22:242–249
Renzini GG, Ravagnan G, Piccolomini R, Nicoletti M, Oliva B (1982) Comparison of different chinolonic compounds as extra-chromosomal transfer inhibitors. Chemotherapia 1:451–453
Roberts CM, Batten J, Hodson ME (1985) Ciprofloxacin-resistant pseudomonas. Lancet 1(8443):1442
Salles B, Paoletti C (1983) Control of uv induction of *rec* A protein. Proc Natl Acad Sci USA 80:65–69
Salles E, Defrais M (1984) Signal of induction of *rec*A protein in *E. coli.* Mutat Res 131:53–59
Sanders CC, Watanakunakorn C (1986) Emergence of resistance to beta-lactams, aminoglycosides and quinolones during combination therapy for infection due to *Serratia marcescens.* J Infect Dis 153:617–619
Sanders CC, Sanders WE, Goering RV, Werner V (1984) Selection of multiple antibiotic resistance by quinolones, beta-lactams, and aminoglycosides with special reference to cross-resistance between unrelated drug classes. Antimicrob Agents Chemother 26:797–801
Sato K, Inoue Y, Fjuii T, Aoyama H, Inoue M, Mitsuhashi S (1987) Purification and properties of DNA gyrase from a fluoroquinolone resistant strain of *Escherichia coli.* Antimicrob Agents Chemother 30:777–780
Setlow JK, Cabrera-Juarez, Albritton NL, Spikes D, Mutschler A (1986) Mutations affecting gyrase in *Haemophilus influenza.* J Bact 164:525–534
Slack R (1984) Review of bacterial resistance – a challenge to the treatment of urinary infection. J Antimicrob Chemother [Suppl B] 13:1–7
Smith GM, Cashmore C, Leyland MJ (1985) Ciprofloxacin-resistant staphylococci. Lancet 2(8461):949
Smith JT (1984) Mutational resistance to 4 quinolone antibacterial agents. Eur J Clin Microbiol 3:347–350
Sugino A, Bott KF (1980) *Bacillus subtilis* deoxyribonucleic acid gyrase. J Bacteriol 141:1331–1339
Sugino A, Cozzarelli NR (1980) The intrinsic ATPase of DNA gyrase. J Biol Chem 255:6299–6306

Sugino A, Peebles K, Krenzer K, Cozzarelli N (1977) Mechanism of action of nalidixic acid: purification of *Escherichia coli nal* A gene product and its relationship to DNA gyrase and a novel nicking-closing enzyme. Proc Natl Acad Sci USA 74:4767–4771
Tenney JH, Maack RW, Chippendale GR (1983) Rapid selection of organisms with increasing resistance on subinhibitory concentrations of norfloxacin in agar. Antimicrob Agents Chemother 23:188–189
Traub WH, Kleber I (1973) Isolation of two strains of *Klebsiella pneumonae* with transferable determinants against ten antimicrobial drugs from clinical material. Zentralbl Bakteriol Mikrobiol Hyg [A] 229:80–88
Vasquez-Ramos JM, Mandelstram J (1981) Oxilinic acid-resistant mutants of *Bacillus subtilis*. J Gen Microbiol 127:1–9
Wagenvoort JH, van-der-Willgen AH, van Vliet HJ, Michel MF, van Klingeren B (1986) Resistance of *Neisseria gonorrhoeae* to enoxacin. J Antimicrob Chemother 18:429
Walker GC (1984) Mutagenesis and inducible responses to deoxyribonucleic acid damage in *Escherichia coli*. Microbiol Rev 48:60–93
Wang JC (1985) DNA topoisomerases. Annu Rev Biochem 54:665–697
Wang JC, Gumport RI, Javaherian K, Kirkegaard K, Klevan L, Katewicz ML, Tse YC (1981) In: Alberts BM, Fox CF (eds) Mechanistic studies of DNA replication and genetic recombination. Academic, New York
Weisser J, Weidemann B (1985) Elimination of plasmids by new 4-quinolones. Antimicrob Agents Chemother 28:700–702
Weisser J, Weidemann B (1987) Inhibition of R-plasmid transfer in *Escherichia coli* by 4-quinolones. Antimicrob Agents Chemother 31:531–534
Wise R, Baker SL, Misra M, Griggs D (1987) The pharmacokinetics of enoxacin in elderly patients. J Antimicrob Chemother 19:343–350
Witkin EM (1976) Ultraviolet mutagenesis and inducible DNA repair in *Escherichia coli*. Bacteriol Rev 40:869–907
Wolfson J, Hooper DC (1985) The fluoroquinolones: structures, mechanisms of action and resistance and spectra of activity in vitro. Antimicrob Agents Chemother 28:581–586
Yamagishi J, Furutani Y, Inoue S, Ohue T, Nakamura S, Shimizu M (1981) New nalidixic acid resistance mutations related to deoxynitonucleic acid gyrase activity. J Bacteriol 148:450–458
Yamagishi J, Yoshida H, Yamaycshi M, Nakamura S (1986) Nalidixic acid-resistant mutations of the *gyr* B gene of *Escherichia coli*. Mol Gen Genet 204:367–373
Yamashita S, Inone Y, Sato K, Inone M, Mitsuhashi S (1986) DNA gyrase from fluoroquinolone resistant *E. cloacae*. Proc 1st Int Symp New Quinolones:13

CHAPTER 9

Ribosomal Changes Resulting in Antimicrobial Resistance

H. HUMMEL and A. BÖCK

A. Introduction

Numerous antibiotics inhibit growth of prokaryotic and/or eukaryotic cells by specifically interfering with protein synthesis, either at the level of soluble protein synthesis factors or at the ribosome. The response of susceptible cells to these compounds may be altered by mutational changes of the primary structure of some component of the translational system or by the enzymatic activity of a gene product which introduces a covalent modification at a specific site. The analysis of such changes has been of eminent importance both for elucidating the mechanism of action of the antibiotics themselves and for understanding the genetic organization, the synthesis and the function of the translational system: (i) The first genes coding for ribosomal proteins were localized with the help of streptomycin-, erythromycin- and spectinomycin-resistant mutants from *E. coli* (for review see NOMURA et al. 1977). Antibiotic resistance mutations were also indispensable tools for cloning the respective genes and for studying their structure and expression. (ii) Antibiotics have been extremely useful in the delineation of the different partial reactions of the translation process. Thus, the isolation and structural characterization of an antibiotic resistant mutant in several instances permitted the correlation of the biochemical reaction, which is blocked by that compound, with a specific site or component of the ribosome. (iii) Many protein synthesis inhibitors are specific either for the 70S eubacterial or the 80S cytoplasmic eukaryotic ribosome. There is increasing evidence which suggests that the structural changes of ribosomal components with occur as a consequence of antibiotic resistance mutations parallel the evolutionary changes differentiating susceptible and non-susceptible cell lineages (HUMMEL et al. 1986).

It is self-evident that ribosomal changes resulting in antimicrobial resistance also aid greatly in the elucidation of the mechanism of action of the respective compound. It is the only means, for example, to demonstrate that an antibiotic acts at a single site in vivo. Furthermore, cross-resistance analysis yields information as to whether several drugs share a common or overlapping binding site.

However, although attractive and plausible, there are some restrictions to this latter approach. First, an alteration in a ribosomal component responsible for the resistance phenotype is not necessarily involved in binding of the antibiotic. A well known example for such a situation is ribosomal protein S12 (*E. coli* nomenclature). S12 mutations confer high-level streptomycin resistance (OZAKI et al. 1969); however, protein S12 is not required for the binding of the aminoglycoside (SCHREINER and NIERHAUS 1973). Second, there are only very few examples where clear-cut, single-step ribosomal mutations confer antibiotic resistance. Frequently, several mutations contribute to resistance, and in some cases, resistant mutants are impossible to obtain.

B. Changes in Ribosomal Proteins

Ribosomal proteins – in contrast to ribosomal RNAs (rRNA) – are encoded by single copy genes (for review see LINDAHL and ZENGEL 1986). Since ribosomal antibiotic resistance mutations are recessive this is the reason why, initially, antibiotic-resistant mutants were obtained with lesions solely in ribosomal proteins. For many years the general view was dominated by the results generated by the analysis of streptomycin resistance mutations. From such studies, it was conceived that ribosomal proteins play a major role in the interaction of antibiotics with the ribosome. With the exception of a single report (GARVIN et al. 1974), the role of rRNA was neglected and considered to be purely structural.

Experimentally, the proof of a causal connection between an antibiotic resistance mutation and a structurally changed ribosomal protein is difficult. Two approaches have been followed in the past. The first one consists of in vitro reconstitution of ribosomal subunits, taking one protein from the resistant mutant and the residual ones from the sensitive wild type and testing the reconstituted particles for their response to the antibiotic in binding or activity assays. This laborious approach was first employed in the characterization of streptomycin resistant mutants (OZAKI et al. 1969). An alternative approach involves the transductional transfer of the resistance mutation into a non-mutagenized genetic background. A statistically significant number of transductants must be analyzed subsequently to determine whether the structural change of the respective protein – visualized, e.g. by two-dimensional gel electrophoresis – is present in all resistant transductants. This approach proved very useful for the analysis of mutants in which the resistance character is caused by more than a single mutational event. The contribution of each single mutation to the overall resistance phenotype can be assessed in this way (DE WILDE et al. 1975; BUCKEL et al. 1977).

I. Protein Changes in the Eubacterial Small Ribosomal Subunit

1. Misreading Inducing Aminoglycosides

On the basis of their mechanism of action aminoglycosides are a heterogeneous class of components. Overall, three groups can be differentiated: (i) Compounds which act bacteriostatically and which do not induce misreading of the genetic code; spectinomycin is an example. (ii) Compounds (like kasugamycin) which act bacteriostatically and which improve the fidelity of protein synthesis. (iii) Bactericidal compounds which impair the fidelity of protein synthesis. The latter group includes those drugs generally conceived as classical aminoglycosides, which can be chemically differentiated into antibiotics with a substituted streptidine and into such with a substituted 2-desoxystreptamine residue (UMEZAWA 1975).

Figure 1 summarizes the events taking place when a sensitive bacterium is confronted with one of the misreading inducing aminoglycosides. After a rapid

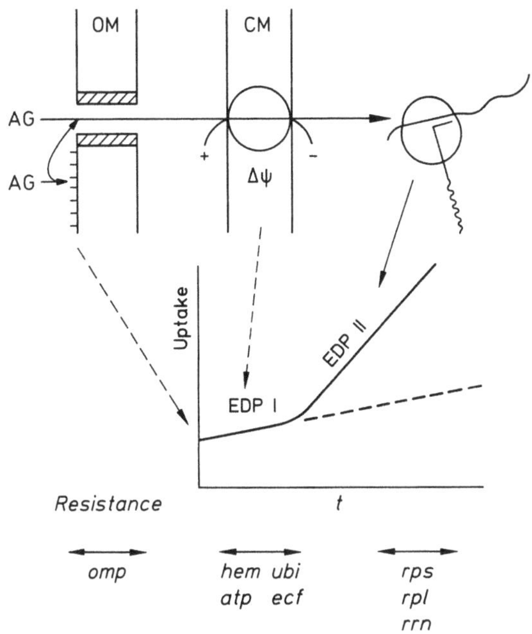

Fig. 1. Scheme of aminoglycoside (*AG*) antibiotic uptake by gram-negative bacteria. The *upper part* indicates the passage of the antibiotic through outer (*OM*) and cytoplasmic (*CM*) membrane; the *lower part* denotes the different phases of uptake together with genetic loci which when mutated confer resistance. For details see text

adsorption phase of the antibiotic to negatively charged groups at the bacterial cell surface (BRYAN and VAN DEN ELZEN 1977; MORRIS and JENNINGS 1975) the compound diffuses into the periplasmic space, possibly by the way of hydrophilic pores (NIKAIDO 1976). It is then taken up across the cytoplasmic membrane by $\Delta\psi$ driven active transport. This phase of uptake [energy dependent phase I (EDPI)] (BRYAN and VAN DEN ELZEN 1977) is slow; the carrier involved is unknown although redox components of the respiratory chain have been implicated in the process (BRYAN and VAN DEN ELZEN 1975, 1976). When the intracellular concentration of the antibiotic is high enough to saturate most of the ribosomes (AHMAD et al. 1980; HANCOCK 1981 b), uptake accelerates dramatically (EDPII). Commencement of this EDPII phase requires protein synthesis (PLOTZ and DAVIS 1962), irrespective of whether the polypeptides made are functional or not (AHMAD et al. 1980). The time course of bactericidal action extrapolates back to the time point of the onset of EDPII (BRYAN and VAN DEN ELZEN 1977).

Recently, DAVIS (1987) postulated an intriguing model which provides a causal relationship between the action of the aminoglycosides at the ribosome and the events occurring at the cytoplasmic membrane. He proposes that misread membrane proteins formed in the presence of aminoglycosides create membrane channels due to aberrant integration or fit. These channels – although not proven to exist – are proposed to be responsible for the increased antibiotic influx during EDPII.

According to the scheme of Fig. 1 mutations conferring resistance to aminoglycosides can affect either the outer membrane (e.g. *omp* mutations) or the capacity for electron transport-mediated membrane energization (*hem*, *ubi*, *atp*, *ecf* mutations) or the affinity of the ribosome for the antibiotic (*rps*, *rpl* and *rrn* mutations).

According to the model of DAVIS (1987) it is the affinity of the ribosome which is crucial for the onset and the rate of killing of bacteria by aminoglycosides. The different types of mutants with altered response to these antibiotics are listed in Table 1. Only a summary is given here since the relevant phenotypes and the biochemical and physiological properties have been presented in extensive reviews recently (PIEPERSBERG et al. 1980; HANCOCK 1981 a, b). In the case of streptomycin, the mutations fall into three classes: (i) Alterations of ribosomal proteins S4 and S5 which cause hypersensitivity (ROSSET and GORINI 1969; PIEPERSBERG et al. 1979) due to an increased affinity of the ribosome (BÖCK et al. 1979) for the drug. S4 and S5 are *ram* (ribosomal ambiguity) mutations since they raise the error frequency in protein synthesis (GORINI 1974; PIEPERSBERG et al. 1975 a). (ii) Mutations in the gene for ribosomal protein S12 which – dependent on the type of amino acid exchange – lead to resistance at a high but different level (sm^R) (BRYAN and VAN DEN ELZEN 1977). These mutations decrease the error frequency in protein synthesis (GORINI 1974). (iii) Specific mutations in ribosomal protein S12 (BIRGE and KURLAND 1969) and S8 (DABBS and WITTMANN 1976) which lead to growth dependence on aminoglycosides (Sm^D).

The differentiation between the Sm^R and Sm^D mutant phenotypes is not strict; so-called pseudodependent strains have been described which can grow in the absence of the aminoglycoside but which exhibit a higher growth rate when the drug is present (ZENGEL et al. 1977). It is plausible to assume that the Sm^D phenotype is a combined trait of two mutations, one conferring resistance and a second dependence. This situation holds for mutants dependent in their growth on spectinomycin (HENKIN et al. 1979; DABBS 1977), erythromycin (SPARLING and BLACKMAN 1973) and kasugamycin (DABBS 1978 a) but this has never been demonstrated conclusively for Sm^D mutations.

Two models have been put forward to explain the intriguing phenotype of Sm^D strains. One postulates that Sm^D mutants require the antibiotic for correct assembly of the ribosome. Organelles synthesized in the absence of the antibiotic are inactive; the linear growth observed when the drug is withdrawn from the medium of a Sm^D strain (SPOTTS 1962) is explained by the residual capacity for protein synthesis of pre-existing ribosomes (SPOTTS 1962; SPOTTS and STANIER 1961; GARVIN et al. 1973). The second model reasons that ribosomes from Sm^D strains are hyperaccurate proof-readers and that they require the presence of an agent like aminoglycosides which increases translational ambiguity (RUUSALA et al. 1984).

There are two observations which argue in favor of the first mechanism. One is the property of "phenotypic masking" displayed by Sm^D mutants (GORINI et al. 1967). Ribosomes from an Sm^D strain grown in the presence of a certain aminoglycoside, like streptomycin, are inhibited by a second related compound, e.g. paromomycin (ZIMMERMANN et al. 1971 a; HUMMEL and BÖCK 1983). When the same strain is grown in the presence of paromomycin they, conversely, exhibit

Table 1. Changes in small ribosomal subunit proteins resulting in altered antibiotic sensitivity

Antiobiotic	Protein[a]	Phenotype[b]	Remarks	Clinical relevance[c]	Reference
Streptomycin	Ec S12	R or D	Restrict misreading	+	Traub and Nomura (1968); Ozaki et al. (1969)
	S8	D	Assembly defect	–	Dabbs and Wittmann (1976)
	S4	HS, I	Increase misreading	–	Rosset and Gorini (1969)
	S5	HS, I	Increase misreading	–	Piepersberg et al. (1975a)
Spectinomycin	Ec S5	R		+	Bollen et al. (1969)
	S5	R and Suc^D	Membrane alteration	–	Dombou et al. (1977)
Neamine	Ec S17	R	Restrict misreading	–	Bollen et al. (1975)
	S5+S12	R	S5 increases, S12 decreases misreading	–	De Wilde et al. (1975)
Gentamicin	Ec L6	R	Restrict misreading; general R	–	Buckel et al. (1977)
Kasugamycin	Ec S2	R		–	Okuyama et al. (1974)
	S9, S13, S18, L11, L14	R/D		–	Dabbs (1978a)
Tetracycline	Sf C additional protein	R	Plasmid encoded	+	Burdett (1986)
Emetine	CHO S14	R	Cross-resistance to other alkaloids	–	Boersma et al. (1979a, b); Reichenbecher and Caskey (1979)
	Pa: S14/S13+S17	R	Hypersensitivity to anisomycin	–	Crouzet and Bégueret (1982)

[a] Denotes the nomenclature of the ribosomal protein change in Ec (*E. coli*), Sf (*Streptococcus faecalis*), C (*Campylobacter*), CHO (chinese hamster ovary cells), Pa (*Podospora anserina*)

[b] R, resistance; D, dependence; Hs, hypersensitivity; I, reversion of dependence; Suc^D, sucrose dependence

[c] +, involved in clinical resistance; –, relevance not demonstrated

sensitivity against streptomycin. This means that the development of an inhibitory site depends upon which compound was present during pre-growth, i.e. that particular antibiotic apparently must have exerted an effect on ribosome formation. The second argument comes from studies of mutants which are streptomycin-dependent due to an altered S8 protein (DABBS and WITTMANN 1976). Secondary mutations in almost any other protein, from the 30S and 50S subunit, can revert dependence to independence (DABBS and WITTMANN 1976; DABBS 1978 b). It appears that the S8 mutation leads to the distorted formation of the ribosome and that mutations at many different sites, even at the other subunit, can revert it genetically to the correct state in the same way as aminoglycoside binding to some site either during (HUMMEL et al. 1983) or after assembly does it phenotypically.

Despite these arguments, however, it is still open which of the two models actually meets the situation. In the light of the extreme genetic and physiological heterogeneity of the Sm^D mutants characterized (MOMOSE and GORINI 1971), it is possible that both mechanisms could be involved.

Ribosomes from Sm^D strains bind streptomycin with a significantly higher affinity than those from Sm^R mutants; association constants are 2×10^5 M^{-1} in equilibrium dialysis experiments compared to about 6×10^3 M^{-1} for Sm^R mutants (CHANG and FLAKS 1972; BÖCK et al. 1979). *ram* mutant ribosomes exhibit a 2–3 fold higher affinity for the drug than wild-type ribosomes (K_A: $1\text{–}2 \times 10^7$ M^{-1}) (BÖCK et al. 1979). The binding constants directly parallel the in vivo sensitivity pattern of the respective mutants. When *ram* mutations are genetically combined with either Sm^D and Sm^R mutations the resultant double mutants display an intermediate phenotype: (i) the restriction of translational misreading is reduced (BJARE and GORINI 1971; PIEPERSBERG et al. 1979); (ii) the sensitivity to streptomycin is decreased (ROSSET and GORINI 1969); and (iii) the ribosomes bind streptomycin with a higher affinity than those from the parental Sm^D and Sm^R strains (BÖCK et al. 1979).

As previously emphasized (DAVIS 1987) there is thus a quantitative correlation between induction of misreading and bactericidal activity. This correlation and the fact that protein synthesis is required for cidal action is in accord with the model put forward by DAVIS (1987), which states that it is the synthesis of faulty proteins which kills the cells. In fact, the onset of killing in *S4* and *S5 ram* mutants occurs earlier and the rate is higher than in wild-type cells (AHMAD et al. 1980), which supports the notion of misreading being related to cell killing.

On the basis of the mutant phenotypes described above there has been much dispute as to the contribution of proteins S4, S5 and S12 with regard to the site of streptomycin binding. Protein S12 does not appear to be required for binding as demonstrated by reconstitution experiments (SCHREINER and NIERHAUS 1973). Anti-S12 antibodies also have no effect on the binding process (LELONG et al. 1974). A positive role has been ascribed to ribosomal proteins S3 and S5 by in vitro assembly studies (SCHREINER and NIERHAUS 1973). The recent results obtained with 16S rRNA (MONTANDON et al. 1985; ETZOLD et al. 1987) mutants and with ribosomes from aminoglycoside producing organisms (CUNDLIFFE, this volume) provide strong support for ribosomal RNA participating, in at least, in the formation of the binding site (see below). The most plausible role for proteins S12, S4 and S5 could then reside in determining the accessibility or the shape of the binding site at the RNA. In this regard it is mandatory to mention that the proposal of RNA as being the primary binding component was suggested by Gorini and coworkers in 1974 (GARVIN et al. 1974).

There have been many attempts to isolate single-step mutants of bacteria with high-level resistance to 2-desoxystreptamine containing aminoglycosides, but without success (APIRION and SCHLESSINGER 1968; HULL et al. 1976; BUCKEL et al. 1977; THORBJARNARDÓTTIR et al. 1978). Reasons for the failure could be: (i) that these compounds have multiple binding sites at the ribosome; (ii) that they bind exclusively to rRNA (which is encoded by several genes); (iii) that the mutations would be lethal; or (iv) that no single mutational event can "close" the binding site completely.

The analysis of mutants of *E. coli* resistant to gentamicin revealed that they harbor at least two mutations. One of them interferes with the accumulation of gentamicin and was identified as an *unc* (ATPase) lesion (AHMAD et al. 1980); the other was in the gene for a large subunit protein of the ribosome, L6 (Table 1) (BUCKEL et al. 1977). Both mutations acted cooperatively in causing generalized aminoglycoside resistance. The different L6 alterations identified restricted translational ambiguity (KÜHBERGER et al. 1979) and their effect was counteracted by specific S4 mutations (HUMMEL et al. 1980). Again, a correlation was observed between the inhibitory potential of the antibiotic and the ability to induce misreading. Binding studies revealed that the L6 mutation reduced, but did not completely prevent, gentamicin binding (LE GOFFIC et al. 1980).

Multiple mutations were also demonstrated by THORBJARNADÓTTIR et al. (1978) to generate aminoglycoside resistance. These authors showed that a mutation in a gene coding for an energy coupling factor (*ecf*) prevented kanamycin accumulation. An additional mutation at the ribosome cooperatively raised the resistance level.

Mutants from *E. coli* resistant to the neomycin cleavage product neamine were isolated and characterized by Bollen and collaborators (DE WILDE et al. 1975; BOLLEN et al. 1975). Two classes could be distinguished, one possessing an altered ribosomal protein S17, the other exhibiting alterations in two proteins, S5 and S12. The mutated proteins were characterized protein chemically (YAGUCHI et al. 1975, 1976) and it was shown that the increase in resistance was paralleled by improved fidelity of protein synthesis.

2. Kasugamycin

Kasugamycin is a specific inhibitor of the initiation step of protein synthesis both at 70S and 80S ribosomes (TANAKA et al. 1966). Interestingly, this antibiotic reduces translational ambiguity of ribosomes (VAN BUUL et al. 1984). In accordance with this result is the finding that kasugamycin-resistant ribosomes display an increased misreading frequency (VAN BUUL et al. 1984). This effect of kasugamycin on the fidelity of protein synthesis may contribute to the high effectiveness of this drug in the treatment of the rice blast disease caused by *Piricularia oryzae*, since translational fidelity seems to be involved in the differentiation of fungal cells; it was, for example, demonstrated that an increase in fidelity prevents sporulation by *Podospora anserina* (DEQUARD-CHABLAT and COPPIN-RAYNAL 1984). *E. coli* mutants resistant to kasugamycin which display alterations in proteins S2, S9, S13, S18, L11 or L14 have been described (OKUYAMA et al. 1974; DABBS 1978a). Their ribosomes exhibit an altered kasugamycin-phenotype in vitro (OKUYAMA et al. 1974; DABBS et al. 1980).

3. Spectinomycin

Mutations in *rpsE*, the gene for ribosomal protein S5, can result in three different phenotypes: (i) high-level spectinomycin-resistance (DEKIO and TANAKA 1969; BOLLEN et al. 1969); (ii) a *ram* phenotype (PIEPERSBERG et al. 1975a) (see above); and (iii) a temperature conditional assembly defect (WITTMANN et al. 1974). Each class of mutation could be allocated to a specific primary structure region of the protein. Spectinomycin resistance is due to alterations close to the N-terminus (FUNATSU et al. 1971) while the *ram* mutations are clustered in the center of the gene sequence (ITOH and WITTMANN 1973) and the assembly defect is the consequence of a change at the C-terminus (PIEPERSBERG et al. 1975b).

Spectinomycin-dependent strains were shown to possess two mutations, one in *rpsE* and the other in an unidentified gene close to the *rif* locus (DABBS 1977). They can be suppressed by altered L1 or L5 genes, i.e. by mutations in the large ribosomal subunit.

Mizushima and coworkers characterized mutants showing resistance to spectinomycin only in the presence of 20% sucrose (DOMBOU et al. 1977). They lack at least one cytoplasmic membrane protein (MIZUMO et al. 1976). It is unknown whether this membrane alteration is the result of a close interaction between ribosomes and the cytoplasmic membrane or of a polarity effect exerted by the S5 mutation on the transcription of the *sec* gene(s) (SHULTZ et al. 1982; ITO et al. 1983) located in the *spc* transcriptional unit downstream from *rpsE*.

4. Tetracycline

Considerable efforts have been made in an attempt to isolate tetracycline resistant mutants of gram-positive or gram-negative bacteria, but without success (PESTKA 1977). A ribosome-associated factor (presumably a protein capable of binding tetracycline) was, however, reported to confer antibiotic resistance to the producer organisms *Streptomyces* (*S.*) *rimosus* and *S. aureofaciens* (OHNUKI et al. 1985; MIKULÍK et al. 1983). This factor can be removed from the ribosomes by washing with 1 *M* NH_4Cl.

Three resistance determinants have been described for *Streptococcus* spp.: *tetL* prevents tetracycline accumulation; *tetM*- and *tetN*-containing cells still accumulate the antibiotic but exhibit a tetracycline insensitive protein synthesis in vitro (BURDETT 1986). Superficially, at least, they resemble the producer organisms in this property. A recent report indicates that tetracycline resistance in *Campylobacter* may have the same biochemical basis (SOUGAKOFF et al. 1987).

II. Protein Changes in the Small Subunit from Eukaryotic Ribosomes

There are only few reports on mutational changes in the 40S subunit from eukaryotic ribosomes which deliver an antibiotic resistant phenotype. Resistance to cryptopleurine in *Saccharomyces cerevisiae* is brought about by recessive mutations (*cryl*) which are located on chromosome III (SKOGERSON et al. 1973; GRANT et al. 1974). *cryl* mutants possess an altered 40S subunit and exhibit cross-resistance to the phenanthrene alkaloids tylocrebrine, tubulosine, tylophorine and the benzoisoquinoline emetine (SÁNCHEZ et al. 1977; JIMÉNEZ et al. 1977). Similar mutants have been obtained with CHO cell lines. They arose with a frequency of 1.5×10^{-7} and displayed an identical cross-resistance pattern (GUPTA and SIMINOVITCH 1977a).

CHO cells were also used for the analysis of mutants with resistance to emetine. Several complementation groups were identified; one of them comprised three different loci providing high-level emetine resistance both in vivo and in vitro (GUPTA and SIMINOVITCH 1977b; REICHENBECHER and CASKEY 1979; BOERSMA et al. 1979a). Several of these mutations correlated with an electrophoretic change of ribosomal protein S14 (REICHENBECHER and CASKEY 1979; BOERSMA et al. 1979b). These mutations caused the loss of several other ribosomal proteins upon isolation of the 40S particle in the presence of 0.5 *M* KCl. From these results it has been concluded that protein S14 does not directly represent the primary binding site of emetine but that it may be part of a very complex and structurally interdependent binding domain (WEJKSNORA and WARNER 1982).

Emetine resistant mutants from *Podospora anserina* have been reported to carry lesions in one of two gene loci, *erml* and *erm2* (CROUZET and BÉGUERET 1982). *erm2* mutations correlate with an alteration of ribosomal protein S14 while those in *erml* correlate with changes in proteins S13 or S17 (CROUZET and BÉGUERET 1982).

III. Protein Changes in the Eubacterial 50S Subunit

Two functional domains of the 50S subunit are the primary targets for antibiotics, namely (i) the peptidyltransferase center and (ii) the GTPase center. Table 2 summarizes the information.

1. Macrolides-Lincosamides-Synergimycins (MLS)

MLS compounds interfere with the peptidyltransfer reaction (for review see VÁZQUEZ 1979). From the macrolides, erythromycin has been studied most extensively and has been found to stimulate the dissociation of peptidyl-tRNA from the ribosome (MENNINGER and OTTO 1982). A mutant with thermosensitive peptidylhydrolase activity, which exhibits a fivefold reduced dissociation rate, concomitantly shows increased erythromycin resistance (ANDERSON and MENNINGER 1987).

High-level erythromycin-resistant mutants from *E. coli* possess alterations in either one of two ribosomal proteins, L4 or L22 (DEKIO et al. 1970). The L4 mu-

Table 2. Changes in the large ribosomal subunit proteins resulting in altered antibiotic sensitivity

Antibiotic	Protein[a]	Phenotype	Remarks	Reference
Erythromycin	Ec L4	R	Reduced affinity	DEKIO et al. (1970); WITTMANN et al. (1973)
	Ec L22	R	Affinity not reduced	WITTMANN et al. (1973)
Spiramycin	Ec L4	R	No cross-resistance to other macrolides	TANAKA et al. (1971)
Tiamulin	Ec L3 or L4	R	Cross-resistance to erythromycin	BÖCK et al. (1982)
Lincomycin	Ec L14 or L15	R	Affinity labeled with lincomycin	HUMMEL et al. (1979)
Thiostrepton	Bs L11 lacking	R	Cross-resistance to micrococcin	WIENEN et al. (1979)
Micrococcin	Bs L11	R	No cross-resistance to thiostrepton	SPEDDING and CUNDLIFFE (1984)
Cycloheximide	Sc L24	R	Reduced binding	STÖCKLEIN and PIEPERSBERG (1980a)
Trichodermin	Sc L3	R	Cross-resistance to other peptidyl-transferase inhibitors	FRIED and WARNER (1981)

[a] Denotes the nomenclature of the ribosomal protein change in Ec, *E. coli*; Bs, *Bacillus subtilis*; Sc, *Saccharomyces cerevisiae*
For other abbreviations see footnotes to Table 1

tation leads to a greatly reduced affinity of the 50S subunits for erythromycin. However, no change in binding constants could be found for the L22 mutants (WITTMANN et al. 1973). It remains an intriguing question as to how resistance is mediated by a mutation which does not affect binding of the inhibitor at all.

When erythromycin-resistant strains acquire an additional locus (*mac*) which is linked to the *tyr*R-*lin*B markers on the *E. coli* chromosome, they become dependent upon the presence of these antibiotics for their growth (SPARLING and BLACKMAN 1973). The growth requirement can be fulfilled by other 50S inhibitors in the following order of efficiency: erythromycin > oleandomycin > lincomycin > chloramphenicol (SPARLING and BLACKMAN 1973). Revertants to independence arise with rather high frequency (10^{-4}).

An early, interesting observation by APIRION and SALTZMAN (1974) is that the expression of erythromycin resistance in strains with an altered L4 protein is masked by mutations in proteins S5 which confer spectinomycin resistance. 70S ribosomes of these double mutants bind erythromycin with nearly the same affinity as those from the wild type (SALTZMAN and APIRION 1976). Isolated 50S subunits with the altered L4, however, display the characteristically reduced affinity. It has to be concluded from these results that alterations in one of the subunits can be counteracted by changes at the other. This is also strongly supported by the analysis of revertants of streptomycin-dependent mutants from *E. coli* with an altered S8 protein. Reversion to streptomycin independent growth could be brought about by changes in almost any protein of the small or large subunit (DABBS 1978 b). Therefore, the two subunits must exhibit conformational interaction.

Mutants resistant to macrolides other than erythromycin have been less well studied. One report deals with the analysis of strains selected for resistance to either 300 µg/ml of leucomycin, tylosin or spiramycin (TANAKA et al. 1971). These mutants display heterogeneous cross-resistance patterns: Class I is resistant to leucomycin, tylosin and spiramycin but sensitive to erythromycin. Class II, on the other hand, is solely resistant to spiramycin; the respective strains possess a mutationally altered L4 protein (TANAKA et al. 1971).

There are several 50S-targeted inhibitors which possess a binding site which overlaps with that for erythromycin. The semisynthetic compound tiamulin is one example (HÖGENAUER 1979). The notion of overlapping binding sites is supported by the phenotypes of tiamulin-resistant mutants from *E. coli* obtained by stepwise selection for resistance to increasing antibiotic concentrations (one-step, high-level resistant mutants did not arise). Mutants with altered L3 or L4 proteins were obtained which display an increase in their resistance to erythromycin. The K_A of these mutants for tiamulin was reduced by a factor of 20–200 (BÖCK et al. 1982).

Lincomycin binding to the ribosome can be competed for by erythromycin (FÉRNANDEZ-MUÑOZ et al. 1971). Mutants from *E. coli* partially resistant to this antibiotic possess electrophoretically altered proteins L14 or L15 (HUMMEL et al. 1979). Binding experiments provided evidence which suggests that these proteins may be located at the binding site for lincomycin (COOPERMAN 1980). Proteins L14 and L15 were specifically labeled in experiments in which a lincomycin derivative was bound to the ribosome by carbene-dependent mechanisms (COOPERMAN

1980). In addition, protein L15 appears to be a component directly or indirectly involved in the formation of the peptidyltransferase center (COOPERMAN 1980; NIERHAUS 1980), along with proteins L2, L16 and L18.

2. Thiostrepton and Micrococcin

Thiostrepton and the structurally related compounds thiopeptin, siomycin and micrococcin are modified peptide antibiotics which interfere with the GTPase activity of the eubacterial large ribosomal subunit (GALE et al. 1981). This functional domain is rather well defined and consists of 23S rRNA, one molecule each of the proteins L10 and L11 and two dimers of the protein L7/L12 (BEAUCLERK et al. 1984). Besides GTP hydrolysis, the GTPase center has an important regulatory role since it is the site at which the ribosome interacts with the so-called stringency factor (PARKER et al. 1976; STARK and CUNDLIFFE 1979a; SMITH et al. 1978). Thiostrepton binds with very high affinity ($K_A > 10^9$ M^{-1}) to a clearly defined region consisting of about 60 nucleotides of the 23S rRNA and of protein L11 (THOMPSON et al. 1979; CUNDLIFFE 1986).

Mutants from gram-positive bacteria resistant to thiostrepton (the drug cannot permeate the membranes of gram-negative organisms) lack ribosomal protein L11 (CUNDLIFFE et al. 1979; WIENEN et al. 1979). They exhibit a decreased growth rate and an impaired protein synthesis capacity in vitro (STARK and CUNDLIFFE 1979b; CUNDLIFFE et al. 1979). Consistent with the fact that their ribosomes still bind thiostrepton, albeit with reduced affinity (K_A: 5×10^6 M^{-1}) (CUNDLIFFE 1986), they are only partially resistant in vivo and their ribosomes display considerable sensitivity in vitro (CUNDLIFFE 1983). Mutants lacking L11 exhibit a relaxed phenotype, i.e. due to the lack of formation of ppGpp the synthesis of rRNA proceeds when protein synthesis is blocked (SMITH et al. 1978; STARK and CUNDLIFFE 1979a). Reversion of the underlying mutation in vivo or complementation of L11 deficient ribosomes with purified L11 in vitro restores thiostrepton sensitivity and the stringent phenotype.

Micrococcin binds to the same 23S rRNA/L11 complex as thiostrepton (CUNDLIFFE and THOMPSON 1981). An important difference, however, is that the elongation factor G-dependent GTP hydrolysis is stimulated rather than inhibited. Mutants selected for resistance to thiostrepton are usually cross-resistant to micrococcin whereas those selected for micrococcin are still inhibited by thiostrepton (SPEDDING and CUNDLIFFE 1984). This, and the fact that ribosomes of methanogenic archaebacteria are highly sensitive to thiostrepton but completely resistant to micrococcin (BEAUCLERK et al. 1985), indicate that the two compounds share overlapping but not identical binding sites. The difference in their interaction with the ribosome is also indicated by the fact that the mutation conferring micrococcin resistance involves a single amino acid exchange in protein L11 whereas all the thiostrepton resistant mutants analysed so far lack this protein.

IV. Protein Changes in the Eukaryotic 60S Subunit

The first antibiotic for which an inhibitory action on eukaryotic 80S ribosomes has been demonstrated is cycloheximide. This antibiotic affects all energy-dependent steps of protein synthesis with initation being the most susceptible reaction (VAZQUEZ 1979). Resistant mutants have been described for many organisms and, in all cases, resistance has been allocated to the 60S subunit and in a few cases to one of the large subunit proteins (BÉGUERET et al. 1977; CODDINGTON and FLURI 1977; STÖCKLEIN and PIEPERSBERG 1980 a). In yeast, for example, resistance is correlated with an electrophoretically changed protein YL24 (STÖCKLEIN and PIEPERSBERG 1980 a, b). YL24 from the mutants differs from the wild-type protein by an amino acid exchange in the tryptic decapeptide T24 in which a Gln residue (wild type) is exchanged for a Glu or Lys (STÖCKLEIN et al. 1981). Different single amino acid exchanges in the same position are therefore responsible for the acquisition of different resistance phenotypes.

The YL24 mutation reduces the binding affinity of 80S ribosomes by about 10-fold, from 2×10^7 M^{-1} to 2×10^6 M^{-1}. Addition of a protein factor, which can be removed by washing with 0.5 M NH_4Cl, increases both the affinity and binding capacity of high-salt washed 80S ribosomes for cycloheximide from wild-type yeast but not from the mutant (STÖCKLEIN and PIEPERSBERG 1980 b). Its function is not known.

1. Anisomycin and Functionally Homologous Compounds

Most of the anti-60S targeted compounds analysed interfere with the peptidyl-transfer reaction of eukaryotic ribosomes. This group comprises structurally unrelated drugs like anisomycin, the 12,13-epoxytrichothecenes (trichodermin, verrucarin A, T-2 toxin, nivalenol, crotocin) and various alkaloids (narciclasine, haemanthamine, pretazettine) (JIMÉNEZ and VÁZQUEZ 1979). One-step and high-level resistant mutants arise spontaneously; they display resistance in vitro. Mutants selected for resistance to one of the above listed drugs are normally cross-resistant to the other ones and they are hypersensitive to sparsomycin (JIMÉNEZ et al. 1975; JIMÉNEZ and VÁZQUEZ 1975).

In *Saccharomyces*, a single recessive mutation (*tcm*l) conferring resistance to trichodermin, verrucarin A and anisomycin, has been localized on the right arm of chromosome XV (GRANT et al. 1976). The respective gene has been cloned and its product identified as ribosomal protein YL3 (FRIED and WARNER 1981), which is the largest protein of yeast ribosomes.

C. Changes in Ribosomal RNA Which Result in Antimicrobial Resistance

I. RNA Changes in the Small Ribosomal Subunit

For almost two decades it was the generally accepted view that protein synthesis inhibitors interact preferentially, or even solely, with the protein components of the ribosome. This opinion has undergone a dramatic change, due mainly to studies conducted on antibiotic resistance mutations in mitochondria (for review see NOLLER 1984), chloroplasts (MONTANDON et al. 1985; ETZOLD et al. 1987) and in bacteria harboring plasmids which carry genes for ribosomal RNA (STEEN et al.

1986). It can be concluded from the results that rRNA appears to be the primary target of translational inhibitors (CUNDLIFFE 1986).

This notion has been strongly supported by recent biochemical studies in which certain antibiotics were shown to protect specific nucleotides of ribosomal RNA against chemical modification (kethoxal; dimethylsulfate) (MOAZED and NOLLER 1987). The modified bases were visualized in primer extension experiments as a premature termination of cDNA synthesis by reverse transcriptase. A surprisingly strict correlation was observed between (i) bases which are protected from modification by antibiotics, (ii) bases which are altered in antibiotic resistant ribosomes, and (iii) nucleotides which are involved in binding of tRNA (MOAZED and NOLLER 1986).

A number of experimental observations indicate that the 3′ terminal region of 16S rRNA is involved in the binding of tRNA (for review see NOLLER et al. 1986). Colicin E3, for example, inactivates ribosomes by a single split of the phosphodiester bond between A-1493 and G-1494 (*E. coli* nomenclature) of the 16S rRNA (BOWMAN et al. 1971). Its action can be competed for by bound aminoacyl-tRNA or by antibiotics like streptomycin, gentamicin or tetracycline which themselves interfere with aminoacyl-tRNA binding (NOMURA et al. 1974). Recently, the anticodon binding region of 16S rRNA could be precisely defined by the photochemical cross-linkage of the 5′-base of the anticodon of valyl-tRNA attached to the ribosomal P-site with C-1400 of the rRNA (PRINCE et al. 1982). The essential functional role of this part of the 16S rRNA in the initiation step of protein synthesis and in the control of translational fidelity was strongly supported by the analysis of modified or mutationally altered ribosomal RNA from antibiotic resistant organelles. Figure 2 summarizes these results; the base positions are given in the *E. coli* nomenclature.

Mutations in the *ksgA* gene, which codes for a methyltransferase, confer kasugamycin resistance (HELSER et al. 1971). This enzyme catalyses the posttranscriptional dimethylation of the two adjacent adenosine residues in positions 1518 and 1519 (HELSER et al. 1971). *ksgA* mutant ribosomes phenotypically resemble *ram* ribosomes since they exhibit an increased translational misreading (VAN BUUL et al. 1984).

Self-protection in aminoglycoside producing organisms is mediated by modification of the 16S rRNA (for review see CUNDLIFFE 1986). Detailed studies showed that *Micromonospora (M.) purpurea*, *Streptomyces (S.) tenjimariensis* and *S. tenebrarius* possess specific methyltransferases which, by modification of a specific base in 16S rRNA, confer resistance to the respective product (PIENDL et al. 1984; BEAUCLERK and CUNDLIFFE 1987; SKEGGS et al. 1987). Resistance to gentamicin and kanamycin in the gentamicin-producing organism *M. purpurea* is the result of N7-methylation of G-1405. 1-Methylation of A-1408 of 16S rRNA from the istamycin producer *S. tenjimariensis* causes resistance to apramycin and kanamycin. *S. tenebrarius* (producer of the nebramycin complex) appears to possess at least two resistance determinants which, by methylation of 16S rRNA, cause resistance either to kanamycin and apramycin or to kanamycin and gentamicin (SKEGGS et al. 1987).

Resistance to aminoglycosides can also be brought about by specific mutations within the 16S rRNA gene. A C/G transversion at position 1409 in the 15S

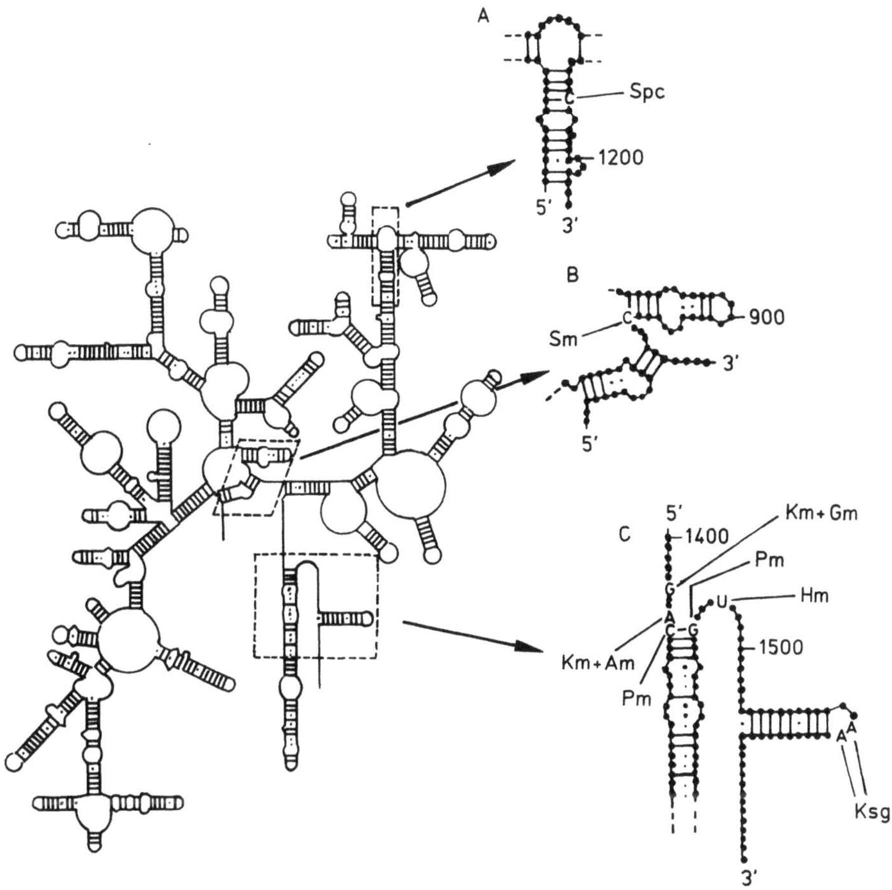

Fig. 2. Secondary structure model of 16S rRNA with an expanded view of domains implicated in interaction with spectinomycin (*Spc*) (*A*), streptomycin (*Sm*) (*B*) and the 2-desoxystreptamin containing aminoglycosides kanamycin (*Km*), gentamicin (*Gm*), paromomycin (*Pm*), hygromycin B (*Hm*), amikacin (*Am*) and kasugamycin (*Ksg*) (*C*)

rRNA of yeast mitochondria and a G/A transition at position 1491 in the 17S rRNA from *Tetrahymena* (*T.*) *thermophila* correlate with high-level resistance to paromomycin (Li et al. 1982; Spangler and Blackburn 1985). Both alterations disrupt basepairing and lead to destabilization of the secondary structure of the 3′-terminal helix of 16S rRNA (Noller 1984). In *T. thermophila*, a base change in this particular region of 17S rRNA (U-1495 to C) has been implicated in resistance to hygromycin B (Spangler and Blackburn 1985). These mutant studies and also the 16S rRNA modification pattern in aminoglycoside producing organisms are in excellent agreement with the results from the chemical modification experiments. They showed that neomycin, paromomycin, gentamicin, kanamycin and hygromycin B interact mainly with nucleotides A-1408 and G-1494 (Moazed and Noller 1987). A-1408, A-1492 and A-1493 have also been ascribed a function in A-site binding of tRNA (Moazed and Noller 1986). One may conclude, therefore, that this group of antibiotics has its primary action in the disruption of the structure of the aminoacyl-tRNA acceptor site.

Previous genetic (for review see PIEPERSBERG et al. 1980) and biochemical analyses (ZIERHUT et al. 1979) demonstrated that streptomycin differs in its mode of action from all the 2-desoxystreptamin containing aminoglycosides. This notion is in accord with the fact that mutations in a different region of the 16S rRNA are involved in causing resistance. In *Euglena gracilis* chloroplasts and in *E. coli*, resistance correlates with a C to U change in position 912 of 16S rRNA (MONTANDON et al. 1985, 1986). C-912 is exchanged for an A in *Nicotiana tabacum* chloroplasts exhibiting streptomycin resistance (ETZOLD et al. 1987). Again, these genetic data are in excellent agreement with the results obtained with chemical modification experiments which indicated binding to A-913, A-914, A-915 and, to a lesser degree, to C-912 and U-911 (MOAZED and NOLLER 1987).

Spectinomycin, in contrast to other aminoglycosides, does not interfere with translational fidelity; its main action is the inhibition of the initiation step of protein synthesis (VÁZQUEZ 1979). Spectinomycin resistance could be correlated with a C/U transition at position 1192 of 16S rRNA (SIGMUND et al. 1984) and it has been shown to protect, specifically, nucleotides C-1063 and G-1064 against chemical modification (MOAZED and NOLLER 1987). Interestingly, G-1064 is involved in base-pairing with 1192; the C-1192 to U-1192 transition, therefore, disrupts the local geometry of that specific helix. Its involvement in the initiation reaction, however, still remains to be demonstrated.

II. RNA Changes in the Large Ribosomal Subunit

The primary target of the 50S inhibitor thiostrepton has been elucidated mainly in studies with ribosomes from the producing organism, *S. azureus* (for review see CUNDLIFFE 1986). The binding domain is well analyzed; the antibiotic binds to 23S rRNA with a K_A of 2×10^6 M^{-1} and in the presence of protein L11 the affinity is increased at least 1000-fold (CUNDLIFFE 1986). Resistance can be conferred by alterations in the protein (lack of protein L11, see above) part as well as in the RNA part. Ribosomes from *S. azureus* are completely resistant due to the action of a RNA-methyltransferase whose product is a 2′-0-methyladenosine at position 1067 in domain II of the 5′ half of the 23S rRNA molecule (Fig. 3) (CUNDLIFFE and THOMPSON 1979). This modified nucleotide is within the L11 binding region (positions 1052-1112) (THOMPSON et al. 1982). The important function of A-1067 in the interaction with thiostrepton is emphasized by the results obtained with mutants from *Halobacterium* species. These archaebacteria contain a single set of rRNA genes. High-level thiostrepton-resistant mutants arise spontaneously; the A at the position equivalent to A-1067 of *E. coli* is changed to either a G or a U (HUMMEL and BÖCK 1987 b).

Resistance to antibiotics of the MLS group and to chloramphenicol can also be brought about by modification or by mutational alterations of 23S rRNA. The nucleotides involved are localized almost exclusively within the so-called peptidyltransferase loop in domain V of the 3′ half of the 23S rRNA molecule (Fig. 4).

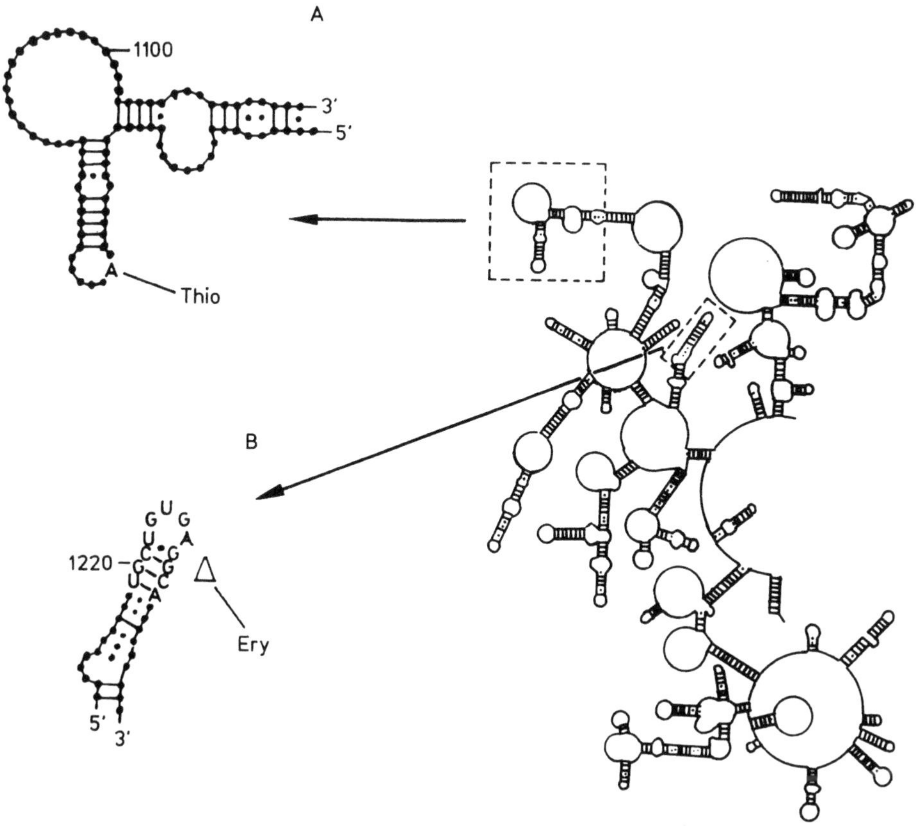

Fig. 3. Secondary structure model of the 5′ half of 23S rRNA with an expanded view of domains implicated in the interaction with thiostrepton (*Thio*) (*A*) and erythromycin (*Ery*) (*B*)

Inducible resistance to MLS antibiotics due to 23S rRNA modification is widespread amongst gram-positive and gram-negative clinical isolates. WEISBLUM and coworkers demonstrated for erythromycin-resistant *S. aureus* strains that a plasmid-encoded RNA-methyltransferase catalyzes a post-transcriptional modification (for review see WEISBLUM 1985) which results in a significant decrease of the affinity of the ribosomes for the antibiotic (LAI and WEISBLUM 1971; SAITO et al. 1969). The product of the modification is N^6,N^6-dimethyladenine at position 2058. Induction of resistance can be brought about by different antibiotics of the MLS group, although to different degrees depending upon the type of *erm* (*e*rythromycin-*r*esistance rRNA *m*ethylase) allele involved (WEISBLUM 1985). Self-protection of the erythromycin producer, *S. erythraeus*, also involves N^6-dimethylation of A-2058 (SKINNER et al. 1983).

The importance of residue A-2058 in the expression of the MLS phenotype is further supported by mutant studies. It has been shown that the conversion of A-2058 to G in yeast mitochondrial 21S rRNA causes erythromycin resistance (SOR and FUKUHARA 1982). Exchange of A-2058 for U in the *rrnH* operon from

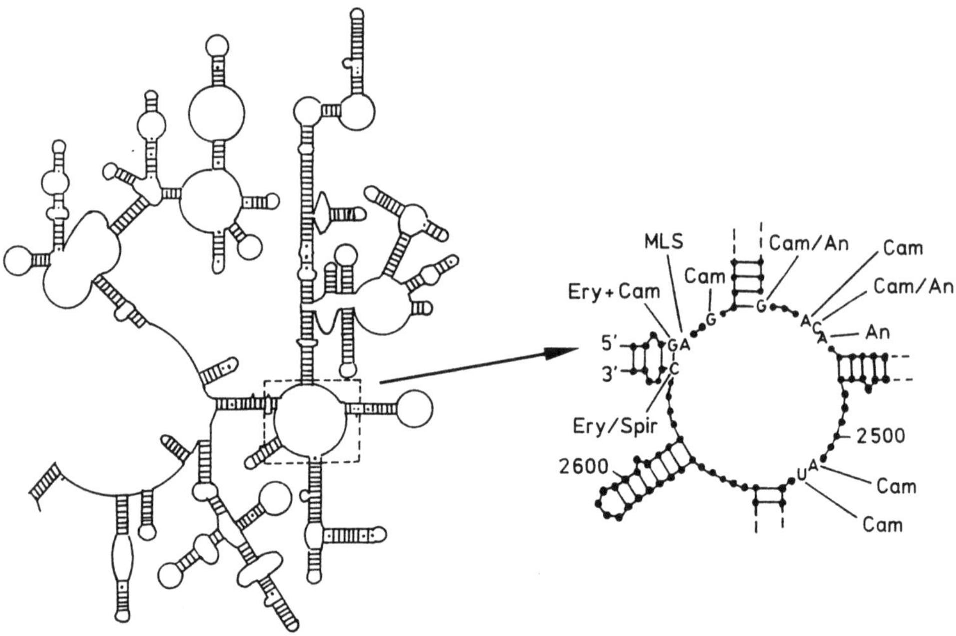

Fig. 4. Secondary structure model of the 3′ half of 23S rRNA with an expanded view of the "peptidyltransferase loop." Nucleotide positions are indicated which are altered in mutants resistant to chloramphenicol (*Cam*), erythromycin (*Ery*), spiramycin (*Spir*), anisomycin (*An*) and MLS group antibiotics

E. coli cloned on a multicopy plasmid leads to multiple resistance to the macrolides erythromycin, oleandomycin, niddamycin, tylosin and spiramycin, to the lincosamides lincomycin and clindamycin and to some streptogramin B-type compounds (SIGMUND et al. 1984).

A C/G transversion of base C-2611, which is in close proximity in the secondary structure model of 23S rRNA (Fig. 3), is correlated with resistance to erythromycin and spiramycin in yeast mitochondria; a C/U transition of the same base generates resistance to spiramycin only (SOR and FUKUHARA 1984).

Recently, MORGAN and coworkers described mutants of *E. coli* possessing a G to A transition of base 2057 of 23S rRNA which acquired resistance both to 14-membered macrolides (erythromycin, oleandomycin) and to chloramphenicol (ETTAYEBI et al. 1985). They were sensitive to 16-membered macrolides. Their phenotype is remarkable since (i) it suggests an overlap of the binding sites of these inhibitors of the peptidyltransferase reaction and (ii) any mutant isolated previously displayed exclusive resistance to either of these compounds. For example, chloramphenicol resistance with unaffected MLS phenotype has been correlated with the following base changes in mitochondrial large ribosomal subunit RNA: G-2061 to A in rat (KOIKE et al. 1983), G-2447 to A (yeast) (DUJON 1980), A-2451 to U (mouse) (SLOTT et al. 1983), C-2452 to A (man) (KEARNEY and CRAIG 1981) or U (mouse) (SLOTT et al. 1983), A-2503 to C (yeast) (DUJON 1980) and U-2504 to C (man, mouse) (BLANC et al. 1981; KEARNEY and CRAIG 1981) (see Fig. 4).

Hydroxylamine mutagenesis of the cloned *rrnB* operon from *E. coli* resulted in a plasmid conferring low-level erythromycin resistance after transformation (DOUTHWAITE et al. 1985). A deletion of position 1219–1230 in domain II of the 23S rRNA was shown to be responsible for resistance. This site is remote from those altered in any of the other erythromycin-resistant mutants (domain V) and may indicate a functional tertiary-structure interaction between these two domains (STIEGE et al. 1983).

The mode of inhibition of protein synthesis by chloramphenicol at 70S ribosomes resembles closely the action of the anti-80S targeted inhibitor anisomycin. Anisomycin resistant mutants could be isolated from *Halobacterium* species which possess a single set of rRNA genes (HOFMAN et al. 1979). Three base alterations in the "peptidyltransferase loop" of 23S rRNA were correlated with resistance; substitution of C-2452 for U conferred high-level resistance, A-2453 for C low-level resistance and G-2447 for C an intermediary level resistance (HUMMEL and BÖCK 1987a). Interestingly, the C-2471 to U transition was demonstrated to cause chloramphenicol resistance in murine mitochondria (SLOTT et al. 1983). This provides evidence which indicates that the two antibiotics bind to functionally homologous sites at the ribosome and that 23S rRNA participates in binding.

D. Antibiotics and Phylogeny

Many protein synthesis inhibitors act specifically on eubacterial 70S or eukaryotic 80S ribosomes (for review see VÁZQUEZ 1979). The structural basis of this differential sensitivity was, until recently, unresolved. During the last few years, however, rRNA sequences from numerous organisms have been accumulated and, by means of mutant studies, those primary and secondary structure details determining the antibiotic sensitivity phenotype have been elucidated. These facts allow a correlation analysis as to whether sequence traits important for antibiotic susceptibility are phylogenetically conserved in the different cell lineages. The discovery of the archaebacterial branch of prokaryotes (FOX et al. 1977) and their unusual mosaic pattern of antibiotic sensitivity (for review see BÖCK and KANDLER 1985) make such a comparision statistically even more significant.

Archaebacteria appear to be generally resistant to streptomycin (BÖCK et al. 1983; HUMMEL et al. 1985; AMILS and SANZ 1986) and their ribosomes lack a streptomycin binding site (SCHMID et al. 1982). A comparision of the 16S rRNA sequences around nucleotide position 912, which has been implicated in streptomycin binding (see above), is given in Table 3. With the exception of *Desulfurococcus* (*D.*) *mobilis*, archaebacteria possess a U-912 instead of C-912. They resemble, in this instance, the small ribosomal RNAs from streptomycin resistant chloroplasts and from eukaryotic cytoplasmic ribosomes.

The 2-deoxystreptamine containing aminoglycosides provide another example (Table 4). Nucleotide A-1408 is methylated by *S. tenjimariensis* to provide self-protection against kanamycin and apramycin (BEAUCLERK and CUNDLIFFE 987). Sensitive eubacteria and archaebacteria have an A in this position whereas the intrinsically resistant archaebacteria (extreme thermophiles) and eukaryotes possess a G-1408.

Table 3. Primary structure of 16S rRNA domain involved in streptomycin resistance

Position (*E. coli* nomenclature)	Organism[a]	Phenotype[b]	Reference
911 912 915			
5′ UAAAACU C AAAUG 3′	*E. coli*	S	BROSIUS et al. (1978)
UGAAACU C AAAGG	*B. brevis*	S	KOP et al. (1984b)
UGAAACU C AAAGG	*E. gracilis*, chloroplast	S	MONTANDON et al. (1985)
------- U -----	*E. gracilis*, chloroplast	R	MONTANDON et al. (1985)
UGAAACU C AAAGG	*N. tabacum*, chloroplast	S	ETZOLD et al. (1987)
------- A -----	*N. tabacum*, chloroplast	R	ETZOLD et al. (1987)
UGAAACU U AAAGG	*S. cerevisiae*, cytoplasm	R	RUBTSOV et al. (1980)
UGAAACU U AAAGG	*T. thermophila*	R	SPANGLER and BLACKBURN (1[illegible]
UGAAACU U AAAGG	*D. discoideum*	R	MCCARROLL et al. (1983)
UGAAACU U AAAGG	*M. vannielii*	R	JARSCH and BÖCK (1985a)
UGAAACU U AAAGG	*M. hungatei*	R	YANG et al. (1985)
UGAAACU U AAAGG	*M. formicium*	R	LECHNER et al. (1985)
UGAAACU U AAAGG	*H. volcanii*	R	GUPTA et al. (1983)
UGAAACU U AAAGG	*T. tenax*	R	LEINFELDER et al. (1985)
UGAAACU C AAAGG	*D. mobilis*	R	KJEMS et al. (1987a)
UGAAACU U AAAGG	*S. solfataricus*	R	OLSEN et al. (1985)

[a] *Escherichia (E.) coli, Bacillus (B.) brevis, Euglena (E.) gracilis, Nicotiana (N.) tabacum, Saccharomyces (S.) cerevisiae, Tetrahymena (T.) thermophila, Dictyostelium (D.) discoideum, Methanococcus (M.) vannielii, Methanospirillum (M.) hungatei, Methanobacterium (M.) formicicum, Halobacterium (H.) volcanii, Thermoproteus (T.) tenax, Desulfurococcus (D.) mobilis, Sulfolobus (S.) solfataricus*

[b] Streptomycin phenotype: S, sensitive; R, resistant

Furthermore, disruption of base-pairing between position 1409 and 1491 is associated with resistance to paromomycin as elucidated by analysis of resistance mutations. Any organism in which base 1409 is paired with base 1491 displays sensitivity (see Table 4). The response of yeast and rat cytoplasmic ribosomes to paromomycin is not known but from the fact that *mitchondrial* mutations can be easily obtained one has to conclude that the *cytoplasmic* ribosomes are resistant. This correlates with the lack of base-pairing between 1409 and 1491 (Table 4). Table 4 also indicates that nucleotide U-1495, which is correlated with inhibition by hygromycin B, is present in all small rRNA sequences. Accordingly, hygromycin B has been shown to affect ribosomes from all cell lineage.

Among the 50S subunit-targeted inhibitors there are several examples which suggest a correlation between the phylogenetic diversity of the 23S rRNA sequences and the antibiotic phenotype: (i) A-1067 of 23S rRNA (eubacteria and archaebacteria) is essential for inhibition by thiostrepton. 2′-O-methylation or change to G and U provides resistance. All eukaryotic sequences analyzed thus far have a G at position 1067. (ii) The rate of inactivation of 50S subunits by α-sarcin depends on the partial 23S rRNA sequence between positions 2654 and 2667 (WOOL 1984). Archaebacterial ribosomes, which are as sensitive as eukary-

Table 4. Sequence of 3′ end of 16S rRNA involved in resistance to aminoglycosides

Organism[a]	Phenotype[b]	5′ 1400	1405		1408	1409				1491		1495	3′	Reference
E. coli	S	ACCGCCC	G	UC	A	C	ACC	...	GGU	G	AAG	U	CGUAACAA	Brosius et al. (1978)
M. capricolum		ACCGCCC	G	UC	A	C	ACC	...	GGU	G	AAG	U	CGUAACAA	Iwami et al. (1984)
M. vannielii	S	ACCGCCC	G	UC	A	C	ACC	...	GGU	G	AAG	U	CGUAACAA	Jarsch and Böck (1985a)
M. formicicum	S	ACCGCCC	G	UC	A	C	GGG	...	GGC	G	AAG	U	CGUAACAA	Lechner et al. (1985)
H. volcanii		ACCGCCC	G	UC	A	A	AGC	...	GCU	U	AAG	U	CGUAACAA	Gupta et al. (1983)
T. tenax	R	ACCGCCC	G	UC	G	C	ACC	...	GGU	G	AAG	U	CGUAACAA	Leinfelder et al. (1985)
S. solfataricus	R	ACCGCCC	G	UC	G	C	UCC	...	GGA	G	AAG	U	CGUAACAA	Olsen et al. (1985)
S. cerevisiae, mitochondria	Pm[S]	AUCACUC	A	UC	A	C	GC	.....	GC	G	AAG	U	UGAAAUAC	Sor and Fukuhara (1980)
S. cerevisiae, mitochondria	Pm[R]	-------	-	--	-	G	--	.....	--	-	---	-	--------	Li et al. (1982)
D. discoideum	S	ACCGCCC	G	UC	G	C	UCC	...	GGA	G	AAG	U	CGUAACAA	McCarroll et al. (1983)
T. thermophila	S	ACCGCCC	G	UC	G	C	UUG	...	CAA	G	AAG	U	CGUAACAA	Spangler and Blackburn (1985)
T. thermophila	Hm[R]	-------	-	--	-	-	--	.....	--	-	---	C	--------	Spangler and Blackburn (1985)
T. thermophila	Pm[R]	-------	-	--	-	-	--	.....	--	A	---	-	--------	Spangler and Blackburn (1985)
S. cerevisiae, cytoplasm		ACCGCCC	G	UC	G	C	UAG	...	CUA	A	AAG	U	CGUAACAA	Rubtsov et al. (1980)
Rat		ACCGCCC	G	UC	G	C	UAC	...	GUA	A	AAG	U	CGUAACAA	Chang et al. (1984); Torczynski et al. (1983)

[a] *Mycoplasma* (*M.*) *capricolum*, the other organisms are the same as in Table 3

[b] S, sensitive; R, resistant; Pm, paromomycin; Hm, hygromycin

Table 5. Primary structure of the 23S rRNA domain involved in MLS resistance

Organism[a]	Phenotype[b]	23S rRNA sequence (*E. coli* nomenclature) 5′	2057	2058				2611	3′	Reference
E. coli	S	GACG	G	A	AAG	....	UC	C	CUAUC	SIGMUND et al. (1984)
E. coli	MLS^R	----	-	U	---	....	--	-	-----	SIGMUND et al. (1984)
E. coli	Cam^R/Ery^R	----	A	-	---	....	--	-	-----	ETTAYEBI et al. (1985)
B. stearothermophilus	S	ACG	G	A	AAG	....	UC	C	CUAUC	KOP et al. (1984a)
Paramecium, mitochondria	S	GACG	G	A	AAG	....	UC	C	CUAUC	SEILHAMER and CUMMINGS (1981)
Yeast, mitochondria	S	GACG	G	A	AAG	....	UU	C	CUAUC	SOR and FUKUHARA (1984)
Yeast, mitochondria	Ery^R	----	-	G	---	....	--	-	-----	SOR and FUKUHARA (1982)
Yeast, mitochondria	Spir^R/Ery^S	----	-	-	---	....	--	U	-----	SOR and FUKUHARA (1984)
Yeast, mitochondria	Spir^R/Ery^R	----	-	-	---	....	--	G	-----	SOR and FUKUHARA (1984)
Yeast, cytoplasm	R	GGAA	A	G	AAG	....	UU	U	UUCC	GEORGIEV et al. (1981)
Murine mitochondria	R	GACG	A	G	AAG	....	UU	U	CUAUC	BIBB et al. (1981)
T. tenax	R	GCG	A	G	AAG	....	UC	U	CUAC	KJEMS et al. (1987b)
D. mobilis	R	GCG	A	U	AAG	....	AC	U	CUAC	LEFFERS et al. (1987)
M. thermoautotrophicum	R	AAG	C	G	AAG	....	UU	G	CUAU	ØSTERGAARD et al. (1987)
M. vannielii	R	AAG	C	G	AAG	....	UU	G	CUAU	JARSCH and BÖCK (1985b)
H. halobium	R	AAG	C	G	AAG	....	CU	G	CUAU	MANKIN and KAGRAMANOVA (1986)

[a] *Bacillus* (*B.*) *stearothermophilus*, *Methanobacterium* (*M.*) *thermoautotrophicum*, *Halobacterium* (*H.*) *halobium*
[b] According to SOR and FUKUHARA 1984: MLS, macrolide-lincosamide-streptogramin B antibiotics; Ery, erythromycin; Spir, spiramycin; Cam, chloramphenicol; R, resistant; S, sensitive

otic 80S ribosomes, have the eukaryotic sequence version (HUMMEL et al. 1986). (iii) Resistance to MLS group antibiotics can be correlated with the primary structure of the so-called peptidyltransferase loop of 23S rRNA. The relevant positions and partial sequences are given in Table 5. A full correlation can be noted between the bases at positions 2057 and 2058 and the response to macrolides.

Thus, antibiotic sensitivity or resistance of organisms belonging to different cell lineages may be a consequence of the structure of their particular rRNA. However, it cannot be precluded that other components are also involved.

E. Ribosomal Antibiotic Resistance in Clinical Isolates

There are only few rigorously proven examples for ribosomal mutations being the cause of antibiotic resistance in clinical isolates. In *Neisseria gonorrhoeae* ribosomal mutations have been shown to be responsible for streptomycin or spectinomycin resistance (MANESS et al. 1974); there are also reports that clinical isolates of enterococci (ZIMMERMANN et al. 1971 b), of *Pseudomonas aeruginosa* (TSENG et al. 1972), *S. aureus* (LACEY and CHOPRA 1972) and *Mycobacterium* (*M.*) *tuberculosis* (BRYAN 1982) possess streptomycin-resistant ribosomes. Viomycin and capreomycin resistance of *M. tuberculosis* strains, as well as low-level resistance to kanamycin, was also attributed to altered 30S or 50S ribosomal subunits (BRYAN 1982).

Tetracycline resistance caused by the *tetM* or *tetN* determinants seems to be due to the synthesis of a protein by streptococci which is associated with the ribosome and, by some unknown mechanism, desensitizes protein synthesis (BURDETT 1986).

Ribosomal resistance due to the action of an rRNA methylase, in contrast to resistance mutations, is much more widespread amongst clinical isolates, e.g. in those resistant to MLS antibiotics (see also CUNDLIFFE, this volume). Both plasmid (*S. aureus*, *Bacteroides* sp., *Streptococcus* sp.) (FOSTER 1983) and chromosomal genes (*S. pneumoniae*) (CLEWELL 1981) have been reported. Formation of the methylase which modifies A-2058 of 23S rRNA is induced by subinhibitory doses of MLS compounds or it is constitutive (see CUNDLIFFE, this volume).

F. Conclusions and Perspectives

Important progress has been achieved during the last few years in the understanding of how antibiotics interact with the ribosome and inhibit protein synthesis. (i) There is now a general consensus that the main target of most, if not all, of the protein synthesis inhibitors is ribosomal RNA (CUNDLIFFE 1986). (ii) The changes at the rRNA – either by mutation or by modification – which confer resistance, are at the site where the antibiotics bind (MOAZED and NOLLER 1987). (iii) The phylogenetic differences in the susceptibility to protein synthesis inhibitors, in many cases, can be correlated with the evolutionary path of rRNA.

Many questions, however, remain to be answered. What is the contribution of ribosomal proteins to antibiotic binding? Are proteins like S12, S4, S5 or L4 and L22 which modulate binding of streptomycin and erythromycin, respectively, at the actual contact site or do they have an indirect role in shaping the geometry of the actual binding site? Certainly, for many ribosomal inhibitors, we know very little concerning the three-dimensional structure of their binding sites and their mode of action.

Another open question concerns the evolution of resistance determined by rRNA methylases. It is unknown at present why methylation of 23S rRNA, causing MLS resistance, has been spread into almost all clinically relevant organisms, whereas 16S rRNA methylation, conferring aminoglycoside resistance, has not been observed yet in pathogenic organisms.

Acknowledgment. We thank Gary Sawers for many helpful suggestions in preparation of the manuscript. We are indebted to Margit Geier for editorial help. The author's experimental work cited in this review has been supported by grants from the Deutsche Forschungsgemeinschaft and the Fonds der Chemischen Industrie.

References

Ahmad MH, Rechenmacher A, Böck A (1980) Interaction between aminoglycoside uptake and ribosomal resistance mutation. Antimicrob Agents Chemother 18:798–806

Amils R, Sanz JL (1986) Inhibitors of protein synthesis as phylogenetic markers. In: Hardesty B, Kramer G (eds) Structure, function, and genetics of ribosomes. Springer, Berlin Heidelberg New York, Tokyo, p 605

Anderson RP, Menninger JR (1987) Tests of the ribosome editor hypothesis. III. A mutant *Escherichia coli* with a defective ribosome editor. Mol Gen Genet 209:313–318

Apirion D, Saltzman L (1974) Functional interdependence of 50S and 30S ribosomal subunits. Mol Gen Genet 135:11–18

Apirion D, Schlessinger D (1968) Coresistance to neomycin and kanamycin by mutations in an *Escherichia coli* locus that affects ribosomes. J Bacteriol 96:768–776

Beauclerk AAD, Cundliffe E (1987) Sites of action of two ribosomal RNA methylases responsible for resistance to aminoglycosides. J Mol Biol 193:661–671

Beauclerk AAD, Cundliffe E, Dijk J (1984) The binding site for ribosomal protein complex L8 within 23S ribosomal RNA of *Escherichia coli.* J Biol Chem 259:6559–6563

Beauclerk AAD, Hummel H, Holmes DJ, Böck A, Cundliffe E (1985) Studies of the GTPase domain of archaebacterial ribosomes. Eur J Biochem 151:245–255

Bégueret J, Perrot M, Crouzet M (1977) Ribosomal proteins in the fungus *Podospora anserina*: evidence for an electrophoretically altered 60S protein in a cycloheximide resistant mutant. Mol Gen Genet 156:141–144

Bibb MJ, van Etten RA, Wright CT, Warberg MW, Clayton DA (1981) Sequence and gene organization of mouse mitochondrial DNA. Cell 26:167–180

Birge EG, Kurland CG (1969) Altered ribosomal protein in streptomycin-dependent *Escherichia coli.* Science 166:1282–1284

Bjare U, Gorini L (1971) Drug dependence reversed by a ribosomal ambiguity mutation, *ram*, in *Escherichia coli.* J Mol Biol 57:423–435

Blanc H, Adams CA, Wallace DC (1981) Different nucleotide changes in the large rRNA gene of the mitochondrial DNA confer chloramphenicol resistance on two human cell lines. Nucleic Acids Res 9:5785–5795

Böck A, Kandler O (1985) Antibiotic sensitivity of archaebacteria. In: Woese CR, Wolfe RS (eds) The bacteria VIII. Archaebacteria. Academic, New York, p 525

Böck A, Petzet A, Piepersberg W (1979) Ribosomal ambiguity (*ram*) mutations facilitate dihydrostreptomycin binding to ribosomes. FEBS Lett 104:317–321

Böck A, Turnowsky F, Högenauer G (1982) Tiamulin resistance mutations in *Escherichia coli.* J Bacteriol 151:1253–1260

Böck A, Bär U, Schmid G, Hummel H (1983) Aminoglycoside sensitivity of ribosomes from the archaebacterium *Methanococcus vannielii*: structure-activity relationship. FEMS Microbiol Lett 20:435–438
Boersma D, McGill SM, Mollenkamp JW, Roufa DJ (1979a) Emetine resistance in Chinese hamster cells. Analysis of ribosomal proteins prepared from mutant cells. J Biol Chem 254:559–567
Boersma D, McGill SM, Mollenkamp JW, Roufa DJ (1979b) Emetine resistance in Chinese hamster cells is linked genetically with an altered 40S ribosomal subunit protein, S20. Proc Natl Acad Sci USA 76:415–419
Bollen A, Davies J, Ozaki M, Mizushima S (1969) Ribosomal protein conferring sensitivity to the antibiotic spectinomycin in *Escherichia coli*. Science 165:85–86
Bollen A, Cabezón T, de Wilde M, Villarroel R, Herzog A (1975) Alteration of ribosomal protein S17 by mutation linked to neamine resistance in *Escherichia coli*. I. General properties of *neaA* mutants. J Mol Biol 99:795–806
Bowman CM, Dahlberg JE, Ikemura T, Konisky J, Nomura M (1971) Specific inactivation of 16S ribosomal RNA induced by Colicin E3 in vivo. Proc Natl Acad Sci USA 68:964–968
Brosius J, Palmer ML, Kennedy JP, Noller HF (1978) Gene organization and primary structure of a ribosomal RNA operon from *Escherichia coli*. Proc Natl Acad Sci USA 75:4801–4805
Bryan LE (1982) Bacterial resistance and susceptibility to chemotherapeutic agents. Cambridge University Press, Cambridge
Bryan LE, van den Elzen HM (1975) Gentamicin accumulation by sensitive strains of *Escherichia coli* and *Pseudomonas aeruginosa*. J Antibiot 28:696–703
Bryan LE, van den Elzen (1976) Streptomycin accumulation in susceptible and resistant strains of *Escherichia coli* and *Pseudomonas aeruginosa*. Antimicrob Agents Chemother 9:928–938
Bryan LE, van den Elzen HM (1977) Effects of membrane-energy mutations and cations on streptomycin and gentamicin accumulation by bacteria: a model for entry of streptomycin and gentamicin in susceptible and resistant bacteria. Antimicrob Agents Chemother 12:163–177
Buckel P, Buchberger A, Böck A, Wittmann HG (1977) Alteration of ribosomal protein L6 in mutants of *Escherichia coli* resistant to gentamicin. Mol Gen Genet 158:47–54
Burdett V (1986) Streptococcal tetracycline resistance mediated at the level of protein synthesis. J Bacteriol 165:564–569
Chang FN, Flaks JG (1972) Binding of dihydrostreptomycin to *Escherichia coli* ribosomes. Characteristics and equilibrium of the reaction. Antimicrob Agents Chemother 2:294–307
Chang YL, Gutell R, Noller H, Wool IG (1984) The nucleotide sequence of a rat 18S ribosomal ribonucleic acid gene and a proposal for the secondary structure of 18S ribosomal ribonucleic acid. J Biol Chem 259:224–230
Clewell DB (1981) Plasmids, drug resistance, and gene transfer in the genus *Streptococcus*. Microbiol Rev 45:409–436
Coddington A, Fluri R (1977) Characterization of the ribosomal proteins from *Schizosaccharomyces pombe* by two-dimensional polyacrylamide gel electrophoresis. Mol Gen Genet 158:93–100
Cooperman BS (1980) Functional sites on the *E. coli* ribosome as defined by affinity labeling. In: Chambliss G, Craven GR, Davies J, Davis K, Kahan L, Nomura M (eds) Ribosomes. Structure, function, and genetics. University Park Press, Baltimore, p 531
Crouzet M, Bégueret J (1982) Altered ribosomal proteins in emetine resistant strains in the fungus *Podospora anserina*. Curr Genet 6:39–42
Cundliffe E (1983) Antibiotics as probes of ribosomal structure and function. In: Edwards DI, Hiscock DR (eds) Chemotherapeutic strategy. Macmillan, London, p 65
Cundliffe E (1986) Involvement of specific portions of ribosomal RNA in defined ribosomal functions: a study utilizing antibiotics. In: Hardesty B, Kramer G (eds) Structure, function, and genetics of ribosomes. Springer, Berlin Heidelberg New York, Tokyo, p 586

Cundliffe E, Thompson J (1979) Ribose methylation and resistance to thiostrepton. Nature 278:859–861
Cundliffe E, Thompson J (1981) Concerning the mode of action of micrococcin upon bacterial protein synthesis. Eur J Biochem 118:47–52
Cundliffe E, Dixon P, Stark M, Stöffler G, Ehrlich R, Stöffler-Meilicke M, Cannon M (1979) Ribosomes in thiostrepton-resistant mutants of *Bacillus megaterium* lacking a single 50S subunit protein. J Mol Biol 132:235–252
Dabbs ER (1977) A spectinomycin dependent mutant of *Escherichia coli*. Mol Gen Genet 151:261–267
Dabbs ER (1978a) Kasugamycin-dependent mutants of *Escherichia coli*. J Bacteriol 136:994–1001
Dabbs ER (1978b) Mutational alterations in 50 proteins of the *Escherichia coli* ribosome. Mol Gen Genet 165:73–78
Dabbs ER, Wittmann HG (1976) A strain of *Escherichia coli* which gives rise to mutations in a large number of ribosomal proteins. Mol Gen Genet 149:303–309
Dabbs ER, Poldermans B, Bakker H, van Knippenberg PH (1980) Biochemical characterization of ribosomes of kasugamycin-dependent mutants of *Escherichia coli*. FEBS Lett 117:164–166
Davis BD (1987) Mechanism of bactericidal action of aminoglycosides. Microbiol Rev 51:341–350
Dekio S, Tanaka R (1969) Genetic studies of the ribosomal proteins in *Escherichia coli*. II. Altered 30S ribosomal protein component specific to spectinomycin resistant mutants. Mol Gen Genet 105:219–224
Dekio S, Takata R, Osawa S, Tanaka K, Tanaki M (1970) Genetic studies of the ribosomal proteins in *Escherichia coli*. IV. Pattern of the alterations of ribosomal protein components in mutants resistant to spectinomycin or erythromycin in different strains of *Escherichia coli*. Mol Gen Genet 107:39–49
Dequard-Chablat M, Coppin-Raynal E (1984) Increase of translational fidelity blocks sporulation in the fungus *Podospora anserina*. Mol Gen Genet 195:294–299
De Wilde M, Cabezón T, Villarroel R, Herzog A, Bollen A (1975) Cooperative control of translational fidelity by ribosomal proteins in *Escherichia coli*. I. Properties of ribosomal mutants whose resistance to neamine is the cumulative effect of two distinct mutations. Mol Gen Genet 142:19–33
Dombou M, Mizuno T, Mizushima S (1977) Interaction of the cytoplasmic membrane and ribosomes in *Escherichia coli*: altered ribosomal proteins in sucrose-dependent spectinomycin-resistant mutants. Mol Gen Genet 155:53–60
Douthwaite S, Prince JB, Noller HF (1985) Evidence for functional interaction between domain II and V of 23S ribosomal RNA from an erythromycin-resistant mutant. Proc Natl Acad Sci USA 82:8330–8334
Dujon B (1980) Sequences of the intron and flanking exons of the mitochondrial 21S rRNA gene of yeast strains having different alleles at the *W* and *rib-1* loci. Cell 20:185–197
Ettayebi M, Prasad SM, Morgan EA (1985) Chloramphenicol-erythromycin resistance mutations in a 23S rRNA gene of *Escherichia coli*. J Bacteriol 162:551–557
Etzold T, Fritz CC, Schell J, Schreier PH (1987) A point mutation in the chloroplast 16S rRNA gene of a streptomycin resistant *Nicotiana tabacum*. FEBS Lett 219:343–346
Fernández-Muñoz R, Monro RE, Torres-Pinedo R, Vázquez D (1971) Substrate- and antibiotic-binding sites at the peptidyl-transferase centre of *Escherichia coli* ribosomes. Studies on the chloramphenicol, lincomycin and erythromycin sites. Eur J Biochem 23:185–193
Foster TJ (1983) Plasmid-determined resistance to antimicrobial drugs and toxic metal ions in bacteria. Microbiol Rev 47:361–409
Fox GE, Magrum LJ, Balch WE, Wolfe RS, Woese CR (1977) Classification of methanogenic bacteria by 16S ribosomal RNA characterization. Proc Natl Acad Sci USA 74:4537–4541
Fried HM, Warner JR (1981) Cloning of yeast gene for trichodermin resistance and ribosomal protein L3. Proc Natl Acad Sci USA 78:238–242

Funatsu G, Schiltz E, Wittmann HG (1971) Ribosomal proteins XXVII. Localization of the amino acid exchanges in protein S5 from two *Escherichia coli* mutants resistant to spectinomycin. Mol Gen Genet 114:106–111
Gale EF, Cundliffe E, Reynolds PE, Richmond MH, Warning MJ (1981) The molecular basis of antibiotic action, 2nd edn. Wiley, London
Garvin RT, Rosset R, Gorini L (1973) Ribosomal assembly influenced by growth in the presence of streptomycin. Proc Natl Acad Sci USA 70:2762–2766
Garvin RT, Biswas DK, Gorini L (1974) The effects of streptomycin or dihydrostreptomycin binding to 16S rRNA or to 30S ribosomal subunits. Proc Natl Acad Sci USA 71:3814–3818
Georgiev OI, Nikolaev N, Hadjiolov AA, Skryabin KG, Zakharyev VM, Bayev AA (1981) The structure of the yeast ribosomal RNA genes. 4. Complete sequence of the 25S rRNA gene from *Saccharomyces cerevisiae*. Nucleic Acids Res 9:6953–6958
Gorini L (1974) Streptomycin and misreading of the genetic code. In: Nomura M, Tissières A, Lengyel P (eds) Ribosomes. Cold Spring Harbor Laboratory, New York, p 791
Gorini L, Rosset R, Zimmermann RA (1967) Phenotypic masking and streptomycin dependence. Science 157:1314–1317
Grant P, Sánchez , Jiménez A (1974) Cryptopleurine resistance: genetic locus for a 40S ribosomal component in *Saccharomyces cerevisiae*. J Bacteriol 120:1308–1314
Grant PG, Schindler D, Davies JE (1976) Mapping of trichodermin resistance in *Saccharomyces cerevisiae*: a genetic locus for a component of the 60S ribosomal subunit. Genetics 83:667–673
Gupta RS, Siminovitch L (1977a) Mutants of CHO cells resistant to the protein synthesis inhibitors, cryptopleurine and tylocrebrine: genetic and biochemical evidence for common site of action of emetine, cryptopleurine, tylocrebrine, and tubulosine. Biochemistry 16:3209–3214
Gupta RS, Siminovitch L (1977b) The molecular basis of emetine resistance in Chinese hamster ovary cells: alteration in the 40S ribosomal subunit. Cell 10:61–66
Gupta R, Lanter JM, Woese CR (1983) Sequence of the 16S ribosomal RNA from *Halobacterium volcanii*, an archaebacterium. Science 221:656–659
Hancock REW (1981a) Aminoglycoside uptake and mode of action – with special reference to streptomycin and gentamicin. I. Antagonists and mutants. J Antimicrob Chemother 8:249–276
Hancock REW (1981b) Aminoglycoside uptake and mode of action – with special reference to streptomycin and gentamicin. II. Effects of aminoglycosides on cells. J Antimicrob Chemother 8:429–445
Helser TL, Davies JE, Dahlberg JE (1971) Change in methylation of 16S ribosomal RNA associated with mutation to kasugamycin resistance in *Escherichia coli*. Nature New Biol 233:12–14
Henkin TM, Campbell KM, Chambliss GH (1979) Spectinomycin dependence in *Bacillus subtilis*. J Bacteriol 137:1452–1455
Hofman JD, Lau RH, Doolittle WF (1979) The number, physical organization and transcription of ribosomal RNA cistrons in an archaebacterium: *Halobacterium halobium*. Nucleic Acids Res 7:1321–1333
Högenauer G (1979) Tiamulin and pleuromutilin. In: Hahn FE (ed) Mechanism of action of antibacterial agents. Springer, Berlin Heidelberg New York, p 344 (Antibiotics, vol 5 part 1)
Hull R, Klinger JD, Moody EEM (1976) Isolation and characterization of mutants of *Escherichia coli* K12 resistant to the new aminoglycoside antibiotic, amikacin. J Gen Microbiol 94:389–394
Hummel H, Böck A (1983) On the basis of aminoglycoside-dependent growth of mutants from *E. coli*: physiological studies. Mol Gen Genet 191:167–175
Hummel H, Böck A (1987a) 23S ribosomal RNA mutations in *Halobacteria* conferring resistance to the anti-80S ribosome targeted antibiotic anisomycin. Nucleic Acids Res 15:2431–2443
Hummel H, Böck A (1987b) Thiostrepton resistance mutations in the gene for 23S ribosomal RNA of halobacteria. Biochimie 69:857–861

Hummel H, Piepersberg W, Böck A (1979) Analysis of lincomycin resistance mutations in *Escherichia coli*. Mol Gen Genet 169:345–347
Hummel H, Piepersberg W, Böck A (1980) 30S subunit mutations relieving restriction of ribosomal misreading caused by L6 mutations. Mol Gen Genet 179:147–153
Hummel H, Ahmad MH, Böck A (1983) On the basis of aminoglycoside-dependent growth of mutants of *Escherichia coli*: in vitro studies and the model. Mol Gen Genet 191:176–181
Hummel H, Bär U, Heller G, Böck A (1985) Antibiotic sensitivity pattern of in vitro polypeptide synthesis systems from *Methanosarcina barkeri* and *Methanospirillum hungatei*. Syst Appl Microbiol 6:125–131
Hummel H, Jarsch M, Böck A (1986) Unique antibiotic sensitivity of protein synthesis in archaebacteria and the possible structural basis. In: Schlessinger D (ed) Microbiology. American Society for Microbiology, Washington DC, p 370
Ito K, Wittekind M, Nomura M, Shiba K, Yura T, Miuza A, Nashimoto N (1983) A temperature-sensitive mutant of *E. coli* exhibiting slow processing of exported proteins. Cell 32:789–797
Itoh T, Wittmann HG (1973) Amino acid replacements in protein S5 and S12 of two *Escherichia coli* revertants from streptomycin dependence to independence. Mol Gen Genet 127:19–32
Iwami M, Muto A, Yamao F, Osawa S (1984) Nucleotide sequence of the *rrnB* 16S ribosomal RNA gene from *Mycoplasma capricolum*. Mol Gen Genet 196:317–322
Jarsch M, Böck A (1985a) Sequence of the 16S ribosomal RNA gene from *Methanococcus vannielii*: evolutionary implications. Syst Appl Microbiol 6:54–59
Jarsch M, Böck A (1985b) Sequence of the 23S rRNA gene from the archaebacterium *Methanococcus vannielii*: evolutionary and functional implications. Mol Gen Genet 200:305–312
Jiménez A, Vázquez D (1975) Quantitative binding of antibiotics to ribosomes from a yeast mutant altered on the peptidyl transferase center. Eur J Biochem 54:483–492
Jiménez A, Vázquez D (1979) Anisomycin and related antibiotics. In: Hahn FE (ed) Mechanism of action of anti-eukaryotic and antiviral compounds. Springer, Berlin Heidelberg New York, p 1 (Antibiotics, vol 5, part 2)
Jiménez A, Sánchez L, Vázquez D (1975) Simultaneous ribosomal resistance to trichodermin and anisomycin in *Saccharomyces cerevisiae* mutants. Biochim Biophys Acta 383:427–434
Jiménez A, Carrasco C, Vázquez D (1977) Enzymatic and non-enzymatic translocation by yeast polysomes. Site of action of a number of inhibitors. Biochemistry 16:4727–4730
Kearney SE, Craig IW (1981) Altered ribosomal RNA genes in mitochondria from mammalian cells with chloramphenicol resistance. Nature 290:607–608
Kjems J, Garrett RA, Ansorge W (1987a) The sequence of the 16S RNA gene and its flanking region from the archaebacterium *D. mobilis*. Syst Appl Microbiol 9:22–28
Kjems J, Leffers H, Garrett RA, Wich G, Leinfelder W, Böck A (1987b) Gene organization, transcription signals and processing of the single ribosomal RNA operon of the archaebacterium *Thermoproteus tenax*. Nucleic Acids Res 15:4821–4835
Koike K, Tair M, Kuchino Y, Yaginuma K, Sekiguchi T, Kobayashi M (1983) Mutations of the rat mitochondrial genome. In: Schweyen RJ, Wolf K, Kaudewitz F (eds) Mitochondria 1983: nuclear-cytoplasmic interactions. de Gruyter, Berlin, p 371
Kop J, Wheaton V, Gupta R, Woese CR, Noller HF (1984a) Complete nucleotide sequence of a 23S ribosomal RNA gene from *Bacillus stearothermophilus*. DNA 3:347–357
Kop J, Kopylov AM, Magrum L, Siegel R, Gupta R, Woese CR, Noller HF (1984b) Probing the structure of 16S ribosomal RNA from *Bacillus brevis*. J Biol Chem 259:15287–15293
Kühberger R, Piepersberg W, Petzet A, Buckel P, Böck A (1979) Alteration of ribosomal protein L6 in gentamicin-resistant strains of *Escherichia coli*. Effects on fidelity of protein synthesis. Biochemistry 18:187–193
Lacey RW, Chopra I (1972) Evidence for mutation to streptomycin resistance in clinical strains of *Staphylococcus aureus*. J Gen Microbiol 73:175–180

Lai CJ, Weisblum B (1971) Altered methylation of ribosomal RNA in an erythromycin-resistant strain of *Staphylococcus aureus*. Proc Natl Acad Sci USA 68:856–860

Lechner K, Wich G, Böck A (1985) The nucleotide sequence of the 16S rRNA gene and flanking regions from *Methanobacterium formicicum*: the phylogenetic relationship between methanogenic and halophilic archaebacteria. Syst Appl Microbiol 6:157–163

Leffers H, Kjems J, Østergaard L, Larsen N, Garrett RA (1987) Evolutionary relationship amongst archaebacteria: a comparative study of 23S ribosomal RNAs of a sulphur-dependent extreme thermophile, an extreme halophile and a thermophilic methanogen. J Mol Biol 195:43–61

Le Goffic P, Capmau M, Tangy F, Caminade E (1980) Have deoxystreptamine aminoglycoside antibiotics the same binding site on bacterial ribosomes? J Antibiot 33:895–899

Leinfelder W, Jarsch M, Böck A (1985) The phylogenetic position of the sulfur-dependent archaebacterium *Thermoproteus tenax*: sequence of the 16S rRNA gene. Syst Appl Microbiol 6:164–170

Lelong JC, Gros D, Gros F, Bollen A, Maschler R, Stöffler G (1974) Function of individual 30S subunit proteins of *Escherichia coli*. Effect of specific immunoglobin fragments (Fab) on activities of ribosomal decoding sites. Proc Natl Acad Sci USA 71:248–252

Li M, Tzagoloff A, Underbrink-Lyon K, Martin NC (1982) Identification of the paromomycin resistance mutation in the 15S rRNA of yeast mitochondria. J Biol Chem 257:5921–5928

Lindahl L, Zengel JM (1986) Ribosomal genes in *Escherichia coli*. Annu Rev Genet 20:297–326

Maness MJ, Foster GC, Sparling PF (1974) Ribosomal resistance to streptomycin and spectinomycin in *Neisseria gonorrhoeae*. J Bacteriol 120:1293–1299

Mankin AS, Kagramanova VK (1986) Complete nucleotide sequence of the single ribosomal RNA operon of *Halobacterium halobium*: Secondary structure of the archaebacterial 23S rRNA. Mol Gen Genet 202:152–161

McCarroll R, Olsen GJ, Stahl YD, Woese CR, Sogin ML (1983) Nucleotide sequence of *Dictyostelium discoideum* small-subunit rRNA inferred from the gene sequence: evolutionary implications. Biochemistry 22:5828–5868

Menninger JR, Otto DP (1982) Erythromycin, carbomycin, and spiromycin inhibit protein synthesis by stimulating the dissociation of peptidyl-tRNA from ribosomes. Antimicrob Agents Chemother 21:810–818

Mikulík K, Jiránová A, Janda I, Weiser J (1983) Susceptibility of ribosomes of the tetracycline-producing strain of *Streptomyces aureofaciens* to tetracycline. FEBS Lett 152:125–130

Mizumo T, Yamada H, Yamagata H, Mizushima S (1976) Coordinated alterations in ribosomes and cytoplasmic membrane in sucrose-dependent, spectinomycin-resistant mutants of *Escherichia coli*. J Bacteriol 125:524–530

Moazed D, Noller HF (1986) Transfer RNA shields specific nucleotides in 16S ribosomal RNA from attack by chemical probes. Cell 47:985–994

Moazed D, Noller HF (1987) Interaction of antibiotics with functional sites in 16S ribosomal RNA. Nature 327:389–394

Momose H, Gorini L (1971) Genetic analysis of streptomycin dependence in *Escherichia coli*. Genetics 67:19–38

Montandon PE, Nicolas P, Schürmann P, Stutz E (1985) Streptomycin-resistance of *Euglena gracilis* chloroplasts: identification of a point mutation in the 16S rRNA gene in an invariant position. Nucleic Acids Res 13:4299–4310

Montandon PE, Wagner R, Stutz E (1986) *E. coli* ribosomes with C912 to U base change in the 16S rRNA are streptomycin resistant. EMBO J 5:3705–3708

Morris VJ, Jennings BR (1975) The effect of neomycin and streptomycin on the electrical polarisability of aqueous suspensions of *Escherichia coli*. Biochim Biophys Acta 392:328–334

Nierhaus KH (1980) Analysis of the assembly and function of the 50S subunit from *Escherichia coli* ribosomes by reconstitution. In: Chambliss G, Craven GR, Davies J, Davis K, Kahan L, Nomura M (eds) Ribosomes. Structure, function and genetics. University Park Press, Baltimore, p 267

Nikaido H (1976) Outer membrane of *Salmonella typhimurium*: transmembrane diffusion of some hydrophobic substances. Biochim Biophys Acta 433:118–132
Noller HF (1984) Structure of ribosomal RNA. Annu Rev Biochem 53:119–162
Noller HF, Asire M, Barta A, Douthewaite S, Goldstein T, Gutell RR, Moazed D, Normanly J, Prince JB, Sterm S, Triman K, Turner S, van Stalk B, Wheaton V, Weiser B, Woese CR (1986) Studies on the structure and function of ribosomal RNA. In: Hardesty B, Kramer G (eds) Structure, function, and genetics of ribosomes. Springer, Berlin Heidelberg New York, Tokyo, p 143
Nomura M, Sidikaro J, Jakes K, Zinder N (1974) Effects of colicin E3 on bacterial ribosomes. In: Nomura M, Tissiéres A, Lengyel P (eds) Ribosomes. Cold Spring Harbor Laboratory, New York, p 804
Nomura M, Morgan EA, Jaskunas SR (1977) Genetics of bacterial ribosomes. Annu Rev Genet 11:297–347
Ohnuki T, Katoh T, Imanaka T, Aiba S (1985) Molecular cloning of tetracycline resistance genes from *Streptomyces rimosus* in *Streptomyces griseus* and characterization of the cloned genes. J Bacteriol 161:1010–1016
Okuyama A, Yoshikawa M, Tanaka N (1974) Alteration of ribosomal protein S2 in kasugamycin-resistant mutant derived from *Escherichia coli* AB312. Biochem Biophys Res Commun 60:1163–1169
Olsen GJ, Pace NR, Nuell M, Kaine BP, Gupta R, Woese CR (1985) Nucleotide sequence of the 16S rRNA gene from the thermoacidophilic archaebacterium *Sulfolobus solfataricus*. J Mol Evol 22:301–308
Østergaard L, Larsen N, Leffers H, Kjems J, Garrett RA (1987) A ribosomal RNA operon and its flanking region from the archaebacterium *Methanobacterium thermoautotrophicum*, Marburg strain: transcription signals, RNA structure and evolutionary implications. Syst Appl Microbiol 9:199–209
Ozaki M, Mizushima S, Nomura M (1969) Identification and functional characterization of the protein controlled by the streptomycin-resistant locus in *E. coli*. Nature 222:333–339
Parker J, Watson RJ, Friesen JD, Fiil NP (1976) A relaxed mutant with an altered ribosomal protein L11. Mol Gen Genet 144:111–114
Pestka S (1977) Inhibitors of protein synthesis. In: Weissbach H, Pestka S (eds) Molecular mechanisms of protein synthesis. Academic, New York, p 467
Piendl W, Böck A, Cundliffe E (1984) Involvement of 16S ribosomal RNA in resistance of the aminoglycoside-producers *Streptomyces tenjimariensis*, *Streptomyces tenebrarius* and *Micromonospora purpurea*. Mol Gen Genet 197:24–29
Piepersberg W, Böck A, Wittmann HG (1975 a) Effect of different mutations in ribosomal protein S5 of *Escherichia coli* on translational fidelity. Mol Gen Genet 140:91–100
Piepersberg W, Böck A, Yaguchi M, Wittmann HG (1975 b) Genetic position and amino acid replacements of several mutations in ribosomal protein S5 from *Escherichia coli*. Mol Gen Genet 143:43–52
Piepersberg W, Noseda V, Böck A (1979) Bacterial ribosomes with ambiguity mutations: effects on translational fidelity, on the response to aminoglycosides and on the rate of protein synthesis. Mol Gen Genet 171:23–34
Piepersberg W, Geyl D, Hummel H, Böck A (1980) Physiology and biochemistry of bacterial ribosomal mutants. In: Osawa S, Ozeki H, Uchida H, Yura T (eds) Genetics and evolution of RNA polymerase, tRNA and ribosomes. University of Tokyo Press, Tokyo, p 359
Plotz PH, Davis BD (1962) Absence of a chloramphenicol-insensitive phase of streptomycin action. J Bacteriol 83:802–805
Prince JB, Taylor BH, Thurlow DL, Ofengand J, Zimmermann RA (1982) Covalent crosslinking of $tRNA^{Val}$ to 16S RNA at the ribosomal P site: identification of crosslinked residues. Proc Natl Acad Sci USA 79:5450–5454
Reichenbecher VE, Caskey CT (1979) Emetine-resistant Chinese hamster cells. The identification of an electrophoretically altered protein of the 40S ribosomal subunit. J Biol Chem 254:6207–6210
Rosset R, Gorini L (1969) A ribosomal ambiguity mutation. J Mol Biol 39:95–112

Rubtsov PM, Musakhanov MM, Zakharyev VM, Krayev AS, Skryabin CG, Bayev AA (1980) The structure of the yeast ribosomal RNA genes. I. The complete nucleotide sequence of the 18S ribosomal RNA gene from *Saccharomyces cerevisiae*. Nucleic Acids Res 8:5779–5794

Ruusala T, Andersson DI, Ehrenberg M, Kurland CG (1984) Hyperaccurate ribosomes inhibit growth. EMBO J 3:2575–2580

Saito T, Hashimoto H, Mitsuhashi S (1969) Drug resistance of *Staphylococci*. Decrease in the formation of erythromycin-ribosomes complex in erythromycin-resistant strains. Jpn J Microbiol 13:119–121

Saltzman L, Apirion D (1976) Binding of erythromycin to the 50S ribosomal subunit is affected by alteration in the 30S ribosomal subunit. Mol Gen Genet 143:301–306

Sánchez L, Vázquez D, Jiménez A (1977) Genetics and biochemistry of cryptopleurine resistance in the yeast *Saccharomyces cerevisiae*. Mol Gen Genet 156:319–326

Schmid G, Pecher T, Böck A (1982) Properties of the translational apparatus of archaebacteria. Zentralbl Bakteriol Hyg I. Abt. Orig C3:209–217

Schreiner G, Nierhaus KH (1973) Protein involved in the binding of dihydrostreptomycin to ribosomes of *Escherichia coli*. J Mol Biol 81:71–82

Seilhamer JJ, Cummings DJ (1981) Structure and sequence of the mitochondrial 20S rRNA and tRNA *tyr* gene of *Paramecium primaurelia*. Nucleic Acids Res 9:6391–6409

Shultz J, Silhavy TJ, Berman ML, Fiil N, Emr SD (1982) A previously unidentified gene in the *spc* operon of *Escherichia coli* K12 specifies a component of the protein export machinery. Cell 31:227–235

Sigmund CD, Ettayebi M, Morgan EA (1984) Antibiotic resistance mutations in the 16S and 23S ribosomal RNA genes of *Escherichia coli*. Nucleic Acids Res 12:4653–4663

Skeggs PA, Holmes DJ, Cundliffe E (1987) Cloning of aminoglycoside-resistance determinants from *Streptomyces tenebrarius* and comparison with related genes from other actinomycetes. J Gen Microbiol 133:915–923

Skinner R, Cundliffe E, Schmidt FJ (1983) Site of action of a ribosomal RNA methylase responsible for resistance to erythromycin and other antibiotics. J Biol Chem 258:12702–12706

Skogerson L, McLaughlin C, Wakatama E (1973) Modification of ribosomes in cryptopleurine-resistant mutants of yeast. J Bacteriol 116:812–822

Slott EF Jr, Shade RO, Lansman RA (1983) Sequence analysis of mitochondrial DNA in a mouse cell line resistant to chloramphenicol and oligomycin. Mol Cell Biol 3:1694–1702

Smith I, Paress P, Pestka S (1978) Thiostrepton-resistant mutants exhibit relaxed synthesis of RNA. Proc Natl Acad Sci USA 75:5993–5997

Sor F, Fukuhara H (1980) Nucleotide sequence of the genes for the mitochondrial 15S ribosomal RNA of yeast. CR Acad Sci 291:933–936

Sor F, Fukuhara H (1982) Identification of two erythromycin resistance mutations in the mitochondrial gene coding for the large ribosomal RNA in yeast. Nucleic Acids Res 10:6571–6577

Sor F, Fukuhara H (1984) Erythromycin and spiramycin resistance mutations in yeast mitochondria: nature of the *rib2* locus in the large ribosomal RNA gene. Nucleic Acids Res 12:8313–8318

Sougakoff W, Papadopoulou B, Nordmann P, Courvalin P (1987) Nucleotide sequence and distribution of gene *tet0* encoding tetracycline resistance in *Campylobacter coli*. FEMS Microbiol Lett 44:153–159

Spangler EA, Blackburn EH (1985) The nucleotide sequence of the 17S ribosomal RNA gene of *Tetrahymena thermophila* and the identification of point mutations resulting in resistance to the antibiotics paromomycin and hygromycin. J Biol Chem 26:6334–6340

Sparling PF, Blackman E (1973) Mutation to erythromycin dependence in *Escherichia coli* K-12. J Bacteriol 116:74–83

Spedding G, Cundliffe E (1984) Identification of the altered ribosomal component responsible for resistance to micrococcin in mutants of *Bacillus megaterium*. Eur J Biochem 140:453–459

Spotts CR (1962) Physiological and biochemical studies on streptomycin dependence in *Escherichia coli*. J Gen Microbiol 28:347–365

Spotts CR, Stanier RY (1961) Mechanism of streptomycin action on bacteria, a unitary hypothesis. Nature 192:633–637

Stark MJR, Cundliffe E (1979a) Requirement for ribosomal protein BM-L11 in stringent control of RNA synthesis in *Bacillus megaterium*. Eur J Biochem 102:101–105

Stark MJR, Cundliffe E (1979b) On the biological role of ribosomal protein BM-L11 of *Bacillus megaterium*, homologous with *Escherichia coli* ribosomal protein L11. J Mol Biol 134:767–779

Steen R, Jemiolo DK, Skinner RH, Dunn JJ, Dahlberg AE (1986) Expression of plasmid-coded mutant ribosomal RNA in *E. coli*: choice of plasmid vectors and gene expression systems. Proc Nucleic Acids Res Mol Biol 33:1–18

Stiege W, Glotz C, Brimacombe R (1983) Localization of a series of intra-RNA cross-links in the secondary structure of 23S RNA induced by ultraviolet irradiation of *Escherichia coli* 50S ribosomal subunits. Nucleic Acids Res 11:1687–1706

Stöcklein W, Piepersberg W (1980a) Altered ribosomal protein L29 in a cycloheximide-resistant strain of *Saccharomyces cerevisiae*. Curr Genet 1:177–183

Stöcklein W, Piepersberg W (1980b) Binding of cycloheximide to ribosomes from wild-type and mutant strains of *Saccharomyces cerevisiae*. Antimicrob Agents Chemother 18:863–867

Stöcklein W, Piepersberg W, Böck A (1981) Amino acid replacements in ribosomal protein YL24 of *Saccharomyces cerevisiae* causing resistance to cycloheximide. FEBS Lett 136:265–268

Tanaka N, Yamaguchi H, Umezawa H (1966) Mechanism of kasugamycin action on polypeptide synthesis. J Biochem 60:429–434

Tanaka K, Tamaki M, Itoh T, Otaka E, Osawa S (1971) Ribosomes from spiramycin resistant mutants of *Escherichia coli* Q13. Mol Gen Genet 114:23–30

Thompson J, Cundliffe E, Stark M (1979) Binding of thiostrepton to a complex of 23S rRNA with ribosomal protein L11. Eur J Biochem 98:261–265

Thompson J, Schmidt F, Cundliffe E (1982) Site of action of a ribosomal RNA methylase conferring resistance to thiostrepton. J Biol Chem 257:7915–7917

Thorbjarnardóttir SH, Magnusdóttir RA, Eggertsson G (1978) Mutations determining generalized resistance to aminoglycoside antibiotics in *Escherichia coli*. Mol Gen Genet 161:89–98

Torczynski R, Bollon AP, Fuke M (1983) The complete nucleotide sequence of the rat 18S ribosomal RNA gene and comparison with the respective yeast and frog genes. Nucleic Acids Res 11:4879–4890

Traub P, Nomura M (1968) Streptomycin resistance mutation in *Escherichia coli*: altered ribosomal protein. Science 160:198–199

Tseng JL, Bryan LE, van den Elzen HM (1972) Mechanisms and spectrum of streptomycin resistance in a natural population of *Pseudomonas aeruginosa*. Antimicrob Agents Chemother 2:136–141

Umezawa S (1975) The chemistry and conformation of aminoglycoside antibiotics. In: Mitsuhashi S (ed) Drug action and drug resistance in bacteria. Vol 2: Aminoglycoside antibiotics. University of Tokyo Press, Tokyo

Van Buul CPJJ, Vissert W, van Knippenberg PH (1984) Increased translational fidelity caused by the antibiotic kasugamycin and ribosomal ambiguity in mutants harbouring the *ksgA* gene. FEBS Lett 177:119–124

Vázquez D (1979) Inhibitors of protein biosynthesis. Springer, Berlin Heidelberg New York (molecular biology, biochemistry, and biophysics, vol 30)

Weisblum B (1985) Inducible resistance to macrolides, lincosamides, and streptogramin type B antibiotics: the resistance phenotype, its biological diversity, and structural elements that regulate expression – a review. J Antimicrob Chemother [Suppl A] 16:63–90

Wejksnora PJ, Warner JR (1982) Mutation-induced instability of antibiotic-resistant mammalian ribosomes. Eur J Biochem 128:239–242

Wienen B, Ehrlich R, Stöffler-Meilicke M, Stöffler G, Smit I, Weiss D, Vince R, Pestka S (1979) Ribosomal protein alterations in thiostrepton- and micrococcin-resistant mutants of *Bacillus subtilis*. J Biol Chem 254:8031–8041

Wittmann HG, Stöffler G, Apirion D, Rosen L, Tanaka K, Tamaki M, Takata R, Dekio S, Otaka E, Osawa S (1973) Biochemical and genetic studies on two different types of erythromycin resistant mutants of *Escherichia coli* with altered ribosomal proteins. Mol Gen Genet 127:175–189

Wittmann HG, Stöffler G, Piepersberg W, Buckel P, Ruffler D, Böck A (1974) Altered S5 and S20 ribosomal proteins in revertants of an alanyl-tRNA synthetase mutant of *Escherichia coli*. Mol Gen Genet 134:225–236

Wool IG (1984) The mechanism of action of the cytotoxic nuclease α-sarcin and its use to analyse ribosome structure. Trends Biochem Sci 9:14–17

Yaguchi M, Wittmann HG, Cabezón T, de Wilde M, Villarroel R, Herzog A, Bollen A (1975) Cooperative control of translational fidelity by ribosomal proteins in *Escherichia coli*. II. Localization of amino acid replacements in proteins S5 and S12 altered in double mutants resistant to neamine. Mol Gen Genet 142:35–43

Yaguchi M, Wittmann HG, Cabezón T, de Wilde M, Villarroel R, Herzog A, Bollen A (1976) Alteration of ribosomal protein S17 by mutation linked to neamine resistance in *Escherichia coli*. II. Localization of the amino acid replacement in protein S17 from a *neaA* mutant. J Mol Biol 104:617–620

Yang D, Kaine BP, Woese CR (1985) The phylogeny of archaebacteria. Syst Appl Microbiol 6:251–256

Zengel JM, Young R, Dennis PP, Nomura M (1977) Role of ribosomal protein S12 in peptide chain elongation: analysis of pleiotropic, streptomycin-resistant mutants of *Escherichia coli*. J Bacteriol 129:1320–1329

Zierhut G, Piepersberg W, Böck A (1979) Comparative analysis of the effect of aminoglycosides on bacterial protein synthesis in vitro. Eur J Biochem 98:577–583

Zimmermann RA, Rosset R, Gorini L (1971 a) Nature of phenotypic masking exhibited by drug-dependent streptomycin mutants of *Escherichia coli*. J Mol Biol 57:403–422

Zimmermann RA, Moellering RC, Weniberg AN (1971 b) Mechanism of resistance to antibiotic synergism in enterococci. J Bacteriol 105:873–879

CHAPTER 10

Methylation of RNA and Resistance to Antibiotics

E. CUNDLIFFE

A. Introduction

Microorganisms have evolved or acquired various modes of resistance to antibiotics, as discussed in depth in this volume. In some cases, active drug molecules may be physically prevented from encountering the target site(s) at which they normally act, either by direct exclusion at membrane barriers or by chemical inactivation due to extracellular enzymes (e.g. β-lactamases). In other instances, where total exclusion of the drug from the cytoplasm cannot be achieved, resistance may depend upon the operation of antibiotic efflux mechanisms (e.g. for tetracycline) or upon drug inactivation by intracellular enzymes and cofactors (e.g. for aminoglycosides). Thus, in some organisms, a critical balance may be struck between drug accumulation on the one hand and its removal or inactivation on the other, so that inhibitory drug concentrations are not established intracellularly.

The present article deals with a radical alternative to the above strategies, according to which the normal target(s) for inhibitory action are modified and thereby rendered unavailable to specific antibiotics.

B. Resistance Due to Target Site Modification

In various micro-organisms, mutational alteration of specific cellular components has been shown to result in resistance to antibiotics and, in some instances, such observations were instrumental in identifying the targets for specific drugs. To cite just a few examples, resistance to nalidixic acid and novobiocin results from alteration of the A and B subunits (respectively) of DNA gyrase, the action of rifamycin is attenuated in mutants possessing an altered β-subunit of RNA polymerase and the ribosomes of streptomycin-resistant bacteria are specifically altered in protein S12. Yet again, transpeptidase-carboxypeptidase enzymes of the cell surface (the so-called "penicillin binding proteins" or PBPs) can be altered by mutation so as to confer collateral resistance to specific β-lactams. As can readily be appreciated since mutations occur randomly, a collection of mutants resistant to any given drug is likely to display a range of phenotypes (perhaps ranging from highly resistant to only marginally so) depending upon the nature and location of the lesions. In contrast, antibiotic resistance in other organisms may be caused by deliberate modification of the target structures at which drugs normally act. Several resistance mechanisms of this genre have been detected in antibiotic-producing actinomycetes, which may turn out to be a rich source of additional examples (for review, see CUNDLIFFE 1984) although, as will be seen, target site modification is by no means restricted to producers. As yet, the systems that have been most extensively characterised all involve ribosomal modification at defined sites leading to high level resistance to specific drugs that normally inhibit protein synthesis. Such resistance mechanisms are the subject of this article.

I. Resistance to Aminoglycosides

Members of the kanamycin, gentamicin and neomycin families of antibiotics are, variously, substrates for a coherent group of drug-modifying enzymes most of which inactivate their substrates. The overlapping substrate profiles of those enzymes can therefore be used to define the "aminoglycoside" group of antibiotics in a purely functional sense. Thus, for the present purposes, "aminoglycosides" comprise the three families of antibiotics listed above together with other compounds (in the present context, apramycin and istamycin) upon which the "aminoglycoside-modifying enzymes" also act. This classification specifically excludes certain other compounds (such as streptomycin, hygromycin B, spectinomycin and kasugamycin) to which the term "aminoglycoside" has been applied in the past but which are quite different in structure and activity from those considered here, despite the fact that these are all inhibitors of protein synthesis and some of them, like aminoglycosides, cause misreading of mRNA codons (for review, see GALE et al. 1981).

Various actinomycetes that produce aminoglycosides have long been known also to produce enzymes capable of modifying and (usually) inactivating such drugs (BENVENISTE and DAVIES 1973; HOTTA et al. 1981; for review, see CUNDLIFFE 1984). Moreover, unequivocal evidence that some of those enzymes can confer resistance to their substrates (at varying levels) has been obtained by cloning the respective genes in a normally sensitive host, e.g. *Streptomyces lividans* (C.J. THOMPSON et al. 1982; CRAMERI and DAVIES 1986). This, together with the observation that some aminoglycoside-producers possess ribosomes that are apparently sensitive to the autogenous antibiotics (SUGIYAMA et al. 1980; HOTTA et al. 1981), leads one to suppose that drug-modifying enzymes may well be involved in the survival of some of those organisms. Nevertheless, the presence of multiple drug-modification enzymes in some strains has complicated the analysis of their likely physiological roles (C.J. THOMPSON et al. 1982). In contrast, certain other aminoglycoside-producing organisms have recently been shown to possess resistant ribosomes, regardless of whether they also possess drug-modifying enzymes. Such strains include *Streptomyces tenjimariensis* (YAMAMOTO et al. 1981), *Micromonospora purpurea* (PIENDL and BÖCK 1982), *Streptomyces tenebrarius* (YAMAMOTO et al. 1982) and *Streptomyces kanamyceticus* (MURAKAMI et al. 1983; NAKANO et al. 1984). Respectively these organisms produce istamycin, gentamicin, the nebramycin complex (i.e. various derivatives of kanamycin B, including tobramycin, plus the novel compound apramycin) and kanamycin. The latter two organisms in the above list also possess aminoglycoside-modification enzymes and, in the case of *S. kanamyceticus*, ribosomal resistance to kanamycin is evidently inducible (NAKANO et al. 1984).

Organisms that produce aminoglycosides typically possess complex resistance phenotypes and, in the four strains featured here, that complexity is mirrored by the resistance characteristics of their ribosomes (see below). The principal exception here concerns *S. tenebrarius*, whose ribosomes do not seem to be sufficiently resistant to neomycin to account for the phenotype (more of this later).

In order to elucidate the mechanism(s) responsible for ribosomal resistance to any given drug, it is first necessary to identify the altered constituent(s) of the particle. Such analysis can be definitive only if the state of defined ribosomal components (ideally, a single component in any given case) can be shown to determine the response of the entire particle to the drug. Ultimately, this must involve reconstitution analysis in which hybrid ribosomal particles are constructed in vitro containing mixtures of RNA and proteins derived from sensitive and resistant ribosomes. As a first step, however, it is usually convenient to carry out conceptually similar "crossover" experiments using 50S and 30S ribonucleoprotein subunits derived from sensitive and resistant ribosomes. In this way, it was ascertained that the smaller (30S) subparticle was the source of ribosomal resistance to aminoglycosides in *M. purpurea* (PIENDL and BÖCK 1982), *S. tenjimariensis* and *S. tenebrarius* (PIENDL et al. 1984) and various other species of *Micromonospora* (MATKOVIĆ et al. 1984). Thereafter, reconstitution analysis revealed that the state of 16S rRNA in the 30S particles was the critical parameter in each of those three strains (PIENDL et al. 1984). As yet, ribosomes from *S. kanamyceticus* have not been subjected to reconstitution analysis but there are good reasons to believe that, again, ribosomal resistance in that strain is determined by 16S RNA (see below). Certainly, resistant clones containing DNA from *S. kanamyceticus* possess altered 30S ribosomal subunits (NAKANO and OGAWARA 1987; see below).

Given the complexity of the resistance profiles of the ribosomes from these various strains, further analysis of the mechanisms involved was not attempted directly. Rather, resistance determinants from all four strains have been cloned and the effects of their products have been studied in a "clean" background (i.e. in *Streptomyces lividans*).

1. Resistance in Clones Containing DNA from *M. purpurea*

Shotgun cloning of *M. purpurea* DNA in *S. lividans* yielded several gentamicin resistant strains, one of which (*S. lividans* JR14) was subjected to detailed analysis (J. THOMPSON et al. 1985). The minimal inhibitory concentrations (MIC values) of various aminoglycosides for this clone are given in Table 1 together with those for the parental *S. lividans* strain and for *M. purpurea*. As can be seen, the phenotype of strain JR14 closely resembled that of *M. purpurea* and it soon became apparent that ribosomes from the two strains were also closely similar in their responses to antibiotics in vitro. Furthermore, as might have been expected from previous studies involving *M. purpurea* (PIENDL et al. 1984), reconstitution analysis revealed that resistance in strain JR14 was due to the state of 16S RNA contained within the 30S ribosomal subunit. Additionally, extracts from strain JR14 were shown to contain methylase activity not present in the parental *S. lividans* strain and a causal connection was established linking the action of that methylase to resistance (J. THOMPSON et al. 1985). Thus, when 30S ribosomal subunits

Table 1. MIC values (μg per ml) of various aminoglycoside antibiotics for *S. lividans* strains and for *M. purpurea* together with the ribosomal resistance levels in vitro

Antibiotic	MIC values (ribosomal resistance levels)		
	S. lividans parental strain	*S. lividans* JR 14 clone	*M. purpurea*
Kanamycin	10–30 (–)	>1000 (+++)	>1000 (+++)
Gentamicin	3–10 (–)	>1000 (+++)	>1000 (+++)
Apramycin	<1 (–)	<1 *	<1 *
Neomycin	1–3 (–)	3–10 *	1 (–)

MIC values were determined on nutrient plates containing antibiotics. Ribosomal resistance levels were determined in cell-free protein synthesising systems directed by poly U
(+++), ribosomes highly resistant to antibiotic; (–), ribosomes fully sensitive to antibiotic (*S. lividans* wild type taken as standard); (*), strain highly sensitive to drug and implies ribosomes are also sensitive
Data taken from Piendl and Böck (1982) and J. Thompson et al. (1985)

from *E. coli* were incubated with extracts from clone JR14, with and without S-adenosyl-methionine (cofactor for methylation), before being introduced into a protein-synthesising system, acquisition of the kanamycin-gentamicin resistance character typical of ribosomes from strain JR14 (or *M. purpurea*) was shown to be absolutely dependent upon inclusion of the methylation cofactor in the pre-incubation mixture. Subsequently, 16S RNA within the 30S ribosomal particles was shown to be the substrate for methylation, which occurred with a stoichiometry close to unity (J. Thompson et al. 1985). Proof that only a single methylation event was involved in ribosomal resistance to kanamycin plus gentamicin was furnished when a fragment of DNA (originally from *M. purpurea*) of about 1.1 kb was subcloned and expressed in *E. coli* (D. J. Holmes and E. Cundliffe, manuscript in preparation). Extracts from the resultant strain incorporated a single methyl group into 16S rRNA from the parental *E. coli* strain, thereby generating a residue of 7-methylguanosine at position 1405 within the RNA sequence (Beauclerk and Cundliffe 1987).

The kanamycin-gentamicin resistance methylase gene (for which the designation *kgm* is proposed) has recently been sequenced (D. J. Holmes and E. Cundliffe, manuscript in preparation). This gene is of interest since it is probably the first one from the genus *Micromonospora* to have been cloned and analysed in such detail. As with *Streptomyces* genes, there is a strong (~95%) preference for G or C in the third codon position although, as yet, no data concerning the promoter(s) are available. The predicted length of the methylase protein is 281 amino acid residues which would give a subunit molecular weight for the methylase of about 31 200 daltons. Precisely such a clone-specific protein band has been observed (D. J. HOLMES, unpublished data), following SDS-PAGE analysis when plasmid containing the *kgm* gene was introduced into the *Streptomyces* coupled transcription-translation system (J. THOMPSON et al. 1984).

2. Resistance in Clones Containing DNA from *S. tenjimariensis*

When DNA fragments from *S. tenjimariensis* were introduced into *S. lividans* and kanamycin-resistant transformants were selected, the progeny were found also to be highly resistant to apramycin, moderately so to sisomicin but only marginally so to gentamicin (Table 2). In that initial study (SKEGGS et al. 1985), low level resistance to neomycin was also evident but, when the phenotype of one of the clones (*S. lividans* TSK 412) was further characterised (SKEGGS et al. 1987), it was interesting to observe that the strain was highly resistant to neamine and ribostamycin which comprise, respectively, two and three rings of the four-ring neomycin molecule (Table 2). Thus, the complex resistance-phenotype of the clone mirrored that of *S. tenjimariensis* and, since strain TSK 412 contained only about 0.9 kb of *S. tenjimariensis* DNA, it seemed likely that only a single resistance determinant was involved. This was confirmed when ribosomes from the clone were subjected to detailed examination, culminating in reconstitution analysis, in vitro. In short, ribosomes from strain TSK 412 were essentially indistinguishable from those of *S. tenjimariensis* (Table 2) and they reflected, in a qualitative sense, the phenotype of the strain. Again, resistance in strain TSK 412 was due to some property of the ribosomal 16S RNA and extracts from the clone possessed meth-

Table 2. MIC values (μg per ml) of various aminoglycosides for *S. lividans* strains and for *S. tenjimariensis* together with ribosomal resistance levels in vitro

Antibiotic	MIC values (ribosomal resistance levels)		
	S. lividans parental strain	*S. lividans* TSK 412 clone	*S. tenjimariensis*
Kanamycin	10–30 (–)	>1000 (+ + +)	>1000 (+ + +)
Gentamicin	3–10 (–)	10–30 (+)	5–10 (+)
Apramycin	<1 (–)	300–1000 (+ + +)	300–1000 (+ + +)
Neamine	10–30 (–)	>1000	
Ribostamycin	3–10 (–)	>1000 (+ + +)[a]	
Neomycin	1–3 (–)	30–100 (+)[a]	10–30 (+)

For details see caption to Table 1
Ribosomal resistances are represented as: (+ + +), high level resistance; (+), low level resistance; (–), full sensitivity
Data taken from SKEGGS et al. (1985; 1987)
[a] P. A. SKEGGS (unpublished data)

ylase activity that was absent from the parental *S. lividans* strain. Thus, in the presence of *S*-adenosyl-[^{3}H-methyl] methionine as cofactor, extracts from strain TSK 412 supported the incorporation of radiolabelled methyl groups into the 16S RNA moiety of 30S ribosomal subunits from the parental *S. lividans* and a causal connection was established between such methylation and acquisition of the complex resistance character typical of *S. tenjimariensis* ribosomes (SKEGGS et al. 1985). Subsequently, using *E. coli* ribosomal particles as substrates for methylation, resistance was shown to result from the generation of a single residue of 1-methyladenosine at position 1408 within 16S rRNA (BEAUCLERK and CUNDLIFFE 1987). As yet, the *k*anamycin-*a*pramycin resistance *m*ethylase gene (provisionally *kam*) has not been sequenced, although a restriction map is available (more of this later).

Throughout the above work carried out in the author's laboratory, istamycin (the natural product of *S. tenjimariensis*) was not available for inclusion in the analyses. Thus, it is not known whether clones such as *S. lividans* TSK 412 are resistant to istamycin and, therefore, whether the *kam* gene is the sole determinant of resistance in *S. tenjimariensis*. (Indeed, had istamycin been available and had strain TSK 412 been resistant to it, the proposed designation of the resistance gene might have been different.) However, *S. tenjimariensis* does not appear to possess aminoglycoside-modifying activity (YAMAMOTO et al. 1981) and there is, at present, no reason to suppose that this organism possesses more than one resistance determinant.

3. Resistance in Clones Containing DNA from *S. tenebrarius*

The resistance phenotype of *S. tenebrarius* is extremely broad so far as aminoglycoside antibiotics are concerned and, in vitro, ribosomes from the strain are likewise resistant to a broad spectrum of aminoglycosides, including both gentamicin and apramycin (Table 3). Accordingly, when DNA fragments from *S. tenebrarius* were introduced into *S. lividans* and transformants resistant to either of these antibiotics were selected (SKEGGS et al. 1987), two groups of clones were obtained. One class (typified by *S. lividans* TSK 31) was selected on gentamicin and proved to be indistinguishable in phenotype from *S. lividans* clones (e.g. JR 14) that contained DNA from *M. purpurea* (of Tables 1, 3). The others (typified by strain TSK 51 and selected on apramycin) closely resembled the clones that contained DNA from *S. tenjimariensis* (e.g. strain TSK 412; cf. Tables 2, 3). These similarities were confirmed and extended when ribosomes from strains TSK 31 and TSK 51 were examined in vitro (Table 3) and when the DNA fragments cloned in strains TSK 51 and TSK 412 on the one hand and strains TSK 31 and JR 14 on the other hand were compared by restriction and cross-hybridisation analysis. Thus, it became evident that *S. tenebrarius* contains two rRNA methylase genes, homologous with the *kgm* and *kam* genes from *M. purpurea* and *S. tenjimariensis* respectively (SKEGGS et al. 1987) and that in *S. lividans* clones TSK 31 and TSK 51 resistance is due to methylation of 16S rRNA at residues G-1405 and A-1408 respectively (A. A. D. BEAUCLERK, personal communication). Presumably, therefore, 16S rRNA in *S. tenebrarius* is doubly modified to give aminoglycoside resistance.

Table 3. MIC values of aminoglycosides for *S. lividans* strains and for *S. tenebrarius* together with ribosomal resistance levels

Antibiotic	MIC values (ribosomal resistance levels)			
	S. lividans parental strain	*S. lividans* TSK 31 clone	*S. lividans* TSK 51 clone	*S. tenebrarius*
Kanamycin	10–30 (–)	>1000 (+++)	>1000 (+++)	>1000 (+++)
Tobramycin	3–10 (–)	300–1000 (++)	100–300 (++)	>1000
Gentamicin	3–10 (–)	>1000 (+++)	10–30 (+)	>1000 (+++)
Apramycin	<1 (–)	1–3 (–)	300–1000 (+++)	>1000 (+++)
Neamine	10–30 (–)	10–30 (–)[a]	>1000 (+++)[a]	>1000 (+++)[a]
Ribostamycin	3–10 (–)	3–10 (–)	>1000 (+++)	>1000 (+++)
Neomycin	1– 3 (–)	3–10 (–)	30–100 (+)	>1000 (+)

For details, see Table 1
Ribosomal resistance levels are expressed as: (+++), high level; (++), moderate to high level; (+), low level; (–), full sensitivity
Data taken from Skeggs et al. (1987)
[a] P. A. Skeggs (unpublished data)

Double methylation of 16S RNA, as above, adequately accounts for all the known resistance characteristics of *S. tenebrarius* ribosomes but not for the phenotype – particularly with respect to neomycin (see Table 3). Therefore, it may be significant that aminoglycoside-modifying activity has also been detected in extracts of *S. tenebrarius* (Davies 1980; Yamamoto et al. 1982) and this could well contribute to the phenotype, as could the (as yet, undetermined) permeability properties of the mycelial surface.

4. Resistance in Clones Containing DNA from *S. kanamyceticus*

Until DNA from *S. kanamyceticus* was first cloned in *S. lividans* (Murakami et al. 1983; Nakano et al. 1984) it was believed that resistance in the donor strain was due to the presence of aminoglycoside-modifying activity, the ribosomes having been reported to be sensitive to kanamycin (Hotta et al. 1981). However, as it turned out, certain clones of *S. lividans* were constitutively resistant to kanamycin and contained resistant ribosomes (Nakano et al. 1984; Matsuhashi et al. 1985). The paradox was resolved when *S. kanamyceticus* was grown in kanamycin-production medium, under which conditions it was also shown to contain resistant ribosomes (Nakano et al. 1984). Evidently, in the *S. lividans* clones, the ribosomal-resistance gene from *S. kanamyceticus* had been separated from its native control element and was no longer inducible.

In common with the ribosomal resistance mechanisms in other aminoglycoside producers, that in *S. kanamyceticus* (or rather, in clones of *S. lividans* harbouring *S. kanamyceticus* DNA, e.g. strain CMA5) operates via the 30S subparticle (NAKANO and OGAWARA 1987). Indeed, although ribosomes from such clones (or from *S. kanamyceticus*) have not yet been subjected to reconstitution analysis, it is tempting to suggest that the resistance mechanism is similar to that specified by the *kgm* gene from *M. purpurea*. Thus, the phenotypes of *S. lividans* strains CMA5 and JR14 (which contains the *kgm* gene – Table 1) are closely similar and their ribosomes share similar resistance profiles (NAKANO et al. 1984; J. THOMPSON et al. 1985). Moreover, detailed examination of 16S rRNA from a strain of *S. lividans* equivalent to CMA5 (transformed with plasmid pMCP5 kindly provided by M. Nakano) revealed that residue G-1405 was modified (and was probably 7 methyl G) as in strains containing *kgm* (A. A. D. BEAUCLERK and E. CUNDLIFFE, manuscript in preparation). Interestingly, however, attempts to demonstrate cross-hybridisation between the respective resistance genes cloned in strains CMA5 and JR 14 have repeatedly failed (P. A. SKEGGS, personal communication). Accordingly, the extent to which the ribosomal-resistance gene from *S. kanamyceticus* (designated *kan* by NAKANO and OGAWARA 1987) and the *kgm* gene from *M. purpurea* might resemble each other remains obscure.

As a result of S1 mapping experiments, it has been established that *kan* expression is regulated at the level of transcription in *S. kanamyceticus* (NAKANO and OGAWARA 1987) although the inducer has not been identified. One obvious candidate can possibly be eliminated: growth of *S. kanamyceticus* in medium containing kanamycin does not induce expression of *kan* (M. J. CALCUTT, personal communication).

II. Resistance to Thiostrepton

Thiostrepton is a modified peptide antibiotic of unusual molecular size (Mr about 1660) that is active against gram-positive bacteria. However, in vitro, thiostrepton binds to bacterial ribosomes from whatever source and inhibits protein synthesis. In various assay systems, several ribosome-dependent processes have been shown to be affected by the drug (for details, see CUNDLIFFE 1979) although, as will be discussed below, the inhibitory effects of thiostrepton are believed to result from binding of the drug to a single ribosomal site. This seemingly complex state of affairs was rationalised by the observation that all thiostrepton-sensitive reactions appear to involve the binding of soluble protein factors to the ribosome and the consequent hydrolysis of GTP (e.g. with initiation factor IF2 or the elongation factors EF Tu and EF G) or the manipulation of guanine nucleotides, as in the presence of stringency factor, which mediates the stringent control of metabolism via the production of (p)ppGpp. Evidently, related ribosomal sites are involved in these various processes since there is persuasive evidence that the protein factors cited above compete with each other for mutually exclusive ribosomal binding sites. Thus, although the details are not yet clear, it seems that thiostrepton blockades a ribosomal domain that is utilised in common by several protein factors and which constitutes one of the active sites of the ribosomal enzyme. That domain clearly contains at least part of the aminoacyl-tRNA binding site known as the A site and is involved in some (probably all) of the ribosome-associated GTPase events that occur during protein synthesis (for a review of the mode of action of thiostrepton, see GALE et al. 1981). Thus, thiostrepton has come to be known as an inhibitor of the GTPase centre of the bacterial ribosome.

In exerting its inhibitory effects, thiostrepton binds with quite extraordinary affinity (K_A greater than 10^9 M^{-1}) to a single site on the larger (50S) subunit of the bacterial ribosome. (For comparison, the ribosome-binding constants for most other inhibitors of protein synthesis yet studied fall within the range of 10^5 to 10^6 M^{-1}: chloramphenicol would be one such example; for further details, see CUNDLIFFE 1980). This general statement holds true for ribosomes from a wide range of bacterial types, including gram-positives plus gram-negatives, and certainly includes a large number of actinomycetes. Exceptionally, however, organisms that produce thiostrepton or one of its close relatives possess ribosomes that are highly refractory (probably totally so) to those compounds. The best studied example relates to *Streptomyces azureus* (producer of thiostrepton), an organism which is indifferent to thiostrepton and whose ribosomes function perfectly well in saturated aqueous solutions of the drug (E. CUNDLIFFE, unpublished data). Such ribosomes do not bind thiostrepton even as assayed by equilibrium dialysis (M.J.R. STARK and E. CUNDLIFFE, unpublished data) and a detailed examination of their components first suggested the likely nature of thiostrepton resistance in that strain. The crucial experiments involved "cross-over reconstitution" analysis according to which 50S ribosomal subunits from *S. azureus* and from a control strain (sensitive to thiostrepton) were dissociated to yield proteins plus 23S RNA. These were then re-associated in vitro in the various possible combinations to yield hybrid ribosomal particles which were tested for their response to thiostrepton. The results were unequivocal: particles containing ribosomal proteins from *S. azureus* bound thiostrepton normally whereas those containing 23S rRNA from that strain did not (CUNDLIFFE 1978). Also at that time, extracts from *S. azureus* were found to contain a methylase enzyme that acted upon free 23S rRNA from other strains and was evidently the source of thiostrepton resistance in *S. azureus*. The enzyme was purified 11000-fold (THOMPSON and CUNDLIFFE 1981), and its action was shown to result in the appearance of a single residue of 2′-O-methyladenosine within the substrate (CUNDLIFFE and THOMPSON 1979) and ribosomal particles containing such specifically methylated RNA were shown to be resistant to thiostrepton.

The site of action of the "thiostrepton-resistance" methylase within 23S rRNA was determined in studies utilising ribosomal protein L11, which had previously been shown to promote the high affinity binding of thiostrepton to protein-deficient ribosomal "core" particles (HIGHLAND et al. 1975). (By hindsight, it is now apparent that core particles can bind thiostrepton with respectable affinity in the absence of protein L11, but such binding is not readily detected for purely technical reasons.) Protein L11 binds directly to 23S rRNA in vitro under which conditions it protects a specific oligonucleotide (about 60 residues long) from nuclease digestion (SCHMIDT et al. 1981). When the RNA fragment protected by protein L11 was generated from *E. coli* 23S rRNA, previously methylated in vitro using [^{3}H-methyl] *S*-adenosyl-methionine as cofactor for the enzyme from *S. azureus*, it was found to contain a radiolabelled methyl group. By conventional fingerprint analysis, this was subsequently located (on pentose) within residue A-1067 (J. THOMPSON et al. 1982).

As assayed by equilibrium dialysis, thiostrepton binds directly to *E. coli* 23S rRNA in free solution (K_A about 2×10^6 M^{-1}; M. J. R. STARK and E. CUNDLIFFE, unpublished data) but not, apparently, to protein L11. Binding of the drug to 23S rRNA is strongly promoted by protein L11 and thiostrepton still binds tightly to the [23S RNA-L11] complex even after nuclease digestion of the latter (J. THOMPSON et al. 1979). Evidently, therefore, the thiostrepton-binding site lies within the L11-protected oligonucleotide and, significantly, 23S rRNA from *S. azureus* does not bind the drug (M. J. R. STARK and E. CUNDLIFFE, unpublished data). Thus, there must be an intimate relationship between the binding site for thiostrepton and residue 1067 within 23S rRNA. Although they are unlikely to be one and the same (since the drug must recognise enough binding elements to generate a unique site within the 23S rRNA polymer of about 2900 nucleotides), it is quite feasible that residue 1067 might lie within the drug-binding site and that methylation might block thiostrepton binding directly at the target. Alternatively, methylation of A-1067 might block access of thiostrepton to an adjacent "pocket" in the tertiary-folded RNA molecule. In any event, protein L11 probably promotes thiostrepton binding by stabilising a particular folded conformation of 23S rRNA. Further analysis of the thiostrepton-binding site is currently being carried out using site-directed mutagenesis of the 23S rRNA gene. Interestingly, in *E. coli*, an A→G substitution at position 1067 within 23S rRNA has only a marginal effect on thiostrepton binding to ribosomes whereas A→U or A→C reduces the binding to undetectable levels (J. THOMPSON et al. 1988). While the full implications of these findings are unclear, there is one interesting comment to be made concerning phylogeny, given that rRNA genes from a wide range of organisms have now been sequenced (NOLLER 1984). Thus far, thiostrepton-sensitive ribosomes (in prokaryotes and archaebacteria) appear always to possess an A residue at position 1067 within 23S rRNA (BEAUCLERK et al. 1985), whereas in those that are insensitive to the drug (as in eukaryotes) the equivalent position in 23S-like rRNA is occupied by G. This reinforces the obvious point, made above, that thiostrepton recognises more than one residue within its target site and indicates that the insensitivity of eukaryotic ribosomes to the drug cannot be ascribed entirely to the nature of the nucleoside at any single site within rRNA.

Thiostrepton is an extremely powerful inhibitor of the growth of gram-positive bacteria – particularly actinomycetes. Thus, the thiostrepton-resistance gene (*tsr*) from *S. azureus* has found considerable application in the development of vector plasmids to facilitate interspecific gene cloning among *Streptomyces* (and other actinomycetes). The *tsr* gene was first cloned at the John Innes Institute, Norwich (C. J. THOMPSON et al. 1980, 1982) and has since become the selectable marker on most of the cloning vectors developed there (the pIJ series of vectors) and elsewhere. The *tsr* gene has also been sequenced (BIBB et al. 1985) and clearly resembles other *Streptomyces* genes in two characteristic respects. The nucleotide sequence of the coding region is heavily biased towards the use of G or C in the third codon position, in keeping with the very high G+C content (about 73%) of *Streptomyces* DNA, and is preceded by a tandem pair of promoters (for review, see HOPWOOD et al. 1986).

In conclusion, thiostrepton is the only ribosomally directed antibiotic for which the target macromolecule is known and the thiostrepton-resistance mechanism was the first such process involving ribosomal modification to be fully characterised. As will be alluded to later, the data obtained in this context have important implications for the understanding of antibiotic action and ribosomal function.

III. Resistance to Macrolides, Lincosamides, and Antibiotics Related to Streptogramin B

In the mid 1950s, *Staphylococcus aureus* was first reported to display inducible resistance to macrolide antibiotics, most notably erythromycin (CHABBERT 1956; JONES et al. 1956; GARROD 1957). Thereafter, it soon became clear that resistance in such strains was also directed against lincosamides and antibiotics related to streptogramin B in addition to the macrolides. Hence, the collective term "MLS antibiotics" was eventually coined to embrace the three groups of compounds against which collateral resistance was expressed (WEISBLUM 1975).

In the early literature, certain strains of *Staph. aureus* were reported to display "dissociated" resistance to macrolides such as erythromycin and spiramycin. Thus, in conventional Kirby-Bauer disc assays, spiramycin would produce large clear zones of inhibition whereas erythromycin gave much smaller zones. By hindsight, we now realise that resistance in such strains was being induced by erythromycin but not by spiramycin and this serves also to explain the so-called "antagonism" between such compounds (i.e. the ability of erythromycin to induce resistance to spiramycin). Indeed, MLS resistance in *Staphylococcus* is induced only by erythromycin and the closely related compound oleandomycin (WEAVER and PATTEE 1964) among the macrolides (of which there are many) and by the lincosamide, celesticetin (ALLEN 1977). Other macrolides, such as spiramycin, tylosin, or carbomycin, do not normally induce nor does lincomycin or streptogramin B, although the range of MLS inducers is expanded in certain mutants of *Staph. aureus* (more of this later). It is also possible to select constitutively resistant strains by plating *Staph. aureus* onto growth medium containing MLS antibiotics that do not normally induce. Various such mutants have featured prominently in tests of the "attenuation" model that has been proposed to explain the mechanism of induction (see later). Crucial in this respect is the concept that all known inducers of MLS resistance are also inhibitors of protein synthesis. This point was established most clearly with 57 congeners of erythromycin (PESTKA et al. 1976).

The MLS resistance phenotype is not restricted to *Staph. aureus* nor is it universally inducible. Such resistance is fairly widespread among bacteria (both gram positives and gram negatives) and is particularly evident among *Streptomyces*, including strains that produce MLS antibiotics. In several organisms, MLS resistance (*erm*) genes are located on plasmids, most prominently the *ermC* gene which is contained within pE194, a plasmid first isolated from *Staph. aureus*. That plasmid has since been introduced into *Bacillus subtilis* and studies of *ermC* in that background have dominated the field. In other organisms, *erm* genes may be chromosomal or located on transposons. To date, several MLS resistance deter-

Table 4. Comparison of MLS resistance determinants and their predicted products

Gene	Origin	Expression	Predicted size of product (Da)	% G+C of *erm*	Reference
ermA	*Staph. aureus* Tn 554	Inducible	28,380	32.5	MURPHY (1985)
ermC	Staph. aureus pE 194	Inducible	29,000	25	GRYCZAN et al. (1980); HORINOUCHI and WEISBLUM (1980)
ermAM	*Streptococcus sanguis* pAM77	Inducible	29,400	32	HORINOUCHI et al. (1983)
ermD	*Bacillus licheniformis* chromosome	Inducible	32,800	39	GRYCZAN et al. (1984)
ermE	*Streptomyces erthraeus* (chromosome?)	Constitutive	41,600	72	UCHIYAMA and WEISBLUM (1985)
ermA'	*Arthrobacter* sp.	?	37,450	76	ROBERTS et al. (1985)
ermF	*Bacteroides fragilis* pBF4	Constitutive	30,360	34	RASMUSSEN et al. (1986)

minants have been sequenced and extensive homologies have been revealed in the predicted amino acid sequences of their products (Table 4).

1. Mechanism of MLS Resistance

The MLS antibiotics are all inhibitors of bacterial protein synthesis and act by binding to the larger (50S) subunit of the ribosome (for a review, see GALE et al. 1981). Normally, ribosomes from *Staphylococcus* are highly sensitive to erythromycin but in induced MLS strains the ribosomal affinity for the drug is reduced (KONO et al. 1966). Together with the finding that erythromycin was not apparently inactivated by resistant strains (NAKAJIMA et al. 1968), this suggested that MLS resistance in *Staph. aureus* involved some form of ribosomal modification. The details began to emerge when Weisblum and colleagues compared the states of methylation of 23S RNA (derived from the 50S ribosomal subunit) in resistant and sensitive *Staphylococcus* and discovered that 23S rRNA from induced or constitutively resistant strains contained N^6,N^6-dimethyladenine whereas that from uninduced or sensitive cells did not (LAI and WEISBLUM 1971; LAI et al. 1973a). Then, a causal connection linking the state of 23S rRNA to the MLS resistance phenotype was established as a result of reconstitution analysis carried out in vitro. In those studies, 50S particles were reconstructed using 5S RNA and total ribosomal proteins from *Bacillus stearothermophilus* (chosen for purely technical reasons) together with 23S RNA from uninduced, induced or constitutively resistant *Staph. aureus* (LAI et al. 1973b). When assayed for their response to MLS antibiotics in protein-synthesising systems, such reconstituted 50S particles were found to reflect the phenotype of the strain from which the 23S rRNA had been derived. Thus, assuming that the various RNA species differed from each other only in the state of methylation, the introduction of dimethyladenine into 23S rRNA was hypothesised to be both necessary and sufficient for expression of the MLS resistance phenotype (LAI et al. 1973b).

Initially, the precise stoichiometry of methylation resulting in MLS resistance was not unequivocally determined, although the possibility was raised that more than one GAAAG sequence within 23S rRNA might have been methylated (LAI et al. 1973a). However, the subsequent isolation of a single methylated octanucleotide indicated that a unique site was probably involved (RANZINI and DUBIN 1983). The matter was finally resolved as a result of studies involving *Streptomyces erythraeus*, the producer of erythromycin. That strain possesses ribosomes to which erythromycin does not bind (TERAOKA and TANAKA 1974) and the presence of N^6,N^6-dimethyladenine in 23S rRNA derived therefrom had first prompted the hypothesis that MLS resistance in *S. erythraeus* was due to specific methylation of 23S rRNA, as in *Staphylococcus* (GRAHAM and WEISBLUM 1979).

That hypothesis was confirmed (SKINNER and CUNDLIFFE 1982) as a result of studies in which 23S rRNA from *B. stearothermophilus* (again chosen for purely technical reasons to facilitate subsequent reconstitution of 50S particles) was methylated in vitro, using extracts from *S. erythraeus*, before being incorporated into ribosomal particles. As predicted, methylation of 23S RNA caused resistance to MLS antibiotics. Moreover, in those and subsequent studies, it became clear that N^6,N^6-dimethylation of 23S rRNA was occurring at a single site (i.e. the stoichiometry of methylation was 2) and that the unique residue corresponded to A-2058 in the *E. coli* numbering system (SKINNER et al. 1983). It was also ascertained at that time that the methylase from *S. erythraeus* was unable to act on 23S RNA from induced *Bacillus subtilis* that contained the *ermC* gene, originally from *Staph. aureus*. Evidently, a family of *erm* gene products share a common site of action within 23S rRNA (see also THAKKER-VARIA et al. 1985).

Thus far, the MLS resistance methylase enzyme has been partially purified from two sources and its properties studied in vitro. On the one hand, the enzyme from *Streptomyces erythraeus* was shown to act exclusively upon free 23S rRNA and did not methylate 50S ribosomal subunits or intact 70S ribosomes (SKINNER et al. 1983). In *S. erythraeus*, the enzyme is produced constitutively and the ribosomes are maximally methylated (at residue 2058) at all times. However, when the *ermC* methylase was obtained from *B. subtilis* containing pE 194, 50S ribosomal subunits were reported to be targets for its action although 23S rRNA was by far the preferred substrate (SHIVAKUMAR and DUBNAU 1981). Thus, it may be that there is a real difference in substrate preference between these two homologous enzymes so that, following induction of *Staphylococcus* or *Bacillus*, pre-existing ribosomes might become modified and resistance might be acquired more rapidly than if ribosomal RNA could be methylated only during transcription. Against this, however, when ribosomal RNA in growing cells was pre-labelled with [^{3}H]adenine followed by a chase with unlabelled adenine before resistance was induced with erythromycin, methylation of the labelled adenine was not detected (LAI 1972), suggesting that methylation of 23S rRNA occurs prior to ribosomal assembly even in induced strains.

2. Control of Expression of MLS Resistance (*ermC*)

In the case of *ermC*, it gradually became apparent that control of expression was exerted not at the level of transcriptional initiation nor via transcriptional attenuation but, rather, that induction involved post-transcriptional events. Thus, the rate of transcription of *ermC* was similar in induced and uninduced minicells of *B. subtilis* and functional mRNA could be produced (evidently from non-functional, pre-existing mRNA) when inducer was added in the absence of RNA synthesis, i.e. following the prior addition of rifampicin (SHIVAKUMAR et al. 1980). These data suggested that *ermC* mRNA is produced constitutively and activated (by induction) post-transcriptionally. Moreover, since a chromosomal mutation that affected the ribosomal affinity for erythromycin also affected the ability of the drug to induce *ermC*, it seemed inescapable that post-transcriptional activation of *ermC* mRNA must involve binding of erythromycin to the ribosome. How so?

The *ermC* gene of pE194 has been fragmented and subcloned so that the MLS resistance determinant and its control element could be physically and functionally mapped. The gene has also been sequenced in two laboratories (GRYCZAN et al. 1980; HORINOUCHI and WEISBLUM 1980) and shown to contain an open reading frame (ORF) potentially capable of encoding a 29KDa polypeptide. Such a protein was also produced in *B. subtilis* minicells containing pE 194 under inducing conditions (SHIVAKUMAR et al. 1979) and a methylase of comparable size was par-

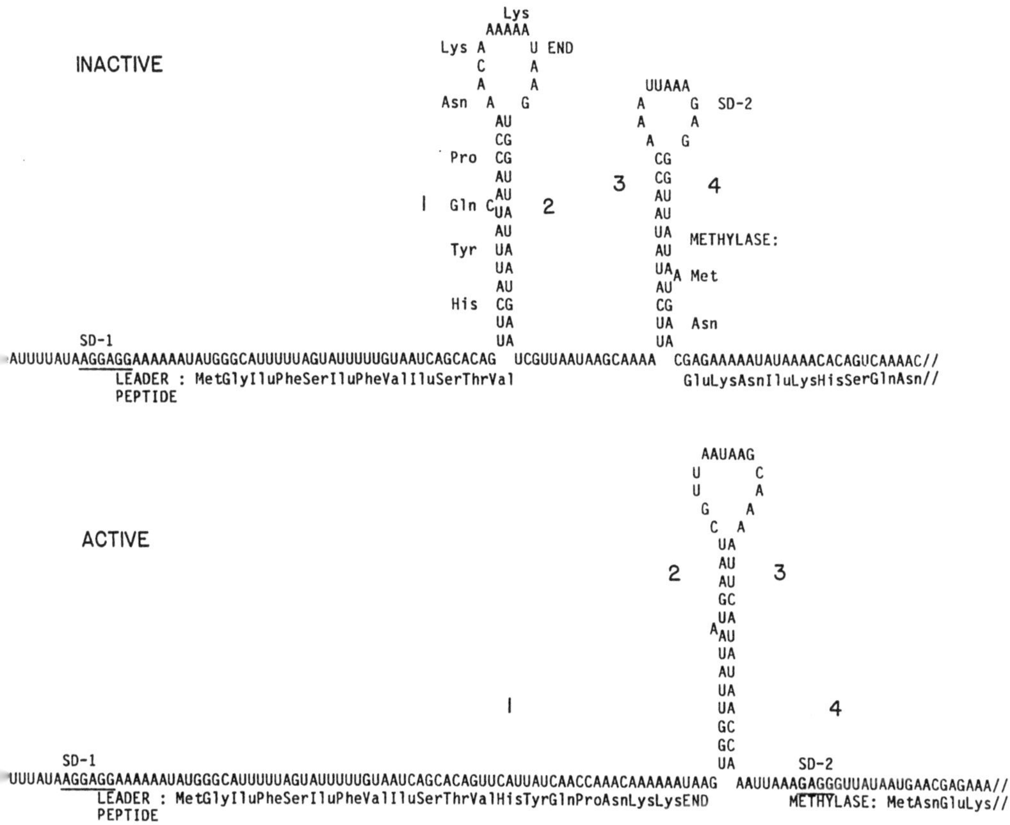

Fig. 1 a, b. Model for control of *ermC* expression. The mRNA control region transcribed from *ermC* and deduced from the DNA sequence is shown (**a**) in an inactive conformation (**b**) in an active conformation. SD-1 and SD-2 are the Shine-Dalgano sequences at which ribosomes attach to synthesise leader peptide and methylase (29K protein) respectively. Complementary inverted sequences are designated *1, 2, 3* and *4*. Diagram kindly provided by B. Weisblum

tially purified from MLS resistant (i.e. induced) *B. subtilis* (SHIVAKUMAR and DUBNAU 1981). Upstream from the methylase coding sequence, within that portion of the transcript that is derived from the control region of *ermC*, the mRNA leader sequence contains complementary inverted repeat sequences that are potentially capable of assuming alternative stem-and-loop structures. Accordingly, it has been proposed that translation of *ermC* mRNA is regulated by the ability of the leader sequence to undergo conformational re-arrangements. Two conceptually similar models have been proposed (on the one hand by GRYCZAN et al. 1980; HAHN et al. 1982 and on the other by HORINOUCHI and WEISBLUM 1980, 1981) the essential features of which are represented schematically in Fig. 1. Four inverted complementary sequences, designated 1, 2, 3 and 4 can base-pair to give 1+2 with 3+4 (as in Fig. 1 a) or 2+3, as in Fig. 1 b. [Other conformations are also possible, and this is where the two models differ slightly, but those represented in Fig. 1 are common and crucial to both. For comprehensive reviews, see Dubnau (1984) and Weisblum (1985).] Prior to induction, the control region of *ermC* mRNA is proposed to adopt the 1+2 with 3+4 conformation which is inactive because the ribosome-recognition site (the so-called Shine-Dalgarno sequence, here SD-2) preceding the 29K methylase coding sequence is partially occluded by base-pairing between 3 and 4 (see Fig. 1 a). Activation of the mRNA requires unmasking of SD-2 via a conformational transition to the 2+3 state (Fig. 1 b). That is brought about by the action of erythromycin on ribosomes engaged in production of a so called "leader" peptide (19 amino acid residues long) encoded by sequence 1 and residues surrounding it. If a ribosome stops during translation of the leader sequence, the model postulates that 2 will be physically displaced from 1 and will pair with 3 instead, thus activating the mRNA. Such "stalling" of the ribosome is caused by erythromycin at concentrations low enough to allow other ribosomes to engage at SD-2 and translate the methylase coding sequence. This model resembles to some extent the transcriptional attenuation models for regulation of amino acid production (for review, see Yanofsky 1981) in that both involve interference with the synthesis of a control (or leader) peptide and consequent conformational re-arrangements within mRNA. In one case, the result is continued transcription; in the other (here), the effect is to allow translation. Hence, *ermC* is said to be regulated via translational attenuation. Experimental evidence consistent with the contention that translation of *ermC* mRNA is governed by alternative pairings between complementary inverted repeats in the leader sequence has come from studies of mutants that are altered within the leader sequence (Horinouchi and Weisblum 1980, 1981; Gryczan et al. 1980; Hahn et al. 1982). To cite just one example, a deletion that removed the whole of sequence 1 and the control peptide sequence but did not affect sequences 2, 3 and 4 resulted in constitutive MLS resistance. According to the model, in this strain nascent *ermC* mRNA would immediately adopt the active 2+3 conformation (Fig. 1 b) and the methylase would be produced directly.

Not all *erm* genes are inducible and not all are plasmid encoded (Table 4) but, among those that *are* inducible, translational attenuation regulation has been proposed for *ermA* of *Staph. aureus* (Murphy 1985), *ermAM* of pAM77 from *Streptococcus sanguis* (Horinouchi et al. 1983) and *ermD* from the chromosome of *Bacillus licheniformis* (Gryczan et al. 1984). In these various systems, the length of the proposed control peptide can vary from 14 (*ermD*) to 36 (*ermAM*) amino acid residues and the number of alternative conformational states available to some of the mRNA control sequences may be much greater than for *ermC*. Given this level of complexity it is perhaps not surprising that critical tests of the attenuator model in these other systems have not (yet) been possible and *ermC* remains as the paradigm for this fascinating aspect of the regulation of gene expression.

Before concluding the discussion of translational attenuation in the context of MLS resistance, the specificity of induction must be considered since, a priori, it might be thought that *any* inhibitor of protein synthesis should cause ribosomes to stop ("stall") during attempted translation of the leader sequence and should thereby induce methylase production. Manifestly, this is not so and it therefore remains to be determined how the range of antibiotics that will induce a given

MLS resistance gene is determined. For example, in *Staph. aureus* MLS resistance is normally induced only by erythromycin, oleandomycin and celesticetin although in certain mutant strains lincomycin or other macrolides (such as carbomycin or leucomycin) can induce (SAITO et al. 1970; TANAKA and WEISBLUM 1974). In contrast, *ermAM* from *Streptococcus* is apparently induced by all MLS antibiotics. Yet again, in *Streptomyces*, expression of resistance to sub-sets of MLS antibiotics may, depending upon the strain, be induced by the autogenous MLS antibiotic or by a "foreign" drug added exogenously (FUJISAWA and WEISBLUM 1981). In attempting to explain these phenomena it will be essential (as proposed by Weisblum) to establish whether different MLS antibiotics inhibit the incorporation of different amino acids into peptide linkage with differing potencies and whether, on that basis, the efficiency with which a given drug induces a given system will depend upon the amino acid composition (or even sequence?) of the leader peptide (see KAMIMIYA and WEISBLUM 1987).

In conclusion, there is one further aspect of *ermC* control that deserves comment. According to the foregoing model, methylase induction will lead to a progressive increase in the proportion of resistant ribosomes within the cell and, eventually, this will trigger a breakdown in the induction mechanism since ribosomes will no longer respond to erythromycin by stalling in the leader sequence. However, it now appears that there is a more direct mechanism for shutting down methylase production, namely translational autoregulation by the methylase protein itself. Generally, in strains containing mutant *ermC* alleles (e.g. those specifying inactive truncated "methylases") induction leads to overproduction of the defective product (SHIVAKUMAR et al. 1980) and this could be explained by continued ability of sensitive ribosomes to translate the message. However, in one strain containing an *ermC* allele in which a point mutation within the methylase-coding sequence gave rise to a full-size (but inactive) protein, the kinetics of accumulation of that product were normal (DENOYA et al. 1986). Since, in that strain, translation of *ermC* mRNA cannot be limited by the decreased availability of sensitive ribosomes (because they all remain sensitive), something else must shut down translation. Accordingly, it has been suggested that the *ermC* gene product (normally, active methylase) can regulate its own production by binding to *ermC* mRNA and preventing excess utilisation of the latter by ribosomes. Since ribosomes normally attach at SD-2 prior to producing the methylase, it is postulated that this portion of *ermC* mRNA might resemble in its conformation and sequence that region of 23S rRNA within which methylation leads to MLS resistance (DENOYA et al. 1986). Indeed, this possibility had been hinted at previously (SHIVAKUMAR et al. 1980; HORINOUCHI and WEISBLUM 1981). As yet there is no direct evidence that the *ermC* methylase can, indeed, recognise its own mRNA either at the SD-2 sequence or elsewhere. Nevertheless, it would be pertinent to know whether mutations (random or directed) affecting the SD-2 sequence (perhaps rendering it more like SD-1) would break the proposed translational autoregulatory loop without impairing ribosome attachment at SD-2 and methylase production.

C. Concluding Remarks

In comparison with the typical effects of random mutations affecting ribosomal components, the RNA methylation systems described above render ribosomes (and therefore cells) very highly resistant, or even insensitive, to specific antibiotics. Moreover, at least in some cases (e.g. with thiostrepton and erythromycin; pertinent studies with the other drugs have not yet been reported), resistance results from failure of the drugs to bind to the modified ribosomes, which points to a direct relationship between methylation sites and antibiotic targets. Indeed, the simplest model to account for such data (and, in the case of thiostrepton, the correct model) would invoke direct binding of the drugs to rRNA. That, in itself, is no light statement since nucleic acids are not renowned for their ability to bind small molecules non-covalently and with high specificity. (The interaction of 23S RNA with thiostrepton is novel in that respect.) Also, other drugs that might also interact directly with rRNA (e.g. aminoglycosides, lincosamides, macrolides etc.) are quite dissimilar in structure from thiostrepton and from each other. Thus, it seems quite feasible that RNA might have an unsuspected capacity to bind a chemically diverse range of small molecules. And there is more.

The ribosome is an enzyme, enzymes have active sites, and antibiotics that block ribosomal function can be considered as inhibitors or regulators of that enzyme. Thus, the very strong suggestion that rRNA is crucially involved in the binding of various antibiotics carries with it the implication that RNA must therefore be involved in active sites of the ribosome. This conclusion is entirely consistent with growing speculation that RNA is not "merely" a structural component of the ribosome (for review, see CUNDLIFFE 1986). The remarkable extent to which the secondary structure of rRNA has been conserved during evolution, together with the logical truism that the original translation machinery must have been protein-free, raises the interesting possibility that rRNA might have been (and might still be) fundamentally involved in the mechanism of mRNA translation. In other words, the ribosome may be an RNA-driven machine for decoding mRNA. Studies of antibiotic resistance mechanisms involving rRNA methylation have contributed significantly to the development of that concept and seem likely to generate continued interest among clinicians (resistance in clinical isolates), biochemists (the mechanism of RNA catalysis) and microbial physiologists (the relationship between antibiotic production and resistance, e.g. in actinomycetes).

Acknowledgements. Work carried out in the author's laboratory and cited herein was funded by MRC, SERC and the Wellcome Trust and involved the skilled efforts of Alan Beauclerk, Jan Dijk, David Holmes, Wolfgang Piendl, Frank Schmidt, Tricia Skeggs, Michael Stark and Jill Thompson, inspired as always by Dino Bedlington.

References

Allen NE (1977) Macrolide resistance in *Staphylococcus aureus*: inducers of macrolide resistance. Antimicrob Agents Chemother 11:669–674

Beauclerk AAD, Cundliffe E (1987) Sites of action of two ribosomal RNA methylases responsible for resistance to aminoglycosides. J Mol Biol 193:661–671

Beauclerk AAD, Hummel H, Holmes DJ, Böck A, Cundliffe E (1985) Studies of the GTPase domain of archaebacterial ribosomes. Eur J Biochem 151:245–255
Benveniste R, Davies J (1973) Aminoglycoside antibiotic-inactivating enzymes in actinomycetes similar to those present in clinical isolates of antibiotic-resistant bacteria. Proc Natl Acad Sci USA 70:2276–2280
Bibb MJ, Bibb MJ, Ward JM, Cohen SN (1985) Nucleotide sequences encoding and promoting expression of three antibiotic resistance genes indigenous to *Streptomyces*. Mol Gen Genet 199:26–36
Chabbert Y (1956) Antagonisme in vitro entre l'erythromycine et la spiramycine. Ann Inst Pasteur 90:787–790
Crameri R, Davies JE (1986) Increased production of aminoglycosides associated with amplified antibiotic resistance genes. J Antibiot (Tokyo) 39:128–135
Cundliffe E (1978) Mechanism of resistance to thiostrepton in the producing-organism, *Streptomyces azureus*. Nature 272:792–795
Cundliffe E (1979) Thiostrepton and related antibiotics. In: Hahn FE (ed) Antibiotics V/I. Mechanism of action of antibacterial agents. Springer, Berlin Heidelberg New York, pp 329–343
Cundliffe E (1980) Antibiotics and prokaryotic ribosomes: action, interaction and resistance. In: Chambliss G, Craven GR, Davies J, Davis K, Kahan L, Nomura M (eds) Ribosomes: structure, function and genetics. University Park Press, Baltimore, pp 555–581
Cundliffe E (1984) Self defence in antibiotic-producing organisms. Br Med Bull 40:61–67
Cundliffe E (1986) Involvement of specific portions of ribosomal RNA in defined ribosomal functions: a study utilising antibiotics. In: Hardesty B, Kramer G (eds) Structure, function and genetics of ribosomes. Springer, Berlin Heidelberg New York Tokyo, pp 586–604
Cundliffe E, Thompson J (1979) Ribose methylation and resistance to thiostrepton. Nature 278:859–861
Davies J (1980) Enzymes modifying aminocyclitol antibiotics and their roles in resistance determination and biosynthesis. In: Rinehart KL Jr, Suami T (eds) Aminocyclitol antibiotics. American Chemical Society, Washington DC, pp 323–334
Denoya CD, Bechhofer DH, Dubnau D (1986) Translational autoregulation of *ermC* 23S rRNA methyltransferase expression in *Bacillus subtilis*. J Bacteriol 168:1133–1141
Dubnau D (1984) Translational attenuation: the regulation of bacterial resistance to the macrolide-lincosamide-streptogramin B antibiotics. CRC Crit Rev Biochem 16:103–132
Fujisawa Y, Weisblum B (1981) A family of r-determinants in *Streptomyces* spp that specifies inducible resistance to macrolide, lincosamide, and streptogramin type B antibiotics. J Bacteriol 146:621–631
Gale EF, Cundliffe E, Reynolds PE, Richmond MH, Waring MJ (1981) The molecular basis of antibiotic action. Wiley, London
Garrod LP (1957) The erythromycin group of antibiotics. Br Med J 2:57–63
Graham MY, Weisblum B (1979) 23S ribosomal ribonucleic acid of macrolide-producing streptomycetes contains methylated adenine. J Bacteriol 137:1464–1467
Gryczan TJ, Grandi G, Hahn J, Grandi R, Dubnau D (1980) Conformational alteration of mRNA structure and the post-transcriptional regulation of erythromycin-induced drug resistance. Nucleic Acids Res 8:6081–6097
Gryczan T, Israeli-Reches M, Del Bue M, Dubnau D (1984) DNA sequence and regulation of *ermD*, a macrolide-lincosamide-streptogramin B resistance element from *Bacillus licheniformis*. Mol Gen Genet 194:349–356
Hahn J, Grandi G, Gryczan TJ, Dubnau D (1982) Translational attenuation of *ermC*: a deletion analysis. Mol Gen Genet 186:204–216
Highland JH, Howard GA, Ochsner E, Stöffler G, Hasenbank R, Gordon J (1975) Identification of a ribosomal protein necessary for thiostrepton binding to *E. coli* ribosomes. J Biol Chem 250:1141–1145
Hopwood DA, Bibb MJ, Chater KF, Janssen GR, Malpartida F, Smith CP (1986) Regulation of gene expression in antibiotic-producing *Streptomyces*. Symp Soc Gen Microbiol 39:251–276

Horinouchi S, Weisblum B (1980) Posttranscriptional modification of mRNA conformation: mechanism that regulates erythromycin-induced resistance. Proc Natl Acad Sci USA 77:7079–7083
Horinouchi S, Weisblum B (1981) The control region for erythromycin resistance: free energy changes related to induction and mutation to constitutive expression. Mol Gen Genet 182:341–348
Horinouchi S, Byeon WH, Weisblum B (1983) A complex attenuator regulates inducible resistance to macrolides, lincosamides, and streptogramin type B antibiotics in *Streptococcus sanguis*. J Bacteriol 154:1252–1262
Hotta K, Yamamoto H, Okami Y, Umezawa H (1981) Resistance mechanisms of kanamycin-, neomycin-, and streptomycin-producing streptomycetes to aminoglycoside antibiotics. J Antibiot (Tokyo) 34:1175–1182
Jones WF Jr, Nichols RL, Finland M (1956) Development of resistance and cross resistance in vivo to erythromycin, carbomycin, oleandomycin, and streptogramin. Proc Soc Exp Biol Med 93:388–393
Kamimiya S, Weisblum B (1987) Inducible macrolide-lincosamide-streptogramin resistance in *Streptomyces*: cloning and characterization of inducible *erm* from *Streptomyces viridochromogenes* and *Streptomyces fradiae*. In: Alačević M, Hranueli D, Toman Z (eds) Genetics of industrial microorganisms – 86: part B. Pliva, Zagreb, pp 169–175
Kono M, Hashimoto H, Matsuhashi S (1966) Drug resistance of staphylococci. III. Resistance to some macrolide antibiotics and inducible system. Jpn J Microbiol 10:59–66
Lai CJ (1972) Erythromycin-inducible resistance in *Staphylococcus aureus*. PhD thesis, University of Wisconsin
Lai CJ, Weisblum B (1971) Altered methylation of ribosomal RNA in an erythromycin-resistant strain of *Staphylococcus aureus*. Proc Natl Acad Sci USA 68:856–860
Lai CJ, Dahlberg JE, Weisblum B (1973a) Structure of an inducibly methylatable nucleotide sequence in 23S ribosomal ribonucleic acid from erythromycin-resistant *Staphylococcus aureus*. Biochemistry 12:457–460
Lai CJ, Weisblum B, Fahnestock SR, Nomura M (1973b) Alteration of 23S ribosomal ribonucleic acid and erythromycin-induced resistance to lincomycin and spiramycin in *Staphylococcus aureus*. J Mol Biol 74:67–72
Matković B, Piendl W, Böck A (1984) Ribosomal resistance as a widespread self-defence mechanism in aminoglycoside-producing *Micromonospora* species. FEMS Microbiol Lett 24:273–276
Matsuhashi Y, Murakami T, Nojiri C, Toyama H, Anzai H, Nagaoka K (1985) Mechanisms of aminoglycoside-resistance of *Streptomyces* harbouring resistant genes obtained from antibiotic-producers. J Antibiot (Tokyo) 38:279–282
Murakami T, Nojiri C, Toyama H, Hayashi E, Katumata K, Anzai H, Matsuhashi Y, Yamada Y, Nagaoka K (1983) Cloning of antibiotic-resistance genes in Streptomyces. J Antibiot (Tokyo) 36:1305–1311
Murphy E (1985) Nucleotide sequence of *ermA*, a macrolide-lincosamide-streptogramin B determinant in *Staphylococcus aureus*. J Bacteriol 162:633–640
Nakajima Y, Inoue M, Oka Y, Yamagishi S (1968) A mode of resistance to macrolide antibiotics in *Staphylococcus aureus*. Jpn J Microbiol 12:248–250
Nakano MM, Ogawara H (1987) Isolation and characterization of ribosome resistance gene from *Streptomyces kanamyceticus*. In: Alačević M, Hranueli D, Toman Z (eds) Genetics of industrial microorganisms – 86. Pliva, Zagreb, pp 177–184
Nakano MM, Mashiko H, Ogawara H (1984) Cloning of the kanamycin resistance gene from a kanamycin-producing *Streptomyces* species. J Bacteriol 157:79–83
Noller HF (1984) Structure of ribosomal RNA. Annu Rev Biochem 53:119–162
Pestka S, Vince R, LeMahieu R, Weiss F, Fern L, Unowsky J (1976) Induction of erythromycin resistance in *Staphylococcus aureus* by erythromycin derivatives. Antimicrob Agents Chemother 9:128–130
Piendl W, Böck A (1982) Ribosomal resistance in the gentamicin producer organism *Micromonospora purpurea*. Antimicrob Agents Chemother 22:231–236

Piendl W, Böck A, Cundliffe E (1984) Involvement of 16S ribosomal RNA in resistance of the aminoglycoside-producers *Streptomyces tenjimariensis*, *Streptomyces tenebrarius* and *Micromonospora purpurea*. Mol Gen Genet 197:24–29
Ranzini AC, Dubin DT (1983) The "erythromycin-resistance" methylated sequence of *Staphylococcus aureus* ribosomal RNA. Plasmid 10:293–295
Rasmussen JL, Odelson DA, Macrina FL (1986) Complete nucleotide sequence and transcription of *ermF*, a macrolide-lincosamide-streptogramin B resistance determinant from *Bacteroides fragilis*. J Bacteriol 168:523–533
Roberts AN, Hudson GS, Brenner S (1985) An erythromycin-resistance gene from an erythromycin-producing strain of *Arthrobacter* sp. Gene 35:259–270
Saito T, Hashimoto H, Mitsuhashi S (1970) Macrolide resistance in *Staphylococcus aureus*. Isolation of a mutant in which leucomycin is an active inducer. Jpn J Microbiol 14:473–478
Schmidt FJ, Thompson J, Lee K, Dijk J, Cundliffe E (1981) The binding site for ribosomal protein L11 within 23S ribosomal RNA of *Escherichia coli*. J Biol Chem 256:12301–12305
Shivakumar AG, Dubnau D (1981) Characterization of a plasmid-encoded ribosome methylase associated with macrolide resistance. Nucleic Acids Res 9:2549–2562
Shivakumar AG, Hahn J, Dubnau D (1979) Studies on the synthesis of plasmid-coded proteins and their control in *Bacillus subtilis* minicells. Plasmid 2:279–289
Shivakumar AG, Hahn J, Grandi G, Kozlov Y, Dubnau D (1980) Posttranscriptional regulation of an erythromycin resistance protein specified by plasmid pE 194. Proc Natl Acad Sci USA 77:3903–3907
Skeggs PA, Thompson J, Cundliffe E (1985) Methylation of 16S ribosomal RNA and resistance to aminoglycoside antibiotics in clones of *Streptomyces lividans* carrying DNA from *Streptomyces tenjimariensis*. Mol Gen Genet 200:415–421
Skeggs PA, Holmes DJ, Cundliffe E (1987) Cloning of aminoglycoside-resistance determinants from *Streptomyces tenebrarius* and comparison with related genes from other actinomycetes. J Gen Microbiol 133:915–923
Skinner RH, Cundliffe E (1982) Dimethylation of adenine and the resistance of *Streptomyces erythraeus* to erythromycin. J Gen Microbiol 128:2411–2416
Skinner R, Cundliffe E, Schmidt FJ (1983) Site of action of a ribosomal RNA methylase responsible for resistance to erythromycin and other antibiotics. J Biol Chem 258:12702–12706
Sugiyama M, Nimi O, Nomi R (1980) Susceptibility of protein synthesis to neomycin in neomycin-producing *Streptomyces fradiae*. J Gen Microbiol 121:477–478
Tanaka T, Weisblum B (1974) Mutant of *Staphylococcus aureus* with lincomycin – and carbomycin – inducible resistance to erythromycin. Antimicrob Agents Chemother 5:538–540
Teraoka H, Tanaka K (1974) Properties of ribosomes from *Streptomyces erythreus* and *Streptomyces griseus*. J Bacteriol 120:316–321
Thakker-Varia S, Ranzini AC, Dubin DT (1985) Ribosomal RNA methylation in *Staphylococcus aureus* and *Escherichia coli*: effect of the "MLS" (erythromycin resistance) methylase. Plasmid 14:152–161
Thompson CJ, Ward JM, Hopwood DA (1980) DNA cloning in *Streptomyces*: resistance genes from antibiotic-producing species. Nature 286:525–527
Thompson CJ, Skinner RH, Thompson J, Ward JM, Hopwood DA, Cundliffe E (1982) Biochemical characterization of resistance determinants cloned from antibiotic-producing streptomycetes. J Bacteriol 151:678–685
Thompson J, Cundliffe E (1981) Purification and properties of an RNA methylase produced by *Streptomyces azureus* and involved in resistance to thiostrepton. J Gen Microbiol 124:291–297
Thompson J, Cundliffe E, Stark M (1979) Binding of thiostrepton to a complex of 23S rRNA with ribosomal protein L11. Eur J Biochem 98:261–265
Thompson J, Schmidt F, Cundliffe E (1982) Site of action of a ribosomal RNA methylase conferring resistance to thiostrepton. J Biol Chem 257:7915–7917

Thompson J, Rae S, Cundliffe E (1984) Coupled transcription-translation in extracts of *Streptomyces lividans*. Mol Gen Genet 195:39–43

Thompson J, Skeggs PA, Cundliffe E (1985) Methylation of 16S ribosomal RNA and resistance to the aminoglycoside antibiotics gentamicin and kanamycin determined by DNA from the gentamicin-producer, *Micromonospora purpurea*. Mol Gen Genet 201:168–173

Thompson J, Cundliffe E, Dahlberg AE (1988) Site-directed mutagenesis of *Escherichia coli* 23S ribosomal RNA at position 1067 within the GTP hydrolysis centre. J Mol Biol 203:457–465

Uchiyama H, Weisblum B (1985) *N*-methyl transferase of *Streptomyces erythraeus* that confers resistance to the macrolide-lincosamide-streptogramin B antibiotics: amino acid sequence and its homology to cognate R-factor enzymes from pathogenic bacilli and cocci. Gene 38:103–110

Weaver JR, Pattee PA (1964) Inducible resistance to erythromycin in *Staphylococcus aureus*. J Bacteriol 88:574–580

Weisblum B (1975) Altered methylation of ribosomal ribonucleic acid in erythromycin-resistant *Staphylococcus aureus*. In: Schlessinger D (ed) Microbiology – 1974. American Society for Microbiology, Washington DC, pp 199–206

Weisblum B (1985) Inducible resistance to macrolides, lincosamides and streptogramin type B antibiotics: the resistance phenotype, its biological diversity, and structural elements that regulate expression – A review. J Antimicrob Chemother [Suppl A] 16:63–90

Yamamoto H, Hotta K, Okami Y, Umezawa H (1981) Ribosomal resistance of an istamycin producer, *Streptomyces tenjimariensis*, to aminoglycoside antibiotics. Biochem Biophys Res Commun 100:1396–1401

Yamamoto H, Hotta K, Okami Y, Umezawa H (1982) Mechanism of resistance to aminoglycoside antibiotics in nebramycin-producing *Streptomyces tenebrarius*. J Antibiot [Tokyo] 35:1020–1025

Yanofsky C (1981) Attenuation in the control of expression of bacterial operons. Nature 289:751–758

CHAPTER 11

Resistance to Trimethoprim

L. P. ELWELL and M. E. FLING

A. Introduction

Trimethoprim (2,4-diamino-5-(3′,4′5′-trimethoxybenzyl)pyrimidine) is one of a series of compounds first fully described by ROTH et al. (1962). These compounds possess both antimalarial and antibacterial activity, the former activity exemplified by pyrimethamine and the latter activity by trimethoprim (Tp). Tp is a potent inhibitor of dihydrofolate reductase (5,6,7,8-tetrahydrofolate: $NADP^+$ oxidoreductase EC 1.5.1.3; DHFR), an enzyme that catalyzes the NADPH-dependent reduction of dihydrofolate to tetrahydrofolate, a cofactor required for the metabolism of some amino acids, purines and thymidine. The structure of trimethoprim and one of its clinically used structural analogs, tetroxoprim, is shown in Fig. 1. Tp has a several thousand-fold higher affinity for bacterial DHFR than for mammalian DHFR; the bacterial synthesis of tetrahydrofolate is preferentially diminished as a consequence of this selective binding (BURCHALL 1973; HITCHINGS 1973).

Tp has been historically used in combination with sulfamethoxazole (SMX). For example, the combination known as co-trimoxazole (as well as Septra and Bactrim) has been widely used in the United Kingdom since 1969. Combinations of sulfonamides and Tp act at different sites in the biosynthetic pathway of tetrahydrofolate (Fig. 2), and this sequential blockade is thought to be responsible for the observed potentiation of the action by the combination of Tp and sulfonamide over the action of each component alone (synergy).

During the last 15 years, outbreaks of disease due to multiply drug-resistant strains of enteric bacterial pathogens have occurred with increasing frequency in the so-called "developing" countries of the world. These outbreaks have involved most of the important etiologic agents of bacterial diarrhea, and the resistance patterns exhibited by these organisms have generally included those antibiotics that were being used most heavily at the time of the outbreak. Resistance to Tp (and SMX) can be included in this emerging world-wide picture (FARRAR 1985).

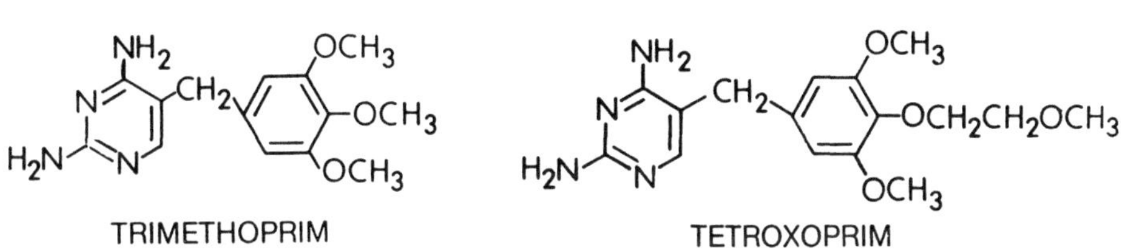

Fig. 1. Structures of trimethoprim and tetroxoprim

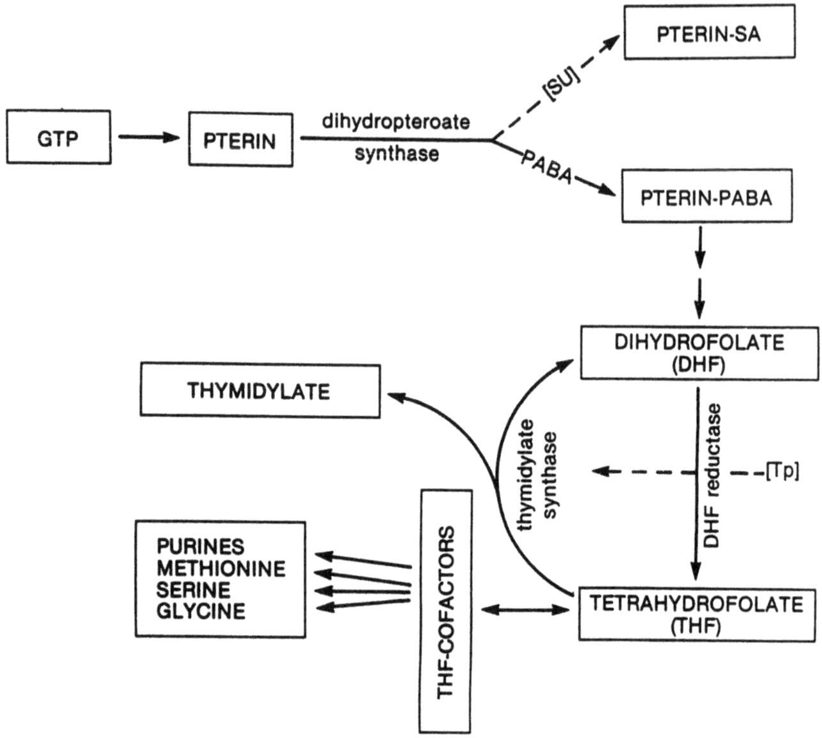

Fig. 2. Schematic diagram for the biosynthetic pathway of tetrahydrofolate and for the interference of sulfonamides (SU) and trimethoprim (Tp)

For example, MURRAY et al. (1985) have reported the incidence of Tp/SMX-resistance among strains of *E. coli* isolated during 1983–1984 in Chile, Thailand, Honduras, Costa Rica and Brazil to be 38–50%. Resistance to Tp/SMX was found in only 4%–6% of *E. coli* isolates tested at several medical centers in the U.S. during the same period.

SHAHID et al. (1985) have recently shown that *S. dysenteriae* type I, which returned to Bangladesh in 1971, has now overtaken *S. flexneri* as the primary cause of bacillary dysentery in that country. Approximately 99% of isolated strains of *S. dysenteriae* were multi-resistant, the predominant pattern being Tp/SMX, streptomycin, tetracycline and chloramphenicol. In contrast, only one of 26 strains isolated 2 years earlier (December, 1982) was resistant to Tp/SMX. The authors suggest that these findings are the reflection of a major change in antibiotic use in Bangladesh. During 1981–1982 there was a 10-fold increase in use of ampicillin, with very little use of Tp/SMX. By 1983 Tp/SMX had largely replaced ampicillin in Bangladesh due to its lower price, longer shelf-life and less-frequent dosage.

Finally, MACADEN and BHAT (1985) have studied the resistance of *Shigella* serotypes to Tp/SMX and ampicillin in Bangladesh and southern India and found that prior to 1981, strains of *S. dysenteriae* were uniformly sensitive to Tp/SMX.

In 1981, resistance suddenly increased to 84%, and, by 1983, approximately 94% of *S. dysenteriae* isolates were resistant. Tp/SMX had been used extensively in southern India in 1976–1978 to control an outbreak of *S. dysenteriae* infections in which the strains were resistant to ampicillin, streptomycin, tetracycline, and chloramphenicol.

The common theme of these three studies is that the introduction of Tp/SMX into certain developing countries has resulted in a rapid increase in the prevalence of resistance in certain bacterial species. This stands in marked contrast to the situation in many industrialized countries, where the prevalence of resistance has remained low despite more than a decade of use. Hence, the results of several studies in the U.S. have shown little development of resistance to Tp/SMX following administration of the drug combination for treatment of urinary tract infections or for therapy or prophylaxis of granulocytopenia (GURWITH et al. 1979; PANCOAST et al. 1980; STAMM et al. 1980; GUERRANT et al. 1981). This is not a unanimous finding, however, since MURRAY et al. (1982) have observed rapid emergence of resistance to Tp/SMX among strains of fecal *E. coli* isolated from American college students who took Tp/SMX daily for two weeks while in Guadalajara, Mexico.

Increasing resistance to trimethoprim is viewed as particularly significant because in many parts of the world more gram-negative bacilli have remained susceptible to Tp than to any other orally administered systemic antibacterial agent and because no comparably inexpensive substitute has been available (O'BRIEN 1987).

B. Mechanisms of Resistance

Resistance to Tp may be intrinsic, the result of a chromosomal mutation(s) (Table 1), or it may be plasmid-associated. High-level resistance to Tp [minimum inhibitory concentration (MIC), greater than 1 mg/ml] is generally due to the presence of a plasmid- or transposon-encoded Tp-resistant DHFR. This resistance mechanism is by far the most clinically important one and fluctuates a great deal according to bacterial species and geographical source. Chromosomal mutations, which are reflected by MICs in the range of 4–500 μg/ml, can also result in clinically significant resistance. In contrast to R plasmid-mediated resistance, chromosomal mutations account for a relatively low proportion (2%–10%) of resistance, and the incidence of these isolates has remained relatively stable over the years.

In the first part of this chapter we will discuss the various mutational strategies that gram-negative bacteria have "devised" to thwart the effectiveness of trimethoprim.

I. Thymine-Requiring Strains

The use of a folic acid antagonist to isolate thymine-requiring (thy^-) mutants was first employed by OKADA et al. (1960) with *E. coli*. Thy^- mutants arise when wild type bacteria are grown in medium containing the drug (aminopterin or Tp) and thymine (or thymidine). The mutation that occurs in response to Tp is an alteration in the gene coding for thymidylate synthase, an enzyme which converts deoxyuridylate (dUMP) to thymidylate (dTMP) (BARNER and COHEN 1959). *Thy*$^-$ mutants can no longer synthesize thymidylate from folates, and therefore require exogenous thymine for DNA synthesis. Such mutants are also resistant to trimethoprim (BERTINO and STACY 1966). These initial mutants are termed "high thymine"-requiring strains, since 40–50 μg/ml of thymine is needed to satisfy the growth requirement. Second-step mutations can occur which result in a lower-level thymine requirement. These map in the *deo* operon. Thus, *deo* C mutants lack the enzyme deoxyribose-5-phosphate aldolase, whereas *deo* B mutants lack the enzyme phosphodeoxyribomutase (LOMAX and GREENBERG 1968). Thymine combines with deoxyribose-1-phosphate to form thymidine; deoxyribose-1-phosphate is also catabolized to breakdown products by the agency of phosphodeoxyribomutase and deoxyribose-5-phosphate aldolase (HOFFEE and ROBERTSON 1969). If the catabolism of deoxyribose-1-phosphate is blocked by mutation of one or both of these enzymes, a pool will accumulate, and thereby lower the concentration of thymine necessary for a steady-state supply of intracellular thymidine (BREITMAN and BRADFORD 1967). In this way, *thy*$^-$ mutants with a considerably lower thymine requirement could theoretically (and apparently do) emerge.

Since 1972 there have been several reports of the isolation of thymine- or thymidine-requiring mutants of bacteria from patients undergoing both long-term and short-term treatment with co-trimoxazole (BARKER et al. 1972; LEWIS and LACEY 1973; OKUBADEJO and MASKELL 1973; TAPSALL et al. 1974; HAYEK and NETHERWAY 1976). In addition, evidence from two independent studies suggests that these mutant strains have retained their pathogenicity (TANNER and BULLIN 1974; MASKELL et al. 1977). On the other hand, thymine-requiring mutants of *Salmonella* have been reported to exhibit reduced virulence (SMITH and TUCKER 1976). MASKELL et al. (1977) presented clinical details of 16 patients from whom *thy*$^-$ mutants of pathogenic microorganisms were isolated. All of the patients had been treated with co-trimoxazole. Interestingly, the urine of six patients infected with *thy*$^-$ mutants contained levels of a "thymine-like" compound sufficient to support their growth. It has been suggested that measurable levels of thymine in the urine of selected patients with renal calculi and urinary tract infection might result either from the breakdown of pus cells or from thymine production by living bacteria persisting in the stones (MASKELL et al. 1976). In addition, some of the organisms isolated in this survey had a low thymine requirement, suggesting that these strains had undergone a secondary mutation(s), presumably in the *deo* operon. MASKELL et al. (1977) reported isolating these mutants at a rate of around one per month. From 1972 to 1979, ACAR and GOLDSTEIN (1982) tested 43,696 isolates of enterobacteria for susceptibility to Tp. *Thy*$^-$ organisms were isolated predominantly from patients being treated with co-trimoxazole for urinary tract infections and represented 1.5% of the Tp-resistant strains isolated per year. It is important that clinical laboratories be aware of the existence of *thy*$^-$ mutants and that patients on long-term co-trimoxazole therapy have regular bacteriological monitoring.

II. Decreased Permeability

In 1976, H. WILLIAMS SMITH described mutants of *Klebsiella pneumoniae* with combined resistance to nalidixic acid, trimethoprim, and chloramphenicol (NTC mutants) after either in vitro or in vivo (gastrointestinal tract of chickens) exposure to any of these three drugs (SMITH 1976). This combined resistance could not be transferred to *E. coli* K12 recipients by bacterial conjugation. A year later, TRAUB and KLEBER (1977) demonstrated the same phenomenon in strains of *Serratia marcescens* either as a spontaneous event or as the result of exposure to increasing concentrations of either chloramphenicol or Tp. *K. pneumoniae*, *Serratia* and *Enterobacter* mutate to this triple resistance, in vitro at a frequency of 10^{-6} to 10^{-7} (ACAR and GOLDSTEIN 1982). A similar mutation in *E. coli* or *Proteus mirabilis* has not been observed.

Because the three antibiotics have totally different modes of action, the simplest mechanism one can invoke to explain NTC resistance is an alteration in the permeability of the bacteria to these antibiotics. In order to systematically test this possibility, GUTMANN et al. (1985) examined the outer membrane protein profiles of one-step NTC mutants of *K. pneumoniae*, *E. aerogenes*, *S. marcescens*, and *E. cloacea*. The profiles of these mutant strains differed from their wild-type counterparts in that the NTC strains had significantly smaller amounts of outer membrane proteins in the size range of 37–41 kilodaltons (kd). In the case of *S. marcescens*, the 40–41 kd proteins have been shown to be porins and are also involved in resistance to β-lactam antibiotics (GOLDSTEIN et al. 1983a). Porins in *E. coli* have a molecular weight of approximately 40 kd. More direct support for the hypothesis of reduced permeability was provided by demonstrating a slower uptake of [^{3}H]glucose and [^{14}C]chloramphenicol in NTC mutants compared with the parental strains and by the almost identical binding of [^{14}C]chloramphenicol to the ribosomes in the wild-type strains and the NTC mutants (GUTMANN et al. 1985). All of the mutants showed a slight, but reproducible increase (generally two-fold) in resistance to ampicillin or carbenicillin. In addition, they showed significant decreases in susceptibility to the new quinolones such as norfloxacin and ciprofloxacin. Thus, it appears likely that cross-resistance to trimethoprim, nalidixic acid, chloramphenicol (and, to a lesser extent, β-lactams and the newer quinolones) is the result of a mutation leading to a reduction in the quantity of outer membrane proteins (probably porins) in the mutant bacteria, rendering them less permeable to the three antibiotics.

With respect to the clinical significance of these isolates, GUTMANN et al. (1985) have found 30 NTC mutants among patients being treated with co-trimoxazole or nalidixic acid for urinary tract infections. Three patients also had concomitant bacteremia.

III. Mutations in Dihydrofolate Reductase Structural Gene

The gene encoding dihydrofolate reductase (DHFR), *fol*A, resides at minute 1 as determined by the analysis of Tp-resistant mutants of *E. coli* K12 (BREEZE et al. 1975; BACHMANN 1983). Such mutants can easily be obtained in the laboratory after chemical mutagenesis. In general, these mutants are one of two types; (i) those that contain an altered enzyme with an approximate 25-fold decreased affinity for Tp or (ii) those in which the regulation of DHFR synthesis is altered to result in a 2- to 200-fold increase in the intracellular concentration of enzyme. SHELDON and BRENNER (1976) demonstrated that in *E. coli* the mutations which caused enzyme overproduction (*fol* regulatory mutations) are *cis*-acting. Although such mutations usually occur in non-diffusible regulatory elements such as operators and promoters, some of the *fol* regulatory mutants were found to be temperature-sensitive for enzyme regulation. Earlier SIROTNAK et al. (1969) had reported that DHFRs from some regulatory mutants had slightly altered kinetic properties compared to those of the wild-type enzyme. In light of these findings, it seemed important to determine whether any of these mutations also affected the structure of DHFR itself. Accordingly, SHELDON (1977) isolated and purified (100-fold) enzyme from three spontaneously occurring *fol* regulatory mutants. He showed that the mutant enzymes differed in their affinity for Tp (10- to 25-fold higher I_{50} values) as well as in their thermolability at 51 °C compared to wild-type DHFR. Thus, these results suggested that some spontaneous mutations resulted in both altered DHFR levels as well as alterations in the structure of the enzyme itself. Earlier, GOLDBERGER (1974) had interpreted this observation to mean that DHFR regulates its own synthesis. However, since the *fol* mutations act in *cis* (SHELDON and BRENNER 1976) autogenous regulation is unlikely to operate in this case (unless DHFR is a *cis*-acting regulator). SMITH et al. (1982) used a more direct strategy to show that Ki (structural) mutations could occur in the *fol* gene. Recombinant plasmids carrying the *fol* gene from *E. coli* were mutagenized in vitro and in vivo and then used to transform recipient strains. Twenty-three transformants were isolated that were able to grow in the presence of high levels of Tp. Eighteen strains had DHFR levels 10- to 30-fold higher than those of the control strain whereas the remaining three strains produced DHFRs with increased Ki values for trimethoprim.

DNA sequence analysis revealed that the plasmids in these three strains had undergone mutations in the DHFR structural gene in a conserved region of the polypeptide that forms part of the dihydrofolate binding site. Specifically, the mutations in these plasmids were shown to affect two amino acids (proline 21 and alanine 26) in a short, highly conserved region of the enzyme. The region Pro 21-Trp 22-X 23-Leu 24-Pro 25-X26-Asp 27 is conserved in DHFRs from *E. coli, Lactobacillus casei*, and *Streptococcus faecium* (FREISHEIM et al. 1978). Analysis of the three-dimensional structure of the enzyme indicated that this sequence forms part of the lower and inner surfaces of the substrate-binding pocket (MATTHEWS et al. 1977). Thus, a change at position 21 from proline to serine understandably affects the binding of Tp to the enzyme. Although alanine 26 is not conserved in bacterial DHFRs, it is adjacent to aspartic acid 27, which is thought to play a role in the catalytic mechanism of the enzyme (MATTHEWS et al. 1977). Thus, the change in position 26 from alanine to threonine could easily have an effect on Tp-binding because the threonine side chain is more bulky and hydrophilic than that of alanine, and the change occurs immediately adjacent to the active site (SMITH et al. 1982).

There are very few published studies that discuss the incidence of these particular kinds of mutants among clinical isolates. GREY et al. (1979) analyzed 133 strains of gram-negative bacteria with acquired resistance to Tp isolated from infected urines in a single London hospital (R plasmid-containing strains were omitted from the analysis). In this particular survey, Tp-resistant *K. aerogenes* and *Enterobacter* spp. predominated. The main mechanism of resistance in the majority of *E. coli* and *K. aerogenes* appeared to be the production of an altered DHFR with a decreased sensitivity to trimethoprim. In the majority of strains there was a good correlation between the MIC for trimethoprim and the I_{50} of Tp for the crude DHFR preparations. The MICs of these isolates ranged from 4 to 100 µg/ml trimethoprim. Unfortunately, these resistant DHFRs were not further purified and definitively shown to be structural mutants. It is clear, however, that Ki mutations, leading to a reasonably high level of Tp resistance, do occur in clinical bacterial isolates.

IV. Mutations Affecting Dihydrofolate Reductase Expression

Hyperproduction of DHFR (3- to 80-fold) was reported in pneumococci resistant to methotrexate (McCuen and Sirotnak 1974) and in *E. coli* K12 (up to 26-fold) resistant to Tp (Breeze et al. 1975). Sheldon and Brenner (1976) using NG-mutagenized cells, described mutants of *E. coli* K12 that contained about 25-fold more DHFR molecules than their wild-type counterparts. Similarly, Smith and Calvo (1979) described an *E. coli* mutant that produced elevated levels of DHFR in response to an increased rate of synthesis of *fol* mRNA. The DHFR from a *fol* regulatory mutant of *E. coli* described by Sheldon (1977) was *both* hyperproduced (10-fold) and had decreased affinity for Tp (20- to 25-fold; see last section).

In spite of the widespread use of Tp over the past 15 years, organisms with chromosomally specified overproduction of DHFR did not seem to occur in clinical material. One reason invoked to explain this was that deregulation of the tetrahydrofolic acid pathway would severely compromise other bacterial functions (Koch 1981). However, Tennhammar-Ekman and Skold (1979) and Steen and Skold (1985) have isolated 3 Tp-resistant clinical isolates (2 *E. coli* and 1 *P. vulgaris*) in which the overproduction (80- to 200-fold) of chromosomal DHFR was found to account for high-level trimethoprim resistance. *E. coli* 1810, a 200-fold DHFR overproducer, has been analyzed in great detail. The overproduced enzyme in *E. coli* 1810 was shown to be similar to the *E. coli* K12 DHFR with respect to heat stability and pH optimum, but different from its K12 counterpart in two respects: the electrophoretic mobility in a non-denaturing polyacrylamide gel is somewhat slower, and the Ki value for Tp is approximately three times higher (Tennhammar-Ekman and Skold 1979).

The high level of DHFR activity in strain 1810 could be the result of enhanced enzyme synthesis (i.e., simply more enzyme molecules) or might be explained in terms of the synthesis of a modified enzyme having a higher turnover number. Turnover numbers for strain 1810 DHFR and K12 enzyme were determined by enzyme titrations using methotrexate. The difference in turnover numbers was relatively small; thus, the 200-fold higher enzyme activity in strain 1810 was most likely explained by the presence of an increased number of enzyme molecules. Thus, Flensburg and Skold (1984) determined the levels of *fol* mRNA in *E. coli*

1810 and HB101 by hybridization techniques, and they found that the relative rate of *fol* mRNA production in the overproducing strain was 15 to 20 times higher than in HB101, which contains a normally regulated K12 *fol* gene.

In order to investigate the precise molecular mechanism responsible for the overproduction of DHFR, FLENSBURG and SKOLD (1987) cloned the Tp-resistance determinant from strain 1810, and its nucleotide sequence was compared with the corresponding *fol* gene in *E. coli* K12. In the −35 region of the promoter to the DHFR gene of the overproducing strain there was a C→T transition (position −34) compared to that of *E. coli* K12. This change increases the homology with the *E. coli* consensus promoter sequence (ROSENBERG and COURT 1979). An identical transition has been shown to exist in mutagenically changed *E. coli* strains mediating about a 15-fold increase in DHFR production (SMITH and CALVO 1982).

Regarding its ribosome-binding site, the *fol* gene from strain 1810 differed in two respects from its *E. coli* K12 counterpart. First, the overproducing strain showed two transitions in the ribosome-binding site to make a five-base continuous sequence of complementarity with the 16S ribosomal RNA. Second, an insertion of one base had occurred, lengthening the sequence between the ribosome-binding site and the start codon. This change would most likely result in a more efficient translation of the DHFR gene in *E. coli* strain 1810. This, together with the more efficient promoter, would explain the overproduction of DHFR. The nucleotide sequence of the strain 1810 DHFR structural gene was identical to that of *E. coli* K12 with nine exceptions, two of which resulted in amino acid changes. At amino acid position 30, glycine was substituted for tryptophan, and at position 154 glutamine occurred instead of glutamate. Neither of these changes are thought to significantly interfere with enzyme function (FLENSBURG and SKOLD 1987). Of the seven base changes that did not alter the amino acid sequence of the overproduced DHFR compared to the *E. coli* K12 enzyme, five resulted in codons that are more commonly used in highly expressed proteins and that correspond to tRNA species that are more abundant in the cell (GOUY and GAUTIER 1982). Thus, the selective pressure of antifolates seems to have resulted in the evolution of a mutated DHFR gene with a more efficient promoter and one capable of more efficient translation than its *E. coli* K12 counterpart.

These observations closely compared with those of SMITH and CALVO (1982) and SMITH et al. (1982), who constructed recombinant plasmids carrying mutagenized *E. coli fol* genes. Sequence analysis showed that 11 of 12 promoter mutations occurred in the −35 region (C→T transitions) and resulted in greater homology of the *fol* promoter sequence with the consensus *E. coli* promoter sequences. SMITH et al. (1982) speculate that the closer homology to the consensus sequence will result in more efficient initiation of mRNA synthesis by RNA polymerase. These transitions all resulted in promoter-up mutations leading to an increase in *fol* mRNA of about 15-fold. This result agrees closely with the aforementioned findings of FLENSBURG and SKOLD (1984, 1987), who studied a Tp-resistant clinical isolate of *E. coli* that had presumably undergone a spontaneous mutation.

In conclusion, chromosomally mediated resistance to Tp in clinically isolated gram-negative bacteria is not very common, despite the fact that co-trimoxazole

Table 1. Mechanisms of chromosomally mediated resistance to trimethoprim

Type of resistance mechanism	Organisms involved	References
Acquired		
Mutation to thymine auxotrophy	Many species, including *S. aureus*	MASKELL et al. (1977) GILLIGAN et al. (1987)
Mutation to decreased permeability	*Serratia, Klebsiella* and *Enterobacter*	TAUB and KLEBER (1977) GUTMANN et al. (1985)
Mutation in DHFR structural gene	Many species	SHELDON (1977) SMITH et al. (1982)
Increased synthesis of DHFR	*E. coli, K. aerogenes P. vulgaris, P. mirabilis*	SHELDON and BRENNER (1976) SMITH and CALVO (1982) STEEN and SKOLD (1985) FLENSBURG and SKOLD (1987)
Intrinsic		
Inherently insensitive DHFR	*Neisseria, Brucella, Bacteroides, Clostridium, Nocardia, Candida, Trypanosoma cruzi*	AVERETT et al. (1979) Then (1982)
Cell envelope impermeability	*Ps. aeruginosa*	BURCHALL et al. (1982) SCUDAMORE and GOLDNER (1982) WERNER and GOETH (1984)

has been widely used for over 18 years. Studies on Tp-resistant bacterial mutants isolated in the laboratory as well as those occasional resistant strains found in clinical material suggest the existence of at least four distinct mechanisms of resistance: (1) a mutation to thymine auxotrophy, (2) overproduction of the target enzyme, DHFR, (3) presence of an altered chromosomally specified DHFR which has a decreased affinity for Tp and (4) decreased outer membrane permeability to Tp (as well as nalidixic acid and chloramphenicol), a mechanism apparently limited to certain strains of *Enterobacter, Klebsiella* and *Serratia* (Table 1).

Due to the small number of thorough and/or reliable surveys, it is very difficult to say which of the four mechanisms of chromosomally mediated resistance is the most prevalent among clinical bacterial isolates. Two studies, one done in the UK (GREY et al. 1979) and the other in Finland (THEN and HERMANN 1981), suggest that the most common mutational mechanism is the production of an altered, Tp-insensitive DHFR, produced either in normal or slightly elevated amounts. Such mutants were found among clinical isolates of *P. mirabilis, K. aerogenes* and *E. coli.* It is interesting to note that, in this relatively small collection of strains, several mechanisms of resistance occur, sometimes singly, but sometimes simultaneously within one strain. Thus, strains have been characterized that contain an altered, as well as overproduced, chromosomal DHFR. It is also likely that impaired penetration is often involved in addition to alterations in the level of DHFR synthesis and/or enzyme structure; however, this possibility has not been thoroughly documented (THEN 1982). In addition, THEN and HERMANN (1981) described three *P. mirabilis* strains that harbored a plasmid-borne resistant DHFR as well as an altered chromosomal reductase. The authors speculate that mutation to low-level Tp insensitivity was the first to occur, followed by the acquisition of an R plasmid conferring high-level Tp resistance. This sequence of events is perhaps made more likely in hospital environments in which antibiotic pressure is most intense. What is not speculation, however, is the fact that many clinically important gram-negative bacteria have responded to the increasing use of trimethoprim with a variety of mutational responses.

V. Trimethoprim Resistance in *Staphylococcus aureus*

Tp resistance in *Staphylococcus aureus* can be chromosomally mediated (LEWIS and LACEY 1973; LACEY 1975) or can be encoded by large R plasmids (see last section of this chapter). In the majority of multiresistant *S. aureus* recently isolated in Australia, the determinants for resistance to clindamycin, erythromycin, fusidic acid, penicillin, rifampicin, streptomycin, tetracycline, and low-level Tp resistance were found to be chromosomally situated (LYON et al. 1984a; GILLESPIE and SKURRAY 1986). As in the gram-negative bacteria, chromosomal and plasmid-specified Tp resistance can often be distinguished on the basis of MICs (LYON and SKURRAY 1987). Unlike the situation in gram-negatives, however, the mechanisms of chromosomally mediated Tp resistance in *S. aureus* are not well understood.

Perhaps the best understood, and most clinically significant, chromosomal resistance mechanisms is the mutation to thymidine (thymine) auxotrophy. Although most strains of *S. aureus* are exquisitely susceptible to Tp/SMX (ELWELL et al. 1986), several investigators (HOWDEN 1981; SPARHAM et al. 1978) have described the emergence of thymidine-requiring strains of *S. aureus* in cystic fibrosis (CF) patients during or after therapy with Tp/SMX. Recently, GILLIGAN et al. (1987) conducted a 1-year survey of the prevalence of thy^- *S. aureus* in patients in two CF centers in the US. Of 200 CF patients who had their respiratory secretions cultured, 95 harbored *S. aureus*, and 20 (21%) had thy^- mutants as their predominant staphylococcal isolate. All 20 of these patients had received Tp/SMX for an average of 31 months. The authors speculate that the survival of these mutant organisms in the lungs of CF patients is not surprising because the bronchial secretions in these patients are purulent and contain many microscopic, deteriorating cells. In addition, the ability of *S. aureus* to synthesize DNase would faciliate their survival by insuring sufficient levels of thymidine in their microenvironment. Presumably, these levels are in excess of 5 μg/ml since STOKES and LACEY (1978) have shown that thy^- *S. aureus* strains undergo thymineless death in vitro at thymidine concentrations of less than 5 μg/ml.

The precise role these Tp/SMX-resistant *S. aureus* mutants play in pulmonary disease of CF patients has not been established. In the meantime, laboratories in CF centers in which Tp/SMX is used as a long-term prophylactic agent should be on the look-out for these resistant organisms.

VI. Intrinsic Resistance

1. Inherently Resistant Dihydrofolate Reductase

Among the bacterial and fungal species in which susceptibility to Tp has been reported, some have relatively high MICs (THEN 1982). These species, including *Neisseria, Brucella, Bacteroides, Clostridium, Candida,* and *Nocardia*, appear to be naturally more resistant to Tp (but not necessarily resistant to the sulfonamides or combination Tp/SMX). These organisms have been shown to contain DHFRs that are relatively insensitive to Tp, often more than 100-fold less susceptible to Tp than the DHFR of *E. coli* B or K12 (THEN 1982; AVERETT et al. 1979).

2. Nonspecific Cell Envelope Impermeability

Impermeability no doubt explains the observed resistance of *Ps. aeruginosa* to Tp as well as the insensitivity of most bacteria (except lactic acid bacteria) to methotrexate. *Ps. aeruginosa* strains generally have Tp MICs in the range of 100–500 μg/ml and yet harbor DHFRs as sensitive as those of *E. coli* (BURCHALL 1973). In addition, permeability mutants of *Ps. aeruginosa* have been shown to have significantly lower Tp MICs than their wild-type counterparts (WERNER and GOETH 1984). Thus, drug impermeability has been invoked to explain high-level Tp resistance in *Ps. aeruginosa* although conclusive experiments measuring the uptake of radiolabeled drug have not been performed (or at least published). For a somewhat contrary view regarding the contribution of the outer-membrane barrier towards intrinsic antibiotic resistance in *Ps. aeruginosa*, the reader is referred to SCUDAMORE and GOLDNER (1982).

VII. R-Plasmid Resistance in Gram-Negative Organisms

1. Introduction

Trimethoprim-resistant gram-negative bacteria were detected shortly after the introduction of the combination Tp/SMX in the UK in 1969 and in France in 1971. As discussed in the previous section, Tp-resistant clinical strains have been isolated in which one or a combination of chromosomal mutations have been implicated in their resistance. However, the mechanism of greatest clinical importance with respect to Tp resistance among pathogenic gram-negative bacteria is the acquisition of R plasmids (BURCHALL et al. 1982). R plasmids that mediated high-level resistance to Tp were first described by FLEMING et al. (1972). Tp-resistant R plasmids encode additional DHFRs with lower affinities for Tp than that of the bacterial chromosomal enzyme. Characterization of the DHFR content of cells containing the R plasmids, R483 (SKOLD and WIDH 1974) or R388 (AMYES and SMITH 1974), showed that each strain contained a DHFR with a lower affinity for Tp. Further characterization of these and other drug-resistant enzymes resulted in the identification of two types of DHFR on the basis of their differing affinities for several reductase inhibitors (PATTISHALL et al. 1977). In addition to these two distinct types of R plasmid-encoded reductases, a third type of DHFR has also been very well characterized (JOYNER et al. 1984). Other candidates for

Table 2. Comparison of R-plasmid dihydrofolate reductases to the *E. coli* chromosomal enzyme

Dihydrofolate reductase	Source	Tp MIC	Molecular weight		DHF K_m (μM)	Tp K_i (μM)
			Native	Denatured		
Chromosomal	J5-3	0.2	18000	18000	2.7	0.0004
Type I	R483	>1000	35000	17577	5.6	6.4
Type II	R67	>2000	34000	8444	4.1	6100
Type III	pAZ1	64	16900	16900	0.4	0.019
Type IV	pUK1123	160	46700	nd	37	0.063

distinct DHFRs include the incompletely characterized enzymes produced by plasmids pUK1123 (YOUNG and AMYES 1986a) and pLM020 (SUNDSTROM et al. 1987).

Bacteria containing plasmids such as R483 or R388, which specify the type I and II enzymes respectively, are inhibited by Tp only at very high concentrations, (MICs greater than 1 mg/ml, see Table 2). Bacterial strains having a high Tp MIC were thus considered likely to contain plasmids carrying the type I or the type II DHFR genes. Another criterion used for distinguishing these enzymes from the bacterial chromosomal enzyme was that they were approximately twice as large (Table 2). It is also possible to differentiate these enzymes by differences in cross-reactivity to antibodies directed against the bacterial, type I, or type II protein (FLING and ELWELL 1980). Because some of these methods involve time-consuming techniques such as purifying the enzyme or antibody production, the detection of plasmid DHFR genes by DNA-DNA hybridization procedures has permitted the identification of the type I or type II DHFR in many naturally occurring clinical isolates. The DNA probes that have been used will be described later (Sect. B.VII.6).

2. Type I Dihydrofolate Reductase

Initially, biochemical criteria were used to identify different types of enzymes. The type I enzyme binds Tp poorly, exhibiting a *Ki* of 6.4 μM, a value about 10000 times higher than that shown by the *E. coli* chromosomal enzyme (Table 2). Bacterial strains containing a plasmid encoding this enzyme have a Tp MIC of 1000–2000 µg/ml. The type I enzyme consists of a dimer of two identical subunits (FLING and ELWELL 1980; NOVAK et al. 1983) that have a calculated molecular weight of 17577 (FLING and RICHARDS 1983). Thus, the subunit of the type I enzyme is comparable in size to the monomeric *E. coli* enzyme. The amino acid sequences of the type I subunit and the *E. coli* monomer have been aligned on the basis of their 40% amino acid sequence homology (Fig. 3) (FLING and RICHARDS 1983). The type I DHFR gene is present on transposon Tn7, a 14 kb transposon whose role in the dissemination of Tp resistance will be discussed later (Sect. C.IV).

```
                                10                  20                  30
                  * * * * * *   *   *     * *     *     * *     *   *
TYPE III      M L I S L I A A L A H N N L I G K D N L I P W H L P A D L R
E. COLI         M I S L I A A L A V D R V I G M E N A M P W N L P A D L A
N. GONO     M L K I T I I A A C A E N L C I G A G N A M P W H I P E D F A
TYPE I        M K L S L M V A I S K N G V I G N G P D I P W S A K G E Q L

                                40                  50
                * * *   * *   * * *   * * *   *   * *   *     * * * * *
TYPE III      H F K A V T L G K P V V M G R R T F E S I G - R P L P G R R
E. COLI       W F K R N T L N K P V I M G R H T W E S I G - R P L P G R K
N. GONO       F F K V Y T L G K P V I M G R K T W E S L P V K P L P G R R
TYPE I        L F K A I T Y N Q W L L V G R K T F E S M G - - A L P N R K

              60                    70                  80
              *   *   * *                   *         *       * * *
TYPE III      N V V V S R N P - Q W Q A I G V E V A P S L D A A L A L L T
E. COLI       N I I L S S Q P - G T D D R - V T W V K S V D E A I A A C G
N. GONO       N I V I S R Q A D Y C A A G - A E T V A S L E V A L A L C A
TYPE I        Y A V V T R S S F T S D N E N V L I F P S I K D A L T N L K

                90                   100                 110
                      *         * * *     *         *   *     *     *   *
TYPE III      D C E - E A M I I G G G Q L Y A E A L P R A D R L Y L T Y I
E. COLI       D V P - E I M V I G G G R V Y E Q F L P K A Q K L Y L T H I
N. GONO       G A E - E A V I M G G A Q I Y G Q A M P L A T D L R I T E V
TYPE I        K I T D H V I V S G G G E I Y K S L I D Q V D T L H I S T I

                 120                 130                 140
              *       * * *     * *           *                   *
TYPE III      D A Q L N G D T H F P D Y L S L G W Q E L E R S T H P A D D
E. COLI       D A E V E G D T H F P D Y E P D D W E S V F S E F H D A D A
N. GONO       D L S V E G D A F F P E I D R T H W R E A E R T E R R V S S
TYPE I        D I E P E G D V Y F P E I - P S N F R P V F T - Q D F A S N

                 150                 160
                        *   *
TYPE III      K N S Y A C E F V T L S R Q R         162
E. COLI       Q N S H S Y C F E I L E R R           159
N. GONO       K G - V A Y T F V H Y L G K           162
TYPE I        - - - I N Y S Y Q I W Q K G           157
```

Fig. 3. Amino acid sequences of the plasmid type III, *E. coli*, *N. gonorrhoeae*, and plasmid type I DHFRs. The alignment is based on maximizing homology between each sequence and the *E. coli* enzyme using as guidelines the positions of the conserved residues and alignments described by VOLZ et al. (1982) and FLING and RICHARDS (1983). *Dashes* indicate gaps in the alignments imposed to increase identity. The residues that are shared by at least three of the four alignments are indicated by an *asterisk*

3. Type II Dihydrofolate Reductase

The presence of a type II enzyme in bacteria results in an MIC of greater than 2000 μg/ml Tp (Table 2). Type II enzymes are the least sensitive to Tp; a typical Ki is about 6100 μ*M*. The type II enzyme encoded by plasmid R67 is a tetramer consisting of four identical subunits with a subunit molecular weight of 8444 (SMITH et al. 1979; STONE and SMITH 1979). The R67 enzyme bears no obvious sequence similarity to any known DHFR (STONE and SMITH 1979). The DNA sequence of the type II DHFR genes from plasmids R67, R388, and R751 has been determined (BRISSON and HOHN 1984; FLENSBURG and STEEN 1986; SWIFT et al. 1981; ZOLG and HANGGI 1981). The three type II DHFR gene products all have 78 residues and are highly related, having an overall identity of 72% (Fig. 4).

```
       *                     * * *   *     *     * * * *
R67    M E R S S N E V S N P V A G N F V F P S N A T F G M
R388   M G Q S S D E A N A P V A G Q F A L P L S A T F G L
R751   M D Q H N N G V S T L V A G Q F A L P S H A T F G L

       * * * * * * * * * * * * * * *   * * * *   *   * * *
R67    G D R V R K K S G A A W Q G Q I V G W Y C T N L T P
R388   G D R V R K K S G A A W Q G Q V V G W Y C T K L T P
R751   G D R V R K K S G A A W Q G Q V V G W Y K T K L T P

       * * * * * * * *   * * * * * * * * * * * * * * *
R67    E G Y A V E S E A H P G S V Q I Y P V A A L E R E N
R388   E G Y A V E S E S H P G S V Q I Y P V A A L E R V A
R751   E G Y A V E S E S H P G S V Q I Y P V A A L E R V A
```

Fig. 4. Amino acid sequences of the type II DHFRs. The deduced amino acid sequences of the type II DHFR genes from plasmids R67, R388, and R751 are aligned. Each of the proteins contains 78 amino acid residues, and maximal homology involved no gaps. Identical residues in all three enzymes are indicated with an *asterisk* above the sequence

4. Type III Dihydrofolate Reductase

The type III DHFR encoded by plasmid pAZ1 confers a moderate Tp MIC. Plasmid pAZ1 is a non-conjugative plasmid that can be mobilized, and it confers upon its host a Tp MIC of around 64 µg/ml (ANDERSON 1980; FLING et al. 1982). This enzyme has a Ki of 0.019 µ*M*, only 50-fold different from the Ki of 0.0004 µ*M* characteristic of the chromosomal, Tp-sensitive enzyme (Table 2) (JOYNER et al. 1984). Several lines of evidence indicate that the *E. coli* and the type III enzymes are related. Unlike the plasmid types I and II enzymes, the type III DHFR is a monomer. In this respect it is more similar to the bacterial DHFRs. The gene has been cloned and sequenced (FLING et al. 1988). The polypeptide deduced from the DNA sequence had 162 amino acids residues, 50% of which are identical to those of the 159 residue *E. coli* chromosomal enzyme. Alignment of the type III protein with the type I, *E. coli* and *Neisseria gonorrhoeae* DHFRs clearly shows that the type III protein is most highly related to the *E. coli* enzyme (Fig. 3). It bears no apparent relationship to the type I enzyme. It is possible that other type III enzymes are present in strains that have MICs of approximately 256–500 µg/ml (TOWNER and PINN 1981; TOWNER 1983; OBASEIKI-EBOR et al. 1986).

5. Other Dihydrofolate Reductases

Several recently described plasmid DHFRs have properties that suggest they may be significantly different from the type I, II, and III enzymes described above; however, these presumably novel reductases have not been well characterized. The so-called type IV enzyme encoded by plasmid pUK1123 is only slightly resistant to Tp; its MIC is 160 µg/ml (YOUNG and AMYES 1986a). The Tp *Ki* for this enzyme is similar to that of the type III (Table 2); yet the enzyme is more than twice as large as the type III enzyme. In fact, it is considerably larger than any known DHFR except the bacteriophage T4 enzyme. A thorough physical characterization of the protein has not yet been made. An additional feature that distinguishes this enzyme is its inducibility. When bacteria containing pUK1123 are grown in increasing levels of Tp, increasing amounts of DHFR are produced, even though cell viability is greatly reduced at concentrations of Tp at 160 μg/ml. This kind of inducibility has not been observed with other plasmid enzymes. Production of this enzyme also seems to be sensitive to the presence of methionine, adenosine, and glycine in the medium (YOUNG et al. 1986).

The DHFR encoded by plasmid pLM020 (SUNDSTROM et al. 1987) is possibly another example of a new DHFR. In this case, the Tp MICs produced by the plasmid are consistent with the presence of a type I or a type II enzyme. In vitro, this enzyme is approximately 10-fold more sensitive to Tp than is a typical type I DHFR. Even though the kinetics were most similar to those of a type I enzyme, plasmid pPLM020 did not hybridize to a type I DNA probe when stringent conditions were used. Hybridization between pLM020 and the type III gene has not been tested. Hybridization to a 1.77 kb type II DNA probe from R388 was positive; however, a 275 bp probe specific for the 3′ end of the R388 structural gene did not hybridize to the cloned Tp resistance determinant. The authors concluded that the pLM020 enzyme was not typical of type I, type II, or type III enzymes. The possibility that the determinant is a type III- or type I-variant DHFR gene should be considered, since the Tp inhibition kinetics are only about 10-fold different from a type I enzyme. Furthermore, discrimination by DNA-DNA hybridization is limited to about 80% homology when conducted under stringent conditions. Hybridization using low stringency conditions and the type I and type III probes or DNA sequencing will better reveal whether the pLM020 DHFR gene is novel or a member of a family of type I or type III DHFR genes. Regardless of the type of DHFR gene residing on plasmid pLM020, the hybridization results obtained with the larger R388 probe suggest that plasmid evolution has taken some surprising and interesting turns in these plasmids. These results will be discussed in more detail later in the chapter (Sect. B.VII.8.b).

6. Detection of Plasmid-Borne Dihydrofolate Reductase Genes

The usefulness of studying antimicrobial genes using DNA probes has been recently reviewed (TENOVER 1986). A variety of DNA probes has been used to detect type I and II DHFR genes as well as Tn*7* sequences. Thus, DATTA et al. (1980b) have used ColEI : Tn*7* probes and other investigators have used similar constructs (e.g., plasmid pFE506; FLING and ELWELL 1980) (Fig. 5). An inherent problem with these probes is that false positives can arise by hybridization of the ColEI DNA sequences of the probe with ColEI-related, naturally occurring R plasmids. In addition, gene *aad*A sequences (encoding the streptomycin/spectinomycin-inactivating enzyme) of Tn*7* can hybridize with similar, commonly occurring sequences in R plasmids specifying streptomycin resistance. With respect to detecting Tn*7* per se, the problem has been somewhat alleviated by cutting the target DNA with *Hin*dIII. The presence of Tn*7* is inferred by the appearance of two distinctive *Hin*dIII bands (Fig. 5). The 2.2 kb *Hin*dIII fragment has been used successfully as a radiolabeled probe for the presence of Tn*7* (DATTA et al. 1980b). PULKKINEN et al. (1984) have studied the distribution of Tn*7* using either a 5.0 kb *Eco*RI-*Bam*HI fragment or a 1.0 kb *Bam*HI fragment of the transposon as probes for *Hin*dIII-digested target DNA. Another way of avoiding problems of non-specific hybridization has been to use the 2.7 kb AvaI fragment whose only resistance

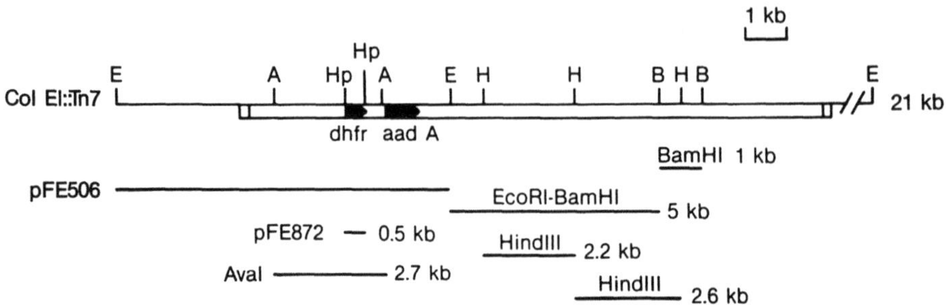

Fig. 5. Restriction endonuclease map of ColE1::Tn7. The *open box* indicates the Tn7 portion, and the *thin line* indicates the ColE1 portion of the plasmid. The position and direction of transcription of the DHFR and *aad*A genes are indicated by the *solid arrows inside the box*. DNA fragments that have been used as hybridization probes or targets are indicated below the restriction map. They are identified using the same designation that appeared in the literature reference (see text). The restriction enzymes are abbreviated as *E*=*Eco*RI, *A*=*Ava*I, *Hp*=*Hpa*I, *H*=*Hind*III, and *B*=*Bam*HI

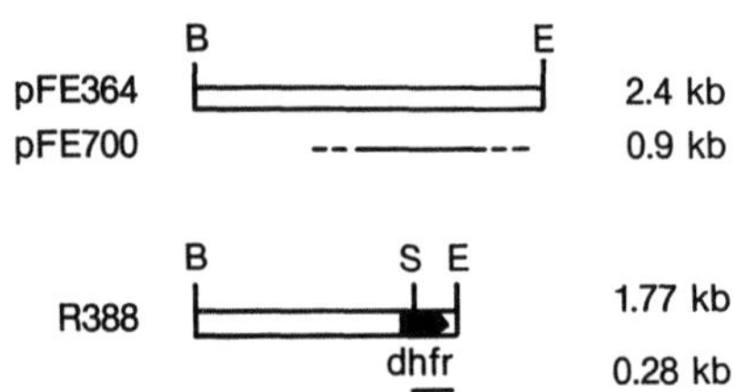

Fig. 6. Restriction endonuclease maps of DNA fragments carrying type II DHFR genes. The location and orientation of the R388 DHFR gene is indicated by the *solid arrow*. Portions that have been subcloned or isolated for use as hybridization probes are indicated by a *thin line below the open box*. The restriction enzymes are abbreviated as *E*=*Eco*RI, *B*=*Bam*HI, *S*=*Sau*3A

marker is the DHFR gene (STEEN and SKOLD 1985) (Fig. 5). A very precise probe for the type I DHFR structural gene is a 499 bp Hpal fragment that can be excised from plasmid pFE872 (FLING and RICHARDS 1983) (Fig. 5).

For the detection of type II DHFR genes, probes have been derived from both of the naturally occurring plasmids R67 and R388. The base sequence homology is 78% within the structural genes. One of the R67-derived probes is a 2.4 kb *Eco*RI-*Bam*HI fragment cloned into pBR322 (plasmid pFE364, FLING and ELWELL 1980) (Fig. 6). A smaller derivative of pFE364 is P700 which contains an 890 bp fragment that was cloned from a partial Sau3A digest (FLING et al. 1982). The precise location of P700 within pFE364 is not known, but the approximate position is shown in Fig. 6. A 1.77 kb *Eco*RI-*Bam*HI fragment of plasmid R388 has also been used as a type II probe. SUNDSTROM et al. (1987) encountered a problem with false-positives using this R388-derived probe when they studied the pLMO plasmids. When they used the very small 275 bp *Sau*3A-*Eco*RI fragment containing only the distal two-thirds of the structural gene (Fig. 6), they avoided the false-positive hybridization result obtained with the larger probe. A similar problem could exist for the pFE364 probe; restriction data suggest that there is similarity between R67 and R388 in the region that provided the hybridization. Plasmid P700 might also include some of the common region which gave rise to false-positive hybridizations. However, there is little DNA sequence homology immediately proximal or distal to the genes. A probe that will be specific for the R67 DHFR gene has been developed by cloning a 277 bp fragment that contains the structural gene and 39 bases upstream. It will also be 78% identical to the R388 DHFR gene and 77% identical to the R751 DHFR gene.

A cloned 822 bp fragment from plasmid pAZ1 encodes the type III structural DHFR gene (FLING et al. 1988). This fragment may be used as a probe for the detection of other type III DHFR genes. It is possible to hybridize the type III probe with the cloned *E. coli* chromosomal DHFR gene under conditions of low stringency, a strategy that produces a faint band on autoradiographs (J. KOPF, unpublished observation).

It is now quite clear that high-level Tp resistance (MICs of 1 mg/ml or higher) can no longer be considered the hallmark of plasmid involvement since the types III and IV DHFR determinants confer only modest resistance upon their host bacterium. On the other hand, a strain like *E. coli* 1810 does not harbor a Tp-resistant R plasmid, or a transposon; yet, it has a high Tp MIC (greater than 1 mg/ml). Strain 1810 was found to have an increased cellular number of DHFR molecules due to a single base substitution in the *fol* promoter. An additional pitfall to the correct interpretation of phenotypic data is that Tn*7* readily transposes into many gram-negative chromosomes. Thus, one can isolate a bacterium with high-level Tp resistance that specifies a type I DHFR, yet is R plasmid-free. DNA-DNA hybridization studies with appropriate DNA probes are required to provide definitive data regarding the nature of plasmid-associated Tp resistance within clinical isolates. It is prudent, in some cases, to use several techniques in combination with DNA-DNA hybridization to exactly define the mechanisms of resistance.

7. Transposition of Dihydrofolate Reductase Genes

Transposable elements (transposons) are discrete pieces of DNA that can insert at many different, nonhomologous sites in the genomes of prokaryotic and eukaryotic cells (for reviews see SHAPIRO 1983). The transposition process occurs independently of "conventional" homology-dependent recombination mediated by the *rec*A system of the host. The current interest in these elements can be attributed to (1) their ubiquity, (2) their postulated role in the evolution of genomes and organisms, (3) the novel mechanisms underlying the transposition event, (4) the regulatory mechanisms that control transposition frequencies and (5) their usefulness in the genetic analysis and engineering of DNA.

Transposons play an important role in the epidemic spread of antibiotic resistances among pathogenic and non-pathogenic bacterial populations. Transposons that have been identified as carriers of DHFR genes are discussed below.

a) Transposon Tn*7*

Transposon Tn*7* is a 14 kb transposable element that encodes resistance to the antibiotics Tp and streptomycin. It was first detected in Britain among Incl plasmids (e.g., R483, BARTH et al. 1976) and has since been reported in plasmids of several other incompatibility groups including IncM, IncC and IncX (DATTA et al. 1979, 1980a; RICHARDS and NUGENT 1979).

The unique transpositional properties of Tn*7* are one of its most interesting aspects. Most transposons are capable of transposition, in either orientation, to a wide variety of sites on bacteriophage, plasmid, and chromosomal DNA molecules. Tn*7*, however, appears to prefer the *E. coli* chromosome, where it inserts efficiently, in a single orientation and at a single site; minute 82 between markers *glm* S and *unc* A (LICHTENSTEIN and BRENNER 1981). Tn*7* also transposes efficiently into the chromosomes of *Ps. aeruginosa*, *K. aeruginosa*, and *A. tumefaciens* (LICHTENSTEIN and BRENNER 1981). Nothing is known about the insertional preferences of Tn*7* (if any) in these particular genomes. Tn*7* is an unusually large transposon (14 kb) harboring two resistance genes on its left-hand flank and its transposition functions in an extensive (6–7.4 kb) internal region (Fig. 5) (FLING and RICHARDS 1983; ROGERS et al. 1986; SMITH and JONES 1984; GOSTI-TESTU et al. 1983; OUARSTI et al. 1985; MCKOWN et al. 1987). Like other transposons, Tn*7* contains terminal inverted repeats, 28 bp in length. In addition, each end contains regions (22 bp long) that occur several times in the same orientation and that are highly conserved with more than 75% homology (LICHTENSTEIN and BRENNER 1982). These direct repeats were found to be contiguous on the right-hand end of Tn*7*, but at the left-hand end they are separated by sequences not found at the other end. This asymmetry at the ends of Tn*7* has been invoked as a possible explanation for the unique orientation at its insertion site (OUARTSI et al. 1985).

b) Transposon Tn*4132*

A 3.2 kb transposon, Tn*4132*, specifying a type I-like DHFR, has been reported by YOUNG and AMYES (1983, 1985). The enzyme associated with Tn*4132* shares many biochemical features with the type I DHFR, but its molecular weight, estimated by gel chromatography, is only 24000 compared to 35000, the size of a typical type I enzyme. Transposition of Tn*4132* into plasmid RP4 was inferred by the resultant increase in molecular mass of the recipient molecule. This transposon has not been physically characterized or systematically compared to Tn*7*.

c) Other Transposons: Tn*402* and Tn*735*

The type II gene of R751 is present on transposon Tn*402*, a 6 kb transposon that has no other markers (SHAPIRO and SPORN 1977). Transposon Tn*402* has a very low frequency of insertion into other replicons. Another transposon that carries a Tp resistance gene is the 13.7 kb transposon Tn*735* (NUGENT et al. 1982). A 2.7 kb *Hin*dIII fragment that expresses the gene has been cloned (M. E. NUGENT, personal communication). The cloned fragment hybridized with pFE364, a derivative plasmid containing a type II DHFR gene (M. FLING, unpublished observation).

8. Origin and Evolution of Plasmid Dihydrofolate Reductase Genes

a) Origin and Evolution of Plasmid Type I Dihydrofolate Reductase Genes

A comparison of the type I DHFR to other DHFRs does not show any special relationship to any other enzyme (Fig. 4). In particular, the subunit structure of the type I enzyme sets it apart from the bacterial DHFRs as well as the type III plasmid DHFR. The only other enzyme that is a dimer is the T4 bacteriophage enzyme. Amino acid sequence identity is very low (18%) between these two enzymes.

The type I DHFR gene is usually, if not always, found associated with Tn*7*. Since many transposons identical or very similar to Tn7 have been isolated from plasmids that are not related to each other (BARTH and DATTA 1977; DATTA et al. 1979; TIETZE et al. 1982) and from bacterial chromosomes (KRAFT et al. 1986; TOWNER 1981), it seems apparent that Tn*7* is a stable element. Only one altered Tn7 (Tn*1825*) has been described in which it appeared that the DHFR gene was substituted by a streptothricin-resistance determinant (TSCHAPE et al. 1984; TIETZE et al. 1987). Restriction site differences involving one of the two distinct *Hin*dIII sites have also been reported. However, the main body of evidence convincingly supports the conclusion that Tn7 is a stable DNA element.

b) Origin and Evolution of Type II Dihydrofolate Reductase Genes

The DNA sequence of several type II DHFR genes has been determined. The considerable similarity displayed by these three type II enzymes (Fig. 4) points to a common ancestral gene and subsequent divergent evolution. Homology between any two enzymes varies from 77% to 85% with the R388- and R751-derived DHFRs being the most similar pair. Most of the differences occur in the first 20 residues. From the crystal structure of the R67 enzyme, we know that the subunits interact in the apoenzyme as dimers (MATTHEWS et al. 1986). These interactions as well as cofactor binding are thought to involve the internal residues. Conservation is therefore a strong force for the central region. Although the three known sequences of the type II DHFRs are highly conserved, this class of enzyme has no DNA sequence or structural similarity to any other known DHFR. An intriguing similarity between the crystal structures of the R67 enzyme and papain has been noted; however, no sequence homology was apparent (MATTHEWS et al. 1986). Speculation about the origin of these apparently unique genes has been considerable (see "Conclusion"), but no convincing evidence in support of any one theory has materialized.

Resistance to the sulfonamides, which have now been in use for more than four decades, is widespread. Depending on the species and geographical location, from 20% to over 40% of strains isolated from clinical material are resistant to the sulfonamides (HAMILTON-MILLER 1979). Thus, the use of combination therapy, Tp plus SMX, essentially guarantees the evolution of linked Tp-sulfonamide (Su) resistance determinants. Plasmid-mediated Su resistance is analogous to the mechanism of Tp resistance in that sulfonamide-resistant R plasmids encode altered dihydropteroate synthases (WISE and ABOU-DONIA 1975). Two different classes of Su-resistant dihydropteroate synthases have been described (types I and II; SWEDBERG 1987). In plasmids such as R388, the type II DHFR gene is tightly

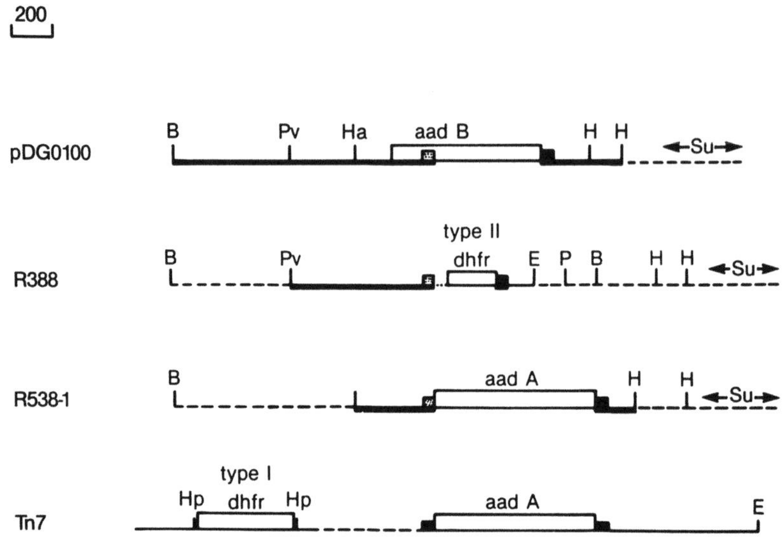

Fig. 7. Restriction endonuclease maps comparing regions of homology among plasmids pDG0100, R388, R538-1, and Tn*7*. *Solid lines, both thick and thin*, indicate regions for which DNA sequence was determined; *dashed lines* indicate regions whose restriction endonuclease maps have been determined. The *thick lines* are identical or nearly identical among all plasmids shown. The *open boxes* identify the known structural genes and their locations. The *small, solid boxes* are elements that are highly homologous or closely related to the 58 bp elements surrounding the Tn*7 aad*A gene. The *small, stippled boxes* represent sequences that retain some partial homology to the 58 bp elements. Abbreviations are *B*= *Bam*HI, *Pv*=*Pvu*II, *Ha*=*Hae*III, *H*=*Hind*III, *P*=*Pst*I, *E*=*Eco*RI, *Hp*=*Hpa*I

linked to a type I Su resistance determinant (Fig. 7). Another plasmid for which this is true is pBWH10 (MAYER et al. 1985; M. FLING, unpublished observation). The linkage of Tp and Su resistance is also suggested by the restriction maps of the FIV plasmids that carry a type II DHFR gene (CAMPBELL and MEE 1987). For plasmid R67 and the determinant of Tn*735*, the proximity or type of Su resistance determinant is unknown. Tn*402* harbors only one resistance determinant, Tp (SHAPIRO and SPORN 1977). Plasmids carrying Tn*7* are also exceptions from the general rule of associated Su resistance, as they do not have a tightly linked Su resistance determinant, and often do not encode Su resistance at all.

The evolution of plasmids such as R388 is likely to be a reflection of the selective pressure of Tp upon plasmids that already have Su resistance genes. Plasmid R388 has two regions that are similar or identical to regions in plasmids pDG0100 and R538-1 (CAMERON et al. 1986; HOLLINGSHEAD and VAPNEK 1985) as revealed by a comparison of the restriction endonuclease maps (Fig. 7). Two other plasmids also have these regions in common, pLM020 (SUNDSTROM et al. 1987) and pSA (TAIT et al. 1985). The common regions are a distal, type I Su resistance gene and a proximal homologous region. In R388, R538-1, pSA, and probably in pLM020, the proximal region is extragenic; however, surprisingly in plasmid pDG0100 it contains much of the amino terminal portion of the *aad*B

```
AACCCTTCCATCGAGGGGGACGTCCAAGGGCTGGCGCCCTTGGCCGCCC-CTCATGTCAAACGTTAGACATCATG aadA gene
AACAATTCATTCAAGCCGACACCGCTT------------CGCGGCGCGG-CTTAATTCAGGAGTTAAACATCATG aadA gene
TATGGAGCAGCAACGATGTTACGCAGC------------AGGGCAGTCGCCCTAAAACAAA-GTTAAACATCATG aadA gene
***************************------------**********************-****GG*CG*ATG aadB gene
***************************------------**********************-****GG*AG*CGT (92 b) ATG dhfr
***************************------------**********************-****GG*TT*ACC (55 b) ATG dhfr

                 CONSENSUS               CCCAANTCAAACGTTAAACNTG
                                          TT T A  GGA    GG  G
```

Fig. 8. Proximal 58 bp element of Tn7. Alignment of the junction sequences of plasmids pSA, R538-1, pDG0100, R388, and R751 to the proximal 58 bp element of Tn7. This region is represented by the *stippled box* in Fig. 7. Each line of DNA sequence represents, in a 5′ to 3′ fashion, the regions corresponding to the Tn7 58 bp element. The alignment was adjusted to maximize the pSA sequence homology to the Tn7 element by inserting a 12 bp gap (*dash*) in the Tn7 and the other sequences. In order to derive the consensus sequence a single base gap was positioned in each sequence as shown. The bases of *aad*B, R388, and R751 that are identical to those in R538-1 are indicated by an *asterisk*

gene product. The proximal homologous region is at least some 380 bp, and, based on the similar restriction maps, might be almost 1 kb in size. It is this region that was apparently involved in the false identification, using the 1.77 kb R388 *Bam*HI-*Eco*RI fragment, of the pLM020 Tp resistance determinant as a type II DHFR gene.

A second element of homology is also involved, namely the directly repeated 58 bp element that is present both immediately 5′ and 3′ to the Tn*7 aad*A gene (Fling et al. 1985) (Fig. 7). This element is seen 3′ to the R388 DHFR gene, the *aad*A gene of plasmids R538-1 and pSA, and the *aad*B gene. Remnants of the 58 bp element are also conserved 5′ to all of these genes (Fig. 8). There is conservation of 50% identity among the last 22 bp of the element. Each of the Tn7 elements is a palindrome. The elements 3′ to the other genes have also retained their palindromic nature. A model for the movement of a gene surrounded by these directly repeated sequences that are also palindromes suggests that the gene can be inserted into a single identical or related element, and that subsequent deletion of the region between any two elements can occur (Wiedemann et al. 1986). In Fig. 9, using this model for modular evolution, the DHFR-Su gene arrangement seen in R388 is derived from a plasmid such as pSA. An alternate model in which *rec*A-dependent recombination via the 380 bp homologous region and the distal Su resistance gene might totally displace the resident *aad*A gene with a different determinant is also feasible. Any determinant residing within the points of recombination could replace the *aad*A gene in this event.

c) Origin and Evolution of the Type III Dihydrofolate Reductase Gene

The type III DHFR gene in plasmid pAZ1 is located very close to a type II Su-determinant; however, the genes are probably convergent (Fling et al. 1988). A model for the origin and evolution of the type III DHFR gene has two aspects. The type III gene probably comes from a gram-negative source closely related to *E. coli*. This assumption is based on the homology exhibited between the type III enzyme and the *E. coli* and *Neisseria* enzymes (Fig. 3). Plasmid pAZ1 belongs to incompatibility group incQ (Hedges 1987). This DHFR gene was inserted into a broad host range incQ plasmid, possibly through a hot spot for recombination.

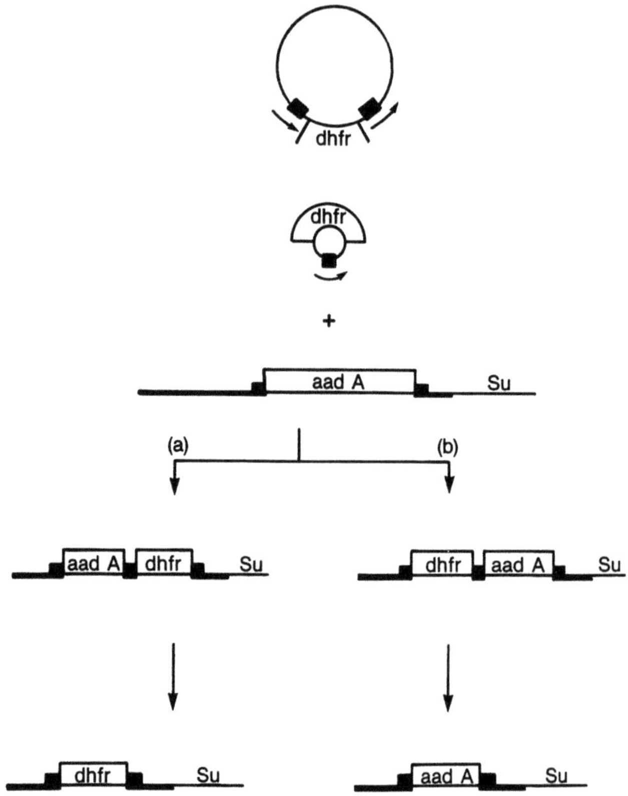

Fig. 9. Model for the modular evolution of resistance determinants. An R plasmid carrying the type II DHFR gene bounded by two directly repeated elements represents the donor molecule. A recipient molecule containing the *aad*A gene and a Su resistance determinant is bounded by the same direct repeats. A *rec*A-independent recombination mechanism would permit the excision of the DHFR gene from the donor and insertion into one of the elements surrounding the *aad*A gene, resulting in the molecules shown in (*a*) or (*b*). Several paths of resolution are possible, depending on which two of the three elements in either molecule are involved. Of the two potential structures shown, the one illustrated in (*a*) would be analogous to the plasmid R388

The similarity of plasmids RSF1010 (BAGDASARIAN et al. 1981) and pAZ1 (FLING et al. 1988) is striking (Fig. 10). The restriction maps of RSF1010 and pFM739, an incQ plasmid from *Neisseria*, are also nearly identical, the difference being that a β-lactamase gene is inserted in pFM739 between the Ava I and Pvu II sites at positions 6.8 kb and 6.9 kb (ROTGER et al. 1986). Among these three plasmids, the only differences appear to be in the right ends. A region important for recombination is suggested by the almost identical positions that the DHFR gene of pAZ1 and the β-lactamase gene of pFM739 occupy with respect to the RSF1010 restriction map. Small plasmids encoding the Su-Sm resistance phenotype are common among the Enterobacteriaceae and have been noted in *Neisseria* and *Pseudomonas* as well (ALBRITTON et al. 1982; BRYAN et al. 1972; BARTH and GRINTER 1974;

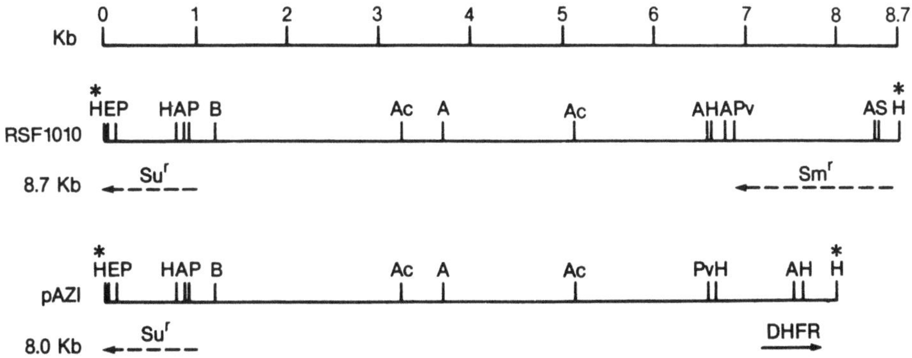

Fig. 10. Comparison of the restriction maps of the incQ plasmids pAZ1 and RSF1010. The restriction maps of both pAZ1 and RSF1010 were determined. The published map of plasmid RSF1010 was revised slightly by repositioning the HpaI/HincII and the HincII sites, as shown. The position and direction of transcription of the type III DHFR gene is indicated by a *solid arrow* labeled Tp. The approximate locations of the sulfonamide (Su) and streptomycin (Sm) resistance determinants are indicated by the *dashed lines*. Abbreviations of restriction enzymes are *A*=*Ava*I, *Ac*=*Acc*I, *B*=*Bst*EII, *E*=*Eco*RI, *H*=*Hinc*II, *H**= *Hpa*I, *P*=*Pst*I, *Pv*=*Pvu*II, *S*=*Sst*I

KORFMANN et al. 1983; BRUNTON et al. 1986). Perhaps it was inevitable to find additional resistance genes, such as Tp-resistant DHFR genes, picked up by this relatively promiscuous class of plasmids after a period of intensive selective pressure.

C. Epidemiology of Trimethoprim Resistance

I. Trimethoprim Resistance in Gram-Negative Organisms

As we mentioned in the "Introduction" to this chapter, Tp resistance among clinical isolates is much more prevalent in developing countries compared to the more industrialized parts of the world. For example, resistance of *E. coli* to Tp/SMX is around 3%–8% at many medical centers within the U.S. (MURRAY et al. 1985); in the UK the incidence is 5.8% among general practice strains (BRUMFITT et al. 1983), and in Sweden the overall frequency of resistance to Tp among enterobacterial strains from UTIs is 3.5% (SELLERS 1982). In contrast, the resistance rate observed among *E. coli* isolated in a pediatric hospital in Santiago, Chile, was 44% and at a general teaching hospital in Bangkok, Thailand, the rate was around 40% (MURRAY et al. 1985). Subsequent investigations in Brazil, Honduras, and Costa Rica suggested that these high resistance rates among clinical *E. coli* strains were not isolated phenomena.

Generalizations about the incidence and dissemination of Tp resistance and Tp-resistant R plasmids are very difficult to make for a variety of reasons. As discussed, the incidence varies greatly from country to country, species to species, and even hospital to hospital. For example, in a Finnish geriatric hospital (Turku City Hospital), 38% of catheter-associated isolates of *E. coli* were found to be Tp-resistant compared to an overall rate of resistance among isolates found in general practice of 4%–10%. Turku City Hospital is known for its heavy use of Tp as a single agent (Tp alone was introduced into clinical use in Finland in 1973) and many of its patients have extended stays (HUOVINEN 1984). These factors help explain the high incidence of resistance in this particular setting. In addition, examination of the incidence of Tp resistance in many areas of the world has been hampered by inappropriate testing procedures (AMYES 1986).

Estimates as to the number of high-level Tp-resistant strains that harbor transferable R plasmids are almost always minimum estimates. This is so because successful conjugation of naturally occurring R plasmids is, in many cases, highly dependent upon the genus of the donor bacterium, the genetic characteristics of the recipient bacterium, the nature of the selective plating medium and the specific mating strategies employed (e.g., conjugation in broth, on membrane filters or in cell pellets) (YOUNG and AMYES 1985; HUOVINEN et al. 1983). This caveat notwithstanding, probably 95% of gram-negative clinical isolates with high-level Tp resistance are resistant by virtue of harboring conjugative or mobilizable R plasmids. The ability of different members of the family Enterobacteriaceae to conjugally transfer Tp resistance varies considerably. Usually, transfer is common among *E. coli* (SELLERS 1982) and uncommon among *Proteus* (HUOVINEN et al. 1983). Resistance transfer among other gram-negative microorganisms such as *Acinetobacter*, *Vibrio* and *Pseudomonas* has also been observed.

In 1980 a new wrinkle appeared in the plasmid-associated Tp resistance picture, that is, low-level (50–100 µg/ml) Tp resistance was shown to be transferable. The implicated plasmid, pAZ1, was 8 kb in molecular mass, non-conjugative but mobilizable, and specified resistances to Tp and Su. It originated in a strain of *S. typhimurium* phage type 179, an organism implicated in epidemics in cattle and sporadic human infections in Great Britain (ANDERSON 1980). Plasmid pAZ1 encodes the prototype type III DHFR (JOYNER et al. 1984). Other, conjugative plasmids that confer low-level Tp MICs upon their recipient hosts have subsequently been described (TOWNER and PINN 1981; TOWNER and WISE 1983; CHIRNSIDE et al. 1985), but the natures of the DHFR genes on these plasmids have yet to be well characterized.

In the following section we present summaries of some recent epidemiological studies of Tp resistance in selected parts of the world.

1. England (London)

a) GRUNEBERG (1984). From 1971–1982 all urinary pathogens sent to a laboratory by general practitioners and all urinary organisms from hospitals in the University College Hospital group were examined. *E. coli* strains represented 340/433 (78%) of general practice strains and 306/552 (55%) of hospital strains. Over this 12-year period, the levels of Tp resistance in *E. coli* increased from 1.5 to 6.6% among the general practice isolates and from 3.2 to 14.3% in the hospital strains.

b) BRUMFITT et al. (1983). Approximately 2700 bacterial strains isolated during 1981 from urine specimens, both from hospitalized patients and general practice, were examined for resistance to Tp. They reported an incidence of 13%

among hospital isolates and 5.8% among general practice strains. The authors noted that the overall incidence of Tp resistance among urinary isolates had changed little since their last survey (1978–1979). What had changed dramatically, however, was the incidence of strains with high-level Tp resistance; 10% in 1975–1977, 60% in 1978–1979 and 78% in 1981.

c) CHIRNSIDE et al. (1985). This survey examined the incidence of Tp resistance and the transferability of that resistance among urinary isolates collected in 1975, 1977, 1979, 1981 and 1983 at Whittington Hospital, London. Overall, Tp resistance remained basically constant, ranging from 9% to 13%. However, between 1975 and 1983, the frequency of transferable, high-level Tp resistance rose from 10% to 40%, caused mainly by increasing numbers of *E. coli* isolates which co-transferred antibiotic resistance to streptomycin and spectinomycin (Tn7?).

2. **Israel** (ALON et al. 1987)

Over 5300 urinary isolates of *E. coli*, "*Klebsiella aerogenes*" and *P. mirabilis* from three medical centers in Haifa, Israel, were examined for resistance to a variety of antibiotics including Tp/SMX. From 1980 to 1985, a gradual increase in Tp/SMX resistance was observed; 63% of the strains from inpatients in 1984 and 51% of those from outpatients in 1985 were resistant to Tp. No significant changes in bacterial susceptibility to cephalosporins and nitrofurantoin were noted over the period studied.

3. **Finland** (HUOVINEN et al. 1986)

Five thousand *E. coli* isolates from urine specimens collected in the Turku City Hospital from 1971–1984 were analyzed. Since 1971, resistance of *E. coli* to Tp/SMX had increased from 8% to around 35% in 1984. The prevalence of DNA sequences in these resistant isolates showing homology with transposon Tn7 sequences was also examined. In 1980–1981, 42% of Tp-resistant *E. coli* isolates showed significant DNA homology with the Tn7 DNA probe, whereas 64% showed similar homology in 1983–1984. Most of these isolates with Tn7-like DNA sequences were unable to conjugally transfer Tp resistance to suitable recipient *E. coli* strains. The authors postulate that these data may indicate the spread of chromosomally situated Tn7 in this particular hospital.

4. **Sweden** (SELLERS 1982)

Tp-alone therapy was registered in Sweden in 1980. A survey of 8986 enterobacterial strains from urinary tract infections was conducted between September, 1980 and June, 1981 in an attempt to discern any shifts in the incidence of Tp resistance as a consequence of the new therapy. The frequency of Tp resistance in *E. coli*, *Klebsiella*, *Enterobacter* and *Citrobacter* ranged from 7.7% in long-term patients to 2.3% in patients from general practice. Transfer frequencies of Tp resistance were similar to those observed in the Finnish isolates; 44% of *E. coli* strains and 22% of the *Klebsiella* strains conjugally transferred their Tp resistance.

5. France (GOLDSTEIN et al. 1986a)

From 1972 to 1984, all Enterobacteriaceae isolated from clinical specimens (73258 strains) at St. Joseph Hospital, Paris, were tested for susceptibility to Tp. During this period, resistance to Tp increased from 18% to 25.5%, the increase being due primarily to strains with high-level resistance. The percentage of strains with high-level resistance increased from 7.2% in 1972 to 34% in 1982 and then decreased to 24% in 1984. Conjugal transfer of resistance was common, varying from 31% of the strains (1974–1975) to 63% (1980–1981). The distribution of the types I and II DHFR genes within 183 strains harboring transferable Tp resistance plasmids was determined using gene-specific DNA probes. Eighty-eight isolates (48%) contained a type I DHFR, 61 (33%) contained a type II reductase, 5 strains (2.7%) apparently harbored both enzymes, and 29 isolates (16%) failed to hybridize with either DNA probe. Type I DHFR was predominant in *E. coli*, *Enterobacter*, and *Serratia*; type II was predominant in *Citrobacter*, *Klebsiella*, and *Proteus*. The distribution was the same in strains isolated from hospitalized patients and those isolates from outpatients.

6. India (AMYES 1986)

The entire clinical enterobacterial population from the Christian Medical Hospital in Vellore, India, was examined from October to December 1984. Sixty-four percent of the urinary enterobacteria were resistant to Tp (MIC greater than 10 μg/ml), whereas 57% of all the strains were highly resistant to Tp (MIC greater than 1000 μg/ml). Fifty-eight (58%) of the high-level Tp-resistant Indian strains were able to conjugally transfer resistance. Interestingly, fewer of the Indian plasmids encoded spectinomycin resistance (55%) compared to United Kingdom plasmids (approximately 80%). The authors postulate that Tn*7*, ubiquitous in the UK, may play a lesser role in the dissemination of Tp resistance in this particular part of India.

II. Trimethoprim Resistance in the Enteric Organisms *Shigella* and *Salmonella*

As mentioned in the "Introduction," Tp resistance in *Shigella* is currently of great concern in certain parts of the world. Up until the late 1970s, Tp-resistance was virtually unknown in clinical isolates of *Shigella*. However, in 1978, BANNATYNE et al. (1980) reported that 3% of *Shigella* strains isolated in Ontario were resistant to Tp. Subsequently, TAYLOR et al. (1980) reported a Tp-resistant strain of *S. sonnei* isolated from a patient who acquired shigellosis in Brazil. This strain harbored a 41 kb conjugative plasmid (pDT200) belonging to incompatibility group N that encoded resistance to Tp, streptomycin, and sulfamethoxazole. Plasmid pDT200 showed significant DNA homology with a type II DHFR gene-specific DNA probe (FLING et al. 1982). Other large, conjugative plasmids capable of transferring Tp resistance from *S. flexneri* have been reported from Brazil (TIEMENS et al. 1984), Thailand (CHATKAEOMORAKOT et al. 1987), and Saudia Arabia (CHINAULT et al. 1986). A *S. flexneri* 2a strain isolated from a patient living in Saudia Arabia was shown to readily transfer its Tp and streptomycin resistance to an *E. coli* recipient. The implicated R plasmid was shown to harbor genes identical to the type I DHFR determinant and the *aad*A gene residing on Tn7 (CHINAULT et al. 1986). In a Korean survey, 85% of the multiply resistant strains were capable of transferring Tp resistance (CHUN et al. 1981). In England and Wales, trimethoprim resistant *Shigella* were first seen in 1979 when they constituted 1.3% of all strains, and by 1983 this number increased to 17%. Interestingly, *Shigella* strains from persons with foreign contacts were less often Tp-resistant than those acquired domestically (GROSS et al. 1984).

Although *Shigella* are usually sensitive to Tp (PANIKER et al. 1978), resistance can increase over a short period of time to include almost all of the population, in contrast to the typical situation with *E. coli*. This phenomenon usually is due to the acquisition by the epidemic strain of a R plasmid that codes for resistance to the chemotherapeutic agents in current use. In Bangladesh, the incidence of Tp resistance among *Shigella* isolates went from 5% in 1979 to 83% in 1983 following the introduction of Tp in 1981 (ZAMAN et al. 1983; SHAHID et al. 1985). The incidence of Tp resistance among clinical isolates in Zaire was also rare until the introduction of Tp. In some medical centers in Zaire, the incidence of Tp resistance is currently 42% (FROST et al. 1982). A detailed analysis of the plasmid content of strains from the African epidemic indicated that a large $IncI_1$ plasmid transferred the Tp resistance determinant (FROST et al. 1985).

In other locations the resistance picture in *Shigella* is quite different. For example, in Spain, *Shigella sonnei* are almost all Tp resistant (89%), but the strain is not an epidemic strain (PALENQUE et al. 1983; LOPEZ-BREA et al. 1983). Resistance was shown to increase sharply in 3 years from 34% to 97%. Transferable Tp resistance could not be demonstrated, and the nature of the resistance determinant was not examined further (LOPEZ-BREA et al. 1983). A similarly high incidence of Tp resistance (83%) was seen among *Shigella flexneri*, *S. boydii*, and *S. sonnei* in a Thai orphanage (CHATKAEOMORAKOT et al. 1987). In slightly over half of the strains, the resistance genes hybridized with type I or type II probes. Almost all of the *S. boydii* and none of the *S. flexneri* or *sonnei* were type I positive. Transferable resistance was infrequently seen, and then only from the type II positive strains. None of the remaining strains (45% of the total) could conjugally transfer their Tp resistance or show homology with types I, II, or III DHFR gene probes.

An extensive survey of *Salmonella* strains of animal and human sources was conducted in the UK between 1970–1981 (THRELFALL et al. 1983). No Tp-resistant *S. typhi* were detected until 1980, and the rate was relatively low (0.4%–0.7%). Strains of *S. typhimurium* resistant to Tp were reported in 1973 (THRELFALL et al. 1980a), and subsequently accounted for 7% of strains of human origin. Subsequently, R plasmids, some of which contained Tn7, were characterized in clinical isolates of *Salmonella* (FINLAYSON and JACKSON 1978; THRELFALL et al. 1983, 1986; RICHARDS et al. 1978; WARD et al. 1982; MURRAY et al. 1985).

A dramatic example of the dissemination of drug resistant pathogenic organisms was the international spread of multiresistant strains of *S. typhimurium* phage types 204 and 193 from Britain to Europe. During 1978 these strains caused numerous outbreaks of salmonellosis in calves on farms throughout the British

Isles (THRELFALL et al. 1978). By 1979, these strains were implicated in over 200 human infections (including one fatality) in the UK, and of these infections 30 occurred in persons on farms where the multiresistant strains had caused outbreaks of salmonellosis among cattle. Eventually, multiresistant strains of *S. typhimurium* phage types 193 and 204 appeared in Belgium presumably by the export of infected calves from Britain (ROWE et al. 1979). One plasmid involved in the phage type 204 epidemic strains specified resistances to ampicillin, chloramphenicol, kanamycin, streptomycin, sulfonamides, tetracycline, and Tp and belonged to incompatibility group I_1. This plasmid was also found in type 204 strains detected in Belgium. As THRELFALL et al. (1983) have pointed out, had these multiresistant *S. typhimurium* strains caused widespread extraintestinal infections in humans, the clinician's choice of antimicrobial treatment would have been severely limited.

In contrast to the propensity of *S. typhimurium* to acquire and disseminate resistance, *S. typhi* seem less likely to acquire Tp resistance (PARAMASIVAN et al. 1977), and even then the determinant seems to be confined to only a few types of plasmids, one of which is of IncHl1 incompatibility group (LING and CHAU 1984; TAYLOR et al. 1985). In one study, the gene was present on transposon Tn*7*; thus, it was probably a type I DHFR (RICHARDS and DATTA 1982). In another, where Tp resistance was detected in 14% of the strains isolated in a 18 month period, it was shown that the resistance determinant was not present on Tn*7* (TAYLOR et al. 1985).

III. Trimethoprim Resistance in Non-enterobacteriaceae

Occasionally, Tp-resistant isolates are encountered among organisms other than Enterobacteriaceae. These organisms include *Acinetobacter* (CAMPBELL et al. 1986; MAYER et al. 1985; GOLDSTEIN et al. 1983b), *Vibrio cholerae* (THRELFALL et al. 1980b; YOUNG and AMYES 1986b; GOLDSTEIN et al. 1986b; MATSUSHITA et al. 1984; FLING et al. 1982; DUPONT et al. 1985), and *Pseudomonas syringae* (LEARY and TROLLINGER 1985).

Isolates of *Acinetobacter* are seldom encountered in samples that are screened for Tp resistance. However, they have been found in the studies from Australia (MEE and NIKOLETTI 1983) and the USA (MAYER et al. 1985). In each location, the plasmids from *Acinetobacter* as well as the *E. coli* were definitively shown to carry the type II DHFR gene. The broader aspects of these studies are described in detail in the following section. A large, self-transmissible plasmid of group Inc 6-C was found in the Tp-resistant *Acinetobacter* isolated in France (GOLDSTEIN et al. 1983b). Hybridization with ColE1::Tn*7* DNA, though positive, was thought to be due only to the presence of *aad*A gene sequences. However, this conclusion was based on the differential hybridization by RNA species transcribed from Tn*7*, and may be subject to more than one interpretation. The incompatibility group 6-C plasmids are frequently found in Saint Joseph's Hospital, Paris, the site from which the Tp-resistant *Acinetobacter* was isolated.

One such Inc6-C R plasmid is R67, from which the first type II Tp-resistant DHFR was detected and characterized (PATTISHALL et al. 1977). Perhaps one of these plasmids found its way into selected members of the *Acinetobacter* genus.

The dissemination of Tp resistance in *Vibrio cholerae* has followed the same dynamics as the dissemination of Tp resistance in other epidemic enteric organisms, such as *Shigella* and *Salmonella*.

Tp resistance was first noted in *Vibrio* in the late 1970s; however, resistance to this drug remains at a relatively low level worldwide (MATSUSHITA et al. 1984). Nonetheless, during some outbreaks, Tp-resistant strains have become the predominant organism. R plasmid involvement in resistance in *Vibrio* spp. is well documented (THRELFALL et al. 1980b; FLING et al. 1982) and Tn*7* has been detected among R plasmids in some isolates (GOLDSTEIN et al. 1986b). In addition, a *Vibrio* plasmid-specified DHFR with biochemical properties and molecular weight very similar to the prototype type I enzyme has been reported (YOUNG and AMYES 1986b).

The discovery of Tp-resistant R plasmids in *Vibrio cholerae* suggests that most gram-negative microorganisms, regardless of their genetic relatedness to *E. coli*, might be candidates for the acquisition of these resistance determinants. What appears to be required is the relatively frequent use of the drug and the existence of broad host range R plasmids harboring a resistant DHFR gene(s) somewhere in the environment.

IV. Role of Transposition in the Dissemination of Plasmid Dihydrofolate Reductase Genes

Of the plasmid DHFR genes, the type I has been most frequently identified as the cause of Tp resistance. Because it can reside on a transposon (Tn*7*) that can have either a plasmid or chromosomal locus, it has a greater propensity for distribution and the potential for greater stability in the gene pool. A number of studies document the dissemination of the type I DHFR gene into many of the plasmid incompatibility groups (BARTH and DATTA 1977; RICHARDS and NUGENT 1979; DATTA et al. 1980a) and show that Tn*7* is the primary mode of dissemination of the type I DHFR gene (DATTA et al. 1979; LABIGNE-ROUSSEL et al. 1982; TIETZE et al. 1982; PULKKINEN et al. 1984; STEEN and SKOLD 1985).

In fact, insertion of Tn*7* into the *E. coli* chromosome occurs at a specific site and in a single orientation (LICHTENSTEIN and BRENNER 1981). Phenotypically, such a strain has nontransferable, high-level Tp resistance. The proportion of enterobacterial isolates with this particular phenotype isolated from the Nottingham area of the UK rose from 4.7% in 1978 to 23% in 1979 (TOWNER et al. 1980). Other recent comparative studies of *E. coli* clinical isolates with high-level Tp resistance also report a significant rise in the number of strains with Tn*7* located exclusively in the chromosome (KRAFT et al. 1986; AMYES et al. 1986). Thus, in some instances, the clinical situation appears to reflect the molecular preference of Tn*7*. Transposon Tn*7* also carries the *aad*A gene which encodes streptomycin/spectinomycin adenyltransferase, a modifying enzyme capable of inactivating the antibiotics streptomycin and spectinomycin. Selection of Tp resistance via the linked *aad*A gene has not been studied.

The type II DHFR gene can also reside on a transposon. The DHFR gene from Tn*402* has been sequenced and shares 77% identity with the R67 DHFR gene (FLENSBURG and STEEN 1986). Transposon Tn*735* probably also has a type

II DHFR gene. However, transposition has not yet been shown to be a significant factor in the dissemination of this particular gene. Dissemination of the type II DHFR seems to occur primarily as a result of its location on plasmids that have a rather broad host range. In some cases, a single plasmid, its close relatives, or a family of related plasmids have been shown to be the primary causes of transmission (MAYER et al. 1985; CAMPBELL et al. 1986). In the latter example, a related series of IncFIV plasmids were seen distributed through various populations. On the basis of a detailed restriction endonuclease analysis, a particular group of these plasmids was postulated to be the transition group for the related, but distinct, plasmid groups from the pig and human populations.

The epidemiology of plasmids carrying the type III, type IV and pLM020 determinants has not yet been examined. There are no data regarding transposition of these determinants, but this fact not withstanding it seems apparent that modular evolution, such as that described in Fig. 10, has played a key role in the selection and arrangement of the resistance determinants on the broad-host range plasmids that carry the type III DHFR genes (and perhaps type II DHFR genes as well?).

D. Mechanism and Epidemiology of Trimethoprim Resistance in Gram-Positive Organisms

Tp, alone or in combination with SMX, has been useful for the therapy and prevention of staphylococcal infections. Tp resistance among gram-positive microorganisms (including *Staphylococcus aureus*, *S. epidermidis*, *S. saprophyticus*, and the enterococci) has been uncommon. In London in 1972, 1.6% of *S. aureus* isolates from hospital sources were resistant to Tp and SMX (NAKHLA 1972). A later study reported similar results, in that 1% of the *S. aureus* strains, both inpatient and outpatient, were resistant to Tp (LEWIS and LACEY 1973). Higher numbers of resistant *S. aureus* were seen in 1977; about 13% of the isolates from a London hospital were resistant to Tp (CHATTOPADHYAY 1977). These resistant strains had MICs of >50 μg/ml, while most of the strains isolated earlier had MICs of <26 μg/ml (LEWIS and LACEY 1973). A later survey (BRUMFITT et al. 1983) reported the incidence of Tp resistance among hospital isolates of *S. aureus* in London to be around 6%.

Other reports included isolates of *S. epidermidis* and *S. saprophyticus*, in addition to *S. aureus* (BRUMFITT et al. 1983; RICHARDSON 1983). An overall resistance frequency of 15% in hospital isolates and 4% in general practice was reported among *S. aureus*, *S. epidermidis*, *S. saprophyticus*, and the enterococci in London (BRUMFITT et al. 1983). No resistance has been reported in *S. saprophyticus*. In contrast, 39% of the *S. epidermidis* strains, the species most frequently isolated, were resistant to Tp. Two surveys, in 1978–1979 and during 1981, showed that resistance levels among *S. epidermidis* isolates had remained essentially constant. RICHARDSON (1983) also reported that the incidence of Tp resistance among gram-positive organisms varied according to species. Thus, among strains of *S. epidermidis* from normal flora, the incidence was about 13%, whereas about 30% of clinical strains of *S. epidermidis* were resistant to >32 μg/

ml Tp whereas all *S. saprophyticus* were sensitive. About 16% of the resistant *S. epidermidis* had Tp MICs >512 μg/ml (RICHARDSON 1983). The reported incidence of Tp resistance in the USA and Canada is 10% for *S. aureus* and 17% for coagulase-negative staphylococci (ARCHER et al. 1986). All of these strains had Tp MICs of >1000 μg/ml, and plasmid-mediated resistance was clearly demonstrated.

Mechanisms of resistance were not investigated in the aforementioned surveys with the exception of the most recent study in which plasmids were responsible for the high level Tp resistance. The fact that some strains had Tp MICs >512 μg/ml suggested plasmid involvement (RICHARDSON 1983). However, it was not shown that plasmids carried Tp resistance until plasmid-mediated Tp resistance was demonstrated among strains of *S. aureus* in Australia (TOWNSEND et al. 1984). Subsequent reports of plasmid-mediated Tp resistance came from Australia (TENNENT et al. 1985), Ireland (COLEMAN et al. 1985), and the USA (ARCHER et al. 1986). In addition to finding Tp resistance on plasmids in gentamicin-resistant *S. aureus* (TOWNSEND et al. 1984), or methicillin-resistant *S. aureus* (COLEMAN et al. 1985), plasmids mediating both Tp and gentamicin resistance were also seen in *S. epidermidis* (ARCHER et al. 1986). Plasmids isolated in Australia and the USA were self-transmissible and carried additional determinants for resistance to quarternary ammonium compounds, ethidium bromide, gentamycin, tobramycin, and kanamycin. The most common plasmid in Australia was found to be approximately 27 kb, whereas, plasmids of 41–55 kb were present in the USA. The plasmids isolated by the different groups have been compared by restriction endonuclease analysis. Plasmids pWG53 (TOWNSEND et al. 1984) and pSK1 (TENNENT et al. 1985) are both about 28 kb and have similar *Eco*RI restriction maps. They differ from the plasmids pGO1 and pGO5 of 50 kb and 55 kb, respectively (ARCHER et al. 1986) with the exception that a small region carrying the Tp resistance determinant seems to be similar by restriction mapping. In Ireland, Tp resistance resided on a plasmid of 33.3 kb that also carried tetracycline, kanamycin, and ethidium bromide resistance (COLEMAN et al. 1985).

Like gram-negative plasmids that mediate Tp resistance, these staphylococcal plasmids encode novel DHFRs that render their host bacterium insensitive to Tp inhibition. A cloned fragment from pGO1, one of the USA staphylococcal plasmids, was used as a probe in hybridization and expression studies (ARCHER et al. 1986; COUGHTER et al. 1987). DNA-DNA hybridization studies at both high and low stringency have shown that the DHFR genes residing on plasmid pGO1 are not closely related to the type I, type II, or type III DHFR genes of gram-negative origin or to the chromosomal genes from staphylococci or *B. subtilis* (ARCHER et al. 1986; COUGHTER et al. 1987). The absence of hybridization under the conditions used indicates that there is less than 70% homology, and therefore a very close relationship probably does not exist with respect to any of the known DHFR genes of gram-negative origin. The IC_{50} of the staphylococcal plasmid protein, now designated the S1 DHFR, is most similar to that of the gram-negative plasmid type III, 1.7 μM compared to 0.65 μM (COUGHTER et al. 1987) (Table 3). Expression of the S1 DHFR in *E. coli*, and analysis of the protein on SDS-polyacrylamide gels, has shown that the protein is about 18500 (COUGHTER et al. 1987) or at most 19700 (LYON and SKURRAY 1987). The size of the cloned

Table 3. Comparison of gram-negative and gram-positive dihydrofolate reductases

Enzyme	Source	IC_{50} (μM)[a]	Tp MIC (μg/ml)
Gram neg.	SK1592	< 0.001 (0.007)[b]	2.5 (0.15)
I	ColE1::Tn7	>1000 (57)	>1000
II	pFE364	>1700 (70000)	>1000
III	pFE1242	0.65 (2.1)	156 (64)
Gram pos.	RN4220	0.038	1
SI	pGO1	7.3	>1000

[a] Numbers derived from COUGHTER et al. (1987)
[b] Numbers in parentheses from PATTISHALL et al. (1977)

fragment correlates with the observed size of the polypeptide. Although it is presumed to be a monomeric enzyme, this has not been unequivocally demonstrated. These data suggest that the Tp resistance determinant on some staphylococcal plasmids is a unique DHFR with a decreased affinity for Tp compared to the chromosomal enzyme (LYON and SKURRAY 1987; COUGHTER et al. 1987).

The question of transposability of the gram-positive DHFR gene remains unresolved. It has been incorrectly reported that Tn*4001* carries resistance to trimethoprim, ethidum bromide and quaternary ammonium compounds (LACEY and KRUCZENYK 1986). In fact, Tn*4001* has determinants only for resistance to gentamicin, tobramycin, and kanamycin (LYON et al. 1984b). In plasmid pSK1, the Tp resistance determinant is bounded by directly repeated sequences of about 920 bp that are indistinguishable from elements (IS257) flanking the *mer* operon in β-lactamase-specifying plasmids (LYON and SKURRAY 1987). The arrangement of these elements suggests that the Tp resistance determinant may form part of a composite transposon. The pGO1 DHFR gene is also flanked by directly repeated DNA sequences; here, the elements appear to be similar, but shorter (COUGHTER et al. 1987). Although no genetic or physical evidence for transposition has been obtained, the hybridization of a pGO1 probe with a chromosomal component in plasmid-free *S. epidermidis* strains suggests that transposition may have occurred (ARCHER et al. 1986). Investigation into this aspect of the dissemination of Tp resistance among the gram-positive organisms continues. Meanwhile, the observations that Tp resistance has surfaced among clinical strains of *S. aureus* and *S. epidermidis* in several geographic locations at about the same time and that the resistance is often located on self-transmissible plasmids suggest that the frequency and the prevalence of Tp resistance will increase among these medically important bacterial species.

E. Conclusion

Less than 20 years have elapsed since trimethoprim was approved for use in human medicine. During the intervening two decades, pathogenic and potentially pathogenic microorganisms have responded with an almost bewildering repertoire of resistance mechanisms; both chromosomal and plasmid-mediated. The first R plasmid specifying Tp resistance was reported in 1972 (FLEMING et al. 1972). Today the clinical microbiologist or molecular biologist is confronted by three authentically distinct plasmid-associated, Tp-resistant DHFRs (and possibly two additional ones) as well as three authentically different transposons harboring Tp resistance determinants (and perhaps others) and there is certainly no reason to expect the discoveries to end here.

In spite of the worldwide use of Tp for an increasing number of indications, the overall incidence of resistance has remained at a relatively low level. However, several disquieting trends have emerged over the past several years that deserve note: (1) Tp resistance among important pathogens (e.g., *S. dysenteriae* type I) in many "developing" countries of the world is extremely high (40%–99%). (2) In many parts of the world, including the industrialized countries, there has been a significant increase in the incidence of strains with *transferable*, high-level Tp resistance. (3) In some medical centers there has been a steady increase in the proportion of clinical isolates with nontransferable, high-level Tp resistance in which a transposon, Tn*7* for the most part, has integrated into the host chromosome.

Much of the work spent on characterizing the various R plasmid-specified DHFRs has only served to deepen the mystery as to the origin(s) of these determinants. As we mentioned earlier, the type III DHFR is obviously a close relative of the Tp-sensitive *E. coli* chromosomal reductase, but what about the type II enzyme that bears no DNA sequence similarity to any characterized DHFR: bacterial, phage or mammalian? It has been suggested that the type II DHFR constitutes a maverick oxidoreductase, hidden somewhere in a gram-negative chromosome, that has been recruited and expressed by a family of R plasmids (J. BURCHALL, personal communication). We have probed a variety of gram-negative chromosomes (including anaerobes) with a radiolabeled, gene-specific type II DNA fragment and have yet to detect a promising signal (L.P. ELWELL and WALTON, unpublished observations). However, a much more thorough and systematic experimental approach will be required before one can dismiss (or accept) this intriguing speculation.

If nothing else we hope that this chapter has convinced the reader that a wealth of interesting research and theory await to be pursued in the area of trimethoprim resistance. Many people will share in this exciting pursuit including clinicians, geneticists, clinical microbiologists, molecular biologists, students and all of those who are interested in the vagaries of molecular evolution.

References

Acar JF, Goldstein FW (1982) Genetic aspects and epidemiologic implications of resistance to trimethoprim. Rev Infect Dis 4:270–275

Albritton WL, Brunton JL, Slaney L, MacLean I (1982) Plasmid-mediated sulfonamide resistance in *Haemophilus ducreyi*. Antimicrob Agents Chemother 21:159–165

Alon U, Davidai G, Berant M, Merzbach D (1987) Five-year survey of changing patterns of susceptibility of bacterial uropathogens to trimethoprim-sulfamethoxazole and other antimicrobial agents. Antimicrob Agents Chemother 31:126–128

Amyes SGB (1986) Epidemiology of trimethoprim resistance. J Antimicrob Chemother [Suppl C] 18:215–221
Amyes SGB, Smith JT (1974) R-factor trimethoprim resistance mechanism: an insusceptible target site. Biochem Biophys Res Commun 58:412–418
Amyes SGB, Doherty CJ, Young HK (1986) High-level trimethoprim resistance in urinary bacteria. Eur J Clin Microbiol 5:287–291
Anderson DM (1980) Plasmid studies of *Salmonella typhimurium* phage type 179 resistant to ampicillin, tetracycline, sulphonamides and trimethoprim. J Hyg 85:293–300
Archer GL, Coughter JP, Johnston JL (1986) Plasmid-encoded trimethoprim resistance in staphylococci. Antimicrob Agents Chemother 29:733–740
Averett DR, Roth B, Burchall JJ, Baccanari DP (1979) Dihydrofolate reductase from *Neisseria* sp. Antimicrob Agents Chemother 15:428–435
Bachmann BJ (1983) Linkage map of *Escherichia coli* K-12, edition 7. Microbiol Rev 47:180–230
Bagdasarian M, Lurz R, Ruckert B, Franklin FCH, Bagdasarian MM, Frey J, Timmis KN (1981) Specific-purpose plasmid cloning vectors. II. Broad host range, high copy number RSF1010-derived vectors, and a host-vector system for gene cloning in *Pseudomonas*. Gene 16:237–247
Bannatyne RM, Toma S, Cheung R, Hu G (1980) Resistance to trimethoprim and other antibiotics in Ontario shigellae. Lancet I:425–426
Barker H, Healing D, Hutchison JG (1972) Characteristics of some co-trimoxazole-resistant Enterobacteriaceae from infected patients. J Clin Pathol 25:1086–1088
Barner HD, Cohen SS (1959) Virus-induced acquisition of metabolic function. IV. Thymidylate synthetase in thymine-requiring *Escherichia coli* infected by T2 and T5 bacteriophages. J Biol Chem 234:2987–2991
Barth PT, Datta N (1977) Two naturally occurring transposons indistinguishable from Tn7. J Gen Microbiol 102:129–134
Barth PT, Grinter NJ (1974) Comparison of the deoxyribonucleic acid molecular weights and homologies of plasmids conferring linked resistance to streptomycin and sulfonamides. J Bacteriol 120:618–630
Barth PT, Datta N, Hedges RW, Grinter NJ (1976) Transposition of a deoxyribonucleic acid sequence encoding trimethoprim and streptomycin resistances from R483 to other replicons. J Bacteriol 125:800–810
Bertino JB, Stacey KA (1966) A suggested mechanism for the selective procedure for isolating thymine requiring mutants of *Escherichia coli*. Biochem J 101:32C–33C
Breeze AS, Sims P, Stacey KA (1975) Trimethoprim-resistant mutants of *E. coli* K12: preliminary genetic mapping. Genet Res 25:207–214
Breitman TR, Bradford RM (1967) The absence of deoxyriboaldolase activity in a thymineless mutant of *Escherichia coli* strain 15: a possible explanation for the low thymine requirement of some thymineless strains. Biochim Biophys Acta 138:217–220
Brisson N, Hohn T (1984) Nucleotide sequence of the dihydrofolate-reductase gene borne by the plasmid R67 and conferring methotrexate resistance. Gene 28:271–275
Brumfitt W, Hamilton-Miller JMT, Wood A (1983) Evidence for a slowing in trimethoprim resistance during 1981 – a comparison with earlier years. J Antimicrob Chemother 11:503–509
Brunton J, Clare D, Meier MA (1986) Molecular epidemiology of antibiotic resistance plasmid of *Haemophilus* species and *Neisseria gonorrhoeae*. Rev Infect Dis 8:713–724
Bryan LE, van den Elzen HM, Tseng JT (1972) Transferable drug resistance in *Pseudomonas aeruginosa*. Antimicrob Agents Chemother 1:22–29
Burchall JJ (1973) Mechanism of action of trimethoprim-sulfamethoxazole – II. J Infect Dis 128:S437–441
Burchall JJ, Elwell LP, Fling ME (1982) Molecular mechanisms of resistance to trimethoprim. Rev Infect Dis 4:246–254
Cameron FH, Groot-Obbink DJ, Ackerman VP, Hall RM (1986) Nucleotide sequence of the AAD(2′) aminoglycoside adenylyltransferase determinant *aad*B. Evolutionary relationship of this region with those surrounding *aad*A in R538-1 and *dhfr*II in R388. Nucleic Acids Res 14:8625–8635

Campbell IG, Mee BJ (1987) Mapping of trimethoprim resistance genes from epidemiologically related plasmids. Antimicrob Agents Chemother 31:1440–1441
Campbell IG, Mee BJ, Nikoletti SM (1986) Evolution and spread of IncFIV plasmids conferring resistance to trimethoprim. Antimicrob Agents Chemother 29:807–813
Chatkaeomorakot A, Echeverria P, Taylor DN, Seriwatana J, Leksomboon U (1987) Trimethoprim resistant *Shigella* and enterotoxigenic *Escherichia coli* strains in children in Thailand. Pediatr Infect Dis 6:735–739
Chattopadhyay BL (1977) Co-trimoxazole resistant *Staphylococcus aureus* in hospital practice. J Antimicrob Chemother 3:371–374
Chinault AC, Blakesley VA, Roessler E, Willis DG, Smith CA, Cook RG, Fenwick RG Jr (1986) Characterization of transferable plasmids from *Shigella flexneri* 2a that confer resistance to trimethoprim, streptomycin, and sulfonamides. Plasmid 15:119–131
Chirnside ED, Emmerson AM, Smith JT (1985) A follow-up survey of transferable, plasmid-encoded trimethoprim resistance in a general hospital (1975–1983). J Antimicrob Chemother 16:419–434
Chun D, Seol SY, Suh MH (1981) Transferable resistance to trimethoprim in *Shigella*. J Infect Dis 143:742
Coleman DC, Pomeroy H, Estridge JK, Keane CT, Cafferkey MT, Hone R, Foster TJ (1985) Susceptibility to antimicrobial agents and analysis of plasmids in gentamicin- and methicillin-resistant *Staphylococcus aureus* from Dublin hospitals. J Med Microbiol 20:157–167
Coughter JP, Johnston AL, Archer GL (1987) Characterization of a staphylococcal trimethoprim resistance gene and its product. Antimicrob Agents Chemother 31:1027–1032
Datta N, Hughes VM, Nugent ME, Richards H (1979) Plasmids and transposons and their stability and mutability in bacteria isolated during an outbreak of hospital infection. Plasmid 2:182–196
Datta N, Dacey S, Hughes V, Knight S, Richards H, Williams G, Casewell M, Shannon KP (1980a) Distribution of genes for trimethoprim and gentamicin resistance in bacteria and their plasmids in a general hospital. J Gen Microbiol 118:495–508
Datta N, Nugent M, Richards H (1980b) Transposons encoding trimethoprim or gentamicin resistance in medically important bacteria. Cold Spring Harbor Symposium Quantitive Biology 45(1):45–51
Dupont MJ, Jouvenot M, Gouetdic G, Michel-Briand Y (1985) Development of plasmid-mediated resistance in *Vibrio cholerae* during treatment with trimethoprim-sulfamethoxazole. Antimicrob Agents Chemother 27:280–281
Elwell LP, Wilson HR, Knick VB, Keith BR (1986) In vitro and in vivo efficacy of the combination trimethoprim-sulfamethoxazole against clinical isolates of methicillin-resistant *Staphylococcus aureus*. Antimicrob Agents Chemother 29:1092–1094
Farrar WE (1985) Antibiotic resistance in developing countries. J Infect Dis 152:1103–1106
Finlayson MC, Jackson FL (1978) Trimethoprim-resistant *Salmonella*. Lancet II:375
Fleming MP, Datta N, Gruneberg RN (1972) Trimethoprim resistance determined by R factors. Br Med J 1:726–728
Flensburg J, Skold O (1984) Regulatory changes in the formation of chromosomal dihydrofolate reductase causing resistance to trimethoprim. J Bacteriol 159:184–190
Flensburg J, Skold O (1987) Massive overproduction of dihydrofolate reductase in bacteria as a response to the use of trimethoprim. Eur J Biochem 162:473–476
Flensburg J, Steen R (1986) Nucleotide sequence analysis of the trimethoprim resistant dihydrofolate reductase encoded by R plasmid R751. Nucleic Acids Res 14:5933
Fling ME, Elwell LP (1980) Protein expression in *Escherichia coli* minicells containing recombinant plasmids specifying trimethoprim-resistant dihydrofolate reductases. J Bacteriol 141:779–785
Fling ME, Richards C (1983) The nucleotide sequence of the trimethoprim-resistant dihydrofolate reductase gene harbored by Tn7. Nucleic Acids Res 11:5147–5158
Fling ME, Walton L, Elwell LP (1982) Monitoring of plasmid-encoded, trimethoprim-resistant dihydrofolate reductase genes: detection of a new resistant enzyme. Antimicrob Agents Chemother 22:882–888

Fling ME, Kopf J, Richards C (1985) Nucleotide sequence of the transposon Tn7 gene encoding an aminoglycoside-modifying enzyme, 3″ (9)-*o*-nucleotidyl transferase. Nucleic Acids Res 13:7095–7106
Fling ME, Kopf J, Richards C (1988) Characterization of plasmid pAZ1 and the type III dihydrofolate reductase gene. Plasmid 19:30–38
Freisheim JH, Bitar KG, Reddy AV, Blankenship DT (1978) Dihydrofolate reductase from amethopterin-resistant *Lactobacillus casei*: sequences of the cyanogen bromide peptides and complete sequences of the enzyme. J Biol Chem 253:6437–6444
Frost JA, Rowe B, Vandepitte J (1982) Acquisition of trimethoprim resistance in epidemic strain of *Shigella dysenteriae* type I from Zaire. Lancet I:963
Frost JA, Willshaw GA, Barclay EA, Rowe B, Lemmens P (1985) Plasmid characterization of drug-resistant *Shigella dysenteriae* 1 from an epidemic in Central Africa. J Hyg 94:163–172
Gillespie MT, Skurray RA (1986) Plasmids in multiresistant *Staphylococcus aureus*. Microbiol Sci 3:53–58
Gilligan PH, Gage PA, Welch DF, Muszynski MJ, Wait KR (1987) Prevalence of thymidine-dependent *Staphylococcus aureus* in patients with cystic fibrosis. J Clin Microbiol 25:1258–1261
Goldberger RF (1974) Autogenous regulation of gene expression. Science 183:810–816
Goldstein FW, Gutmann L, Williamson R, Collatz E, Acar JF (1983a) In vivo and in vitro emergence of simultaneous resistance to both *β*-lactam and aminoglycoside antibiotics in a strain of *Serratia marcescens*. Ann Microbiol (Paris) 134(A):329–337
Goldstein FW, Labigne-Roussel A, Gerbaud G, Carlier C, Collatz E, Courvalin P (1983b) Transferable plasmid-mediated antibiotic resistance in *Acinetobacter*. Plasmid 10:138–147
Goldstein FW, Papadopoulou B, Acar JF (1986a) The changing patterns of trimethoprim resistance in Paris, with a review of worldwide experience. Rev Infect Dis 8:725–737
Goldstein FW, Gerbaud G, Courvalin P (1986b) Transposable resistance to trimethoprim and 0129 in *Vibrio cholerae*. J Antimicrob Agents 17:559–569
Gosti-Testu F, Norris V, Brevet J (1983) Restriction map of Tn7. Plasmid 10:96–99
Gouy M, Gautier C (1982) Codon usage in bacteria: correlation with gene expressivity. Nucleic Acids Res 10:7055–7074
Grey D, Hamilton-Miller JMT, Brumfitt W (1979) Incidence and mechanisms of resistance to trimethoprim in clinically isolated gram-negative bacteria. Chemother 25:147–156
Gross RJ, Threlfall EJ, Ward LR, Rowe B (1984) Drug resistance in *Shigella dysenteriae*, *S. flexneri*, and *S. boydii* in England and Wales: increasing incidence of resistance to trimethoprim. Br Med J 288:784–786
Gruneberg RN (1984) Antibiotic sensitivities of urinary pathogens, 1971–1982. J Antimicrob Chemother 14:17–23
Guerrant RL, Wood SJ, Krongaard L, Reid RA, Hodge RH (1981) Resistance among fecal flora of patients taking sulfamethoxazole-trimethoprim or trimethoprim alone. Antimicrob Agents Chemother 19:33–38
Gurwith MJ, Brunton JL, Lank BA, Harding GKM, Ronald AR (1979) A prospective controlled investigation of prophylactic trimethoprim/sulfamethoxazole in hospitalized granulocytopenic patients. Am J Med 66:248–256
Gutmann L, Williamson R, Moreau N, Kitzis MD, Collatz E, Acar JF, Goldstein FW (1985) Cross-resistance to nalidixic acid, trimethoprim, and chloramphenicol associated with alterations in outer membrane proteins of *Klebsiella*, *Enterobacter*, and *Serratia*. J Infect Dis 151:501–507
Hamilton-Miller JMT (1979) Mechanisms and distribution of bacterial resistance to diamino-pyrimidines and sulfonamides. J Antimicrob Chemother [Suppl B] 5:61–73
Hayek LJ, Netherway J (1976) Thymine-requiring bacteria. Lancet I:1080
Hedges RW (1987) A plasmid of group Q which confers resistance to trimethoprim and sulfonamides. Microbiol Immunol 31:1113–1115
Hitchings GH (1973) Mechanism of action of trimethoprim-sulfamethoxazole – I. J Infect Dis 128:S433–436

Hoffee PA, Robertson BC (1969) 2-Deoxyribose gene-enzyme complex in *Salmonella typhimurium*: regulation of phosphodeoxyribomutase. J Bacteriol 97:1386–1396
Hollingshead S, Vapnek D (1985) Nucleotide sequence analysis of a gene encoding a streptomycin/spectinomycin adenyltransferase. Plasmid 13:17–30
Howden R (1981) A new medium for isolation of *Staphylococcus aureus*, including thymine requiring strains, from sputum. Med Lab Sci 38:29–33
Huovinen P (1984) Trimethoprim resistant *E. coli* in a geriatric hospital. J Infect 8:145–148
Huovinen P, Pulkkinen L, Toivanen P (1983) Transferable trimethoprim resistance in three Finnish hospitals. J Antimicrob Chemother 12:249–256
Huovinen P, Pulkkinen L, Helin HL, Makila M, Toivanen P (1986) Emergence of trimethoprim resistance in relation to drug consumption in a Finnish hosital from 1971 through 1984. Antimicrob Agents Chemother 29:73–76
Joyner SS, Fling ME, Stone D, Baccanari DP (1984) Characterization of an R-plasmid dihydrofolate reductase with a monomeric structure. J Biol Chem 259:5851–5856
Koch AL (1981) Evolution of antibiotic resistance gene function. Microbiol Rev 45:355–378
Korfmann G, Ludtke W, van Treeck U, Wiedemann B (1983) Dissemination of streptomycin and sulfonamide resistant by plasmid pBP1 in *Escherichia coli*. Eur J Clin Microbiol 2:463–468
Kraft CA, Timbury MC, Platt DJ (1986) Distribution and genetic location of Tn7 in trimethoprim-resistant *Escherichia coli*. J Med Microbiol 22:125–131
Labigne-Roussel A, Witchitz J, Courvalin P (1982) Modular evolution of disseminated Inc 7-M plasmids encoding gentamicin resistance. Plasmid 8:215–231
Lacey RW (1975) Antibiotic resistance plasmids of *Staphylococcus aureus* and their clinical importance. Bacteriol Rev 39:1–32
Lacey RW, Kruczenyk (1986) Epidemiology of antibiotic resistance in *Staphylococcus aureus*. J Antimicrob Chemother 18 [Suppl C]:207–214
Leary JV, Trollinger DB (1985) Identification of an indigenous plasmid carrying a gene for trimethoprim resistance in *Pseudomonas syringae* pv. *glycinea*. Mol Gen Genet 201:485–486
Lewis EL, Lacey RW (1973) Present significance of resistance to trimethoprim and sulphonamides in coliforms, *Staphylococcus aureus*, and *Streptococcus faecalis*. J Clin Pathol 26:175–180
Lichtenstein C, Brenner S (1981) Site-specific properties of Tn7 transposition into the *E. coli* chromosome. Mol Gen Genet 183:380–387
Lichtenstein C, Brenner S (1982) Unique insertion site of Tn7 in the *E. coli* chromosome. Nature 297:601–603
Ling J, Chau PY (1984) Plasmids mediating resistance to chloramphenicol, trimethoprim, and ampicillin in *Salmonella typhi* strains isolated in the Southeast Asian region. J Infect Dis 149:652
Lomax MS, Greenberg GR (1968) Characteristics of the *deo* operon: role in thymine utilization and sensitivity to deoxyribonucleosides. J Bacteriol 96:501–514
Lopez-Brea M, Collado L, Vincente F, Perez-Diaz JC (1983) Increasing antimicrobial resistance of *Shigella sonnei*. J Antimicrob Chemother 11:598
Lyon BR, Skurray R (1987) Antimicrobial resistance of *Staphylococcus aureus*: genetic basis. Microbiol Rev 51:88–134
Lyon BR, Iuorio JL, May JW, Skurray RA (1984a) Molecular epidermiology multiresistant *Staphylococcus aureus* in Australian hospitals. J Med Micro Biol 17:79–89
Lyon BR, May JW, Skurray RA (1984b) Tn4001: a gentamicin and kanamycin resistance transposon in *Staphylococcus aureus*. Mol Gen Genet 193:554–556
Macaden R, Bhat P (1985) The changing pattern of resistance to ampicillin and co-trimoxazole in *Shigella* serotypes in Bangalore, southern India. J Infect Dis 152:1348
Maskell R, Okubadejo OA, Payne RH (1976) Thymine-requiring bacteria associated with co-trimoxazole therapy. Lancet I:834–835
Maskell R, Okubadejo OA, Payne RH, Pead L (1977) Human infections with thymine-requiring bacteria. J Med Microbiol 11:33–45

Matsushita S, Kudoh Y, Ohashi M (1984) Transferable resistance to the vibriostatic agent 2,4-diamino-6,7-diisopropyl-pteridine (O/129) in *Vibrio cholerae*. Microbiol Immunol 28:1159–1162

Matthews DA, Alden RA, Bolin JT, Freer ST, Hamlin R, Xuong N, Kraut J, Poe M, Williams M, Hoogsteen K (1977) Dihydrofolate reductase: X-ray structure of the binary complex with methotrexate. Science 197:452–455

Matthews DA, Smith SL, Baccanari DP, Burchall JJ, Oatley SJ, Kraut J (1986) Crystal structure of a novel trimethoprim-resistant dihydrofolate reductase specified in *Escherichia coli* by R-plasmid R67. Biochemistry 25:4194–4204

Mayer KH, Fling ME, Hopkins JD, O'Brien TF (1985) Trimethoprim resistance in multiple genera of Enterobacteriaceae at a U.S. hospital: spread of the type II dihydrofolate reductase gene by a single plasmid. J Infect Dis 151:783–789

McCuen RW, Sirotnak FM (1974) Hyperproduction of dihydrofolate reductase in *Diplococcus pneumoniae* by mutation in the structural gene. The absence of an effect on other enzymes of folate coenzyme biosynthesis. Biochim Biophys Acta 338:540–544

McKown RL, Waddell CS, Arciszewska LK, Craig NL (1987) Identification of a transposon Tn*7*-dependent DNA-binding activity that recognizes the ends of Tn*7*. Proc Natl Acad Sci USA 84:7807–7811

Mee BJ, Nikoletti SM (1983) Plasmids encoding trimethoprim resistance in bacterial isolates from man and pigs. J Appl Bacteriol 54:225–235

Murray BE, Rensimer ER, DuPont HL (1982) Emergence of high-level trimethoprim resistance in fecal *Escherichia coli* during oral administration of trimethoprim or trimethoprim-sulfamethoxazole. N Engl J Med 306:130–135

Murray BE, Alvarado T, Kim KH, Vorachit M, Jayanetra P, Levine MM, Prenzel I, Fling M, Elwell L, McCracken GH, Madrigal G, Odio C, Trabulsi LR (1985) Increasing resistance to trimethoprim-sulfamethoxazole among isolates of *Escherichia coli* in developing countries. J Infect Dis 152:1107–1113

Nakhla LS (1972) Resistance of *Staphylococcus aureus* to sulfamethoxazole and trimethoprim. J Clin Pathol 25:708–712

Novak P, Stone D, Burchall JJ (1983) R plasmid dihydrofolate reductase with a dimeric subunit structure. J Biol Chem 258:10956–10959

Nugent ME, Ellis K, Datta N, Bradley DE (1982) pHH502, a plasmid with IncP and Incδ characters, loses the latter by a specific *rec*A-independent deletion event. J Gen Microbiol 128:2781–2790

Obaseiki-Ebor EE, Abiodun PO, Emina PA (1986) Fecal *Escherichia coli* mediating transferable multi-antibiotic resistance and undesirable extra-chromosomal genes. Ann Trop Paediatr 6:283–286

O'Brien TF (1987) Resistance of bacteria to antibacterial agents: report of task force 2. Rev Infect Dis 9 [Suppl 3]:S244–S260

Okada T, Yanagisawa K, Ryan FJ (1960) Elective production of thymine-less mutants. Nature 188:340–341

Okubadejo OA, Maskell RM (1973) Thymine-requiring mutants of *Proteus mirabilis* selected by co-trimoxazole in vivo. J Gen Microbiol 77:533–535

Ouartsi A, Borowski D, Brevet J (1985) Genetic analysis of Tn7 transposition. Mol Gen Genet 198:221–227

Palenque E, Otero JR, Noriega AR (1983) High prevalence of non-epidemic *Shigella sonnei* resistant to co-trimoxazole. J Antimicrob Chemother 11:196–198

Pancoast SJ, Hyams DM, Neu HC (1980) Effect of trimethoprim and trimethoprim-sulfamethoxazole on development of drug-resistant vaginal and fecal floras. Antimicrob Agents Chemother 17:263–268

Paniker CKJ, Vimala KN, Bhat P, Stephen S (1978) Drug resistant shigellosis in south India. Indian J Med Res 68:413–417

Paramasivan CN, Subramanian S, Shanmugasundaram N (1977) Antimicrobial resistance and incidence of R factor among *Salmonella* isolated from patients with enteric fever and other clinical conditions in Madras, India (1975–1976). J Infect Dis 13:796–800

Pattishall KH, Acar J, Burchall JJ, Goldstein FW, Harvey RJ (1977) Two distinct types of trimethoprim-resistant dihydrofolate reductase specified by R-plasmids of different compatibility groups. J Biol Chem 252:2319–2323
Pulkkinen L, Huovinen P, Vuorio E, Toivanen P (1984) Characterization of trimethoprim resistance by use of probes specific for transposon Tn7. Antimicrob Agents Chemother 26:82–86
Richards H, Datta N (1982) Plasmids and transposons acquired by *Salmonella typhi* in man. Plasmid 8:9–14
Richards H, Nugent M (1979) The incidence and spread of transposon 7. In: Timmis KN, Puhler A (eds) Plasmids of medical, environmental and commercial importance. Elsevier, Amsterdam, pp 195–198
Richards H, Datta N, Sojka WJ, Wray C (1978) Trimethoprim-resistance plasmids and transposons in Salmonella. Lancet II:1194–1195
Richardson JF (1983) Frequency of resistance to trimethoprim among isolates of *Staphylococcus epidermidis* and *Staphylococcus saprophyticus*. J Antimicrob Chemother 11:163–167
Rogers M, Ekaterinaki N, Nimmo E, Sherratt D (1986) Analysis of Tn7 transposition. Mol Gen Genet 205:550–556
Rosenberg M, Court D (1979) Regulatory sequences involved in the promotion and termination of RNA transcription. Annu Rev Genet 13:319–353
Rotger R, Rubio F, Nombela C (1986) A multi-resistance plasmid isolate from commensal *Neisseria* species is closely related to the enterobacterial plasmid RSF1010. J Gen Microbiol 132:2491–2496
Roth B, Falco EA, Hitchings GH (1962) 5-benzyl-2,4-diaminopyrimidines as antibacterial agents. I. Synthesis and antibacterial activity in vitro. J Med Pharm Chem 5:1103–1123
Rowe B, Threlfall EJ, Ward LR, Ashley AS (1979) International spread of multiresistant strains of *Salmonella typhimurium* phage types 204 and 193 from Britain to Europe. Vet Rec 105:468–469
Saad AF, Farrar WE Jr (1977) Antimicrobial resistance and R factors in *Salmonella* isolated from humans and animals in Georgia and South Carolina. South Med J 70:305–308
Scudamore RA, Goldner M (1982) Limited contribution of the outer-membrane penetration barrier towards intrinsic antibiotic resistance of *Pseudomonas aeruginosa*. Can J Microbiol 28:169–175
Sellers J (1982) Frequency and transmissibility of trimethoprim resistance in enterobacteria from urinary infections. Scand J Infect Dis 14:157–158
Shahid NS, Rahaman MM, Haider K, Banu H, Rahman N (1985) Changing pattern of resistant shiga bacillus (SHIGELLA DYSENTERIAE type I) and *Shigella flexneri* in Bangladesh. J Infect Dis 152:1114–1119
Shapiro JA (1983) Mobile genetic elements. Academic Press, New York
Shapiro JA, Sporn P (1977) Tn402: a new transposable element determining trimethoprim resistance that inserts in bacteriophage lambda. J Bacteriol 129:1632–1635
Sheldon R (1977) Altered dihydrofolate reductase in *fol* regulatory mutants of *Escherichia coli* K12. Mol Gen Genet 151:215–219
Sheldon R, Brenner S (1976) Regulatory mutants of dihydrofolate reductase in *Escherichia coli* K12. Mol Gen Genet 147:91–97
Sirotnak FM, McCuen RW (1973) Hyperproduction of dihydrofolate reductase in *Diplococcus pneumoniae* after mutation in the structural gene. Evidence for an effect at the level of transcription. Genetics 74:543–556
Sirotnak FM, Hachtel SL, Williams WA (1969) Increased dihydrofolate reductase synthesis in *Diplococcus pneumoniae* following translatable alteration of the structural gene. II. Individual and dual effects on the properties and rate of synthesis of the enzyme. Genetics 61:313–326
Skold O, Widh A (1974) A new dihydrofolate reductase with low trimethoprim sensitivity induced by an R factor mediating high resistance to trimethoprim. J Biol Chem 249:4324–4325

Smith DR, Calvo JM (1979) Regulation of dihydrofolate reductase synthesis in *Escherichia coli*. Mol Gen Genet 175:31–38
Smith DR, Calvo JM (1982) Nucleotide sequence of dihydrofolate reductase genes from trimethoprim-resistant mutants of *Escherichia coli*. Evidence that dihydrofolate reductase interacts with another essential gene product. Mol Gen Genet 187:72–78
Smith DR, Rood JL, Bird PI, Sneddon MK, Calvo JM, Morrison JF (1982) Amplification and modification of dihydrofolate reductase in *Escherichia coli*. Nucleotide sequence of *fol* genes from mutationally altered plasmids. J Biol Chem 257:9043–9048
Smith GM, Jones P (1984) Effects of deletions in transposon Tn7 on its frequency of transposition. J Bacteriol 157:962–964
Smith HW (1976) Mutants of *Klebsiella pneumoniae* resistant to several antibiotics. Nature 259:307–308
Smith HW, Tucker JF (1976) The virulence of trimethoprim-resistant thymine-requiring strains of *Salmonella*. J Hyg 76:97–108
Smith SL, Stone D, Novak P, Baccanari DP, Burchall JJ (1979) R plasmid dihydrofolate reductase with subunit structure. J Biol Chem 254:6222–6225
Sparham PD, Lobban DI, Speller DC (1978) Isolation of *Staphylococcus aureus* from sputum in cystic fibrosis. J Clin Pathol 31:913–918
Stamm WE, Counts GW, Wagner KF, Martin D, Gregory D, McKevitt M, Turck M, Holmes KK (1980) Antimicrobial prophylaxis of recurrent urinary tract infections: a double-blind, placebo-controlled trial. Ann Intern Med 92:770–775
Steen R, Skold O (1985) Plasmid-borne or chromosomally mediated resistance by Tn7 is the most common response to ubiquitous use of trimethoprim. Antimicrob Agents Chemother 27:933–937
Stokes A, Lacey RW (1978) Effect of thymidine on activity of trimethoprim and sulfamethoxazole. J Clin Pathol 31:165–171
Stone D, Smith SL (1979) The amino acid sequence of the trimethoprim-resistant dihydrofolate reductase specified in *Escherichia coli* by R-plasmid R67. J Biol Chem 254:10857–10861
Sundstrom L, Vinayagamoorthy T, Skold O (1987) Novel type of plasmid-borne resistance to trimethoprim. Antimicrob Agents Chemother 31:60–66
Swedberg G (1987) Organization of two sulfonamide resistance genes on plasmids of gram-negative bacteria. Antimicrob Agents Chemother 31:306–311
Swift G, McCarthy BJ, Heffron F (1981) DNA sequence of a plasmid-encoded dihydrofolate reductase. Mol Gen Genet 181:441–447
Tait RC, Rempel H, Rodriguez RL, Kado CI (1985) The aminoglycoside-resistance operon of the plasmid pSa: nucleotide sequence of the streptomycin-spectinomycin resistance gene. Gene 36:97–104
Tanner EI, Bullin CH (1974) Thymidine-dependent *Escherichia coli* infection and some associated laboratory problems. J Clin Path 27:565–568
Tapsall JW, Wilson E, Harper J (1974) Thymine dependent strains of *Escherichia coli* selected by trimethoprim-sulphamethoxazole therapy. Pathology 6:161
Taylor DE, Keystone JS, Devlin HR (1980) Resistance to trimethoprim and other antibiotics in Ontario shigellae. Lancet I:476
Taylor DE, Chumpitaz JC, Goldstein F (1985) Variability of IncHI1 plasmids from *Salmonella typhi* with special reference to Peruvian plasmids encoding resistance to trimethoprim and other antibiotics. Antimicrob Agents Chemother 28:452–455
Tennent JM, Lyon BR, Gillespie MT, May JW, Skurray RA (1985) Cloning and expression of *Staphylococcus aureus* plasmid-mediated quaternary ammonium resistance in *Escherichia coli*. Antimicrob Agents Chemother 27:79–83
Tennhammar-Ekman B, Skold O (1979) Trimethoprim resistance plasmids of different origin encode different drug-resistant dihydrofolate reductases. Plasmid 2:334–346
Tenover FC (1986) Studies of antimicrobial resistance genes using DNA probes. Antimicrob Agents Chemother 29:721–725
Then RL (1982) Mechanisms of resistance to trimethoprim, the sulfonamides, and trimethoprim-sulfamethoxazole. Rev Infect Dis 4:261–269
Then RL, Hermann F (1981) Mechanisms of trimethoprim resistance in enterobacteria isolated in Finland. Chemotherapy 27:192–199

Threlfall EJ, Ward LR, Rowe B (1978) Spread of multiresistant strains of *Salmonella typhimurium* phage types 204 and 193 in Britain. Br Med J 2:997
Threlfall EJ, Ward LR, Ashley AS, Rowe B (1980 a) Plasmid-encoded trimethoprim resistance in multiresistant epidemic *Salmonella typhimurium* phage types 204 and 193 in Britain. Br Med J 280:1210–1211
Threlfall EJ, Rowe B, Huq I (1980 b) Plasmid-encoded multiple antibiotic resistance in *Vibrio cholerae* el tor from Bangladesh. Lancet II:1247–1248
Threlfall EJ, Frost JA, King HC, Rowe B (1983) Plasmid-encoded trimethoprim resistance in salmonellas isolated in Britain between 1970 and 1981. J Hyg 90:55–60
Threlfall EJ, Ward LR, Rowe B (1986) R plasmids of *Salmonella typhimurium* in the United Kingdom. J Antimicrob Chemother 18 [Suppl C]:175–177
Tiemens KM, Shipley PL, Correia RA, Shields DS, Guerrant RL (1984) Sulfamethoxazole-trimethoprim-resistant *Shigella flexneri* in northeast Brazil. Antimicrob Agents Chemother 25:653–654
Tietze E, Prager R, Tschape H (1982) Characterization of the transposons Tn1822 (Tc) and Tn1824 (TpSm) and the light they throw on the natural spread of resistance genes. Plasmid 8:253–260
Tietze E, Brevet J, Tschape H (1987) Relationships among the streptothricin resistance transposons Tn1825 and Tn1826 and the trimethoprim resistance transposon Tn7. Plasmid 18:246–249
Towner KJ (1981) A clinical isolate of *Escherichia coli* owing its trimethoprim resistance to a chromosomally-located trimethoprim transposon. J Antimicrob Chemother 7:157–162
Towner KJ (1983) Transposon-directed mutagenesis and chromosome mobilization in *Acinetobacter calcoaceticus* EBF65/65. Genet Res 41:97–102
Towner KJ, Pinn PA (1981) A transferable plasmid conferring only a moderate level of resistance to trimethoprim. FEMS Microbiol Lett 10:271–272
Towner KJ, Wise PJ (1983) Transferable resistance plasmids as a contributory cause of increasing trimethoprim resistance in general practice. J Antimicrob Chemother 11:33–39
Towner KJ, Pearson NJ, Pinn PA, O'Grady F (1980) Increasing importance of plasmid-mediated trimethoprim resistance in enterobacteria: two six-month clinical surveys. Br Med J 280:517–519
Townsend DE, Ashdown N, Greed LC, Grubb WB (1984) Analysis of plasmids mediating gentamicin resistance in methicillin-resistant *Staphylococcus aureus*. J Antimicrob Chemother 13:347–352
Traub WH, Kleber I (1977) Selected and spontaneous variants of *Serratia marcescens* with combined resistance against chloramphenicol, nalidixic acid, and trimethoprim. Chemotherapy 23:436–451
Tschape H, Tietze E, Prager R, Voigt W, Wolter E, Seltmann G (1984) Plasmid-borne streptothricin resistance in gram-negative bacteria. Plasmid 12:189–196
Volz KW, Matthews DA, Alden RA, Freer ST, Hansch C, Kaufman BT, Kraut J (1982) Crystal structure of avian dihydrofolate reductase containing phenyltriazine and NADPH. J Biol Chem 257:2528–2536
Ward LR, Rowe B, Threlfall EJ (1982) Incidence of trimethoprim resistance in salmonellae isolated in Britain: a twelve year study. Lancet II:705–706
Werner RG, Goeth H (1984) Trimethoprim failure to penetrate into *Pseudomonas aeruginosa* cells. FEMS Microbiol Lett 23:201–204
Wiedemann B, Meyer JF, Zuhlsdorf MT (1986) Insertions of resistance genes into Tn21-like transposons. J Antimicrob Chemother 18[Suppl C]:85–92
Wise EM, Abou-Donia MM (1975) Sulfonamide resistance mechanism in *E. coli*: R plasmids can determine sulfonamide-resistant dihydropteroate synthases. Proc Natl Acad Sci USA 72:2621–2525
Young HK, Amyes SGB (1983) Trimethoprim-resistance: an epidemic caused by two related transposons. In: Spitzy KH, Karrer K (eds) Proc 13th Int Congr Chemother. Egerman, Vienna, 87:93–96
Young HK, Amyes SGB (1985) Characterization of a new transposon-mediated trimethoprim-resistant dihydrofolate reductase. Biochem Pharmacol 34:4334–4337

Young HK, Amyes SGB (1986a) A new mechanism of plasmid trimethoprim resistance. Characterization of an inducible dihydrofolate reductase. J Biol Chem 261:2503–2505

Young HK, Amyes SGB (1986b) Plasmid trimethoprim resistance in *Vibrio cholerae*: migration of the type I dihydrofolate reductase gene out of the Enterobacteriaceae. J Antimicrob Chemother 17:697–703

Young HK, Jesudason MV, Koshi G, Amyes SGB (1986) Unusual expression of new low-level-trimethoprim-resistance plasmids. J Clin Microbiol 24:61–64

Zaman K, Yunis MD, Baqui AH, Hossain KMB, Khan MU (1983) Cotrimoxazole-resistant *Shigella dysenteriae* type 1 outbreak in a family in rural Bangladesh. Lancet II:796–797

Zolg JW, Hanggi UJ (1981) Characterization of a R plasmid-associated, trimethoprim-resistant dihydrofolate reductase and determination of the nucleotide sequence of the reductase gene. Nucleic Acids Res 9:697–710

CHAPTER 12

Resistance to Sulfonamides

R. L. THEN

A. Introduction

Sulfonamides were the first widely used selective antibacterial drugs, and the report of G. DOMAGK in 1935 on the efficacy of prontosil in streptococcal animal infections paved the way for effective antibacterial chemotherapy. Nowadays sulfonamides alone are hardly the drugs of first choice due to the availability of more active antibiotics and to the prevalence of resistance. Despite their age, however, they maintained importance as alternative drugs or – mostly in combination with dihydrofolate reductase inhibitors – as drugs of first choice for a variety of infections.

Sulfonamides, sulfones such as dapsone (4,4′-diaminodiphenyl-sulfone) as well as *p*-aminosalicyclic acid (pAS) are structural analogs of *p*-aminobenzoic acid (pAB) (see Fig. 1) and hence are among the few examples of classical antimetabolites useful as antimicrobial drugs. They competitively inhibit dihydropteroate synthetase (DHPS, EC 2.5.1.15) and are alternative substrates of this enzyme. Resistance selected with a particular compound generally results in cross-resistance to other sulfonamides. The mechanisms evolved by microorganisms to escape the detrimental effect of sulfonamides are more diverse than those causing resistance to many antibiotics and include metabolic alterations, changes in the target enzyme or the uptake of the drug, as well as the production of novel, drug-resistant bypass-enzymes. It is somewhat surprising that in view of the sulfonamides being the oldest antibacterials, mechanistic and genetic studies on the ba-

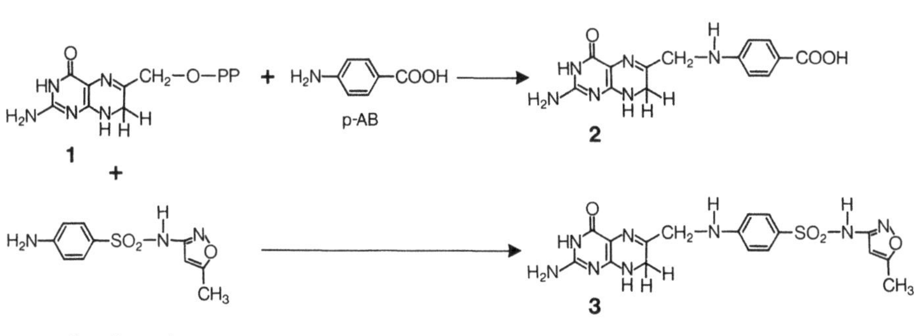

Fig. 1. Reaction of 7,8-dihydro-6-hydroxymethylpteridine-pyrophosphate (*1*) with pAB to form dihydropteroic acid (*2*) as the physiological reaction catalyzed by DHPS and formation of the corresponding sulfamethoxazole-analog (*3*) with sulfamethoxazole

sis of sulfonamide resistance are still very scarce and our knowledge lags behind the detailed knowledge available on the mechanism of resistance to many antibiotics. This chapter focuses on the mechanisms of sulfonamide resistance in bacteria, and as far as knowledge is available, on those prevailing in other microorganisms, especially in plasmodia. Emphasis will be laid on the newer literature and the reader is referred to other recent reviews on resistance mechanisms to sulfonamides in bacteria (THEN 1982; FOSTER 1983; HITCHINGS 1983; HAMILTON-MILLER 1984) or in malarial parasites (PETERS 1985; SPENCER 1985; YUTHAVONG et al. 1985; WARHURST 1986).

B. Sulfonamide Usage Today

Resistance development clearly parallels prescription habits. Withdrawal of a drug from clinical use results in a lowering of the incidence of resistance, especially if it is chromosomally coded. It seems thus necessary to gain some insight into the use of sulfonamides today.

I. Sulfonamides Alone and Combined with Antibiotics

Only a few indications exist today for the use of a sulfonamide, i.e. in chancroid (causative pathogen *Haemophilus ducreyi*), trachoma, actinomycosis, ulcus molle and nocardiosis. Sulfonamides are still frequently prescribed in many countries in acute, mild infections, such as uncomplicated urinary tract infections. They are also used locally in eye infections (often combined with antibiotics) or prophylactically in certain conditions. A large number of sulfonamides are available for these indications in different countries. The use of many of these compounds, however, has drastically decreased since 1980 and the drugs of greatest use today are sulfamethoxazole, sulfisoxazole (sulfafurazole) and sulfadiazine (see Table 1).

One of the most active sulfonamides, sulfadiazine, is sometimes used to treat toxoplasmosis (MILLS 1986). In some areas, such as the Pailin region on the Kampuchea-Thai border, sulfathiazole as a cheap sulfonamide was used to treat malarial fever attacks, which was, however, followed by rapid resistance development (VERDRAGER 1986). There exists a large number of combinations of various antibiotics with sulfonamides for the treatment of systemic or ocular infections in various countries. One such combination, acetylsulfafurazole with erythromycin (Pediazole), is frequently prescribed for otitis media in the US.

II. Sulfonamides in Combination with Dihydrofolate Reductase Inhibitors

Sulfonamides are now much more frequently used in combination with dihydrofolate reductase inhibitors (Table 1), based on the mutual synergism and the prevention of resistance development. In many countries such combinations are consumed in larger amounts than, e.g. ampicillin. Since the first introduction of such

Table 1. Development of the use of several important sulfonamides from 1980 to 1987. (Source: International Medical Statistics)

Market[a]	Sulfonamide		Tons used in		
	Alone	Combined with	1980	1983	1987
USA	All[b]	–	98.8	49.2	33.2
	Sulfafurazole	–	42.2	16.7	12.4
	Acetylsulfafurazole	–	22.2	15.8	13.4
	Sulfadiazine	–	3.4	1.1	1.0
	Sulfapyridine	–	1.5	1.2	1.0
	Sulfamethoxazole	–	21.3	11.2	5.4
	Sulfamethoxazole	Trimethoprim	148.6	199.5	289.3
	Acetylsulfafurazole	Erythromycin	12.5	49.3	66.6
Japan	All	–	62.9	45.6	26.9
	Sulfamethoxazole	–	28.5	17.4	2.2
	Sulfamethoxazole	Trimethoprim	11.8	13.8	8.0
	Sulfadimethoxine	–	7.9	5.6	1.4
	Sulfamonomethoxine	–	6.1	3.5	1.7
	Sulfasomidine	–	7.8	6.1	1.2
Germany	All	–	5.4	2.7	0.9
	Sulfamethoxazole	Trimethoprim	72.6	65.0	61.0
	Sulfadiazine	Trimethoprim	3.9	2.9	0.9
UK	All	–	2.1	1.9	1.1
	Sulfamethoxazole	Trimethoprim	54.8	53.3	42.2
Italy	All	–	1.8	0.9	0.4
	Sulfamethoxazole	Trimethoprim	69.2	95.0	81.8
Brazil	All	–	9.5	7.6	7.0
	Sulfadiazine	–	3.1	3.6	5.0
	Sulfadiazine	Trimethoprim	0	0	9.7
	Sulfamethoxazole	Trimethoprim	45.2	46.4	78.7

[a] Hospital and pharmacy market, except Brazil, where only the pharmacy sales are given
[b] Including sulfasalazine

a combination for the treatment of bacterial infections, viz. sulfamethoxazole plus trimethoprim (TMP) (co-trimoxazole) in the late sixties, a variety of such combinations has become available in various countries. They comprise fixed combinations of TMP with sulfadiazine, sulfamoxole, sulfametrole, sulfamethopyrazine, sulfamerazine, and tetroxoprim with sulfadiazine. These combinations, especially co-trimoxazole are also an effective treatment of some protozoal diseases, e.g. *Pneumocystis carinii* pneumonia. For toxoplasmosis a combination of sulfadiazine plus pyrimethamine is used (Mills 1986).

Nowadays, long-acting sulfonamides are used only in combination with a dihydrofolate reductase inhibitor to treat malaria. The mostly used combination of this type is sulfadimethoxine plus pyrimethamine (Fansidar), another is sulfalene plus pyrimethamine (Metakelfin). The W.H.O. estimate that sulfonamides will play an important and expanding role among the drugs to be used for malaria control (Beales 1988).

III. Sulfones and Other Agents

Leprosy is an important disease in many countries with an estimated 15 million cases worldwide. Besides monotherapy with dapsone, combination therapy with rifampicin and clofazimine is advocated. Acedapsone and sulfamethoxypyridazine have also been used in the therapy of lepromatous leprosy. Atypical mycobacteria are often susceptible to dapsone and several sulfonamides and these compounds are sometimes contained in drug regimens used to treat mycobacterioses.

Local application of silver sulfadiazine is used to prevent infections in burns (HOFFMANN 1984). The mechanism of action of this compound, however, is complex and probably also involves interaction of silver with DNA replication. Sulfasalazine, which is used to treat inflammatory bowel disease, is split by bacteria into sulfapyridine and 5-aminosalicylic acid.

For malaria, a fixed combination of dapsone with pyrimethamine (Maloprim) is available.

IV. Sulfonamides in Veterinary Medicine

Sulfonamides have maintained an important position in the veterinary field. They are used in the treatment of bacterial or protozoal infections or as medicated feed additives. A recent survey lists 18 different sulfonamides, among them sulfaquinoxaline, sulfadimidine, sulfadiazine, sulfadimethoxine, and sulfachloropyridazine (REHM et al. 1986). Several fixed combinations of TMP with sulfonamides are available in various countries to treat bacterial infections in domestic animals. Among these combinations are TMP/sulfadoxine, TMP/sulfadimethoxine, TMP/sulfatroxazole, TMP/sulfadiazine, TMP/sulfachlorpyridazine. Sulfonamides, alone or in combination with TMP, diaveridine or ormetoprim are also used to control bacterial fish diseases, or, as medicated feed additives, to control coccidiosis in the poultry industry. Use of sulfonamides in animals poses the problem of sulfonamide residues in meat, milk, and eggs, a problem which has been discussed by REHM et al. (1986).

The total market for sulfonamides in 1986 in veterinary medicine was estimated at US $ 154 million (excluding centrally planned economies). This includes sulfonamides as well as combinations with other antibiotics. Of these, $ 47 million worth were sold as medicated feed additives, $ 107 million worth as ethical drugs.

The selection of resistant strains by antimicrobial usage in animals is thought to be an important reservoir for the spread of resistant strains to humans (COHEN and TAUXE 1986). An exchange of plasmid-bearing *E. coli* between pigs and humans has been observed (CAMPBELL et al. 1986), and a close molecular relationship between plasmids from human and animal sources exists (TOWNER et al. 1986).

C. Prevalence of Sulfonamide Resistance

I. Bacteria

Sulfonamides were the first antibacterial agents to be marketed and were introduced for clinical use in 1936–1937. At that time they were highly effective in vivo against most strains of *Neisseria gonorrhoeae* and *N. meningitidis*. Subsequently their effectiveness in gonorrhoea decreased and from 1944 to 1948 75%–85% of strains isolated were sulfonamide resistant, *N. meningitidis* remaining susceptible (CATLIN 1967). Meningococci resistant to sulfadiazine were first reported in 1963. In the late seventies epidemics of such strains were reported from northern Africa, Brazil, and Norway. Pneumococci with acquired resistance to sulfonamides had already been reported in the late thirties.

The efficacy of sulfonamides against shigellosis, which provoked heavy use in Japan from 1940, was followed by the spread of sulfonamide resistance. In the early sixties, 90%–95% of *Shigella* and 97%–99% of *S. aureus* were resistant to sulfonamides. Subsequent use of other antimicrobials like chloramphenicol, streptomycin and tetracycline resulted in the selection and spread of multiresistant *Shigella* strains and other species harboring conjugative plasmids.

Sulfonamide resistance in *Shigella* remains a specific and global problem. A comparison of resistance patterns in enteric pathogens from different parts of the world showed marked variability (MURRAY 1986). Seventy to 80% of shigellae were resistant to sulfonamides in Great Britain in 1974–1982. Many were multiresistant. In other places resistance frequencies varied from 19% in Sri Lanka in 1980 to over 80% in Egypt and Brazil. For *Salmonella*, sulfonamide-resistance frequencies were 5% in Australia (1980–1983), 13% in Finland (1980s) but 90% in Egypt (1980). Sulfonamide resistance in enterotoxigenic *E. coli* ranged from 25% to 53% in the US, Africa, and Asia. In Spain, a country with a high consumption of cotrimoxazole, 100% of *S. sonnei* tested in 1982 were resistant to sulfamethoxazole, 81% of those also to TMP (PALENQUE et al. 1983). In northern Norway resistance to antimicrobials in *E. coli* was highest for sulfonamides (20.8%) in 1980 (VORLAND et al. 1985). Over a period from 1971 to 1984 resistance to sulfamethoxazole in *E. coli* in a Finnish hospital remained fairly constant at around 40%, despite changes in the consumption of TMP or co-trimoxazole (HUOVINEN et al. 1986). A recent study from the USSR showed 92.7% sulfonamide resistance in enterobacteria from fecal isolates, most of these being multiresistant (VOSMIRKO 1986).

In the US and other parts of the world salmonellosis due to nontyphoid *Salmonella* is a problem and resistance is increasing (COHEN and TAUXE 1986). Different serotypes differ in resistance frequencies. In a 1984 study 29% of 117 strains of human *Salmonella* isolates were sulfonamide resistant, which was actually lower than resistance to tetracycline (55%) or ampicillin (38%). Animal isolates of *Salmonella* had a 61% frequency of resistance to sulfadiazine from 1978 to 1981. Recently, resistance to sulfonamide, ampicillin, chloramphenicol, and TMP has also been acquired by *Vibrio cholerae* el tor, due to a large, 72 MDa conjugative plasmid (DUPONT et al. 1985). Resistance of *Pseudomonas* and other bacteria to silver sulfadiazine has been reported and is high at some centers (HOFFMANN 1984).

From this background and the still heavy selection pressure it is not surprising that sulfonamide resistance is generally stated as being high. An additional reason for this is that the sulfonamide resistance marker is frequently linked genetically to other resistances and hence sulfonamide-resistant strains are often coselected by other agents.

With regard to the spread of resistance it is of interest that the Su-resistance marker, along with other resistances, is frequently found among different species of fecal coliforms isolated from sewage, surface water or sea water (NIEMI et al. 1983).

However, remarkable differences in the incidence of Su resistance, exist for different pathogens and different geographical areas. Su resistance monitored by a multicenter study in central Europe in 1984 showed a low of 6% resistant *Salmonella*, 7% for *Proteus* ssp., and a high of 34% of *E. coli* (KRESKEN and WIEDEMANN 1986). These frequencies were actually lower than those for ampicillin and tetracycline and were also lower than those reported for the same organisms in 1980/1981. Methodological differences, such as change in media and testing conditions, rather than a significant drop in actual resistance during this period, must be assumed to be the reason for this.

Testing of sulfonamides presents a particular problem. Suitable media with a low thymidine content are required and not too dense inocula have to be applied to guarantee reliable results (HAMILTON-MILLER 1984). Since these requirements are not always met resistance frequencies reported for sulfonamides or to antifolates may tend to be too high.

The main obstacle in studies on resistance in *Mycobacterium leprae* remains that this organism can only be grown in animals. The only available and universally acceptable method for assessing the multiplication of *M. leprae* has been the mouse foot pad model, which requires 6–12 months. The criterion for defining *M. leprae* susceptibility to dapsone is the inability of the organism to multiply in mice administered dapsone incorporated into their diet in a concentration of 0.0001 g/100 g diet (SHEPARD et al. 1986).

The first report on primary dapsone resistance, i.e. resistant isolates from patients without previous treatment, appeared in 1977 (SHEPARD et al. 1986). Secondary resistance to dapsone studied in 1981/1982 in Upper Volta showed a resistance level of around 7% (PATTYN et al. 1984). The number of lepromatous patients developing sulfone resistance has been estimated to be 2.5% in Malaysia, 7% in Costa Rica, and 19% in Ethiopia (GELBER 1984). In other parts of the world 1.1 to 20% resistance levels have been reported (SREEVATSA et al. 1985).

II. Protozoa

Resistance in human malaria is mainly a problem in relation to *P. falciparum*. The number of available drugs against malaria is limited and hence resistance development a serious problem. Resistance to Fansidar has developed rapidly during the past decade. Strains of *P. falciparum* resistant to chloroquine as well as to combinations of sulfonamides and antifols have been reported from Southeast Asia, East and West Africa and South America (SPENCER 1985; PETERS 1985).

Coccidia rapidly acquire resistance to any drug once it is used to control coccidiosis. Hence prevention of resistance is dependent on drug rotation programs and hygienic means. In a recent survey conducted in France resistance to sulfaquinoxaline, used as a mixture with amprolium-ethopabate-pyrimethamine against coccidia in chicken, was 50% to >90% (HAMET 1986).

D. Mode of Action of Sulfonamides

Sulfonamides, sulfones and pAS are structural analogs of pAB and compete with pAB for the active site of DHPS, the enzyme which forms dihydropteroic acid from 2-amino-4-hydroxy-6-hydroxymethyl-7,8-dihydropteridine pyrophosphate and pAB. Besides pAB, *p*-aminobenzoylglutamate is also used as a substrate by this enzyme, but with lower efficiency (SWEDBERG et al. 1979). For a long time sulfonamides were considered as classical competitive inhibitors. Studies in the late seventies and early eighties, however, showed that they are not only competitive inhibitors of DHPS, but also alternative substrates which are processed to sulfonamide analogs of dihydropteroate (BOCK et al. 1974) (Fig. 1). The pteridine precursor does not usually accumulate in inhibited cells, since it is consumed in the presence as well as in the absence of sulfonamide. First evidence that sulfonamides inhibited the incorporation of pAB into dihydropteroate was presented by BROWN (1962), who also strongly suggested the formation of an analog. The dihydropteroate analogs formed are devoid of significant inhibitory activity for a number of folate enzymes and diffuse out of the cell (ROLAND et al. 1979).

Dapsone has also been shown to be an inhibitor of the *E. coli* DHPS, being twofold less active than sulfadiazine (MCCULLOUGH and MAREN 1973). The meningococcal enzyme is three times more susceptible to dapsone than to sulfadiazine (HO et al. 1975). Dapsone is also a potent inhibitor of dihydropteroic acid synthesis in extracts of *M. leprae*. In contrast to *E. coli*, however, no dapsone analog of dihydropteroic acid was found (KULKARNI and SEYDEL 1983). DHPS has not yet been purified to homogeneity and biochemical studies with this enzyme are so far restricted to crude extracts or partially purified preparations. The DHPS-gene from *S. pneumoniae* has, however, recently been cloned and its nucleotide sequence determined (LOPEZ et al. 1987). The enzyme was efficiently expressed in *E. coli*.

E. Mechanisms of Sulfonamide Resistance

I. Bacteria

1. Production of a Plasmid-Coded, Sulfonamide-Resistant Bypass Enzyme

Shortly after plasmid encoded TMP resistance was found to be based on the production of a drug-resistant bypass dihydrofolate reductase in 1974 (see Chap. 11), a similar mechanism was uncovered for sulfonamide resistance. WISE and ABOU-DONIA (1975) and independently SKÖLD (1976) proved the presence of sulfonamide resistant, additional DHPS in sulfonamide-resistant, plasmid-bearing strains of *E. coli* and *Citrobacter*, making the cell diploid for DHPS. Transfer of the plasmid-coded DHPS rescued a temperature sensitive DHPS-mutant from its thermosensitivity (SKÖLD 1976). The plasmids coding for these enzymes carried additional resistance markers and originated from the US, Australia and France. This mechanism was also demonstrated with isolates from Japan (NAGATE et al. 1978) and probably constitutes the most important mechanism of sulfonamide resistance.

The amount of resistant DHPS produced varies in different strains and in general the specific activity of total enzyme in resistant strains is only slightly increased over that of sulfonamide-sensitive strains. In some cases, e.g. with plasmids R388 and R22259, the expression of resistant DHPS is very poor (SWEDBERG and SKÖLD 1983). This depends on the promoter efficiency in different plasmids.

The sulfonamide-resistant DHPS in crude extracts was more sensitive to heat than the chromosomal enzyme. Whereas the latter decreases in the stationary phase the resistant DHPS was constant through the life cycle and was not inducible. Chromosomal and plasmid enzyme can be separated by gel filtration and ion-exchange chromatography and easily distinguished by their different susceptibilities to sulfonamides and heat. Interestingly, other pAB analogs such as pAS discriminated much less between the two enzyme types (WISE and ABOU-DONIA 1975; SWEDBERG and SKÖLD 1980). Some properties of different DHPS are compared in Table 2.

Based on different heat stability observed with several plasmid derived DHPS, two different types were assumed to exist (SWEDBERG and SKÖLD 1980). This notion was confirmed by Southern blot hybridization and restriction mapping, which clearly showed that the genetic determinants for sulfonamide-resistant

Table 2. Properties of dihydropteroate synthetases

Enzyme source	Molecular weight (kDa)	Susceptibility to heat	K_m (μM) for pAB	IC_{50} for sulfathiazole	Satur. concn. for pteridin substrate (μM)	Reference
E. coli, chromosomal	45	Stable	5	$10^{-6}\,M$	15	SWEDBERG an[d] SKÖLD (198[0])
E. coli, chromosomal mutant (C-167ts20)	45	Labile	40	$\gg 10^{-6}\,M$	15	SWEDBERG et a[l.] (1979)
E. coli, plasmid pGS05	41	Labile	5	$10^{-2}\,M$		SWEDBERG an[d] SKÖLD (198[0])
E. coli, plasmid pGS03	41	Labile	5	$10^{-2}\,M$		SWEDBERG an[d] SKÖLD (198[0])
E. coli, plasmid pGS04	41	Labile	5	$10^{-2}\,M$		SWEDBERG an[d] SKÖLD (198[0])
E. coli, plasmid pKT012	–	Very labile[a]	5	$10^{-2}\,M$		SWEDBERG an[d] SKÖLD (198[0])

[a] Stabilized by sucrose, dithiothreitol

DHPS differed. Enzymes coded by plasmid pGS05 and pGS01, which differ in heat stability, belong to different classes. The origin of these enzymes and their genes remains unknown.

2. Mutation of the Target Enzyme

There are several examples of mutational changes in target enzymes known which decrease their affinity for an inhibitor. These enzymes still fulfil their normal function sufficiently well, but render the cell resistant to the inhibitor. During uptake studies with [^{35}S]sulfanilamide, WACKER et al. (1957) observed that the sulfanilamide could be more easily removed from resistant enterococci or *E. coli* cells than from susceptible ones. They interpreted these findings as indicating that the affinity of the "receptor" for the sulfonamide had been decreased. Mutations affecting "folate" synthesis were described early on in *E. coli* (PATO and BROWN 1963) and in pneumococci (ORTIZ and HOTCHKISS 1966). Such mutants, selected over increasing sulfonamide concentrations, were easily obtained in vitro. Extracts of these mutants had similar abilities to synthesize "folate" as the wild type. K_m values for pAB seemed not to be different for resistant and susceptible strains, but in one case (*E. coli*) the resistant enzyme was heat labile.

A comparison of sulfonamide susceptible and resistant meningococci showed that resistant strains did not overproduce pAB and did not differ in the binding of [^{35}S]sulfadiazine. Mutation of DHPS may therefore have been the reason for resistance (VAICHULIS and VEDROS 1971). Clinical isolates of *N. meningitidis* and *N. gonorrhoeae* resistant to sulfanilamide were later shown to have DHPS with reduced affinities for sulfanilamide. K_i for sulfanilamide was two- to more than tenfold higher in the resistant enzymes, whereas the affinity of the substrate pAB was not changed (Ho et al. 1974).

Pneumococcal DHPS from wild type and resistant strains, obtained by transformation, was approximately 30-fold purified and characterized by ORTIZ (1970). Both enzymes had similar K_m values for pAB (1.5 to 7.3 μM), but the mutant enzymes had slightly higher K_m values for *p*-aminobenzoylglutamate. Importantly, the enzymes from the drug-resistant mutants displayed reduced binding of sulfanilamide, as reflected by an approximately 10-fold increase in K_i. Interestingly, the molecular weight of the streptococcal DHPS was found to be 75000 to 95000, which is twice the size of the *E. coli* enzyme.

Mutants of *E. coli*, selected in vitro with sulfathiazole, were shown to owe their resistance to a thermosensitive, sulfonamide-resistant DHPS, which was less active than the normal enzyme (SKÖLD 1976). The mutant enzyme had drastically reduced affinity for the substrate pAB, and also for the alternative substrate *p*-aminobenzoylglutamic acid. The affinity for sulfathiazole was reduced 150-fold (SWEDBERG et al. 1979). Although some of the mutant enzymes were catalytically less efficient than the normal enzyme, they seemed to be able to fulfil the folate-cofactor requirement of the cell. RAPPOLD and BACHER (1976), however, described a mutant of *Aerobacter aerogenes* in which DHPS had been affected to such an extent that a nutritional requirement for pAB resulted. It was not shown whether this mutation caused a drastically reduced catalytic efficiency of DHPS or whether abnormally low levels of a normal enzyme were present.

Based on the limited studies available it seems that mutation to a drug-insensitive DHPS having decreased affinity for sulfonamides (and in part also for pAB) constitutes an important mechanism of sulfonamide resistance found in clinical isolates of pneumococci, neisseriae, and most likely also in other species.

3. Overproduction of Physiological Metabolites

Sulfonamides directly compete with pAB for the active site of DHPS. Hence an increased production of pAB by a mutational change in one or more of the enzymes involved in the biosynthesis of pAB will reduce the activity of sulfonamides. MACLEOD (1940) reported on the production of sulfonamide-antagonizing substances by sulfonamide-resistant pneumococci. The production of these "sulfonamide inhibitors" was much higher in sulfapyridine-resistant pneumococci than in the sensitive parent strains. The nature of these compounds remained unknown. Since these compounds were antagonistic in *E. coli*, a folate nature can be excluded.

In a later study it was found that sulfonamide-resistant staphylococci, selected in vitro by exposure to sulfathiazole, produced an approximately 70-fold increased level of pAB. The responsible mutation was stable (LANDY et al. 1943). Their study of other species such as *E. coli*, *Vibrio*, *Shigella* and *Diplococcus pneumoniae* failed to detect overproduction of pAB. In *S. aureus* and *N. gonorrhoeae* increased production of pAB was later confirmed as a mechanism of resistance to sulfonamides (LANDY and GERSTUNG 1944). The level of pAB produced in gonococci, determined by a microbiological assay, was correlated to in vitro susceptibility and clinical response. In sulfadiazine-resistant isolates of *N. meningitidis* increased production of pAB was also the most likely explanation for resistance (IVLER et al. 1965).

Later, WHITE and WOODS (1965a) found increased production of pAB in laboratory mutants and clinical isolates of *S. aureus*. The relationship between the degree of pAB overproduction and sulfonamide resistance was not always proportional. Some of the strains studied seemed to have undergone other mutations as well, leading to the enhanced synthesis of folic acid, the location of the responsible mutation having not been defined at that time. A sulfonamide-resistant *S. aureus* strain (2102 R) was found to produce five times as much "*L. casei* factor" as the parent strain (LASCELLES and WOODS 1952). The nature of this factor also remained unknown.

Mutants of *Brevibacterium flavum* and *Corynebacterium glutamicum* resistant to sulfaguanidine were found to have higher tryptophan productivities and occurred at high frequency. Deregulation of those steps leading to aromatic amino acids was assumed to be the reason for the elevated tryptophan levels produced and a twofold increased production of chorismate was indeed confirmed. Since chorismate is the precursor of pAB, sulfonamide resistance could reasonably be explained by elevated pAB levels, but these were not determined (SHIIO et al. 1984). *Streptomyces griseus* mutagenized and selected for sulfonamide resistance was found to overproduce pAB. The pAB-synthetase gene transformed into *S. lividans* or *E. coli* also rendered these organisms sulfonamide-resistant (GIL and HOPWOOD 1983).

Thus although overproduction of pAB and perhaps other intermediates in folic acid biosynthesis has been documented in several species, this mechanism has not been further studied recently and its importance in sulfonamide resistance awaits further clarification.

4. Acquisition of Auxotrophies

The toxicity of sulfonamides to the microbial cell depends on the medium composition, since a shortage of tetrahydrofolate cofactors affects the synthesis of purines, methionine and thymidylate. The degree of toxicity is therefore dependent on the presence of these metabolites, which cause a tetrahydrofolate-cofactor-sparing effect. Whereas the presence of purines, methionine and thymidine together largely antagonize the activity of sulfonamides, as well as of antifolates (THEN and ANGEHRN 1973), purines exhibit a sulfonamide-potentiating effect, dependent on the activity of phosphoribosyl transferase (BRUCE et al. 1984).

The conversion of dUMP to thymidylate requires stoichiometric amounts of N^5N^{10}-methylene tetrahydrofolate. Loss or mutation of the catalyzing enzyme, thymidylate synthetase (EC 2.1.1.45), results in a thymidine requirement and renders the cell resistant to sulfonamides, as well as to antifolates. Thymine auxotrophs are easily selected in vitro and have been isolated from patients in whom co-trimoxazole therapy failed (MASKELL et al. 1978; KING et al. 1983). Cystic fibrosis patients seem to be particularly prone to selection of such auxotrophs (GILLIGAN et al. 1987). Thymine-auxotrophic pathogenic variants have been found among a variety of species such as *E. coli*, *Providencia*, *Serratia*, *Proteus*, *Streptococcus*, *Staphylococcus* and *Salmonella*.

In *Neisseriaceae*, low levels of resistance to sulfadiazine in clinical isolates were frequently connected to a deficiency for methionine. Since the biosynthesis of methionine from homocysteine requires 5-methyl-tetrahydrofolate, a tetrahydrofolate-sparing effect is provided, resulting in increased tolerance to sulfonamide (CATLIN 1967). In another study, pro^- isolates of penicillinase-producing *N. gonorrhoeae* were found to be less susceptible to antibiotics and sulfamethoxazole than prototrophic strains (VAN KLINGEREN et al. 1985). Acquisition of auxotrophies in vivo has been reported for a variety of species (BORDERON and HORODNICEANU 1978; KENYON 1978), but the relationship between these auxotrophies and the concomitantly acquired resistance to different antibiotics is not always clear.

5. Resistance Due To Impaired Penetration

Very little is known about the route of penetration of sulfonamides into the cytoplasm of bacteria. They are accumulated two- to sixfold in the bacterial cell, depending on the pH and substance and the physiological state of the cell, and they are assumed to enter via passive diffusion (ROLAND et al. 1979; BÜTTNER and BÜTTNER 1980). No differences in the accumulation of sulfonamides between sensitive and resistant *E. coli* were found (BÜTTNER and BÜTTNER 1972). Similarly, sensitive and resistant staphylococci did not differ in the accumulation of [^{35}S]sulfathiazole (WHITE and WOODS 1965b).

Mutations resulting in an impaired penetration of sulfonamides have often been held responsible for resistance if other mechanisms, such as altered DHPS, overproduction of pAB, etc. could not be detected. PATO and BROWN (1963) thus attributed resistance of some of their *E. coli* mutants to decreased penetration. Besides production of a sulfonamide-resistant DHPS, sulfonamide resistance mediated by plasmids encoding triple or quadruple resistance was assumed to be based on decreased permeability (UNOWSKY and KRAINSKY 1971; NAGATE et al. 1978). However, a suspected plasmid-derived permeability change brought about by plasmids R388 and R22259 could not be confirmed in a more detailed study, and these plasmids were shown to code for drug-resistant DHPS (SWEDBERG and SKÖLD 1983). Thus plasmid-based changes in permeability as a resistance mechanism to sulfonamides remain to be demonstrated.

A strong penetration barrier is the reason for intrinsic resistance of *Pseudomonas aeruginosa* to sulfonamides. This is easily delineated from the fact that phosphanilic acid, another antimetabolite of pAB, is active against *Pseudomonas* (MISIEK et al. 1985). The existence of a penetration barrier in bacteria had already been noticed by BROWN (1962), who found that sulfanilic acid was a good enzyme inhibitor, but poorly active in vitro.

The synergism between polymyxin and sulfonamides in both intact bacteria and L forms also suggests that the cell envelope presents a penetration barrier to sulfonamides (MONTGOMERIE et al. 1973).

Cross resistance to TMP, nalidixic acid, chloramphenicol, tetracyclines and sulfonamides observed in *Klebsiella*, *Enterobacter* and *Serratia* is based on impaired penetration due to modification of outer membrane proteins (GOLDSTEIN et al. 1986). This type of mutant has been shown (for *K. pneumoniae*) to also have slightly diminished susceptibility to sulfafurazole (SMITH 1976). We detected slight changes in the MICs for sulfonamides in strains exhibiting alterations in the porin-protein pattern, but the role of porins in sulfonamide uptake remains to be established.

6. Other Mechanisms

Metabolic degradation by the bacterial cell is an important resistance mechanism for many antibiotics, especially the β-lactams. Few reports are available in which metabolic degradation of sulfonamides to inactive products has been considered. In meningococci resistant to sulfadiazine no inactivation was found, at least not with the methods employed (IVLER et al. 1965; VAICHULIS and VEDROS 1971). Likewise, no evidence for a conversion of sulfadiazine into a noninhibitory compound was found in staphylococci (WHITE and WOODS 1965b). In a study with propionibacteria no degradation of sulfadiazine was found (REDDY et al. 1973). Employing a microbiological disk method, KANAZAWA and KARUMATA (1966) found slight inactivation of sulfisoxazole in both sensitive and resistant strains. The ruminal flora in cows was seen to degrade TMP, and metabolism of sulfonamides may also take place, though this remains an open question (NIELSEN et al. 1978). From all these studies it seems unlikely that inactivation of sulfonamides constitutes an important mechanism of resistance.

Overproduction of the target enzyme, DHPS, has not been established as a means of acquiring resistance to sulfonamides as is the case for dihydrofolate reductase in TMP or methotrexate resistance. In *S. pneumoniae* it has, however, been observed that multiple copies of the *sul*-s gene (coding for wild type DHPS) confer a very low degree of sulfonamide resistance (LOPEZ et al. 1984). The *sul*-d gene, in contrast, coding for a drug-resistant DHPS and present in a single copy, decreased the sulfonamide sensitivity from 0.02 mg/ml to 0.2 mg/ml. The same gene, present in a multicopy plasmid (pLS 80), conveyed resistance to 2 mg/ml sulfonamide. A deleted plasmid (pLS 83), containing the entire sul-d gene and expressing the mutant DHPS product, however, did not confer resistance to sulfonamides (LOPEZ et al. 1987).

Sulfamethoxazole in combination with TMP is standard therapy for *Pneumocystis carinii* pneumonias. Sometimes folinic acid is coadministered to reverse hematological abnormalities. There are anecdotal reports that folinic acid may render *Pneumocystis* resistant to sulfamethoxazole/TMP (NUNN and ALLISTONE 1984), suggesting that this organism, in contrast to most pathogenic bacteria, is able to utilize exogenous folinic acid. However, no evidence for this was obtained in a pneumonia model in rats (D'ANTONIO et al. 1986) and intact organisms did not transport folinic acid (ALLEGRA et al. 1987).

II. Plasmodia

The key enzyme, DHPS, has been detected in several plasmodial species. Studies on sulfonamide resistance are limited, however, and particularly hampered by the fact that some aspects of folate metabolism in different plasmodial species are not yet very clear (GEARY et al. 1985; MILHOUS et al. 1985; YUTHAVONG et al. 1985; WATKINS et al. 1985). *P. falciparum* seems to be able to synthesize pAB de novo (DIECKMANN and JUNG 1986), but poor growth of *P. falciparum* was obtained if the pAB content was less than 25 μg/l (TAN-ARIYA and BROCKELMAN 1983). Based on the method employed for pAB determination, this figure is probably too high and a standard medium now recommended by the WHO contains 0.5 μg pAB/l. Strains with a capacity to use low levels of pAB could easily be selected and reduced susceptibility to sulfonamide was acquired along with this ability (TAN-ARIYA and BROCKELMAN 1983). Synthesis of folic acid derivatives also seems to occur de novo, but exogenous folic acid may be used to some extent (MILHOUS et al. 1985; WATKINS et al. 1985) and different species and strains may behave differently. The possibility of increasing the utilization of exogeneously available folic acid compounds (in the erythrocyte storage pool of polyglutamated ^{5}N-methyl tetrahydrofolate) may explain acquisition of resistance to sulfonamides and pyrimethamine (MILHOUS et al. 1985).

In synchronous cultures of *P. falciparum*, a resistant strain was shown to incorporate less [^{35}S]sulfadoxine than a sensitive strain (DIECKMANN and JUNG 1986). Although the strains were not isogenic, reduced uptake, perhaps via a pAB-transporting system, could play a role in sulfadoxine resistance. In both strains the formation of the sulfadoxine analog of dihydropteroate could be demonstrated. Since the conversion of sulfadoxine to this analog in crude extracts was less efficient in the resistant strain, a mutational change of DHPS, as known from bacteria, could also play a role. Degradation of the sulfonamide was excluded. In an earlier study, TAN-ARIYA and BROCKELMAN (1983) also demonstrated reduced uptake of [^{14}C]sulfadoxine into a sulfadoxine-resistant strain of *P. falciparum* as a mechanism of resistance to the drug.

Acquisition of resistance to either pyrimethamine or sulfonamide usually affects sensitivity to the other drug as well and hence shared or linked mechanisms of resistance may be common (MILHOUS et al. 1985; BEALE 1980). On the other hand, it has been reported that strains resistant to pyrimethamine or other antifols became hypersensitive to sulfonamides and sulfones (BEALE 1980). Chloroquine resistance in a multiply drug resistant strain of *P. falciparum* could be reversed by verapamil, a calcium-channel blocker (MARTIN et al. 1987). Enhanced active efflux of drug was discussed as a possible mechanism of resistance, but this, as well as its relevance for sulfonamide resistance, remains to be established for plasmodia.

Since uptake studies are usually performed with parasitized erythrocytes, it has to be considered that *P. falciparum* also modifies the erythrocyte's plasma membrane (TRIGLIA et al. 1987). Uptake of drugs may thus well be influenced differently in different strains. Progress in the in vitro cultivation of plasmodia over the last 10 years will aid in further studies on the mechanisms of resistance in malarial parasites.

F. Genetics of Sulfonamide Resistance

Most of the mechanisms discussed in the preceding sections are due to mutations located on the chromosome, e.g. in the sulA gene leading to pAB overproduction, or mutations resulting in alterations of the target site, DHPS. Although some of these mechanisms are common, little is known about their frequencies in clinical isolates.

Resistance to sulfonamides due to R factors has been known for a long time and this was one of the first plasmid-borne resistance determinants found. Plasmid-coded sulfonamide resistance certainly constitutes the most important mechanism. Sulfonamide-resistance plasmids differ in size, they belong to different incompatibility groups, and are found all over the world. It is interesting to note that numerous plasmids found in *Pseudomonas aeruginosa* carry the Su^R determinant, although this species is intrinsically sulfonamide-resistant (JACOBY 1984).

Small, nonconjugative plasmids, coding only for sulfonamide resistance were described in *Shigella* from Japan (NAGATE et al. 1978). In *Haemophilus ducreyi*, a small, 4.9 MDa nonconjugative plasmid has been found which carries only the sulfonamide and not the streptomycin resistance gene. It is related to RSF 1010, which is of enteric origin (ALBRITTON et al. 1982). An 8.5 MDa plasmid also coding for sulfonamide but not streptomycin resistance has been detected in *Neisseria meningitidis* (FACINELLI and VARALDO 1987). The sulfonamide resistance trait is, however, frequently genetically linked to other resistances such as ampicillin, chloramphenicol, tetracycline, streptomycin or kanamycin (HOCHMANNOVA et al. 1982). Streptomycin and sulfonamide resistance reside on large, conjugative or on small, nonconjugative plasmids. Plasmid pBP1, a small, nonconjugative plasmid, is for instance found in *E. coli* all over the world, both in human and veterinary isolates (KORFMANN et al. 1983). Efficient interspecific transfer of these widely distributed nonconjugative plasmids was shown to be effected by mobilization with other, conjugative, plasmids (ARAKI et al. 1987). Another well characterized plasmid of this type is RSF1010 (5.5 MDa). A large, 62 MDa plasmid, Rldrd19, carries resistance to ampicillin, chloramphenicol, streptomycin, spectinomycin, kanamycin and sulfonamide (HOCHMANNOVA et al. 1982, SWEDBERG and SKÖLD 1980). A large, 35–39 MDa plasmid, R485 only carried sulfonamide resistance (HOCHMANNOVA et al. 1982).

Among the many sulfonamide-resistance plasmids several have a very broad host range. The Inc P-4 high copy number-plasmid R1162, carrying streptomycin and sulfonamide resistance, is found in many genera, including *E. coli* and *Pseudomonas* species. It is closely related or identical to RSF1010 (MEYER et al. 1985a). pFM739, an R plasmid from *Neisseria sicca*, carrying penicillin, streptomycin and sulfonamide resistance, also showed a close relationship to RSF 1010 (ROTGER et al. 1986). Plasmid pBWH 1 (92 kb, IncM) carrying resistance to gentamicin, tobramycin, kanamycin, ampicillin, chloramphenicol and sulfonamide, has been found in different genera of the Enterobacteriaceae over a 10-year period (HOPKINS et al. 1986).

The sulfonamide resistance marker resides on several transposons, and this is one explanation for its wide distribution. Several of these transposons carry different types of β-lactamases, such as TEM-1, OXA-1, PSE-1, PSE-2, PSE-4 along with sulfonamide and other resistances. A survey of transposons coding for sulfonamide resistance is given in Table 3. The sulfonamide-carrying transposons Tn*2410* and Tn*2411*, isolated from a *Salmonella typhimurium* R factor (R1767), were closely related to each other and also to Tn*2603* and Tn*4*, Tn*21* being the possible ancestral mercury transposon (KRATZ et al. 1983; WIEDEMANN et al. 1986; HALL and VOCKLER 1987).

The type I sulfonamide resistance gene is found on plasmids R1, R6, R100, close to the streptomycin resistance gene. In R388 it is close to the TMP resistance gene. The type II resistance gene is found on small as well as on large conjugative plasmids. Among the small ones are RSF1010 and pBP1, where sulfonamide resistance is linked to streptomycin resistance. The type II gene has its own promoter.

Expression of the type I gene in R388 is also effected by a promoter of its own, whereas in all other plasmids the linked genes were transcribed from a common promoter. Detailed studies with plasmid R6-5 showed that expression of sulfonamide resistance was completely dependent on the linked streptomycin resistance gene (SWEDBERG 1987).

A 6.0 MDa plasmid, isolated from commensal strains of *Neisseria* ssp. and *Branhamella catarrhalis*, resisant to penicillin, streptomycin and sulfamethoxazole, complements a mutation which determines the production of a thermosensitive DHPS and hence this plasmid probably also codes for a drug resistant DHPS (PINTADO et al. 1985). The same mechanism was postulated for the sulfonamide resistance plasmid found in *N. meningitidis* (FACINELLI and VARALDO 1987). The sulfonamide resistance gene from plasmid pSAS R06 of *E. coli* has recently been introduced into a hybrid plasmid able to replicate both in *E. coli* and

Table 3. Transposons carrying the sulfonamide-resistance marker

Transposon	Host plasmid[a]	Resistances on transposon[b]	Reference
Tn*4*	R 1	Ap Sm Sp Su Hg	PHILLIPON et al.(1983)
Tn *21*	R 100	Sm Su Hg	TANAKA et al. (1983)
Tn*536*	pPT 4	Sm Su Hg Sp Tp	TONIN and GRANT (1987)
Tn*1401*	pMG 217	Ap Sm Sp Su Hg	PHILLIPON et al. (1983)
Tn*1402*	pMG 209	Ap Sm Sp Su Hg	PHILLIPON et al. (1983)
Tn*1403*	RPL 11	Cb Cm Sm Sp Su Hg	JACOBY (1984)
Tn*1404*	R 151	Cb Gm Km Sm Sp Su Tm	PHILLIPON et al. (1983)
Tn*1696*	R 1033	Cm Gm Sm Su Hg	JACOBY (1984)
Tn*1831*	R 702	Ap Sm Sp Su Hg	MEYER et al. (1985b)
Tn*2011*	Rms 213	Ap Sm Sp Su Hg	NAKAZAWA and MITSUHASHI (1983)
Tn*2101*	Rms 433	Ap Sm Sp Su Hg	PHILLIPON et al. (1983)
Tn*2353*	R 15	Sm Su Hg	DOBRITSA et al. (1985)
Tn*2410*	R 1767	Ap Su Hg	KRATZ et al. (1983)
Tn*2411*	R 1767	Sm Su Hg	KRATZ et al. (1983)
Zn*2424*	NR 79	Ami Cm Sm Sp Su Hg	MEYER et al. (1985b)
Tn*2425*	pMH 2	Ap Sm Sp Su Hg	MEYER et al. (1985b)
Tn*2521*	chromosome	Cb Sm Sp Su	PHILLIPON et al. (1983)
Tn*2603*	RGN 238	Ap Sm Sp Su Hg	PHILLIPON et al. (1983)
Tn*2607*	RGN 14	Ap Sm Su	TANAKA et al. (1983)
Tn*2608*	RGn 823	Sm Su Hg	TANAKA et al. (1983)
Tn*2610*	pCS 200	Cb Sm Su	YAMAMOTO et al. (1983)

[a] Only examples are given; many transposons reside on several plasmids
[b] *Abbreviations:* Ap, ampicillin; Cb, carbenicillin; Ami, amikacin; Cm, chloramphenicol; Hg, mercuric chloride; Km, kanamycin; Gm, gentamycin; Sm, streptomycin, Sp, spectinomycin; Su, sulfonamide; Tm, tobramycin

Streptomyces lividans, where it is phenotypically expressed (SHARECK et al. 1984).

The genetic background of sulfonamide resistance has so far been studied nearly exclusively in gram-negative species. However, sulfonamide resistance is quite common in staphylococci. Multiple antibiotic resistant *S. aureus* from Australia were uniformly resistant to sulfonamides and TMP. Many of the resistance determinants, which are usually located on plasmids, were associated with the chromosome, including sulfonamide resistance. The presence of a transposable element is therefore inferred (LYON et al. 1983; TOWNSEND et al. 1984). To date only a single sulfonamide resistance plasmid (pWA2) has been identified in *S. aureus* (COURVALIN and FIANDT 1980; LYON and SKURRAY 1987).

Sulfonamides were initially used as single agents. In the late sixties sulfamethoxazole was introduced as a fixed combination with TMP and, later, TMP became available as a single agent in many countries. These changes in prescription habits would be expected to influence the selection and the prevalence of sulfonamide-resistant strains. Many plasmids confer resistance to both sulfonamide and TMP.

Examples are plasmids R388 (SuTp) (for abbreviations see Table 3), R22259 (SuTpTcCm), (SWEDBERG and SKÖLD 1980), R32 (SmCmTcSuTp), R67

(ApSmCmTcSuTp), R67bis, (SmTcSuTp), R27 (SuTp) (PATTISHALL et al. 1977). This linkage would guarantee an efficient protection against the widely used combination of sulfamethoxazole with TMP. A recent study of a novel, plasmid-derived TMP-resistant dihydrofolate reductase, detected in isolates from Sri Lanka, showed that this gene was inserted very close to a sulfonamide resistance gene (SUNDSTRÖM et al. 1987).

Depending on the geographic location and year of isolation, sulfonamide resistance cotransferred with TMP resistance varied from 20% in Boston (1982) to 97% in Paris (1984) (GOLDSTEIN et al. 1986). In a London hospital, 90.7% of *E. coli* resistant to TMP in 1981 were also resistant to sulfonamides. In 1985, interestingly, this figure has dropped to 80%. For *Klebsiella* the situation was static (HAMILTON-MILLER and PURVES 1986). That these changes were due to the changing selection pressure was convincingly documented by TOWNER and SLACK (1986), who observed a steady increase in TMP-resistant, but sulfonamide-susceptible, isolates of *E. coli*, *Klebsiella*, *Enterobacter* and *Proteus* since the use of TMP alone.

The genetic basis of resistance in malarial parasites has so far been followed to a limited extent only in rodent plasmodia. Resistances studied, e.g. to sulfonamides, antifols or chloroquine, were stably inherited and no R factors are involved (BEALE 1980).

References

Albritton WL, Brunton JL, Slaney L, MacLean L (1982) Plasmid-mediated sulfonamide resistance in *Haemophilus ducreyi*. Antimicrob Agents Chemother 21:159–165

Allegra CJ, Kovacs JA, Drake JC, Swan JC, Chabner BA, Masur H (1987) Activity of antifolates against *Pneumocystis carinii* dihydrofolate reductase and identification of a potent new agent. J Exp Med 165:926–931

Araki Y, Inoue M, Hashimoto H (1987) Characterization and mobilization of nonconjugative plasmids encoding resistance to streptomycin and sulfanilamide. Microbiol Immunol 31:1107–1111

Beale GH (1980) The genetics of drug resistance in malaria parasites. Bull WHO 58:799–804

Beales PF (1988) The prevention and control of malaria. Int Pharmacy J 2:16–20

Bock L, Miller GH, Schaper KJ, Seydel JK (1974) Sulfonamide structure-activity relationships in a cell-free system. 2. Proof for the formation of a sulfonamide-containing folate analog. J Med Chem 17:23–28

Borderon E, Horodniceanu T (1978) Metabolically deficient dwarf-colony mutants of *Escherichia coli*: deficiency and resistance to antibiotics of strains isolated from urine culture. J Clin Microbiol 8:629–634

Brown GM (1962) The biosynthesis of folic acid. II. Inhibition by sulfonamides. J Biol Chem 237:536–540

Bruce J, Hardy J, Stacey KA (1984) Potentiation by purines of the growth-inhibitory effects of sulphonamides on *Escherichia coli* K12 and the location of the gene which mediates this effect. J Gen Microbiol 130:2489–2495

Büttner D, Büttner H (1972) Binding of ^{35}S-sulfadiazine to cells and cell fractions of *Escherichia coli*. Chemotherapy 17:309–319

Büttner D, Büttner H (1980) pH Dependency in uptake of sulfonamides by bacteria. Chemotherapy 26:153–163

Campbell IG, Mee BJ, Nikoletti SM (1986) Evolution and spread of Inc FIV plasmids conferring resistance to trimethoprim. Antimicrob Agents Chemother 29:807–813

Catlin BW (1967) Genetic study of sulfadiazine-resistant and methionine-requiring *Neisseria* isolated from clinical material. J Bacteriol 94:719–733
Cohen ML, Tauxe RV (1986) Drug-resistant *Salmonella* in the United States: an epidemiologic perspective. Science 234:964–969
Courvalin D, Fiandt M (1980) Aminoglycoside-modifying enzymes of *Staphylococcus aureus*, expression in *Escherichia coli*. Gene 9:247–269
D'Antonio RG, Johnson DB, Winn RE, Van Dellen AF, Evans ME (1986) Effect of folinic acid on the capacity of trimethoprim-sulfamethoxazole to prevent and treat *Pneumocystis carinii* pneumonia in rats. Antimicrob Agents Chemother 29:327–329
Dieckmann A, Jung A (1986) Mechanisms of sulfadoxine resistance in *Plasmodium falciparum*. Mol Biochem Parasitol 19:143–147
Dobritsa AP, Mikhailova TG, Dubovraya VI (1985) Physical and genetic structure of the Inc N plasmid R15. Plasmid 14:99–105
Dupont MJ, Jouvenot M, Covedic G, Michel-Briand Y (1985) Development of plasmid-mediated resistance in *Vibrio cholerae* during treatment with trimethoprim-sulfamethoxazole. Antimicrob Agents Chemother 27:280–281
Facinelli B, Varaldo PE (1987) Plasmid-mediated sulfonamide resistance in *Neisseria meningitidis*. Antimicrob Agents Chemother 31:1642–1643
Foster TJ (1983) Plasmid-determined resistance to antimicrobial drugs and toxic metal ions in bacteria. Microbiol Rev 47:361–409
Geary TG, Divo AA, Bonanni LC, Jensen JB (1985) Nutritional requirements of *Plasmodium falciparum* in culture. III. Further observations on essential nutrients and antimetabolites. J Protozool 32:608–613
Gelber RH (1984) Primary dapsone-resistant leprosy in San Francisco. Int J Lepr Other Mycobact Dis 52:471–474
Gil JA, Hopwood DA (1983) Cloning and expression of p-aminobenzoic acid synthetase gene of the candicidin-producing *Streptomyces griseus*. Gene 25:119–132
Gilligan PH, Gage PA, Welch DF, Muszynski MJ, Wait KR (1987) Prevalence of thymidine-dependent *Staphylococcus aureus* in patients with cystic fibrosis. J Clin Microbiol 25:1258–1261
Goldstein FW, Papadopoulou B, Acar JF (1986) The changing pattern of trimethoprim resistance in Paris, with a review of worldwide experience. Rev Infect Dis 8:725–737
Hall RM, Vockler C (1987) The region of the IncN plasmid R46 coding for resistance to β-lactam antibiotics, streptomycin, spectinomycin and sulphonamides is closely related to antibiotic resistance segments found in IncW plasmids and in Tn 21-like transposons. Nucleic Acid Res 15:7491–7501
Hamet N (1986) Resistance to anticoccidial drugs in poultry farms in France from 1975–1984. In: McDougald LR, Joyner LP, Long PL (eds) Research in avian coccidiosis. Proc Georgia Coccidiosis Conference 1985. Univ of Georgia Press, Athens, pp 415–420
Hamilton-Miller JMT (1984) Resistance to antibacterial agents acting on folate metabolism. In: Bryan LE (ed) Antimicrobial drug resistance. Academic, Orlando, pp 173–190
Hamilton-Miller JMT, Purves D (1986) Trimethoprim resistance and trimethoprim usage in and around The Royal Free Hospital in 1985. J Antimicrob Chemother 18:643–644
Hitchings GH (1983) Inhibition of folate metabolism in chemotherapy. Springer, Berlin Heidelberg New York Tokyo (Handbook of experimental pharmacology, vol 64)
Ho RI, Corman L, Morse SA, Artenstein MS (1974) Alterations in dihydropteroate synthetase in cell-free extracts of sulfanilamide-resistant *Neisseria meningitidis* and *Neisseria gonorrhoeae*. Antimicrob Agents Chemother 5:388–392
Ho RI, Corman L, Morse SA, Schneider H (1975) Structure-activity of sulfones and sulfonamides on dihydropteroate synthetase from *Neisseria meningitidis*. Antimicrob Agents Chemother 7:758–763
Hochmannova J, Nesvera J, Stokrova J, Stransky J (1982) Molecular and genetic properties of plasmid R485 conferring resistance to sulphonamides. J Gen Microbiol 128:529–537

Hoffmann S (1984) Silver sulfadiazine: an antibacterial agent for topical use in burns. Scand J Plast Reconstr Surg 18:119–126

Hopkins JD, Mayer KH, Gilleece ES, O'Brien TF; Syvanen M (1986) Genetic and physical characterization of IncM plasmid pBWHl and its variance among natural isolates. J Bacteriol 165:47–52

Huovinen P, Pulkkinen L, Helin HL, Mäkilä M, Toivanen P (1986) Emergence of trimethoprim resistance in relation to drug consumption in a Finnish hospital from 1971 through 1984. Antimicrob Agents Chemother 29:73–76

Ivler D, Leedom JM, Thrupp LD, Wehrle PF, Portnoy B, Mathies AW (1965) Naturally occurring sulfadiazine-resistant meningococci. Antimicrob Agents Chemother 1964:444–450

Jacoby GA (1984) Resistance plasmids of *Pseudomonas aeruginosa*. In: Bryan LE (ed) Antimicrobial drug resistance. Academic, Orlando, pp 497–514

Kanazawa Y, Kuramata T (1966) A simple method for determination of ability of bacteria to inactivate chemotherapeutics using sensitivity discs. J Antibiot [A] 19:272–277

Kenyon JE (1978) *Neisseria gonorrhoeae*: acquisition of auxotrophy in the mouse. Curr Microbiol 1:253–256

King C, Shlaes DM, Dul MJ (1983) Infection caused by thymidine-requiring, trimethoprim-resistant bacteria. J Clin Microbiol 18:79–83

Korfmann G, Lüdtke W, van Treek U, Wiedemann B (1983) Dissemination of streptomycin and sulfonamide resistance by plasmid pBPl in *Escherichia coli*. Eur J Clin Microbiol 2:463–468

Kratz J, Schmidt F, Wiedemann B (1983) Characterization of Tn2411 and Tn2410, two transposons derived from R-plasmid R1767, and related to Tn2603 and Tn21. J Bacteriol 155:1333–1342

Kresken M, Wiedemann B (1986) Development of resistance in the past decade in central Europe. J Antimicrob Chemother 18 [Suppl C]:235–242

Kulkarni VM, Seydel JK (1983) Inhibitory activity and mode of action of diaminodiphenyl sulfone in cell-free folate-synthesizing systems prepared from *Mycobacterium lufu* and *Mycobacterium leprae*. Chemotherapy 29:58–67

Landy M, Gerstung RB (1944) p-Aminobenzoic acid synthesis by *Neisseria gonorrhoeae* in relation to clinical and cultural sulfonamide resistance. J Bacteriol 47:448

Landy M, Larkum NW, Oswald EJ, Streightoff F (1943) Increased synthesis of p-aminobenzoic acid associated with the development of sulfonamide resistance in *Staphylococcus aureus*. Science 97:265–267

Lascelles J, Woods DD (1952) The synthesis of "folic acid" by *Bacterium coli* and *Staphylococcus aureus* and its inhibition by sulphonamides. Br J Exp Pathol 33:288–303

Lopez P, Espinosa M, Lacks SA (1984) Physical structure and genetic expression of the sulfonamide-resistance plasmid pLS80 and its derivatives in *Streptococcus pneumoniae* and *Bacillus subtilis*. MGG 195:402–410

Lopez P, Espinosa M, Greenberg B, Lacks SA (1987) Sulfonamide resistance in Streptococcus pneumoniae: DNA sequence of the gene encoding dihydropteroate synthase and characterization of the enzyme. J Bacteriol 169:4320–4326

Lyon BR, Skurray R (1987) Antimicrobial resistance of *Staphylococcus aureus*: genetic basis. Microbiol Rev 51:88–134

Lyon BR, May JW, Skurray RA (1983) Analysis of plasmids in nosocomial strains of multiple-antibiotic-resistant *Staphylococcus aureus*. Antimicrob Agents Chemother 23:817–826

Macleod CM (1940) The inhibition of the bacteriostatic action of sulfonamide drugs by substances of animal and bacterial origin. J Exp Med 72:217–232

Martin SK, Oduola AMJ, Milhous WK (1987) Reversal of chloroquine resistance in *Plasmodium falciparum* by verapamil. Science 235:899–901

Maskell R, Okubadejo OA, Payne RH, Pead L (1978) Human infections with thymine-requiring bacteria. J Med Microbiol 11:33–45

McCullough JL, Maren TH (1973) Inhibition of dihydropteroate synthetase from *Escherichia coli* by sulfones and sulfonamides. Antimicrob Agents Chemother 3:665–669

Meyer RJ, Lin LS, Kim K, Brasch MA (1985a) Broad host-range plasmid R1162: replication, incompatibility, and copy-number control. Basic Life Sci 30:173–188

Meyer JF, Nies BA, Kratz J, Wiedemann B (1985b) Evolution of Tn21-related transposons: isolation of Tn2425, which harbours IS161. J Gen Microbiol 131:1123–1130

Milhous WK, Weatherly NF, Bowdre JH, Desjardins RE (1985) In vitro activities of and mechanisms of resistance to antifol antimalarial drugs. Antimicrob Agents Chemother 27:525–530

Mills J (1986) *Pneumocystis carinii* and *Toxoplasma gondii* infections in patients with AIDS. Rev Infect Dis 8:1001–1011

Misiek M, Buck RE, Pursiano TA, Chisholm DR, Tsai YH, Price KE, Leitner F (1985) Antibacterial activity of phosphanilic acid, alone and in combination with trimethoprim. Antimicrob Agents Chemother 28:761–765

Montgomerie JZ, Kalmanson GM, Guze LB (1973) Synergism of polymyxin and sulfonamides in L-forms of *Staphylococcus aureus* and *Proteus mirabilis*. Antimicrob Agents Chemother 3:523–525

Murray BE (1986) Resistance of *Shigella*, *Salmonella*, and other selected enteric pathogens to antimicrobial agents. Rev Infect Dis 8 [Suppl 2]:S172–S181

Nagate T, Inoue M, Inoue K, Mitsuhashi S (1978) Plasmid-mediated sulfanilamide resistance. Microbiol Immunol 22:367–375

Nakazawa H, Mitsuhashi S (1983) Tn2011, a new transposon encoding oxacillin-hydrolyzing β-lactamase. Antimicrob Agents Chemother 23:407–412

Nielsen P, Romvary A, Rasmussen F (1978) Sulphadoxine and trimethoprim in goats and cows: absorption fraction, half-lives and the degrading effect of the ruminal flora. J Vet Pharmacol Ther 1:37–45

Niemi M, Sibakov M, Niemela S (1983) Antibiotic resistance among different species of fecal coliforms isolates from water samples. Appl Environ Microbiol 45:79–83

Nunn PP, Allistone JC (1984) Resistance to trimethoprim-sulfamethoxazole in the treatment of *Pneumocystis carinii* pneumonia. Implication of folinic acid. Chest 86:149–150

Ortiz PJ (1970) Dihydrofolate and dihydropteroate synthesis by partially purified enzymes from wild-type and sulfonamide-resistant *Pneumococcus*. Biochemistry 9:355–361

Ortiz PJ, Hotchkiss RD (1966) The enzymatic synthesis of dihydrofolate and dihydropteroate in cell-free preparations from wild-type and sulfonamide-resistant pneumococcus. Biochemistry 5:67–74

Palenque E, Otero JR, Noriega AR (1983) High prevalence of non-epidemic *Shigella sonnei* resistant to co-trimoxazole. J Antimicrob Chemother 11:196–198

Pato ML, Brown GM (1963) Mechanisms of resistance of *Escherichia coli* to sulfonamides. Arch Biochem Biophys 103:443–448

Pattishall KH, Acar J, Burchall JJ, Goldstein FW, Harvey RJ (1977) Two distinct types of trimethoprim-resistant dihydrofolate reductase specified by R-plasmids of different compatibility groups. J Biol Chem 252:2319–2323

Pattyn SR, Yada A, Sansarricq H, Van Loo L (1984) Prevalence of secondary dapsone-resistant leprosy in Upper Volta. Lepr Rev 55:361–367

Peters W (1985) The problem of drug resistance in malaria. Parasitology 90:705–715

Philippon AM, Paul GC, Jacoby GA (1983) Properties of PSE-2 β-lactamase and genetic basis for its production in *Pseudomonas aeruginosa*. Antimicrob Agents Chemother 24:362–369

Pintado C, Salvador C, Rotger R, Nombela C (1985) Multiresistance plasmid from commensal *Neisseria* strains. Antimicrob Agents Chemother 27:120–124

Rappold H, Bacher A (1976) Nutritional requirement for 4-aminobenzoate caused by mutation of dihydropteroate synthetase. Z Naturforsch 31c:285–287

Reddy MS, Williams FD, Reinbold GW (1973) Sulfonamide resistance of propionibacteria: nutrition and transport. Antimicrob Agents Chemother 4:254–258

Rehm WF, Teelmann K, Weidekamm E (1986) General aspects of metabolism, residues, and toxicology of sulfonamides and dihydrofolate reductase inhibitors. In: Rico DG (ed) Drug residues in animals. Academic, Orlando, pp 65–109

Roland S, Ferone R, Harvey RJ, Styles VL, Morrison RW (1979) The characteristics and significance of sulfonamides as substrates for *Escherichia coli* dihydropteroate synthetase. J Biol Chem 254:10337–10345
Rotger R, Rubio F, Nombela C (1986) A multi-resistance plasmid isolated from commensal *Neisseria* species is closely related to the enterobacterial plasmid RSF1010. J Gen Microbiol 132:2491–2496
Shareck F, Sasarman A, Vezina C (1984) Construction of a suttle vector and expression in *Streptomyces lividans* of the sulfonamide-resistance gene derived from *Escherichia coli* plasmid pSAS1206. Can J Microbiol 30:515–518
Shepard CC, Rees RJW, Levy L, Pattyn SR, Baohong J, DelaCruz EC (1986) Susceptibility of strains of *Mycobacterium leprae* isolated prior to 1977 from patients with previously untreated lepromatous leprosy. Int J Lepr Other Mycobact Dis 54:11–15
Shiio I, Sugimoto S, Kawamura K (1984) Production of L-tryptophan by sulfonamide-resistant mutants. Agric Biol Chem 48:2073–2080
Sköld O (1976) R-factor-mediated resistance to sulfonamides by a plasmid-borne, drug-resistant dihydropteroate synthetase. Antimicrob Agents Chemother 9:49–54
Smith HW (1976) Mutants of *Klebsiella pneumoniae* resistant to several antibiotics. Nature 259:307–308
Spencer HC (1985) Drug-resistant malaria-changing patterns mean difficult decisions. Trans R Soc Trop Med Hyg 79:748–758
Sreevatsa, Ramu G, Desikan KV (1985) Prevalence of drug resistance in Dharmapuri and A. Pallipatti areas of tamil nadu. Indian J Lepr 57:376–382
Sundström L, Vinayagamoorthy T, Sköld O (1987) Novel type of plasmid-borne resistance to trimethoprim. Antimicrob Agents Chemother 31:60–66
Swedberg G (1987) Organization of two sulfonamide resistance genes on plasmids of gram-negative bacteria. Antimicrob Agents Chemother 31:306–311
Swedberg G, Sköld O (1980) Characterization of different plasmid-borne dihydropteroate synthases mediating bacterial resistance to sulfonamides. J Bacteriol 142:1–7
Swedberg C, Sköld O (1983) Plasmid-borne sulfonamide resistance determinants studied by restriction enzyme analysis. J Bacteriol 153:1228–1237
Swedberg G, Castensson S, Sköld O (1979) Characterization of mutationally altered dihydropteroate synthase and its ability to form a sulfonamide-containing dihydrofolate analog. J Bacteriol 137:129–136
Tanaka M, Yamamoto T, Sawai T (1983) Evolution of complex resistance transposons from an ancestral mercury transposon. J Bacteriol 153:1432–1438
Tan-Ariya P, Brockelman CR (1983) *Plasmodium falciparum*: variations in *p*-aminobenzoic acid requirements as related to sulfadoxine sensitivity. Exp Parasitol 55:364–371
Then RL (1982) Mechanisms of resistance to trimethoprim, the sulfonamides, and trimethoprim-sulfamethoxazole. Rev Infect Dis 4:261–269
Then R, Angehrn P (1973) Sulphonamide-induced "thymineless death" in *Escherichia coli*. J Gen Microbiol 76:255–263
Tonin PN, Grant RB (1987) Genetic and physical characterization of trimethoprim resistance plasmids from *Shigella sonnei* and *Shigella flexneri*. Can J Microbiol 33:905–913
Towner KJ, Slack RCB (1986) Effect of changing selection pressures on trimethoprim resistance in enterobacteriaceae. Eur J Clin Microbiol 5:502–506
Towner KJ, Wise PJ, Lewis MJ (1986) Molecular relationships between trimethoprim R plasmids obtained from human and animal sources. J Appl Bacteriol 61:535–540
Townsend DE, Ashdown N, Greed LC, Grubb WB (1984) Analysis of plasmids mediating gentamicin resistance in methicillin-resistant *Staphylococcus aureus*. J Antimicrob Chemother 13:347–352
Triglia T, Stahl HD, Crewther PE, Scanlon D, Brown GV, Anders RF, Kemp DJ (1987) The complete sequence of the gene for the knob-associated histidine-rich protein from *Plasmodium falciparum*. EMBO J 61:1413–1419
Unowsky J, Krainski ML (1971) Mechanism of R-factor mediated sulfonamide resistance in *Escherichia coli*. Bacteriol Proc 52

Vaichulis EMK, Vedros NA (1971) The uptake of ^{35}S-sulfadiazine by sulfonamide-sensitive and resistant *Neisseria meningitidis* with reference to the mode of action. Chemotherapy 16:153–161
Van Klingeren B, Ansink-Schipper MC, Dessens-Kroon M, Verheuvel M (1985) Relationship between auxotype, plasmid pattern and susceptibility to antibiotics in penicillinase-producing *Neisseria gonorrhoeae*. J Antimicrob Chemother 16:143–147
Verdrager J (1986) Epidemiology of emergence and spread of drug-resistant falciparum malaria in southeast asia. Southeast Asian J Trop Med Public Health 17:111–118
Vorland LH, Carlson K, Aalen O (1985) Antibiotic resistance and small R plasmids among *Escherichia coli* isolates from outpatient urinary tract infections in northern Norway. Antimicrob Agents Chemother 27:107–113
Vosmirko VL (1986) Resistance to antibiotics and sulfanilamides of Enterobacteriaceae strains isolated in the Ulyanovsk region (in Russian). Antibiot Med Biotekhnol 31:863–866
Wacker A, Trebst A, Simon H (1957) Über den Stoffwechsel des Sulfanilamids-[^{35}S] bei empfindlichen und resistenten Bakterien. Z Naturforsch 12b:315–319
Warhurst DC (1986) Antimalarial drugs: mode of action and resistance. J Antimicrob Chemother 18 [Suppl B]:51–59
Watkins WM, Sixsmith DG, Chulay JD, Spencer HC (1985) Antagonism of sulfadoxine and pyrimethamine antimalarial activity in vitro by *p*-aminobenzoic acid, *p*-aminobenzoylglutamic acid and folic acid. Mol Biochem Parasitol 14:55–61
White PJ, Woods DD (1965a) The synthesis of *p*-aminobenzoic acid and folic acid by staphylococci sensitive and resistant to sulphonamides. J Gen Microbiol 40:243–253
White PJ, Woods DD (1965b) Biochemical properties of staphylococci sensitive and resistant to sulphonamides. J Gen Microbiol 40:255–271
Wiedemann B, Meyer JF, Zühlsdorf MT (1986) Insertions of resistance genes into Tn21-like transposons. J Antimicrob Chemother 18 [Suppl C]:85–92
Wise EM, Abou-Donia MM (1975) Sulfonamide resistance mechanism in *Escherichia coli*: R plasmids can determine sulfonamide-resistant dihydropteroate synthetase. Proc Natl Acad Sci USA 72:2621–2625
Yamamoto T, Watanabe M, Matsumoto K, Sawai T (1983) Tn2610, a transposon involved in the spread of the carbenicillin-hydrolyzing β-lactamase gene. MGG 189:282–288
Yuthavong Y, Panijpan B, Ruenwongsa P, Sirawaraporn W (1985) Biochemical aspects of drug action and resistance in malaria parasites. Southeast Asian J Trop Med Public Health 16:459–472

CHAPTER 13

Chloramphenicol Acetyltransferases

W. V. SHAW and A. G. W. LESLIE

A. Chloramphenicol Resistance: General Aspects

I. Introduction

Chloramphenicol became available for clinical use in 1948 and rapidly became accepted as a valuable broad spectrum antibiotic with a number of attractive properties. Although generally accepted to be more often bacteriostatic rather than bactericidal for most micro-organisms sensitive to it, chloramphenicol inhibits virtually all gram-positive and gram-negative bacteria, including rickettsia and enters the cerebrospinal fluid in the absence of inflammation of the meninges. Indeed, its anti-microbial and chemical properties (see below) made it an almost ideal therapeutic agent, and it is probable that it might have remained a first line antibiotic had it not been for the several unusual and life threatening toxicity syndromes, widely appreciated since the mid-1960s, which have restricted its general usefulness. Nonetheless, chloramphenicol remains a valuable antibiotic for certain serious infections and clinical circumstances (SANDE and MANDELL 1985).

II. Chemistry and Properties of Chloramphenicol

The structure of chloramphenicol (Fig. 1) immediately suggests the reasons for its ready access to most of the extra-cellular body compartments and its ability to reach intracellular bacteria. Chloramphenicol is amphiphilic and unionized at physiological pH, possessing both reasonable solubility in aqueous systems and the ability to traverse biological membranes without significant hindrance. The stereochemistry of the propanediol side chain at C-1 and C-2 of chloramphenicol yields four possible diastereoisomers of which only one, (D-threo), is active as an antibiotic via the ability to inhibit the peptidyl transferase centre of prokaryotic ribosomes (GALE et al. 1981). Although early studies suggested that both hydroxyl groups were essential for antimicrobial activity it has been observed that the 3-fluoro (3-deoxy) analogue of chloramphenicol is a potent antibiotic and indifferent to the action of chloramphenicol acetyltransferase (see below) by virtue of the absence of an acetyl acceptor site. A number of substitutions, most notably CH_3SO_2- for NO_2-, are permitted at the para position of the 1-phenyl moiety without loss of activity and various acyl groups can replace Cl_2CHCO- at the 2-amino position but none without some sacrifice in antimicrobial potency (PONGS 1979; SYRIOPOULOU et al. 1981).

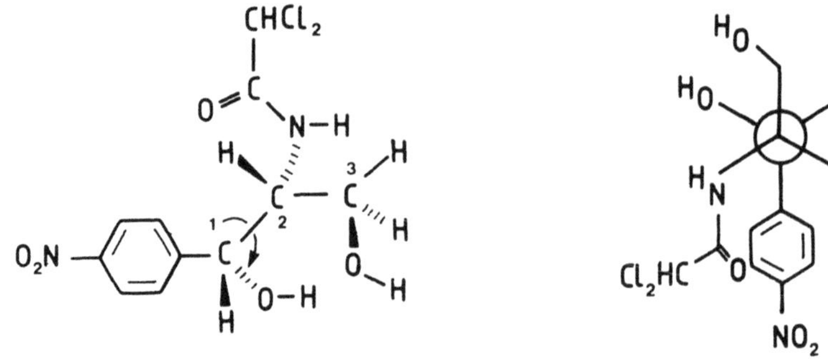

Fig. 1. The structure of chloramphenicol depicted by two conventions. The chiral centres at C-1 and C-2 generate four diastereoisomers of which only the D-threo is active as an antibiotic. Chloramphenicol acetyltransferase (CAT) catalyzes acetylation at the C-3 hydroxyl, and non-enzymic acyl migration to form the C-1 ester generates the substrate for a second acetylation step catalyzed by CAT (see text). The Newman projection emphasizes how rotation around the C-1/C-2 bond can allow the hydroxyls at C-1 and C-3 to approach within hydrogen bonding distance, possibly stabilizing that conformer and facilitating the intramolecular rearrangement in solution. The structure of chloramphenicol bound to CAT is, however, in an extended conformation (Fig. 5)

III. Emergence of Resistance to Chloramphenicol

1. Discovery of Chloramphenicol Acetyltransferase

Within a few years of its introduction into widespread clinical use there were sporadic reports of resistance to chloramphenicol. The explosive appearance in 1955 of epidemic strains of *Shigella* resistant to chloramphenicol and three other unrelated antimicrobial agents led not only to the recognition of plasmid-mediated transmissible antibiotic resistance but also to a greater awareness of the need to delineate the biochemical mechanism conferred by each resistant determinant (WATANABE 1963). It soon became clear that most gram-positive and gram-negative bacteria which were resistant to chloramphenicol are able to inactivate the antibiotic (MIYAMURA 1964). It was noted subsequently that the inactivation phenotype of chloramphenicol resistance could be attributed to enzymic acetylation of the antibiotic by the enzyme chloramphenicol acetyltransferase (CAT) using acetyl-CoA as the acyl donor (SHAW 1967; SUZUKI and OKAMOTO 1967). The general subject of chloramphenicol resistance and CAT in particular has been reviewed previously (SHAW 1983, 1984).

2. Non-enzymic Mechanisms of Chloramphenicol Resistance

Although most clinical isolates of chloramphenicol-resistant bacteria owe their phenotype to genes specifying CAT, either plasmid-borne or chromosomal, it has become clear that at least one other mechanism for chloramphenicol resistance exists. Plasmid-encoded resistance to chloramphenicol in enteric bacteria without detectable CAT has been known for some years (NAGAI and MITSUHASHI 1972). Although the precise mechanism remains unclear, there is evidence that an important non-CAT phenotype involves a gene product which is associated with the bacterial cell membrane and which probably serves to prevent chloramphenicol from gaining access to its ribosomal target at a concentration sufficient to inhibit protein synthesis. In contrast to CAT, which characteristically mediates high level resistance to chloramphenicol, often with minimum inhibitory concentrations in excess of 100 $\mu g\ ml^{-1}$, the non-CAT mechanism usually leads to lower levels of resistance but cannot confer resistance to the 3-fluoro chloramphenicol analog (GAFFNEY et al. 1981, DORMAN and FOSTER 1982). A novel 31 kDa membrane-associated protein associated with the resistance phenotype shows no homology with CAT or with the tetracycline resistance proteins which are known to operate by an active exclusion mechanism (DORMAN et al. 1986). Its synthesis, superficially similar to that of CAT in gram-positive bacteria (see Sect. C.III), depends on the presence of chloramphenicol and also appears to be regulated at a post-transcriptional level (DORMAN and FOSTER 1985).

The matter of chloramphenicol resistance in *Pseudomonas aeruginosa* and *Haemophilus influenzae* appears to be more complicated than is the case for most gram-negative bacteria. CAT variants specified by plasmid-linked or chromosomal genes have been implicated in both cases, but it is also clear that non-CAT mechanisms are also observed. The observation that an apparent permeability barrier for chloramphenicol in *H. influenzae* may be responsible is analogous to the conclusions from the work of Dorman and Foster with *E. coli* but the details appear to be different (BURNS et al. 1985). There is evidence, for example, that non-CAT resistance to chloramphenicol in *P. aeruginosa* is associated with a transposon-related DNA fragment which may possess homology with chromosomal sequences in *H. influenzae* (BURNS et al. 1986). The circumstantial evidence is that the *absence* of outer membrane proteins may be involved in such cases. It remains to be seen how the product of such chloramphenicol resistance genes can be related to more general aspects of the cell envelope, the role of porins in particular, and recent data which suggest that chloramphenicol uptake in gram-negative bacteria may be less passive than has been previously imagined (ABDEL-SAYED 1987).

B. Enzymology of Chloramphenicol-Acetylation

I. Acetylation and Inactivation

Although the reaction catalyzed by CAT is usually written in such a way as to emphasize its role in the inactivation of chloramphenicol, it is reversible in vitro and steady state kinetic parameters have been obtained for both the forward and reverse reactions (KLEANTHOUS and SHAW 1984).

$$\text{Chloramphenicol} + \text{acetyl CoA} \rightleftarrows \text{3-O-acetyl chloramphenicol} + \text{CoA}$$

Since the forward reaction involves the cleavage of a thioester bond and formation of an oxyester product, the equilibrium is safely in the direction of acetylation and inactivation of chloramphenicol. The ultimate disposition of the antibiotic is, however, more complicated since the monoacetyl product undergoes isomerization and is in equilibrium with 1-O-acetyl chloramphenicol. This non-enzymic and intramolecular acyl migration allows CAT to catalyze a second round of acetylation, yielding 1,3-diacetyl chloramphenicol. The apparent rate at which the diacetyl product forms in vivo and in vitro is a complicated function of pH, the nature and amount of CAT present, and the concentration of acetyl CoA. The second acetylation seems not to be necessary since the monoacetyl products are devoid of significant antimicrobial activity by virtue of their lack of affinity for the ribosomal target. A fuller account of the subject appears elsewhere (SHAW 1983). For the purpose of the present discussion, however, it should be noted that naturally occurring variants of CAT may differ with respect to their ability to accomodate 1-O-acetyl chloramphenicol at the active site. For example, it has been demonstrated that a variant of CAT in many isolates of *H. influenzae* may not catalyze the formation of 1,3-diacetyl chloramphenicol or do so at a rate which is not detectable by chemical assays (SMITH and KELSEY, in press). The high resolution three dimensional structure for a plasmid-specified CAT reveals that the "fit" for 1-acetyl chloramphenicol is tight at the antibiotic binding site and that small structural differences between variants could explain such observations (LESLIE et al., 1988).

II. Mechanism of the Reaction

Early efforts to understand the means by which CAT catalyzes the acetylation of chloramphenicol centered on the type I protein typically encoded by Tn9 and F-like resistance plasmids in gram-negative bacteria (ZAIDENZAIG and SHAW 1978; THIBAULT et al. 1980). Subsequently crystals of the type III variant, specified by a non-F enteric plasmid, were shown to be of a quality likely to yield high resolution X-ray diffraction data and a three-dimensional structure for CAT (LIDDELL et al. 1978; LESLIE et al. 1986). Subsequent studies, using steady state kinetic analysis, chemical modification, and, more recently, site-directed mutagenesis have been carried out with the type III enteric variant of CAT (MURRAY et al. 1988). A uniquely reactive and absolutely conserved histidyl residue was detected by an active site directed reagent, 3-bromoacetyl chloramphenicol, an electrophilic analogue of the product of the forward reaction (KLEANTHOUS et al. 1985). Since kinetic studies favoured the view that the reaction proceeds via a ternary complex (sequential) mechanism, without evidence of the formation of an acetyl-enzyme intermediate, the schematic outline shown in Fig. 2 was proposed. All studies to data are compatible with a general base role for the imidazole of His 195 whereby deprotonation of the primary (C-3) hydroxyl of chloramphenicol is followed by attack of the resulting anion on the carbonyl of acetyl CoA. The resultant tetrahedral intermediate would then be expected to collapse to yield 3-acetyl chloramphenicol and CoA. It was observed that alkylation of the imidazole ring of His 195 only occurred at the N-3 position, suggesting a precise and preferred alignment of the side chain, a position likely to be essential for the stabilization of the tautomer with a lone pair of electrons at N-3. The crystallographic data are summarized in the schematic diagram of the active site shown in Fig. 4. The suggested network of hydrogen bonds serves to polarize the imidazole ring of His 195 and the interaction of the side chain of Asp 199 with that of Arg 18 appears to be an important determinant of stability (LEWENDON et al. 1988).

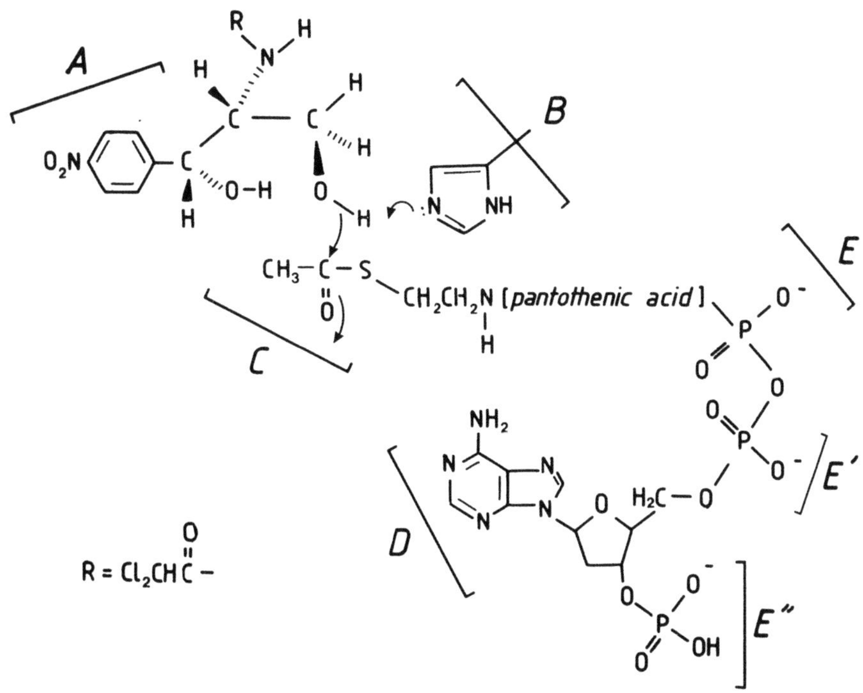

Fig. 2. Diagram of the active site of CAT based on chemical modification and kinetic studies but *before* determination of the structure of the type III variant by X-ray crystallography. The predicted hydrophobic pocket (*A*) for the C-1 substituted phenyl moiety of chloramphenicol has been identified (see Fig. 3) as have the aromatic and other interactions (*D*) promoting the binding of the adenine ring of CoA. The permitted size of the acyl group (*C*) is limited by the geometry of the active site at the cleft between two subunits. The catalytic imidazole (*B*) is that of His 195. Contrary to expectation the phosphoanions (*E*, *E′*, or *E″*) of CoA do *not* appear to be paired with the side chains of protonated lysyl or arginyl residues but are in contact with solvent (LESLIE et al. 1988)

III. Structure of Chloramphenicol Acetyltransferase

1. Quaternary Structure

The results of earlier studies had suggested that each natural variant of CAT was composed of identical subunits and was a tetramer (SHAW et al. 1972; PACKMAN and SHAW 1981; SHAW 1983). The latter conclusion is now known to be erroneous. The X-ray diffraction data and results of hydrodynamic studies are in agreement that CAT is a trimer (LESLIE et al. 1988; HARDING et al. 1987). The symmetrical arrangements of the subunits around the three-fold axis result in three subunit interfaces, each of which contributes to an active site. One subunit contributes most of the binding contacts for chloramphenicol and CoA whereas the other provides the catalytic imidazole (His 195). The ability of the type I and type III variants to form stable and fully functional heteromeric trimers in vivo emphasizes the conservation of complementarity at the subunit interfaces (PACKMAN and SHAW 1981).

2. Tertiary Structure of the Subunits

Each of the three subunits of the type III variant of CAT consists of a compact assembly of five α-helical segments and seven β-strands such that the latter constitute a twisted sheet which involves six strands from one subunit and the seventh from an adjoining one. Figure 3 shows the linear arrangement of the α-helices and β-strands in the type III protein and emphasizes the likelihood that each CAT variant packs in a similar fashion. The residues contributing side chains which are

```
            1   5    10   15   20   25   30   35   40   45   50   55   60   65   70   75   80
I           MEKKITGYTTVDISQWHRKEHFEAFQSVAQCTYNQTVQLDITAFLKTVKKNKHKFYPAFIHILARLMNAHPEFRMAMK D
Proteus     MDTKRVGYTVVDLSQWGRKEHFEAFQSFAQCTFSQTVQLDITSLLKTVKQNGYKFYPTFIYIISLLVNKHAEFRMAMK D
III              MNYTKFDVKNWVRREHFEFYRHRLPCGFSLTSKIDITTLKKSLDDSAYKFYPVMIYLIAQAVNQFDELRMAIK D
Bacillus         M FKQID ENYLRKEHFHHYMTLTRCSYSLVINLDITKLHAILKEKKLKVYPVQIYLLARAVQKIPEFRMDQVND
pC221            MTFNIIKLENWDRKEYFEHY FNQQTTYSITKEIDITLFKDMIKKKGYEIYPSLIYAIMEVVNKNKVFRTGINSE
pC194            MNFNKIDLDNWKRKEIFNHY LNQQTTFSITTEIDISVLYRNIKQEGYKFYPAFIFLVTRVINSNTAFRTGYNSD

              85   90   95  100  105  110  115  120  125  130  135  140  145  150  155  160
I           GELVIWDSVHPCYTVFHEQTETFSSLWSEYHDDFRQFLHIYSQDVACYGENLAYFPKGFI ENMFFVSANPWVSFTSFDL
Proteus     GELVIWDSVNPGYNIFHEQTETFSSLWSYYHKDINRFLKTYSEDIAQYGDDLAYFPKEFI ENMFFVSANPWVSFTSFNL
III         DELIVWDSVDPQFTVFHQETETFSALSCPYSSDIDQFMVNYLSVMERYKSDTKLFPQGVTPENHLNISALPWVNFDSFNL
Bacillus     ELGYWEILHPSYTILNKETKTFSSIWTPFDENFAQFYKSCVADIETFSKSSNLFPKPHMPENMFNISSLPWIDFTSFNL
pC221       NKLGYWDKLNPLYTVFNKQTEKFTNIWTESDNNFTSFYNNYKNDLLEYKDKEEMFPKKPIPENTIPISMIPWIDFSSFNL
pC194       GELGYWDKLEPLYTIFDGVSKTFSGIWTPVKNDFKEFYDLYLSDVEKYNGSGKLFPKTPIPENAFSLSIIPWTSFTGFNL

             165  170  175  180  185  190  195  200  205  210  215  220  225  230  235  240
I           NVANMDNFFAPVFTMGKYYTQGDKVLMPLAIQVHHAVCDGFHVGRMLNELQQYCDEWQGGA
Proteus     NMANINNFFAPVFTIGKYYTQGDKVLMPLAIQVHHAVCDGFHVGRLLNEIQQYCDEGCK
III        _NVANFTDYFAPIITMAKYQQEGDRLLLPLSVQVHHAVCDGFHVARFINRLQELCNSKLK
Bacillus    NVSTDEAYLLPIFTIGKFKVEEGKIILPVAIQVHHAVCDGYHAGQYVEYLRWLIEHCDEWLNDSLHIT
pC221       NIGNNSNFLLPIITIGKFYSENNKIYIPVALQLHHAVCDGYHASLFMNEFQDIIHKVDDWI
pC194       NINNNSNYLLPIITAGKFINKGNSIYLPLSLQVHHSVCDGYHAGLFMNSIQELSDRPNDWLL
```

Fig. 3. Alignment of published sequences for natural variants of CAT after allowances to maximize identities. All are deduced from DNA sequences except that for the type I enzyme, which was determined directly (SHAW et al. 1979). Nucleotide sequences of the cloned genes for the type I CAT, that of *Proteus mirabilis*, the type III enzyme, and variants of CAT from *Bacillus pumilus* and two staphylococcal plasmids were determined respectively by ALTON and VAPNEK (1979), MARCOLI et al. (1980); CHARLES et al. (1985); MURRAY et al. (1988); HARWOOD et al. (1983); HORINOUCHI and WEISBLUM (1982), and BRENNER and SHAW (1985). *Underlining* for the type III variant indicates the segments of primary structure which are α-helical (*solid*) or β-stranded (*dashed*) in the tertiary structure (LESLIE et al., 1988). *Solid triangles* at the bottom of each nest of six structures indicate those residues which are identical in nine sequences for which data are available. *Open triangles* highlight residues which are identical in the illustrated six-fold comparison of published sequences but which differ in one or more of the other three, that of the type II CAT and those from *Bacteroides* and *Streptomyces* (MURRAY, I. A., unpublished data). The *solid diamond* indicates the catalytic His 195 and the *open diamonds* call attention to Arg 18 and Asp 199, absolutely conserved residues involved in the active site network of hydrogen bonds (Fig. 4). The *circles* indicate residues of the type III protein in contact with chloramphenicol, *solid ones* referring to those from the subunit providing His 195 and *open ones* for those of the opposing subunit which constitutes much of the binding surface for chloramphenicol and virtually all of that for CoA

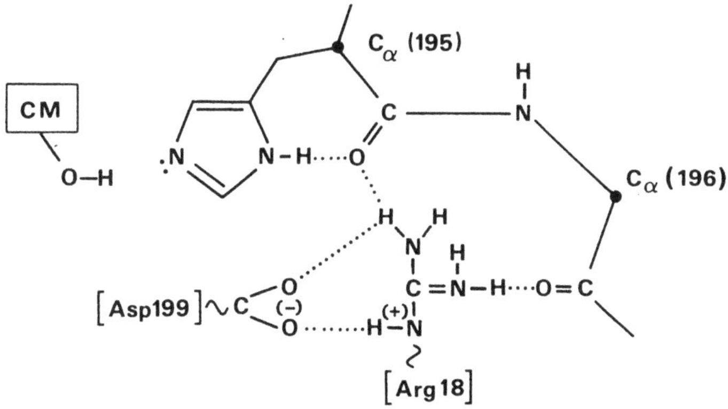

Fig. 4. The probable network of hydrogen bonds at the active site of the type III variant of CAT (LESLIE et al., 1988). Only the C-3 hydroxyl of chloramphenicol (*CM*) is shown. Note the extensive interactions between the side chains of Asp 199 and Arg 18 and back bone carbonyl oxygens. The polarization of the imidazole ring is in accord with chemical modification experiments which reveal alkylation only at the N-3 position (KLEANTHOUS et al. 1985)

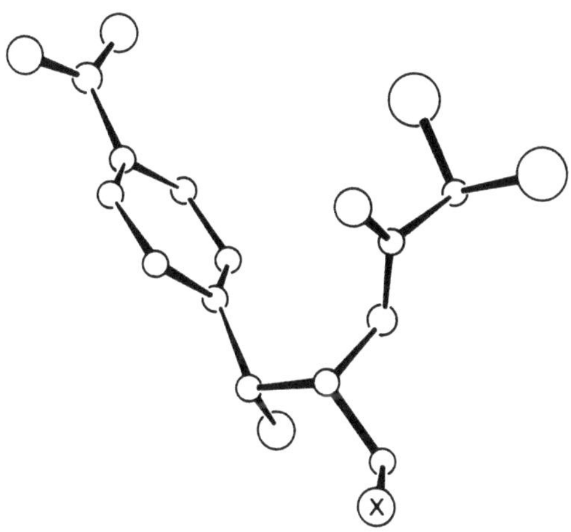

Fig. 5. The extended conformation of chloramphenicol at the active site of the type III CAT as determined by X-ray crystallography (LESLIE et al., 1988). The site of acetylation at the C-3 oxygen is indicated (*X*). This structure should be compared with those in Fig. 1, which depict a more compact conformation based on the results of spectroscopic studies of the free antibiotic in solution

important for the binding of chloramphenicol are shown, as are residues which are highly conserved. One of the unexpected aspects of the structure has been the observation that chloramphenicol is bound in an extended conformation, quite different from those deduced as most likely for the free antibiotic in solution (Fig. 1). The structure shown in Fig. 5 probably maximizes the number of interatomic contacts between the protein and its substrate and therefore the binding energy. It is of interest that for those CAT variants studied the dissociation constant for chloramphenicol approximates to the minimum inhibitory concentration of the antibiotic (~5–10 μ*M*), a concordance which must be a result of natural selection and is in accord with the need of resistant bacteria to bind and inactivate the antibiotic at a concentration of the latter which is a threat to viability.

One of the most striking features of the three dimensional structure of CAT is the "two tunnel" nature of the active site at the interface between subunits. The acyl moiety of acetyl CoA approaches the catalytic centre (near His 195) from one side via a long tunnel (accomodating the pantetheine arm of the coenzyme) and chloramphenicol enters from the opposite side, placing the 3-hydroxyl of the antibiotic deep in the cleft and equidistant with the sulphur of CoA to the N-3 of the imidazole of His 195. The remarkable catalytic efficiency (600 s^{-1}) of the type III variant must depend on a very precise geometry at the catalytic centre which is easily disturbed by relatively minor structural changes due to mutation (LEWENDON et al. 1988).

IV. Sequence Comparisons and Natural Variation

The amino acid sequence data shown in Fig. 3 emphasize the overall conservation of primary structure within the CAT family but also calls attention to the fact that only 25 residues are identical in the nine primary structures for which data are available. Unlike the situation with β-lactamases wherein variations in enzyme structure have been correlated with substrate specificity and may be the result of evolution as new β-lactam antibiotics have been introduced into clinical practice, the CAT story involves considerable variation without an obvious force for selection of substrate (antibiotic) affinity. There are only a few isolated examples of analogues of chloramphenicol which have been used in human or veterinary medicine (SYRIOPOULOU et al. 1981). There is reason to believe therefore that the variation in the CAT family observed must reflect the result of selection for other properties. An intriguing observation is the property of the type I variant of CAT to confer resistance to fusidic acid and to bind bile acids and triphenylmethane dyes (TANAKA et al. 1974; PROCTOR and ROWND 1982; BENNETT and SHAW 1983). Each of the unusual and unexpected ligands binds competitively with respect to chloramphenicol, but there is no evidence of inactivation or chemical modification. Model building and site-directed mutagenesis experiments will be necessary to predict a reasonable type I structure from the data for the type III CAT and deduce the precise contacts and structural features which enable the former to bind fusidate and the other compounds or which *exclude* them from the active sites of all CAT variants *except* the type I protein.

C. Control of Expression of Chloramphenicol Acetyltransferases

I. General Considerations

Bacteria have developed a number of different strategies for coping with general environmental variations and the presence of antibiotics in particular. The CAT system represents a single mechanism, that of enzymic inactivation using a valuable (in energetic terms) metabolic intermediate, acetyl CoA, as the chemical effector. By way of contrast, the hydrolysis of β-lactams by β-lactamase uses water as the reactant. The CAT reaction is, however, an efficient and discriminating one in that acetyl-CoA is hydrolyzed only very slowly in the absence of chloramphenicol (KLEANTHOUS and SHAW 1984). Nonetheless, the rate of hydrolysis of the thioester may be significant, encouraging the bacterium to synthesize CAT only when it is required, namely when chloramphenicol is present. However the latter strategy presents a difficulty in that chloramphenicol is a classic inhibitor of induced enzyme synthesis. To wait for chloramphenicol before synthesizing CAT is to court disaster. The variety of means by which bacteria deal with this dilemma is both interesting and instructive.

II. Gram-Negative Bacteria

It has been pointed out on several occasions that the family of CAT genes constitutes a collection of "cassettes" or "cartridges" which specify more or less the same effector function but do so under the control of very different nucleotide sequences 5′ to the start of the CAT coding sequences (SHAW 1984; SHAW et al. 1984). The conservation of the primary structure of CAT is not mirrored in the upstream sequences. There are as yet no exceptions within gram-negative bacteria to the rule that no two CAT genes have similar regulatory sequences. All are synthesized constitutively and one is under catabolite control mediated by cyclic AMP and its effector protein, a positive control element promoting transcription of a number of important genes (and operons) in *E. coli*. Studies with the type I CAT gene have shown it to be controlled at the transcriptional level by cAMP (LEGRICE and MATZURA 1981). Such is not the case with other CAT genes from gram-negative bacteria wherein all of the upstream sequences are different from that of the type I and from each other and are not subject to cAMP control (SHAW et al. 1984; CHARLES et al. 1985; MURRAY et al. 1988).

III. Gram-Positive Bacteria

The first experiments directed at the control of synthesis of CAT in staphylococci confirmed earlier observations that the resistance phenotype was fully expressed only after prior exposure of bacteria to chloramphenicol and demonstrated further that the induction process bore a striking resemblance to repressor-mediated control systems (WINSHELL and SHAW 1969). The use of an analogue of chloramphenicol without the C-3 hydroxyl target for acetylation made it possible to study the process without the complications caused by the accumulation of products (mono- and diacetyl chloramphenicol) which are *not* inducers. The hypothesis advanced was that CAT synthesis in staphylococci might be dependent upon the interaction of chloramphenicol with a putative apo-repressor, releasing the latter's ability to block transcription. Such a model became untenable when it was shown that all of the information specifying inducibility resides within a segment of DNA which contains the structural gene for CAT and is only slightly longer than the coding sequence for the protein (HORINOUCHI and WEISBLUM 1982).

The story of CAT synthesis in gram-positive bacteria has been extended and developed by several groups, and there are indications that a consensus is not far off. The most extensive and searching analysis has been carried out with *cat-86*, a chromosomal gene for CAT from *Bacillus pumilus*, which yields a transcript with a stem-loop structure which involves the ribosome binding site for translation of the m-RNA for CAT. Chloramphenicol induces translation of pre-formed transcripts when rifampicin is employed to inhibit de novo RNA synthesis, and there is evidence that the release of the block to translation can be effected by antibiotics other than chloramphenicol which interact with the 50S ribosomal subunit or by stalling ribosomes in transit during translation of an upstream leader mRNA specifying a small peptide (DUVALL and LOVETT 1986; DUVALL et al. 1985; DUVALL et al. 1987). The model is best seen as an example of a class of post-transcriptional controls involving sequestration of the ribosomal binding site with release arising by several mechanisms. Analogous results have been observed with staphylococcal plasmids pC194 and pUB112 (BYEON and WEISBLUM 1984; BRUCKNER and MATZURA 1985; BRUCKNER et al. 1987). Taken together the gram-positive systems for controlling *cat* gene expression are best described as pure examples of translational attenuation, in contrast to the transcriptional attenuation observed in the control of amino acid biosynthetic operons (KOLTER and YANOFSKY 1982). For the sake of completeness it should be pointed out that enhanced mRNA stability may also play a contributory role in the induction of *cat* genes from gram-positive bacteria. The fragmentation of *cat-86* mRNA in *B. subtilis* has been shown to involve several discrete steps which lead to RNA fragments which are probably untranslatable and the process is probably inhibited by translation of the full length transcript (AMBULOS et al. 1987). Hence, the already baroque process of induction of CAT synthesis by chloramphenicol, via release of sequestration of the ribosome binding site as noted above, may also involve an indirect stimulation of CAT synthesis via enhanced stability of the mRNA itself. Clearly, the CAT system continues to confound, surprise, and even delight those with patience as well as curiosity. A full understanding of the physiological and evolutionary pressures which have led to such a diversity of control systems for *cat* gene expression is, however, still not at hand.

References

Abdel-Sayed S (1987) Transport of chloramphenicol into sensitive strains of *Escherichia coli* and *Pseudomonas aeruginosa*. J Antimicrob Chemother 19:7–20

Alton NK, Vapnek D (1979) Nucleotide sequence analysis of the chloramphenicol resistance transposon Tn9. Nature 282:864–869

Ambulos NP Jr, Duvall EJ, Lovett PS (1987) The mRNA for an inducible chloramphenicol acetyltransferase gene is cleaved into discrete fragments in *Bacillus subtilis*. J Bacteriol 169:967–972

Bennett AD, Shaw WV (1983) Resistance to fusidic acid in *Escherichia coli* mediated by the type I variant of chloramphenicol acetyltransferase. Biochem J 215:29–38

Brenner DG, Shaw WV (1985) The use of synthetic oligonucleotides with universal templates for rapid DNA sequencing: results with staphylococcal replication pC221. EMBO J 4:561–568

Bruckner R, Matzura H (1985) Regulation of the inducible chloramphenicol acetyltransferase gene of the *Staphylococcus aureus* plasmid of pUB112. EMBO J 4:2295–2300

Bruckner R, Dick T, Matzura H (1987) Dependence of expression of an inducible *Staphylococcus aureus cat* gene on the translation of its leader sequence. Mol Gen Genet 207:486–491

Burns JL, Mendelman PM, Levy J, Stull TL, Smith AL (1985) A permeability barrier as a mechanism of chloramphenicol resistance in *Haemophilus influenzae*. Antimicrob Agents Chemother 27:46–54
Burns JL, Rubens CE, Mendelman PM, Smith AL (1986) Cloning and expression in *Escherichia coli* of a gene encoding non-enzymatic chloramphenicol resistance from *Pseudomonas aeruginosa*. Antimicrob Agents Chemother 29:445–450
Byeon WH, Weisblum B (1984) Post-transcriptional regulation of chloramphenicol acetyltransferase. J Bacteriol 158:543–550
Charles IG, Keyte JW, Shaw WV (1984) Nucleotide sequence analysis of the *cat* gene of *Proteus mirabilis*: comparison with the type I (Tn9) *cat* gene. J Bacteriol 164:123–129
Charles IG, Keyte IW, Shaw WV (1985) Nucleotide sequence analysis of the *cat* gene of *Proteus mirabilis*: comparison with the type I (Tn9) *cat* gene. J Bacteriol 164:123–129
Dorman CJ, Foster TJ (1982) Nonenzymatic chloramphenicol resistance determinants specified by plasmids R26 and R55-1 in *Escherichia coli* K-12 do not confer high level resistance to fluorinated analogs. Antimicrob Agents Chemother 19:294–297
Dorman CJ, Foster TJ (1985) Posttranscriptional regulation of the inducible non-enzymatic chloramphenicol resistance determinant of IncP plasmid R26. J Bacteriol 161:147–152
Dorman CJ, Foster TJ, Shaw WV (1986) Nucleotide sequence of the R26 chloramphenicol resistance determinant and identification of its gene product. Gene 41:349–353
Duvall EJ, Lovett PS (1986) Chloramphenicol induces translation of the mRNA for a chloramphenicol resistance gene in *Bacillus subtilis*. Proc Natl Acad Sci USA 83:3939–3943
Duvall EJ, Mongkolstuk S, Kim UJ, Lovett PS, Henkin TM, Chambliss GH (1985) Induction of the chloramphenicol acetyltransferase gene *cat-86* through the action of the ribosomal antibiotic amicetin: involvement of a *Bacillus subtilis* ribosomal component in *cat* induction. J Bacteriol 161:665–672
Duvall EJ, Ambulos NP Jr, Lovett PS (1987) Drug-free induction of a chloramphenicol acetyltransferase gene in *Bacillus subtilis* by stalling ribosomes in a regulatory leader. J Bacteriol 169:4235–4241
Fitton JE, Shaw WV (1979) Comparison of chloramphenicol acetyltransferase variants in staphylococci. Biochem J 177:575–582
Gale EF, Cundliffe E, Reynolds PE, Richmond MH, Waring MJ (1981) The molecular basis of antibiotic action, 2nd edn. Wiley, London, pp 462–468
Gaffney DF, Cundliffe E, Foster TJ (1981) Chloramphenicol resistance that does not involve chloramphenicol acetyltransferase encoded by plasmids from gram-negative bacteria. J Gen Microbiol 125:113–121
Harding SE, Rowe AJ, Shaw WV (1987) The molecular mass and trimeric nature of cnloramphenicol transacetylase. Biochem Soc Trans 15:513
Harwood CR, Williams DM, Lovett PS (1983) Nucleotide sequence of a *Bacillus pumilus* gene specifying chloramphenicol resistance. Gene 24:163–169
Horinouchi S, Weisblum B (1982) Nucleotide sequence and functional map of pC194, a plasmid that specifies inducible chloramphenicol resistance. J Bacteriol 150:815–825
Kleanthous C, Shaw WV (1984) Analysis of the mechanism of chloramphenicol acetyltransferase by steady state kinetics. Biochem J 223:211–220
Kleanthous C, Cullis PM, Shaw WV (1985) 3-Bromoacetyl-chloramphenicol: an active site directed inhibitor for chloramphenicol acetyltransferase. Biochemistry 24:5307–5312
Kolter R, Yanofsky (1982) Attenuation in amino acid biosynthetic operons. Annu Rev Genet 16:113–134
LeGrice SFJ, Matzura H (1981) Binding of RNA polymerase and the catabolite gene activator protein within the *cat* promoter in *Escherichia coli*. J Mol Biol 150:185–196
Leslie AGW, Liddell JM, Shaw WV (1986) Crystallization of a type III chloramphenicol acetyltransferase. J Mol Biol 188:283–285
Leslie AGW, Moody PCE, Shaw WV (1988) The structure of chloramphenicol acetyltransferase at 1.75A resolution. Proc Natl Acad Sci USA 85:4133–4137
Lewendon A, Murray IA, Kleanthous C, Shaw WV (1988) Substitutions in the active site of chloramphenicol acetyltransferase: role of a conserved aspartate. Biochemistry 27:7385–7390

Liddell JM, Shaw WV, Swan IDA (1978) Preliminary crystallographic data for a chloramphenicol acetyltransferase from *Escherichia coli*. J Mol Biol 124:285–286
Marcoli R, Iida S, Bickle TA (1980) The DNA sequence of an IS1-flanked transposon coding for resistance to chloramphenicol and fusidic acid. FEBS Lett 110:11–14
Miyamura S (1964) Inactivation of chloramphenicol by chloramphenicol-resistant bacteria. J Pharm Sci 53:604–607
Murray IA, Hawkins AR, Keyte JW, Shaw WV (1988) Nucleotide sequence analysis and overexpression of the gene encoding a type III chloramphenicol acetyltransferase. Biochem J 252:173–179
Nagai Y, Mitsuhashi S (1972) New type of R factors incapable of inactivating chloramphenicol. J Bacteriol 109:1–7
Packman LC, Shaw WV (1981) The use of naturally occurring hybrid variants of chloramphenicol acetyltransferase to identify subunit contact domains. Biochem J 193:541–552
Pongs O (1979) Chloramphenicol. In: Hahn FE (ed) Mechanism of action of antibacterial agents. Springer, Berlin Heidelberg New York, pp 26–42
Proctor GN, Rownd RH (1982) Rosanalins: indicator dyes for chloramphenicol-resistant enterobacteria containing chloramphenicol acetyltransferase. J Bacteriol 150:1375–1382
Sande MA, Mandell GL (1985) Chloramphenicol. In: Gilman AG, Goodman LS, Rall TW, Murad F (eds) The pharmacologic basis of therapeutics, 7th edn. Macmillan, New York, pp 1179–1184
Shaw WV (1967) The enzymatic acetylation of chloramphenicol by extracts of R factor-resistant *Escherichia coli*. J Biol Chem 242:687–693
Shaw WV (1983) Chloramphenicol acetyltransferase: enzymology and molecular biopsy. CRC Crit Rev Biochem 14:1–46
Shaw WV (1984) Bacterial resistance to chloramphenicol. Br Med Bull 40:36–41
Shaw WV, Hopwood DA (1976) Chloramphenicol acetylation in *Streptomyces*. J Gen Microbiol 94:159–166
Shaw WV, Sands L, Datta N (1972) Hybridization of variants of chloramphenicol acetyltransferase specified by fi^+ and fi^- R factors. Proc Natl Acad Sci USA 69:3049–3053
Shaw WV, Packmann LC, Burleigh BD, Dell A, Morris HR, Hartley BS (1979) Primary structure of a chloramphenicol acetyltransferase specified by R plasmids. Nature 282:870–872
Shaw WV, Brenner DG, Murray IA (1984) Regulation of antibiotic resistance in bacteria: the chloramphenicol acetyltransferase system. Curr Top Cell Regul 26:455–468
Smith MD, Kelsey MC (in press) Demonstration of a functional variant of chloramphenicol acetyltransferase in *Haemophilus influenzae*. J Med Microbiol
Suzuki Y, Okamoto S (1967) The enzymatic acetylation of chloramphenicol by the multiple drug resistant *Escherichia coli* carrying R factor. J Biol Chem 242:4722–4730
Syriopoulou VP, Harding AL, Goldmann DA, Smith AL (1981) In vitro antibacterial activity of fluorinated analogs of chloramphenicol and thiamphenicol. Antimicrob Agents Chemother 19:294–297
Tanaka H, Izaki K, Takahashi H (1974) Some properties of chloramphenicol acetyltransferase, with particular reference to the mechanism of inhibition by triphenylmethane dyes. J Biochem 76:1009–1019
Thibault G, Guitard M, Daigneault R (1980) A study of the enzymatic inactivation of chloramphenicol by highly purified chloramphenicol acetyltransferase. Biochim Biophys Acta 614:339–349
Watanabe T (1963) Infective heredity of multiple drug resistance in bacteria. Bacteriol Rev 27:87–115
Winshell E, Shaw WV (1969) Kinetics of induction and purification of chloramphenicol acetyltransferase from chloramphenicol-resistant *Staphylococcus aureus*. J Bacteriol 98:1248–1257
Zaidenzaig Y, Shaw WV (1978) The reactivity of sulfhydryl groups at the active site of an R factor specified variant of chloramphenicol acetyltransferase. Eur J Biochem 83:553–562

CHAPTER 14

General Properties of Resistance Plasmids

D. E. TAYLOR

A. Introduction

Bacterial plasmids are extrachromosomal molecules of circular double-stranded DNA. Those that mediate antibiotic resistance were first discovered in Japan in 1957 (AKIBA et al. 1960). This chapter deals with the general properties of bacterial resistance plasmids and will concentrate primarily on plasmids of the H incompatibility group. Although it is not possible because of space limitations to discuss plasmids of other incompatibility groups in detail, some of their features will be compared with those of H plasmids, when this is appropriate or when information on H plasmids is not available.

In 1972 the first epidemic of chloramphenicol-resistant typhoid fever occurred in Mexico. Resistance to chloramphenicol was particularly serious because this is the most effective drug for treating typhoid fever. The plasmid shown to be responsible for resistance to chloramphenicol and to several other antibiotics belonged to a new incompatibility group designated "H group" (ANDERSON and SMITH 1972). There were at least 10000 cases of typhoid fever in the Mexico epidemic and many deaths occurred, particularly at the beginning of the outbreak before ampicillin was used for treatment (ANDERSON 1975). Subsequent outbreaks of typhoid fever caused by chloramphenicol-resistant *S. typhi* strains containing H plasmids occurred in India, Vietnam and Thailand (ANDERSON 1975). Antibiotic resistance in *S. typhi* is frequently associated with the carriage of H group plasmids (TAYLOR et al. 1985b). Plasmids of the H group are all very large (greater than 100 megadaltons), a characteristic that has made them rather more difficult to analyze physically and genetically than plasmids of other groups. This review summarizes what we know so far about this important group of plasmids. Readers may also wish to refer to a recent review article stressing the environmental aspects of H group plasmids (MAHER and COLLERAN 1987).

B. Plasmid Classification

Antibiotic resistance plasmids from Enterobacteriaceae were initially divided into two classes, fi^+ and fi^- (NAKAYA et al. 1960). The fi^+ property was used to designate fertility inhibition: the ability of a plasmid to inhibit F plasmid transfer when present with the F factor in the same host cell. Members of the fi^+ and fi^- classes could coexist in the same cell with F and with some fi^- plasmids, but plasmids within each class were unable to coexist. Ultimately it was realized that the fi^+ and fi^- classes were too narrow and the classification scheme was extended

Table 1. Plasmid incompatibility groups in Enterobacteriaceae

Inc group[a]	Sub-group[b]	Plasmid[c]	Original host[d]	Phenotype[e]	Size[f]	Reference[g]
B	–	R724	*Shigella flexneri*	CmSmSpSuTcHg	58	Datta and Olarte (1974)
C	–	RA1	*Aeromonas liquefaciens*	SmTc	86	Aoki et al. (1971)
D	–	R7116	*Providencia* spp.	Km	33	Hedges (1974)
FI	–	R455	*Proteus morganii*	ApCmSmSpSu TcHgPhi	63	Hedges et al. (1973)
FII	–	R1	*Salmonella paratyphi* B	ApCmKm	62	Meynell and Datt (1966)
FIII	–	ColB-K98	*Escherichia coli*	ColB	70	Freydman and Meynell (1969)
FIV	–	R124	*Salmonella typhimurium*	TcPhi	82	Hedges and Datta (1972)
HI	1	R27	*Salmonella typhimurium*	Tc	112[h]	Meynell and Datt (1966)
	2	R478	*Serratia marcescens*	CmKmTc HgTePhi	166	Hedges et al. (1975a
	3	MIP233	*Salmonella ohio*	ScrTePhi	150	Roussel and Chabbe (1978)
HII	–	pHH1508a	*Klebsiella aerogenes*	SmSpTp TePhi	100[h]	Bradley et al. (198
I1	–	R64	*Salmonella typhimurium*	SmTcPhi	72	Meynell and Datt (1966)
I2	–	TP114	*Escherichia coli*	Km	41	Grindley et al. (197
Iγ	–	R621a	*Salmonella typhimurium*	Tc	65	Hedges and Datta (1973)
J	–	R391	*Proteus rettgeri*	KmNmHg	ND	Coetzee et al. (1972
K	–	R387	*Shigella flexneri*	CmSm	53	Hedges and Datta (1971)
M	–	R446b	*Proteus morganii*	SmTc	47	Hedges et al. (1973)
N	–	N3	*Shigella* spp.	SmSpSuTc HgPhi	33	Datta and Hedges (1971)
P	α	RP1	*Pseudomonas aeruginosa*	CbKmTcTe[i]	36	Grinsted et al. (197
	β	R751	*Klebsiella aerogenes*	Tp	30	Jobanputra and Datta (1974)
Q	–	R300b	*Salmonella typhimurium*	SmSu	5.7	Barth and Grinter (1974)
T	–	RtS1	*Proteus vulgaris*	KmPhi repts	126	Coetzee et al. (1972
U	–	RA3	*Aeromonas hybrophila*	CmSmSpSu	30	Bradley et al. (198
W	–	S-a	*Shigella flexneri*	CmGmKmSm SpSuTm	23	Grindley et al. (197
X	–	R6K	*Escherichia coli*	ApSm	26	Kontomichalou et (1970)
Y[j]	–	P1Cm	*Escherichia coli*	Cm	60	Hedges et al. (1975b
Com9[k]	–	R71	*Escherichia coli*	ApCmSm SpSuTc	51	Scavizzi (1973)

and refined in several laboratories (GRINDLEY et al. 1972; CHABBERT et al. 1972; DATTA 1975). Letters of the alphabet were used to designate particular incompatibility groups, with F kept for the F factor and related plasmids. Plasmids within the same group are unable to replicate in the same host cell with one another and are said to be incompatible. There are 24 incompatibility groups which are currently recognized in Enterobacteriaceae (Table 1).

I. Incompatibility Testing

To determine the incompatibility group of a plasmid, pairs of plasmids are tested for coexistence after selection for the entry of one of the plasmids by conjugation, transformation or by transduction. In Enterobacteriaceae, conjugation is usually used for transferable plasmids and transformation for non-conjugative plasmids (DATTA 1979). This process is repeated with selection for the entry of the second plasmid. Usually 10 clones are examined for the fate of the two plasmids (TAYLOR and GRANT 1977a). If entry of both plasmids leads to elimination of the resident

[a] Plasmids within the same incompatibility group are unable to coexist in the same host cell

[b] Plasmids within all subgroups of the same incompatibility group are incompatible with one another. Subgroups of H and P groups are defined based on other characteristics; see text for more details

[c] A single plasmid has been chosen to represent each group. If possible the "prototype" plasmid of an Inc group or the one on which most studies have been done has been chosen for inclusion. All plasmids listed, as well as other plasmids of the various Inc groups, are available from the Plasmid section, National Collection of Type Cultures, Central Public Health Laboratory, 61 Colindale Avenue, London NW9 5HT, England

[d] The original host of the plasmid shown in the list is given. Other plasmids from the same group may have originated in other bacterial hosts

[e] Phenotypes are designated as follows. Resistance to the following antibiotics: ampicillin, Ap; carbenicillin, Cb; chloramphenicol, Cm; gentamicin, Gm; kanamycin, Km; neomycin, Nm; spectinomycin, Sp; streptomycin, Sm; sulfonamides, Su; tetracycline, Tc; tobramycin, Tm; trimethoprim, Tp. Resistance to mercury, Hg; potassium tellurite, Te; production and resistance to colicin B, ColB; ability to ferment sucrose, Scr; temperature sensitive replication, repts; phage inhibition, Phi

[f] Sizes of plasmids are given in megadaltons. These have usually been determined by agarose gel electrophoresis of total plasmid DNA with reference to other plasmids of known size or, in some cases, by contour length measurement under the electron microscope

[g] The reference given is usually that in which the plasmid was first described and may not necessarily contain the molecular weight or other significant features. Sometimes in the original reference the plasmid was classified into a different group, for example R478 was originally classified into the S group by HEDGES et al. (1975); see section B.II for more information on discontinued groups

[h] Based on restriction analysis the IncHI plasmid R27 is 182 kb (118 Mdaltons) and the IncHII plasmid pHH1508a is 208 kb (135 Mdal) (TAYLOR et al. 1985; YAN and TAYLOR 1987)

[i] Resistance to potassium tellurite is a "silent" determinant in RP1 (TAYLOR and BRADLEY 1987); for more details see Sect. F.V.II

[j] The Y group contains plasmids incompatible with bacteriophage P1 (see CAPAGE et al. 1982)

[k] R71 is now designated as the single member of the SII group. For further information see Sect. B.V.3

plasmids, then the plasmids are truly incompatible and are members of the same Inc group. If the resident plasmid is eliminated from some of the clones, then continued growth of the clone in absence of antibiotics is used to determine if the plasmids can stably coexist (compatible) or if one is ultimately eliminated (incompatible). If the two plasmids appear to be compatible then confirmatory tests are performed using conjugation, and sometimes agarose gel electrophoresis to detect the presence of the plasmids, and to verify that the plasmids still coexist separately without having undergone recombination. These studies of plasmid incompatibility can represent a formidable amount of work. We owe the present classification scheme to the tireless efforts of Naomi Datta, Bob Hedges and their associates, although many others, some of whom are mentioned in the reference list to Table 1, have contributed to the incompatibility group classification scheme for plasmids in Enterobacteriaceae.

II. Extant and Religated Incompatibility Groups in Enterobacteriaceae

Although more than 26 Inc groups were once recognized in Enterobacteriaceae, a number of the groups have been reorganized and the plasmids within these groups assigned to other groups. In the case of the S group, first designated by HEDGES et al. (1975a), several plasmids were identified in *Serratia marcescens* and designated "S" plasmids. Subsequently we showed that the "S" plasmids were incompatible with H_2 plasmids (TAYLOR and GRANT 1977b). Today these plasmids, which include R478, are all placed within the group HI, subgroup 2. Similarly the RA1 plasmid once placed in the A group (HEDGES and DATTA 1971) is now included in the C group. Those in the L group were placed within the M group (RICHARDS and DATTA 1979). Groups E and V are now no longer recognized. The I groups have undergone a number of reorganizations and there are currently three I groups recognized: I1, I2 and Iγ. The 24 groups shown in Table 1 constitute the Inc groups recognized by the Plasmid section of the National Collection of Type Cultures, U.K. This collection was accumulated by Naomi Datta and her colleagues at Hamemrsmith Hospital between 1960 and 1982.

III. Incompatibility Groups in *Pseudomonas aeruginosa*

In *Pseudomonas aeruginosa* 13 incompatibility groups are currently recognized. These groups were reviewed by JACOBY 1984, who has carried out much of the incompatibility group classification in *Pseudomonas*. Some *Pseudomonas* plasmids have a broad host range (OLSEN and SHIPLEY 1973) and this has resulted in classification of plasmids such as RP1 (equivalent to RP4 and RK2) into the P-1 group in *Pseudomonas* and into the P group in Enterobacteriaceae. Similarly IncP-3 plasmids of *Pseudomonas* (e.g. RIP64) belong to the IncC group in Enterobacteriaceae and IncP-4 plasmids of *Pseudomonas* (e.g. R1162, pUB300, RSF1010) belong to the IncQ group in Enterobacteriaceae.

Table 2. Plasmid incompatibility groups in *Pseudomonas aeruginosa*

Inc group[a]	Plasmid[b]	Phenotype[c]	Size[d]	Reference[e]
P-1[f]	RP1	CbKmTcTe[g]	36	GRINDSTED et al. (1972)
P-2	pMG1	GmSmSuBorHgTe[g]Phi	312	JACOBY (1974)
P-3[h]	RIP64	CbCmGmSuTmHg	95	WITCHITZ and CHABBERT (1971)
P-4[i]	R1162	SmSu	5.5	BRYAN et al. (1972)
P-5	Rms163	CmSuTcBor	145	IYOBE et al. (1974)
P-6	Rms149	CbGmSmSuPhi	36	SAGAI et al. (1975)
P-7	Rms148	SmPhi	120	SAGAI et al. (1975)
P-8	Fp2	HgPmrCma	60	LOUTIT (1970)
P-9	R2	CbKmSmSu	44	KAWAKAMI et al. (1972)
P-10	R91	Cb[j]	35	JACOBY (1978)
P-11	pMG39	CbGmKmSmSuTm	60	JACOBY (1984)
P-12	R716	SmHg	110	JACOBY (1978)
P-13	pMG25	CbCmGmKmSmSuTmBor	66	JACOBY (1985)

[a] Incompatibility groups determined as described in footnote [a] in Table 1
[b] A single plasmid was chosen to represent each Inc group. These plasmids are also available from the National Collection of Type Cultures, for address see footnote [c] in Table 1
[c] Phenotypes are as shown in Table 1, footnote [e] plus resistance to boron, Bor; and to phenyl mercuric acetate, Pmr; chromosome mobilizing ability, Cma
[d] Size given in megadaltons, see Table 1, footnote [f]
[e] Reference is usually that in which the plasmid was first described
[f] The P-1 group is equivalent to IncP in Enterobacteriaceae, as shown in Table 1
[g] In RP1 and other IncP-1α plasmids resistance to potassium tellurite is silent, but is expressed constitutively in IncP-2 plasmids (TAYLOR and BRADLEY 1987, SUMMERS and JACOBY 1977)
[h] IncP-3 in *Pseudomonas* is equivalent to IncC in Enterobacteriaceae
[i] IncP-4 in *Pseudomonas* is equivalent to IncQ in Enterobacteriaceae
[j] R91 encodes resistance to Km and Tc which is expressed only in Enterobacteriaceae

IV. Incompatibility Groups in *Staphylococcus aureus*

Thirteen incompatibility groups have been identified in *S. aureus*, due mainly to the work of R. Novick and S. Iordanescu and their colleagues (Table 3). As plasmids from gram-positive organisms cannot replicate in *E. coli*, there is no overlap between the Enterobacteriaceae and the *S. aureus* groups as seen between the Enterobacteriaceae and *Pseudomonas* groups. In *S. aureus*, incompatibility is tested using plasmid transduction with phage $\phi 11$ or 80α or other suitable phage (NOVICK 1967) or by protoplast transformation (CHANG and COHEN 1979) to place the plasmids in the same host cell.

V. Designation of Incompatibility Subgroups and Complexes

1. IncH subgroups

Plasmids which are members of the same incompatibility group usually exhibit a large amount of DNA homology when tested in DNA-DNA hybridization ex-

Table 3. Plasmid incompatibility groups in *Staphylococcus aureus*

Inc group[a]	Plasmid[b]	Phenotype[c]	Size[d]	Reference
Inc1	pUB108	Asa Hg Col	35	CHOPRA et al. (1973)
Inc2	pII145	Pc Asa Hg Cd Pb Bi	21	RUBY and NOVICK (1975)
Inc3	pT127	Tc	2.7	RUBY and NOVICK (1975)
Inc4	pC221	Cm	30	NOVICK (1976)
Inc5	pS177	Sm	2.7	NOVICK (1976)
Inc6	pK545	KmNm	15	RUBY and NOVICK (1975)
Inc7	pUB101	Pc Cd Fa	14.6	CHOPRA et al. (1973)
Inc8	pC194	Cm	1.8	NOVICK (1976)
Inc9	pUB112	Cm	3.0	NOVICK (1976)
Inc10	pC223	Cm	3.0	NOVICK (1976)
Inc11	pE194	Em	2.3	WEISBLUM et al. (1979)
Inc12	pE1764	Em	1.8	IORDANESCU and SURDEANU (1980)
Inc13	pUB110	KmNmTm	3.0	GRYCZAN et al. (1978)

[a] After NOVICK (1976), IORDANESCU et al. (1978), and IORDANESCU and SURDEANU (1980)
[b] Single plasmid chosen as a representative for each group
[c] Phenotypes designated as in Table 1 and resistance to arsenate, Asa; bismuth, Bi; boron, Bor; cadmium, Cd; erythromycin, Em; fusidic acid, Fa; lead, Pb; penicillin, Pc
[d] Sizes of plasmids given in megadaltons. Determined by various methods including contour length measurement in the electron microscope, comparative sedimentation rates in sucrose gradients, and agarose gel electrophoresis using plasmids of known size as molecular weight standards

periments (GRINDLEY et al. 1973; FALKOW 1975). In contrast, some of the plasmids of the H group were shown to have little homologous DNA, although all plasmids demonstrated incompatibility with one another (GRINDLEY et al. 1973). This led researchers at the Collinale laboratory to divide the H group into two subgroups based on their DNA hybridization results. The H_1 group contained R27 as well as other plasmids which mediated chloramphenicol resistance (Cm^r) in *S. typhi*. The H_2 group contained larger plasmids such as TP116 (GRINDLEY et al. 1973; ANDERSON 1975; ANDERSON et al. 1975). Moreover, Smith and coworkers demonstrated that the H group plasmids could be divided into H_1 and H_2 based on their interaction with the F factor. The H_1 plasmids mediated a unilateral incompatibility with the F factor, such that transfer of an H_1 plasmid into a cell containing F*lac* led to the rapid elimination of the F plasmid. The H_2 plasmids did not exhibit this phenomenon (SMITH et al. 1973).

The existence of a third subgroup of H plasmids was demonstrated by ROUSSEL and CHABBERT (1978). These workers confirmed the work of GRINDLEY et al. (1973), which established the H_1 and H_2 subgroups, and using DNA-DNA hybridization in formamide showed that a third group, H_3, existed, with a single member MIP233. We confirmed these findings using Southern blotting, which enabled us to visualize the very small amount of DNA homology among the various H group plasmids (WHITELEY and TAYLOR 1983).

Although incompatibility and DNA hybridization are useful and important methods for the classification of plasmids, examination of the type of conjugative pilus specified by a plasmid has also been extremely useful. Much of the methodology for these studies have been developed and applied by David E. Bradley. Most plasmids specify one type of pilus and the pilus type corresponds to its incompatibility group. However, a few exceptions to this rule have been identified (TAYLOR et al. 1981a; BRADLEY et al. 1986). Bradley identified H pili as long flexible structures using the electron microscope. Immunoelectron microscopy demonstrated that they were serologically unrelated to any other type of conjugative pilus (BRADLEY 1980). Both H_1 (subsequently referred to as H1) and H_2 (subsequently H2) plasmids appeared to specify the same type of pilus.

2. H Complex

In 1982 BRADLEY et al. identified a new group of plasmids. Members of this group, designated IncHII, which originated in *Klebsiella aerogenes*, specified H pili but were compatible with other previously recognized H plasmids. To accommodate these findings, the original H1, H2 and H3 plasmids were classified as members of three different subgroups within the HI group. The H plasmids were considered by Bradley and coworkers to form part of a complex (H complex), in that they all specified H pili but their incompatibility reactions varied (BRADLEY et al. 1982).

The characteristic features of plasmids of the H complex are shown in Table 4 and will be discussed in detail in subsequent sections. Although the H complex provides a workable classification scheme for the present, it will no doubt require further modification. Bradley has shown that the single member of IncHI subgroup 3 (MIP233) specifies unique pili which are unrelated to H pili (BRADLEY 1986). Thus ultimately it may be necessary to reclassify MIP233. However, as it shares many features in common with the HI2 plasmids it has been included in Table 4.

3. Other Plasmid Complexes

The H complex may be considered to be analogous to the F complex (HEDGES and DATTA 1972), in which plasmids of the FI, FII, FIII, and FIV groups all specify F pili. Members of each group, although incompatible within the group, are compatible with members of other F groups. Plasmids of the I complex, similarly, all specify I pilus production and have analogous incompatibility properties (BRADLEY 1984). More recently the S complex has been described (COETZEE et al. 1986). Four plasmids: EDP208 (or F_0*lac drd*), R71, TP224 :: Tn*10* and pPLS :: Tn*5* determine serologically related pili but are compatible with one another. EDP208 (once erroniously classified as IncFV) is now IncSI; R71, originally Com9 (SCAVIZZI 1973) is now IncSII; TP224 :: Tn*10* which determines heat-stable enterotoxin and Tc^r from Tn*10* insertion (SCOTLAND et al. 1979) is now IncSIII and pPLS : Tn*5* which mobilizes the K88 colonization antigen and carries Km^r from Tn*5* insertion (BRADLEY 1985a) is IncSIV. Since only one plasmid has been assigned to each group, these S groups have not been included in Table 1. The S-complex plasmids are not related to the earlier "S" group of plasmids from *S. marcescens* (HEDGES et al. 1975a), members of which are now included in the IncHI2 group.

Table 4. Characteristic features of plasmids within the H complex[a]

Inc group	Sub-group	Plasmid	Size[b] (kilobases)	Phenotype[c]	Original host	Temperature sensitive transfer[d]	H pili[e]	Inc with F factor[f]	Place and date and origin	Reference
HI	1	R27	182	Tc	*S. typhimurium*	+	+	+	England (1961)	TAYLOR et al. (1985)
HI	1	TP123	193.5	CmSmSpSuTc	*S. typhi*	+	+	+	Mexico (1972)	TAYLOR and BROSE (1985a)
HI	1	R726	210	CmSmSpSu	*S. typhi*	+	+	+	India (1972)	TAYLOR and BROSE (1985a)
HI	2	TP116	220	CmSmSuHgTePhi	*S. typhi*	+	+	–	Spain (1969)	TAYLOR and LEVINE (1980)
HI	2	R478	256	CmKmTcAsHgTePhi	*Ser. marcescens*	+	+	–	USA (1969)	TAYLOR and LEVINE (1980)
HI	2	MIP235	256	LacCmSmSuTePhi	*S. oranienburg*	+	+	–	Brazil (1973)	TAYLOR and LEVINE (1980)
HI	3	MIP233	231	ScrTePhi	*S. ohio*	+	–	–	England (1972)	TAYLOR and LEVINE (1980); Bradley (1986)
HII	–	pHH1508a	208	SmTpTePhi	*Klebsiella aerogenes*	–	+	–	England (1981)	YAN and TAYLOR (1987)
		pHH1457	169	ApCmGmKmSmSu TcTpHgTePhi	*Klebsiella aerogenes*	–	+	–	England (1981)	BRADLEY et al. (1982)

[a] For a definition of H complex see Sect. B.V.2
[b] Determined from the sum of restriction fragments (R27, TP123, R726, pHH1508a) or by conversion from megadaltons (other plasmids)
[c] Resistance to ampicillin, Ap; arsenic, As; chloramphenicol, Cm; gentamicin, Gm; kanamycin, Km; spectinomycin, Sp; streptomycin, Sm; sulfonamides, Su; tetracycline, Tc; tobramycin, Tm; trimethoprim, Tp; mercury, Hg; potassium tellurite, Te; ability to ferment sucrose, Scr; ability to ferment lactose, Lac; phage inhibition, Phi
[d] See Sect. D.II.2
[e] See Sect. D.I.2
[f] See Sect. E.III.1

4. IncP Subgroups

Except for IncH and IncP plasmids, other plasmids in Enterobacteriaceae (Table 1), in *P. aeruginosa* (Table 2) or in *S. aureus* (Table 3) have not been assigned to specific subgroups. The P plasmids have been divided into two subgroups, IncPα and IncPβ, based on DNA homology studies of their transfer origins (YAKOBSON and GUINEY 1983). Similar results were obtained using cloned fragments encoding replication functions (CHIKAMI et al. 1985). Two regions of RK2 (or RP4), a 700-base-pair (bp) *Hae*II fragment containing the origin of replication (*ori*V) and a 1.5 kilobase (kb) pair region designated trfA* (trans-acting replication function) hybridized strongly to IncPα plasmids (pUZ8, R702, R839, R938, R995 and R1033), whereas IncPβ plasmids (R751, R772 and R906) showed a much weaker level of hybridization (CHIKAMI et al. 1985). The IncPα plasmids are generally larger than the IncPβ plasmids and the former encode normally unexpressed resistance to tellurium compounds which can be turned on by growth on medium containing potassium tellurite (BRADLEY 1985b).

C. Structure of Plasmids

I. General Structure

Plasmids are covalently closed circular molecules of DNA which exist autonomously from the bacterial chromosome. They can usually be lost from the bacterial host cell without any obvious detrimental effects. Many useful functions are carried on plasmids which enable their bacterial hosts to exist and even flourish in otherwise hostile environments.

II. Molecular Sizes of Plasmids

Plasmids belonging to the same incompatibility group are usually about the same size. Therefore, it is often helpful before beginning incompatibility testing to compare the size of the unknown plasmid to those of plasmids from other incompatibility groups. Agarose gel electrophoresis using molecular weight markers of known size as standards has often been used to determine plasmid size (HANSEN and OLSEN 1978; CROSA and FALKOW 1981; TAYLOR and LEVINE 1980). Electron microscopy (GRINDLEY et al. 1973); HANSEN and OLSEN 1978) as well as comparative sedimentation rates in sucrose gradients (NOVICK 1976) have also been used to determine molecular sizes. The molecular sizes of representative plasmids from all the various incompatibility groups are given in Tables 1–3 and are expressed in megadaltons.

Since all H plasmids have high molecular weights and these are difficult to determine accurately by agarose gel electrophoresis (HANSEN and OLSEN 1978; TAYLOR and LEVINE 1980), we used restriction endonuclease digestion with *Xba*I to determine the size of a series of IncHI1 plasmids (TAYLOR and BROSE 1985a). Estimations of sizes determined previously by electron microscopy or agarose gel electrophoresis always gave a smaller size than that obtained by addition of *Xba*I restriction fragments. R27 (112 megadaltons) would be expected to have a size of 172.5 kilobases, based on the formula that 1 megadalton = 1.54 kilobases (HELLING and LOMAX 1978). In fact R27 was determined from *Xba*I digestion to be 182 kilobases in length (TAYLOR and BROSE 1985b). A similar phenomenon has been observed with the IncHII plasmid pHH1508a. Although BRADLEY et al. (1982) estimated that this plasmid had a molecular weight of 100 megadaltons by agarose gel electrophoresis, using *Xba*I and *Xho*I digests, we determined that pHH1508a had a molecular size of 208 kilobases or equivalent to 135 megadaltons (YAN and TAYLOR 1987). Similar results have been observed with other plasmids. For example, RP4 was determined to have a molecular size of 36 megadaltons or 54.5 kilobases (see Table 1). Although initial restriction maps of RP4 were based on 56.4 kb (BARTH 1979), the most recent map of RP4 using S*sph*I sites was based on 60 kb (LANKA et al. 1983). In general, the more restriction fragments that are used to determine the plasmid size, the larger the total size appears to be. Since the relationship between molecular weight and migration distance is linear only in the range 10–100 megadaltons (HANSEN and OLSEN 1978), the sum of the restriction fragments is likely to give a more precise estimate of the molecular size for large plasmids.

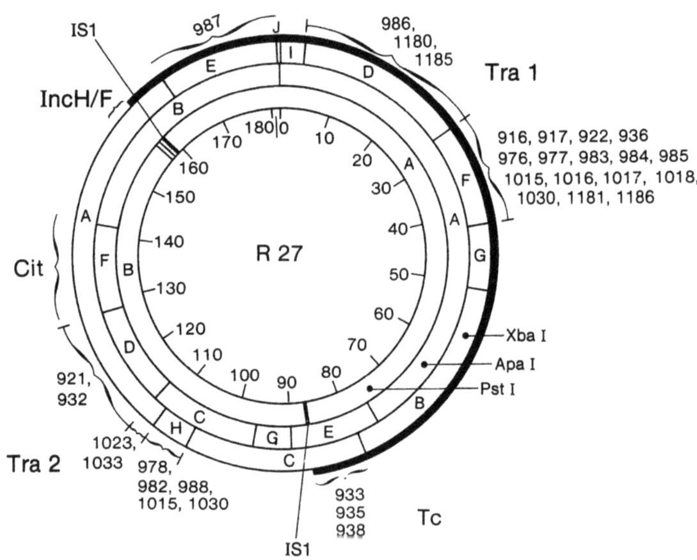

Fig. 1. Physical and genetic map of R27. Restriction endonuclease cleavage sites and fragments are indicated in the outer circles. These sites were oriented with respect to the *Xba*I site at coordinate O and the map numbered by distance (in kilobases) from that site. Tra1 and Tra2 are regions concerned with plasmid transfer which were defined by Tn*5* and Tn*7* insertion mutagenesis as shown by the number designations. Position of the Tc^r region was defined by Tn*7* insertions and hybridization with a Tn*10* probe. The position of the citrate utilization (*Cit*) determinant was inferred by hybridization with Tn*3411*. The positions of the IncH/F region and the IS1 sequences were determined by cloning and by hybridization with ^{32}P-labelled probes. The *dark shaded area on the outer circle* represents the deletion mutant pDT1047

III. Plasmid Organization

Conjugative plasmids encode certain specialized functions for their replication and maintenance in host cells, as well as for conjugative transfer and pilus production. Resistance to antibiotics and metals, as well as determinants for metabolism of sugars or other compounds are often specified by the plasmids. Plasmid transfer and replication will be discussed in more detail in sections D and E and other plasmid-coded properties in section F. A genetic and physical map of the IncHI1 plasmid R27 is shown in Fig. 1. This plasmid, isolated from *S. typhimurium* in England in 1961, was the earliest documented example of an IncHI1 plasmid. Subsequently the IncHI1 plasmids acquired resistance to Cm and HI1 plasmids such as pRG1271 and R726 were found to encode resistance to CmSmSuTc in *S. typhi* (ANDERSON and SMITH 1972). *S. typhi* strains ultimately became resistant to ampicillin, with isolation of plasmids like pRG1251 (ApCmSmSuTc^r) (ANDERSON 1975). Our studies showed that the other resistance determinants appeared to have integrated into R27 adjacent to the Tc^r determinant and all within the *Xba*I B fragment (Fig. 1) (TAYLOR and BROSE 1985 a). Although the detailed organization of these resistance determinants is not yet known, the *Xba*I B fragment contains the insertion sequence IS1 (TAYLOR and Brose unpublished data), which in other plasmids is known to be involved in the insertion of resistance determinants (OHTSUBO and OHTSUBO 1978; HU et al. 1975). These IS elements can mediate transposition of a complete set of resistance determinants to other replicons. Blocks of resistance determinants were transposed from the HI1 plasmid pRG1251 to the bacteriophage P1 (TAYLOR et al. 1981 b). The P1 prophage acquired ApTc markers, or CmSmSu markers or a combination of all markers. Moreover, spontaneous loss of CmSmSu was observed from pRG1251, suggesting that the ApTc determinants are located close together as are the CmSmSu determinants (TAYLOR et al. 1981 b).

D. Plasmid Transfer

I. Conjugative Pili

1. Pilus Structure

All conjugative plasmids in Enterobacteriaceae have the capacity to specify pili (BRADLEY 1980). These are found in two basic forms – flexible and rigid. Pili range in thickness from 6 to 11 nm (BRADLEY 1980). By far the largest number of incompatibility groups specify thick (8–9 mm) flexible pili (C, D, F, HI, HII, J, T, V, X and Com 9), although thin (6 mm) flexible pili are specified by a few groups (B, I1, I2, Iγ, K) (BRADLEY 1980). Several groups (M, N, P and W) encode rigid pili (BRADLEY 1980).

The structure of F pili has been studied most extensively (IPPEN-IHLER and MINKLEY 1986). F pili are made up of a single component, F pilin (molecular weight 7200 daltons). Pili originate in the inner membrane and extend from zones of inner-outer membrane adhesion (BAYER 1975). F pili are thought to retract by disassembly of F pilin subunits so as to establish direct wall-to-wall contact between conjugal donor and recipient cells. The F plasmid then transfers as a single strand of DNA from the donor to the recipient cell, probably via some type of pore structure (WILLETTS and WILKINS 1984).

2. H Pili

H pili specified by the HII plasmid pHH1508 a (Fig. 2 a) are 8 nm in diameter and the average number per cell ranges from 1 to 2 (YAN and TAYLOR in preparation). Analysis of proteins was carried out in *E. coli* cells containing HII plasmids and from partially purified H pili preparations from pHH1508 a by polyacrylamide gel electrophoresis and subsequent immunoblotting using H pilus specific antibody. No small subunit corresponding to F pilin was identified. Instead, a larger molecular weight polypeptide of approximately 40 000 daltons reacted with the H pilus-specific antibody. This protein was absent in *E. coli* cells containing transfer-defective mutants, which did not specify H pili (YAN and TAYLOR in preparation). It is not clear if this protein represents an aggregate of low molecular weight H pilin molecules which were not visible in the gels or if the structure of H pili is completely different from that of F pili.

3. Pilus-Specific Phage

Pili encoded by plasmids of various Inc groups are able to act as receptors for specific bacteriophages and H pili are no exception. An H pilus-specific RNA phage (pilHα) was isolated from South African sewage (COETZEE et al. 1985). The pilHα phage absorbs along the length of the shafts of both IncHI and IncHII plasmid-coded pili (Fig. 2 b). Plaque formation was temperature sensitive in hosts contain-

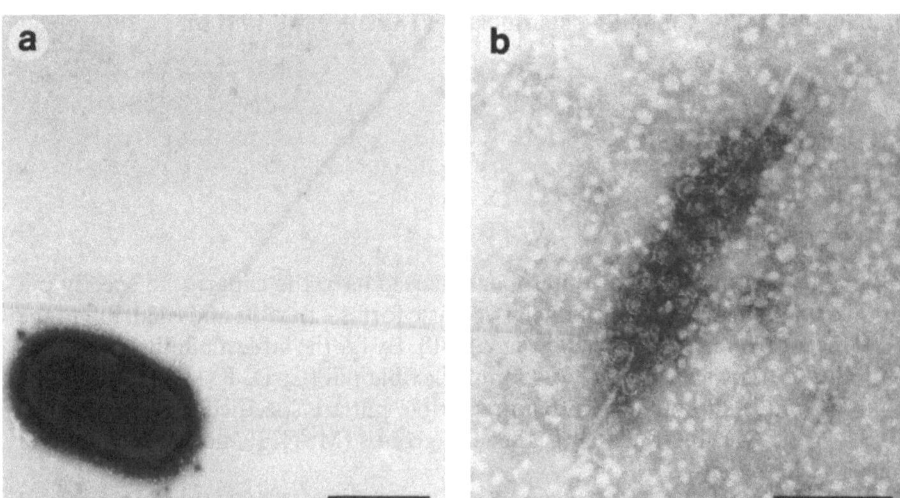

Fig. 2. a Electron micrograph showing *E. coli* JE2571 harbouring IncHII plasmid pHH1508a and producing H conjugative pili. The *bar* represents 1.0 μm. **b** Electron micrograph showing bacteriophage pilHα attached to an H pilus, specified by pHH1508a. The *bar* represents 0.1 μm

ing IncHI and IncHII plasmids, in that plaques formed after incubation of cells at 26 °C but not after incubation at 37 °C. This is unexpected since, although transfer of IncHI plasmids the thermosensitive (see Sect. D.II.2), transfer of HII plasmids is not. This finding suggests that pilHα may have evolved under conditions favoring attachment and replication at 26 °C, such as those in hosts harboring IncHI plasmids, and may only later have encountered hosts containing IncHII plasmids.

Although single-stranded DNA phages (f1, M13, fd) have been isolated which attach to the F pilus tip (IPPEN-IHLER and MINKLEY 1986), DNA phages for which H pili act as receptors have not yet been identified.

II. Transfer Conditions

1. Surface Versus Liquid Matings

Rigid pili such as those encoded by M, N, P and W groups are fairly fragile and are apparently broken by brownian motion or convection forces in liquid (BRADLEY et al. 1980). Thus, plasmids that determine rigid pili transfer at least 2000 times better on plates than in broth and have been described as surface-obligate mating types. Moreover, some plasmids that determine thick flexible pili also transfer somewhat better on plates (from 45 to 470 times better than in broth), and are, therefore, considered to have surface-preferred transfer systems. The IncHII plasmid pHH1508α transferred from 30 to 128 times higher in plates than in broth (BRADLEY et al. 1982; TAYLOR, unpublished) and, therefore, belongs to the surface-preferred group. Plasmids of a number of other groups (including IncHI plasmids) transferred equally well on plates or in broth (BRADLEY et al. 1980). The mechanism responsible for the surface-preferred phenomenon is not clear, but may be related to a relatively weak linkage between the pili and the donor cells during mating pair formation. Examination of transfer frequencies using plates and liquid matings can be useful in classification of an unknown plasmid. These relatively simple tests led to the reclassification of R831 b, once considered to be an IncHI2 plasmid, as IncM (BRADLEY et al. 1980).

2. Thermosensitive Transfer of IncHI Plasmids

Thermosensitive transfer of IncHI plasmids was first reported in 1974 (SMITH 1974). At 37 °C the transfer frequency is reduced by a factor of 10^6 compared with transfer at 26 °C. The process of thermosensitive transfer was investigated for the IncHI1 plasmid pRG1251 and the IncHI2 plasmids pSD114 and R478 in short term (2 h) mating experiments (TAYLOR and LEVINE 1980). The growth temperature of the recipient had little effect on the transfer of the IncH plasmids. In contrast, the growth temperature of the donor culture significantly affected transfer and there was a 10^{-2} to 10^{-3}-fold reduction in the mating frequency at 26 °C when donor preincubation temperatures were increased from 26 ° to 42 °C. The level of transfer achieved during a 2 h mating was also affected by the temperature of the mating mixture. The optimum mating temperature was from 26 °C to 30 °C. At mating temperatures of 37 °C or higher, transfer was not detected. It was not possible to effect transfer of IncHI plasmids in mating mixtures incubated at 37 °C or higher by preincubation of the donor culture at low temperatures (26 ° or 30 °C). Although donor cells containing IncHI plasmids appear to produce fewer pili when incubated at 26 °C than when incubated at 37 °C (YAN and TAYLOR unpublished observation), thermosensitive transfer cannot depend only on production of pili. Other steps in the transfer process have a temperature sensitive component (TAYLOR and LEVINE 1980).

In contrast to IncHI plasmids, IncHII plasmids are not temperature sensitive for transfer (BRADLEY et al. 1982). Moreover, because of their high frequency of transfer (approximately 1×10^{-2} transconjugants in a 1 h mating), and ability to specify more pili than IncHI plasmids, they are considered to be naturally derepressed for transfer (BRADLEY et al. 1982).

III. Transfer Gene Organization

1. Transfer Genes on the IncHI Plasmid R27

Similar to other IncHI plasmids, R27 transfers at a frequency of 1×10^{-2} transconjugants per recipient in an 18 h mating at 26 °C and the transfer frequency is reduced by a factor of 10^6 at 37 °C. A Tn*5* insertion mutant of R27 (pDT933) has an enhanced frequency of transfer of 1.3 transconjugants per recipient in an 18 h mating at 26 °C (TAYLOR et al. 1985c). This apparently derepressed phenotype of pDT933 is thought to result from a 1 kb insertion within the *Xba*I D fragment (4–28 kb) on the R27 map (Fig. 1). In addition pDT933 carries a Tn*5* insertion occupying part of the *Apa*I E fragment between coordinates 79–87 causing it to be Tc^s.

To identify regions of the IncHI1 plasmid R27 that are involved in conjugative transfer, we constructed transfer-defective (Tra^-) mutants of R27 and pDT933 by insertion of Tn*5* and Tn*7* (TAYLOR 1983; TAYLOR et al. 1985c). *E. coli* strains containing Tn*5* or Tn*7* inserted at a chromosomal site and either R27 or pDT933 were used as donors in mating experiments with nalidixic acid resistant recipients. A second mating was used to test for transfer ability (TAYLOR 1983). Almost all Tra^- insertion mutants isolated by this method resulted in complete inhibition of transfer after an 18 h mating at 26 °C. The locations of Tn*5* and Tn*7* insertion sites were determined using *Xba*I and *Apa*I digestion. Figure 1 summarizes the data obtained from these experiments. The Tra^- mutants were clustered into two major regions of the R27 map. The majority of insertions were located within a 22 kb segment comprising coordinates 28 to 42 and 105 to 112. The large size of the *Xba*I and *Apa*I fragments analyzed necessitated an overestimate of the Tra regions shown in Fig. 1. In fact mutants such as pDT921 and pDT932 in *Xba*I fragment D could have inserted very close to the position of those in pDT1023 and pDT1033. Similarly, the insert in pDT986, pDT1180 and pDT1185 could be located close to the large group of inserts within *Xba*I fragment F. The transfer genes on R27 are, therefore, located in two major widely separated transfer regions, Tra1 and Tra2 (Fig. 1).

Only the pDT987 mutant mapped outside these two regions. Moreover, its frequency of transfer was only moderately reduced, from 1.3 from the parent plasmid pDT933 to 3.3×10^{-4} transconjugants per recipient for the mutant. We are continuing our studies of R27 transfer by mapping these mutants in greater detail as well as by analysis of cloned fragments from within the individual transfer regions.

2. Transfer Genes on IncHII Plasmid pHH1508a

The IncHII plasmid pHH1508a has been mapped using the enzymes *Xba*I, *Xho*I and *Not*I. Tra^- derivatives of this plasmid by insertion of Tn*5* have also been obtained (YAN and TAYLOR 1987). Although only seven Tn*5* mutants were mapped, their insertion sites were found to be widely distributed over the plasmid map (Fig. 3). A deletion mutant of pHH1508a, designated pDT1178, was constructed in vitro using *Xba*I (Fig. 3). Immunogold labelling experiments using H pilus specific antiserum demonstrated that pDT1178, despite its Tra^- phenotype, was still capable of synthesizing H pili. Therefore, the genes required for H pilus production and assembly are probably located together in one transfer region close to the trimethoprim and streptomycin resistance determinants which are part of the transposon Tn7. The observation that cells carrying pDT1178 produced fewer pili than cells carrying pHH1508a suggests that other genes located outside this region might be involved in the regulation of the number of pili produced (YAN and TAYLOR 1987). Since IncHI and HII plasmids have little homologous DNA (WHITELEY and TAYLOR 1983), it is likely that homologous H pilin genes account for only a small fraction of DNA present in the H plasmids.

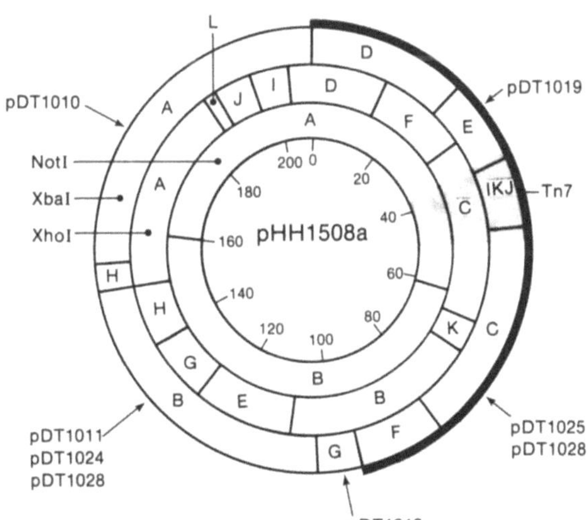

Fig. 3. Physical and genetic map of pHH1508a. Restriction endonuclease cleavage sites and fragments are indicated on the outer circles. These sites were oriented with respect to the *Xba*I site at coordinate O and the map numbered by distance (in kilobases) from that site. Locations of Tn*5* insertion which produced transfer defective mutants are shown by *arrows*. The location of the natural position of Tn7 within the plasmid is shown by the *shaded area*. The *dark shaded area on the outer circle* represents the deletion mutant pDT1178

3. Transfer Genes on Other Plasmids

The transfer genes of F have been characterized most completely, although significant questions still remain to be answered (IPPEN-IHLER and MINKLEY 1986). Genes and sites essential for F plasmid transfer are clustered in a single 33.3 kb contiguous region and a minimum of 22 activities are associated with transfer. A large number of genes are required for expression of F pili; two other genes are required to stabilize mating pairs formed from donor and recipient cells. Other transfer genes are required to nick plasmid DNA at the origin of transfer, to displace the single strand and then transplant it to the recipient cell (WILLETTS and WILKINS 1984; IPPEN-IHLER and MINKLEY 1986).

Like F, the IncN plasmid R46 appears to contain its transfer genes in a single fragment of 22.5 kb (BROWN and WILLETTS 1981). In contrast, transfer genes in other plasmids, such as the IncP-10 plasmid R9 1–4 from *Pseudomonas aeruginosa* and the IncP plasmid RP4, lie in two or three distinct regions (MOORE and KRISHNAPILLAI 1982; BARTH 1979). The arrangement of transfer genes in both the IncHI plasmid R27 and the IncHII plasmid pHH1508a more closely resemble that of IncP plasmids from *Pseudomonas* than the IncF or IncN plasmids.

Ti (tumour inducing plasmids) from *Agrobacterium tumefaciens* which are of approximately the same size as R27 also transfer by a temperature-sensitive mechanism (HOLSTERS et al. 1980). Examination of the Ti plasmid pTiC58 by transposon insertion with Tn*1* and Tn*7* led to the isolation of two Tra$^-$ mutants. On the basis of this study, two widely spaced Tra regions were identified in pTiC58 (HOLSTERS et al. 1980). Since the H plasmids and Ti plasmids all have high molecular weights, the location of the transfer genes in widely separated regions of the plasmid may account for conservation of the relatively large amounts of DNA in these plasmids.

IV. Surface Exclusion Systems

Surface (or entry) exclusion refers to the mechanism by which a plasmid inhibits entry into the host cell of a second closely related plasmid. In the F transfer system, two genes (*tra*T and *tra*S) are involved in entry exclusion and are located next to one another among the F transfer genes. The TraT protein is located in the outer membrane (ACHTMAN et al. 1977) and is thought to act as a specific protein barrier to self-mating, probably by competing with the F pilus tip for binding to an appropriate receptor. The TraS protein is located in the inner membrane and is thought to be the surface exclusion component which prevents triggering of conjugal DNA synthesis by the donor (IPPEN-IHLER and MINKLEY 1986).

Although plasmids of other incompatibility groups exhibit entry exclusion, the mechanisms have not been studied in detail. The IncHI plasmids exhibit strong surface exclusion reactions between highly related plasmids (TAYLOR and GRANT 1977a). The surface exclusion index (defined as the frequency of transfer of a plasmid to a bacterial strain divided by the frequency of transfer of the plasmid under similar conditions to an R$^+$ derivative of the same recipient strain) was 400 when derivatives of the IncHI1 plasmid pRG1251 were tested and was 100 when derivatives of the IncHI2 plasmid pAS251–2 were tested (TAYLOR and GRANT 1977a). In contrast, the surface exclusion between IncHI1 and IncHI2 plasmids was much weaker with surface exclusion indices of 10 for interactions between pRG1251 and pAS251–2 (TAYLOR and GRANT 1977a).

The entry exclusion indices of the transfer-defective Tn*5* and Tn7 insertion mutants discussed in Sect. D.III.1 and D.III.2 were identical to those obtained with wild-type R27, i.e. 10^2 to 10^4. However, a deletion derivative of R27 prepared in vitro from the *Pst*I A fragment of R27 had lost the entry exclusion phenotype characteristic of R27 (TAYLOR et al. 1985c). The deletion in pDT1047 extended from coordinates 87 to 160. If the surface exclusion genes are located near to other transfer genes, as is the case in F, then they would be expected to be located within the Tra2 region (Fig. 1).

E. Plasmid Maintenance and Replication

I. Maintenance of IncH Plasmids

The IncHI plasmids are present in about one copy per chromosome and are generally maintained stably in host cells at 26 °C to 37 °C. At higher temperatures these plasmids appear to be less stable. At 42 °C, 4% of clones of *E. coli* RG192 (R478) lost the plasmid after 20 generations. This rose to 30% plasmid-free clones after incubation at 44 °C. Although some other IncHI1 and IncHI2 plasmids were stable at these temperatures, the IncHI1 plasmid pRG1251 was eliminated from 18% of clones after 20 generations at 44 °C (TAYLOR and LEVINE 1980). Smith has also demonstrated that IncHI plasmids are unstable at high temperature (SMITH et al. 1978a). High temperature elimination of H plasmids, the Hte phenotype, suggests that some HI plasmids may also have temperature sensitive steps in replication and/or maintenance.

We isolated a thermosensitive mutant of the IncHI2 plasmid pDT114 using ethyl methane sulfonate mutagenesis (TAYLOR and LEVINE 1979). This plasmid, designated pDT4, was eliminated from 100% of clones after 20 generations at 37 °C, although it was stable at 30 °c. Moreover, pDT4 was also eliminated by treatment of the host cells with novobiocin or coumermycin A1. Both of these antibiotics inhibit the B subunit of bacterial DNA gyrase (GELLERT et al. 1976). Nalidixic acid, which interferes with the A subunit of DNA gyrase (HIGGINS et al. 1978), had no effect on pDT4. Neither ethidium bromide nor acridine orange, which are curing agents that interfere with DNA replication, were able to eliminate pDT4. Although we did not identify any other IncH plasmids that were susceptible to novobiocin curing, the IncHII plasmid pMG110 and the multicopy ColE1-derived plasmid pBR322 are also eliminated by growth at 37 °C and by coumermycin A1 treatment (WOLFSON et al. 1982).

To determine if novobiocin and coumermycin A1 acted directly on the host DNA gyrase or on an enzyme coded by the plasmid, pDT4 was transferred to *E. coli* K12 NI747 (*cou*^{s} *dna*A$^+$) and NI748 (*cou*^{r} *dnaA*$^+$). Although pDT4 was eliminated from both strains at 37 °C, it was only eliminated from NI747 at 30 °C after novobiocin treatment. The presence of the coumermycin resistant DNA gyrase in NI748 protected the plasmid from being eliminated by novobiocin treatment (TAYLOR and LEVINE 1979). The IncHII plasmid pMG110 was also protected from coumermycin elimination by a similar mutation in the host (WOLFSON et al. 1982). These results suggested to us that the H plasmid uses host DNA gyrase for replication. The mutation in pDT4 may be in another enzyme or DNA site required to interact with DNA gyrase for successful plasmid replication. Moreover, along with thermosensitivity and novobiocin sensitivity, pDT4 also has a reduced transfer frequency compared to the wild type plasmid. Therefore, the defect in pDT4 appears to affect both vegetative replication as well as conjugative DNA replication (TAYLOR and LEVINE 1979).

II. Replication Functions of Mini-plasmids

1. Mini F

Replication and maintenance of several plasmids have been studied by construction of mini-plasmids containing all the genes necessary for replication and maintenance. The mini-F plasmid, for example, consists of the f5 *Eco*R1 restriction fragment of 9 kilobases occupying coordinates 40.3 to 49.3 on the F plasmid map (SCOTT 1984; KLINE 1985). Mini-F (Fig. 4) contains two origins of replication. EICHENLAUB et al. (1977) mapped an origin of replication, *ori*V or *ori*1 at map coordinates 42.6 kb. However, this origin can be deleted and the resulting plasmid retains the same maintenance properties as the parent (MANIS and KLINE 1977). The second origin, *ori*S or *ori*2, is located at 45.07 kb (EICHENLAUB et al. 1981). Replication from *ori*V is bidirectional, whereas replication from *ori*S is leftward and undirectional. A fragment of DNA containing *ori*V (40.8 to 43 kb) cannot form a plasmid, whereas the fragment of DNA containing *ori*S (44 to 46 kb) does form a plasmid (KLINE 1985). The *rep*E gene located at 45.24 to 46.007 kb encodes the essential 29000 dalton gene E protein (MUROTSU et al. 1981, 1984). To the left of the E gene lies a cluster of four 19 base pair direct repeat known as *incB* and to the right a cluster of five more 19 base pair direct repeats known as *incC* (MUROTSU et al. 1984). These repeat sequences constitute the determinants of F incompatibility (KLINE and LANE 1980). Based on the sequence of MUROTSU et al. (1984), it has been observed that the operator region of gene E contains a 10

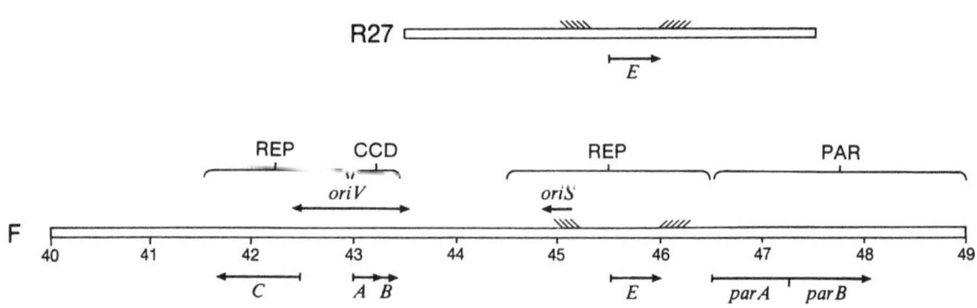

Fig. 4. Comparative maps of mini-F and mini-H plasmids. Maps units are in kilobases. The regions of mini-F shown contain genes involved in replication (REP); coupled cell division (*CCD*), and partitioning (*PAR*). The *oriV* and *oriS* indicate origins of replication, gene products of F are shown at the *bottom of the figure* and the direction of transcription is indicated (→). The *arrows* (\\\\\) and (/////) define the F *incB* and *incC* regions. Each *arrow* represents a 19-bp direct repeat. Similar repeats are found on R27 which control incompatibility between R27 and F (IncH/F)

base pair inverted repeat separated by 9 base pairs. Of the 10 base pairs, 8 are the same as the 8 consecutive bases in the repeats that compose *IncB* and *IncC* (SCOTT 1984). The gene E protein is thought to regulate its own synthesis by binding to its own operator region (i.e. autorepression). It also appears to bind to sites located in the *IncB* and *IncC* regions, thereby reducing the amount of free E protein available for replication and resulting in incompatibility (SCOTT 1984; KLINE 1985).

In addition to protein E, several other proteins are specified by mini-F. These include protein C, a 34000 dalton protein which is required in addition to protein E for replication using *oriV* (EICHENLAUB and WEHLMANN 1980). Two small proteins, which are the products of the *ccdA* (10500 daltons) and *ccdB* genes (11000 daltons), are required to couple cell division to plasmid replication (OGURA and HIRAGA 1983). Proteins A (44000 daltons) and B (37000 daltons) are required for the efficient partitioning of F plasmids to daughter cells (KLINE 1985). These genes are located within the Par region (46.5–49 kb).

2. Other Mini-Plasmids

Mini-P1 (IncY) and Mini-Rts1 (IncT) plasmids have been constructed and both are similar to mini-F in their basic replicon organization (CHATTORAJ et al. 1985; KAMIO et al. 1984). Both consist of a set of five inverted repeats (19 or 24 base pairs) in front of a replication protein gene followed by nine (P1) or three (Rts1) repeats of 19 or 21 base pairs, respectively. In addition, within the same region mini-P1 codes for proteins involved in partitioning and probably also in coupling plasmid replication to cell division.

3. Mini-H Plasmids

We have isolated a mini-plasmid from the IncHI plasmid R27 consisting of the Tc resistance gene from R27 attached to a fragment of approximately 2 kb which encodes replication functions (TAYLOR and BROSE in preparation). A self-replicating mini-plasmid consisting of a 7.6 kb *Eco*R1 fragment of R27 ligated to a DNA fragment conferring spectinomycin resistance has also been isolated by Bergquist and coworkers (SAUL and BERGQUIST 1986). The structure of a portion of the minimal R27 replicon is shown in Fig. 4 for comparison with mini-F. The DNA sequence of a portion of the R27 minimal replicon region has been determined (SAUL and BERGQUIST 1986). A high degree of homology exists between the R27 replicon sequence and the mini-F sequence in the *IncB* and the gene E open reading frame regions. The four direct repeats within the H plasmid *IncB* region are almost identical to the F *IncB* repeats except for two base pairs within the first repeat and one base pair within the third repeat. The 29000 dalton open reading frame of the E protein homologue of R27 gave approximately 88% amino acid sequence homology with the E protein from the F factor.

Homology between the R27 replicon and mini-F was also observed within the *IncC* regions. The first two 19 base pair repeats were identical and the third and fourth repeats differed by 2 and 3 base pairs, respectively. Homology was less pronounced downstream of the first two repeats of *IncC* except within the 19 base pair repeats. Since the mini-R27 plasmids resemble mini-F so closely and are also autonomous replicons, an origin of replication is likely to be present within the region homologous to the *incB* region. Using the mini-R27 plasmid that we obtained as well as probes for the *incB* region and gene E, we were able to identify the location of these determinants on the R27 map (Fig. 1).

As discussed above, F contains two replication origins, *ori*V and *ori*S. Moreover, an additional origin is present within the f7 *Eco*R1 fragment of F as a mini-F plasmid can also be made from this fragment (LANE and GARDNER 1979). It is likely that R27 also has more than one replication origin. The deletion mutant pDT1047 constructed in vitro after *Pst*I digestion which consists of the *Pst*IA fragment (Fig. 1) does not contain the 156–157 kb *incB-repE-incC* region associated with incompatibility or the putative origin of replication. Moreover pDT1047 is compatible with the F factor. Yet it can still replicate autonomously. Therefore, other R27 replication origin(s) still remain to be identified.

III. Incompatibility

1. H Plasmid Incompatibility

Three types of incompatibility reactions appear to be encoded by IncHI plasmids. Strong incompatibility reactions are seen between closely related plasmids such as between two HI1 plasmids or between two HI2 plasmids. Weaker incompatibility reactions are observed between an IncHI1 and an IncHI2 plasmid (TAYLOR and GRANT 1977a). Strong incompatibility (rapid loss of the unselected plasmid) was often accompanied by plasmid recombination. Weak incompatibility (slow loss of one of the plasmids) was not accompanied by recombination. Moreover, incompatibility between HI1 and HI2 plasmids usually resulted in loss of the HI1 plasmid regardless of the order of entry (TAYLOR and GRANT 1977).

The third type of incompatibility displayed only by HI1 plasmids is the unidirectional elimination of the F factor by an IncHI1 plasmids (SMITH et al. 1973). The F/HI1 incompatibility is dependent upon the presence of the *incB-repE-IncC* region in both F and the IncHI1 plasmid described in Sect. E.II. A pair of IncHI1 plasmids pIP166 from *S. typhi* and its derivative pIP522 were isolated by CHABBERT and GERBAUD (1974). The latter had lost 23.5 kb of DNA, including the Tc^r determinant and F/H incompatibility. Whereas pIP166 hybridized to a probe for the *incB* and gene E region (pBK207 comprising F coordinates 44.1–45.88 kb), pIP522 did not (TAYLOR and BROSE 1985a; TAYLOR et al. 1985c). The mini-H plasmids prepared from R27 and described above which contain the *IncB-repE-IncC* region also show the one way incompatibility with the F factor. Therefore, the replication region homologous to the F region is necessary for incompatibility. The one-way incompatibility between IncHI1 and F may reside in the ability of the *repE* protein of the IncHI1 plasmid to attach more tightly to the binding domains on F than on its own DNA. Consequently, replication of the F factor is shut off first leading to elimination of F while the IncHI1 plasmid replication continues unhindered.

The mini-H plasmid which we isolated was compatible with IncHI2 plasmids and was only very weakly incompatible with IncHI1 plasmids (TAYLOR and BROSE unpublished). Therefore, other determinants specifying H incompatibility must be present on R27. Just as there are likely to be more than one origin of replication carried on IncH plasmids, there is also likely to be more than one set of incompatibility determinants. Moreover, the deletion mutant pDT1047 is incompatible with both IncHI1 and IncHI2 plasmids and, therefore, H incompatibility determinants are likely to be located in the region from 161-0-87 kb on the R27 map. The mechanisms controlling the other H incompatibility functions are unknown.

2. Incompatibility Mechanisms Specified by Other Plasmids

The phenomenon of incompatibility appears to be a direct consequence of normal maintenance and replication control functions. Several factors have been shown to be involved in incompatibility, in both low copy and multicopy plasmids. In this section I will review the processes involved with reference to plasmids of several different incompatibility groups.

As is the case with several plasmids, including the F factor, incompatibility is controlled by a diffusible initiator protein which binds to directly repeated oligonucleotide sequences or "iterons" (Novick 1987). These include P1, Rts1, RK2 and R6K (Chattoraj et al. 1985; Kamio et al. 1984; Shafferman et al. 1981; Stalker et al. 1982). Regulation in these plasmids involves binding to the iterons as well as autoregulation. Binding may directly inhibit replication or may regulate the initiator concentration. The initiator protein is believed to gradually fill up the iterons, eventually triggering replication and creating a new set of iterons on the daughter plasmid (Novick 1987).

The primary determinants of incompatibility for all plasmids that contain iterons are the regions that contain the iterons. For mini-F these are the *incB* and *incC* regions (Murotsu et al. 1984). F iterons express incompatibility in direct proportion to their gene dosage (Tolun and Helinski 1981). Moreover, deletions in mini-F in the iterons caused an increase in copy number inversely proportional to the number of iterons present (Kline and Travick 1983).

In contrast, other plasmids use a different regulatory system, known as the "inhibitor-target" system (Novick 1987). These include the ColEI plasmid (Tomizawa et al. 1981); the IncFII plasmid R1 (Light and Molin 1982a) and pT181 from *Staphylococcus aureus* (Kumar and Novick 1985). These plasmids encode a diffusible replication inhibitor which acts by binding to a plasmid-determined target. This binding either inhibits replication directly or inhibits the synthesis of a product required for replication. In the case of ColEI, the replication preprimer is inhibited (Tomizawa et al. 1981). For the IncFII plasmids the messenger RNA for a rate-limiting replication protein (*rep*) which initiates plasmid replication is the target (Light and Molin 1982a). Similarly for pT181 the mRNA for a replication protein (*repC*) is inhibited (Kumar and Novick 1985). For all three types of plasmids the inhibitors are RNA molecules of 80–150 nucleotides that are transcribed from the 5′ end of the target transcript. In each case pairing is thought to occur between the inhibitor and the target transcript to give RNA-RNA duplex molecules. An additional regulatory protein is encoded by ColEI. The ColEI *rop* protein (Cesarini et al. 1982) participates in the RNA-RNA interaction (Tomizawa and Som 1984).

Two plasmids containing regions which specify the same inhibitor RNA molecules are incompatible. The cloned inhibitor RNA determinants also specify strong incompatibility (MOLIN and NORDSTROM 1980; NOVICK et al. 1984; TAMM and POLISKY 1983). The inhibitory RNA acts as the major incompatibility determinant. Mutations that cause changes in the inhibitory RNA, particularly in the loop regions which interact with the target DNA to prevent replication, can alter incompatibility properties (LACATENA and CESARENI 1983).

In some plasmids incompatibility depends on the presence of related replication origins. Replication of plasmids such as ColEI is directly regulated (GRINDLEY et al. 1978), since the inhibitor blocks synthesis of a replication primer (TOMIZAWA et al. 1981). In contrast plasmids such as pT181 are indirectly regulated, since the inhibitor blocks synthesis of the transacting replication protein *repC* (KUMAR and NOVICK 1985). Among those plasmids which are indirectly regulated, plasmids with identical origins of replication are incompatible, even if they share no other replication or maintenance functions (NOVICK 1987). The cloned origin of replication of the iteron-containing plasmids expresses incompatibility (ABELES et al. 1984; SHAFFERMAN et al. 1981; TSUTSUI et al. 1983) as does that of the pT181 plasmid (NOVICK et al. 1984). Those of the directly regulated plasmids ColEI and IncFII do not (HASHIMOTO-GOTOH and INSELBURG 1979; TIMMIS et al. 1978).

Finally, cloned partitioning determinants (*par*) have been shown to cause incompatibility for R1 (NORDSTROM et al. 1980) as well as for the F plasmid (KLINE 1985). Nothing is known of partitioning determinants in IncH plasmids. Although details of incompatibility mechanisms in a few plasmids, particularly ColEI, are well understood, a complete understanding of the phenomenon in high molecular weight plasmids remains elusive.

F. Antibiotic Resistance and Other Plasmid-Encoded Properties

A list of the characteristics encoded by various IncH plasmids is shown in Table 4. Several of these will be discussed in detail.

I. Chloramphenicol Resistance

Most IncHI1 plasmids as well as many IncHI2 plasmids encode chloramphenicol resistance. The determinant in the IncHI1 plasmid R726 as well as the IncHI2 plasmid R478 was shown to be related to Tn*9* (GAFFNEY and FOSTER 1978). A chloramphenicol acetyl transferase gene of type 1 modifies the antibiotic so it is no longer functional. This Cm^r determinant, which is bounded by direct repeats of ISI, is probably responsible for much of IncHI plasmid resistance to chloramphenicol (ALTON and VAPNECK 1979; TAYLOR and BROSE 1985a).

II. Tetracycline Resistance

R27 and most other IncHI1 plasmids encode tetracycline resistance (Table 4). The Tc^r determinant of R27 is located between coordinates 79–87 on the R27 map

(Fig. 1). This TC^r determinant is related to Tn*10* and falls in the *tetB* class as determined by DNA hybridization with various DNA probes (MENDEZ et al. 1980). In Tn*10* specifies a repressor as well as a structural TET protein. This latter protein is incorporated into the cytoplasmic membrane and mediates active efflux of the antibiotic (LEVY 1984). The IncHI1 determinant (*tetB1*) differs from *tetB* in that the minimal inhibitory concentration (MIC) of tetracycline for *E. coli* strains harbouring IncHI1 plasmids is lower than that of strains carying plasmids containing the *tetB* determinant. The MIC of tetracycline for R27 is 64 μg/ml whereas that for R222 is 128 μg/ml (TAYLOR, unpublished). Resistance to tetracycline analogues minocycline and chelocardin is also lower (MENDEZ et al. 1980). The reasons for the difference between the levels of expression of the *tetB* and *tetB1* genes are currently under study in this laboratory.

III. Trimethoprim Resistance

Trimethoprim resistance (Tp^r) in both *Klebsiella aerogenes* and *S. typhi* is specified by the IncHII plasmid pHH1508a (DATTA et al. 1981). The specific determinant has been mapped on pHH1508a (Fig. 3) and its homology with transposon Tn7 was confirmed (YAN and TAYLOR 1987). Tn7 specifies a type 1 dihydrofolate reductase (FLING et al. 1982). In contrast an IncHI plasmid pDT1131 responsible for Tp^r in *S. typhi* isolated in Peru contained a Tp^r determinant unrelated to Tn7 (TAYLOR et al. 1985b). Thus H plasmids continue to acquire new resistance determinants in response to selection pressure brought about by antibiotic usage.

IV. Tellurium Resistance

Tellurium compounds are used in light sensitive industrial processes, in the rubber industry and in the manufacture of batteries. They are toxic to humans, animals and many microorganisms, probably because of their strong oxidizing ability (SUMMERS and JACOBY 1979). Although resistance to tellurium (Te^r) is unusual in Enterobacteriaceae, it is encoded by plasmids of the IncHI2, IncHI3 and IncHII groups (SUMMERS and JACOBY 1977; TAYLOR and SUMMERS 1979; TAYLOR and LEVINE 1980; BRADLEY et al. 1982). In *Pseudomonas aeruginosa* the narrow host range P2 plasmids encode tellurium resistance (SUMMERS and JACOBY 1977). The broad host range IncP1 plasmids such as RP4 can also encode Te^r but it is not usually expressed. It is necessary to expose strains containing RP4 to potassium tellurite before the tellurite resistance gene is turned on (BRADLEY 1985b).

Both resistant and susceptible cells can apparently reduce potassium tellurite with the formation of black metallic tellurium in the cells. The tellurium deposits appear to be prevalent in bacterial cells containing the plasmid pHH1508a and especially in strains containing the Te^r determinant from pHH1508a cloned into pUC8 (Fig. 5). The mechanism of Te^r encoded by IncH or IncP plasmids is not yet clearly understood, but is under active study in our laboratory.

1. Tellurium Resistance Encoded by IncHI2 Plasmid pMER610

The Te^r determinant from pMER610 originally isolated from *Alcaligenes* spp. has been cloned in *E. coli* (JOBLING and RITCHIE 1987). Te^r was inducible and maxicell

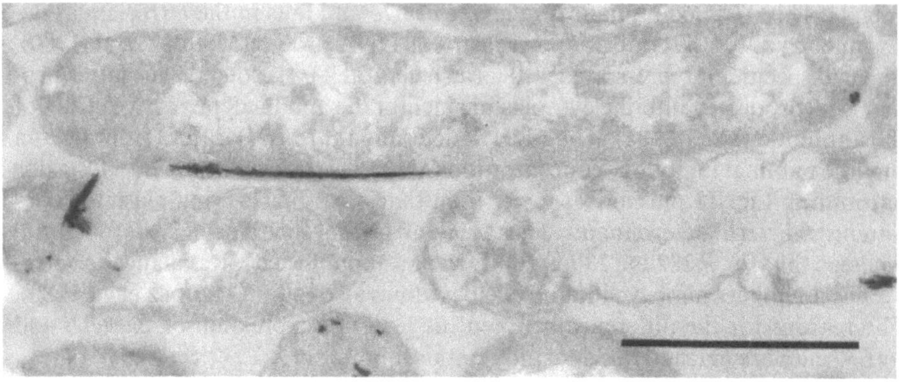

Fig. 5. Electron micrograph of an ultrathin section of *E. coli* strain containing pDT1364, a pUC8 derivative into which the Te^r determinant from pHH1508a was inserted, growing on medium containing potassium tellurite. Reduced metallic tellurium is seen as black deposits within the cells. The *bar* represents 0.1 μm

analysis identified four polypeptides of 15.5, 22, 23 and 41 kilobases specified by the cloned fragment. Analysis using Tn*1000* insertion mutagenesis indicated that the 15.5, 22 and 41 kilodalton proteins were involved in Te^r. Resistance to both tellurite and tellurate appeared to be determined by a single locus and failure to isolate mutants expressing constitutive Te^r suggested that the Te^r operon is positively regulated (Jobling and Ritchie 1987).

2. Tellurium Resistance Encoded by IncHII Plasmid pHH1508a

The Te^r determinant from pHH1508a has been cloned into pUC8. The restriction map of the cloned fragment encoding Te^r in the recombinant plasmid pDT1364 was quite different from that mediating Te^r in pMER610 and from the Te^r determinant from the IncP plasmid RP4 (see below). In vitro transcription-translation of pDT1364 produced two polypeptides of 23 and 12 KD associated with the cloned fragment. Tn*1000* insertion mutants of pDT1364 which were tellurite susceptible lacked the 23 kilodalton polypeptide suggesting that this polypeptide was required for resistance to tellurium compounds. Unlike the IncHI2 Te^r determinant, Tc^r in pHH1508a was expressed constitutively (Walter and Taylor in preparation).

3. Tellurium Resistance Encoded by IncP1 Plasmid RP4

Once turned on by growth on potassium tellurite, Te^r is expressed constitutively by RP4Te^r. The Te^r determinant is located at coordinates 56-0-1.5 kb on the RP4 map between the *korA* and the *kilA* determinants (Taylor and Bradley 1987). The *kil* genes are lethal to host cells and the *kor* (kill override) genes prevent the lethal effects of the kil genes on the host (Figurski et al. 1982). We do not believe that the *kil* and *kor* genes which are involved in plasmid replication and control are directly connected with tellurite resistance since the Te^r determinant can be cloned separately from these determinants (WALTER and TAYLOR in preparation). Unlike the IncH plasmids, the RP4 Te^r system specified a single 40 kilodalton polypeptide in an in vitro transcription/translation system. The Te^r determinant from RP4 is located on a transposon (Tn521) which was transposed to the F factor as well as to other conjugative plasmids (BRADLEY and TAYLOR 1987). Once the DNA sequences of the Te^r genes from IncHI and IncHII and IncP plasmids become available, it will be of interest to compare the degree of homology among the determinants acquired from plasmids of different incompatibility groups. These analyses should allow us to determine the mechanism of Te^r and will give us clues to how Te^r evolved.

V. Bacteriophage Inhibition

Plasmids of the IncHI2, IncHI3 and IncHII groups inhibit the development of double stranded DNA phages lambda, T*1*, T*5* and T*7* (TAYLOR and GRANT 1976, 1977c; BRADLEY et al. 1982). This phage inhibition phenomenon (Phi) has been used to discriminate between IncHI1 and IncHI2 plasmids (TAYLOR and GRANT 1977c; CHASLUS-DUNCLA and LAFONT 1985). The mechanism seems to depend on restriction of phage DNA without associated modification (WATANABE et al. 1966; REVEL and GEORGOPOULOS 1969). In all IncH plasmids examined, bacteriophage inhibition was always associated with resistance to potassium tellurite (TAYLOR and SUMMERS 1979; BRADLEY et al. 1982). The association between Phi and Te^r appears to be coincidental, since when the Te^r determinant pHH1508a was cloned onto pUC8 the recombinant plasmid was not associated with inhibition of bacteriophage development (WALTER and TAYLOR unpublished). Other plasmids also inhibit phage development (Tables 1, 2). For a review of the various types of phage inhibition mediated by plasmids from Enterobacteriaceae, see TAYLOR and GRANT 1977c.

VI. Citrate Utilization

Many IncHI1 plasmids enable their hosts to utilize citrate (SMITH et al. 1978b; ISHIGURO et al. 1979, 1981; TAYLOR and BROSE 1986). The Cit determinant has been cloned from two different IncHI1 plasmids and the DNA sequences determined (ISHIGURO and SATO 1985; SASUTSU et al. 1985). Moreover, one of these determinants was also shown to reside on a transposon designated Tn*3411* (ISHIGURO et al. 1982). The Cit determinant was located between 128.5 and 142 kb on the R27 map (Fig. 1) using a DNA fragment of Tn*3411* as a probe (TAYLOR and BROSE 1986). These plasmids determine a citrate transport system necessary for the uptake of citrate into host cells, although details of its mode of regulation remain to be elucidated.

VII. Lactose Utilization

Several IncHI2 plasmids are able to specify lactose fermentation. These include pWR23 (JOHNSON et al. 1976), MIP235 (ROUSSEL and CHABBERT 1978) and pJI2 (TIMONEY et al. 1980). The pJI2 plasmid was isolated from a strain of *S. typhi*-

murium which caused an outbreak of enteric and septicemic salmonellosis in calves. The ability to metabolize lactose gave the organisms a growth advantage both in the intestines of the calves fed on a milk replacer which contained lactose, or in tanks used to prepare the food for the calves. The lactose marker on pJI2 caused difficulties in the identification of the organism as *S. typhimurium* and the chloramphenicol resistance carried by the plasmid caused problems in treatment of the disease (TIMONEY et al. 1980).

VIII. Determinants of Pathogenicity

Direct determinants of pathogenicity such as invasive ability, serum resistance or toxin production have not been shown to reside on IncH plasmids. However, the IncH plasmids indirectly increase the pathogenicity of their hosts by rendering them resistant to antibiotics and antimetabolites or by enabling them to utilize additional substrates. Moreover, the IncHI2 plasmid pJT4 appeared to increase the persistence of strains of *S. typhimurium* in the intestines of calves. Strains containing the plasmid persisted for 20 days or longer, whereas strains without the plasmid decreased rapidly after 7 days (TIMONEY and LINTON 1982). This phenomenon may be an important factor in the epidemic spread and maintenance of H plasmids in bacterial populations and merits further study.

G. Conclusions and Directions for Future Studies

IncHI plasmids are found predominantly in *Salmonella* spp. (Table 4) but also in *E. coli* (CHASLUS-DUNCLA and LAFONT 1985) and *Ser. marcesens* (HEDGES et al. 1975a). To date IncHII plasmids have been identified in *K. aerogenes* and in *S. typhi* (BRADLEY et al. 1982; DATTA et al. 1981). All H plasmids have high molecular weights and all the IncHI plasmids have a thermosensitive mode of transfer. In some IncH plasmids replication also appears to be thermosensitive.

More detailed studies of HI plasmid transfer genes are required so that we can understand the basis behind the thermosensitive mechanism of transfer. We also need to understand more about the replication of these large plasmids, their incompatibility characteristics and the means by which they are maintained within host bacterial cells. The location of other genes on these large plasmids needs to be investigated, as do unusual characteristics such as tellurite resistance, phage inhibition and ability to increase persistence of the host bacterium within the calf intestines.

Acknowledgements. I thank the following individuals for supplying unpublished data: E. C. Brose, E. G. Walter, W. Yan, R. Sherburne and P. L. Bergquist. I also thank R. Novick for supplying an unpublished manuscript, D. E. Bradley, G. A. Jacoby and E. K. Manavathu for their advice, V. J. Krishnapillai for reading the manuscript and Heather Mitchell for help in preparing the manuscript.

Work quoted from my laboratory was supported by grants from the Medical Research Council of Canada. The Alberta Heritage Foundation for Medical Research provided equipment and additional support. The author is a Heritage Medical Scholar.

References

Abeles AL, Snyder KM, Chattoraj DK (1984) P1 plasmid replication: replicon structure. J Mol Biol 173:307–324

Achtman M, Kennedy N, Skurray R (1977) Cell-cell interactions in conjugatory *Escherichia coli*: role of *traT* protein in surface exclusion. Proc Natl Acad Sci USA 74:104–108

Akiba T, Koyame K, Ishiki Y, Kumira S (1960) On the mechanism of the development of multiple drug-resistance clones of *Shigella*. Jpn J Microbiol 4:219–227

Alton NK, Vapnek D (1979) Nucleotide sequence analysis of the chloramphenicol resistance transposon Tn*9*. Nature 282:864–869

Anderson ES (1975) The problem and implication of chloramphenicol resistance in the typhoid bacillus. J Hyg (Camb) 74:289–299

Anderson ES, Smith HR (1972) Chloramphenicol resistance in the typhoid bacillus. Br Med J 3:329–332

Anderson ES, Humphreys GO, Willshaw GA (1975) The molecular relatedness of R factors in Enterobacteria of human and animal origin. J Gen Microbiol 91:376–382

Aoki T, Egusa S, Ogata Y, Watanabe T (1971) Detection of resistance factors in fish pathogen *Aeromonas liquifaciens*. J Gen Microbiol 65:343–349

Barth PT (1979) RP4 and R300B as wide host-range plasmid cloning vehicles. In: Timmis KN, Puller A (eds) Plasmids of medical, environmental and commercial importance. Elsevier, Amsterdam, pp 399–410

Barth PT, Grinter NJ (1974) Comparison of the DNA molecular weights and homologies of plasmids conferring linked resistance to streptomycin and sulfonamides. J Bacteriol 120:618–630

Bayer ME (1975) Role of adhesion zones in bacterial cell-surface function and biogenesis. In: Tzagaloff A (ed) Membrane biogenesis. Plenum, New York, pp 393–427

Bradley DE (1980) Morphological and serological relationships of conjugative pili. Plasmid 4:155–169

Bradley DE (1984) Characteristics and function of thick and thin conjugative pili determined by transfer derepressed plasmids of incompatibility group I1, I2, I5, B, K and Z. J Gen Microbiol 130:1489–1502

Bradley DE (1985a) Transfer systems of K88 and K99 plasmids. Plasmid 13:118–128

Bradley DE (1985b) Detection of tellurite-resistance determinants in IncP plasmids. J Gen Microbiol 131:3135–3137

Bradley DE (1986) The unique conjugation system of IncHI3 plasmid MIP233. Plasmid 16:63–71

Bradley DE, Taylor DE (1987) Transposition from RP4 to other replicons of a tellurite-resistance determinant not normally expressed in IncPα plasmids. FEMS Microbiol Lett 41:237–240

Bradley DE, Taylor DE, Cohen DR (1980) Specification of surface mating systems among conjugative drug resistance plasmids in *Escherichia coli* K-12. J Bacteriol 143:1400–1470

Bradley DE, Hughes VM, Richards H, Datta N (1982) R plasmids of a new incompatibility group determine constitutive production of H pili. Plasmid 7:230–238

Bradley DE, Taylor DE, Levy SB, Cohen DR, Brose EC, Whelan J (1986) pIN32: a cointegrate plasmid with IncHI2 and IncFII components. J Gen Microbiol 132:1339–1346

Brown AM, Willetts N (1981) A physical and genetic map of the IncN plasmid R46. Plasmid 5:188–201

Bryan LE, van den Elzen HM, Tseng JT (1972) Transferable drug resistance in *Pseudomonas aeruginosa*. Antimicrob Agents Chemother 1:22–29

Capage MA, Goodspeed JK, Scott JR (1982) Incompatibility group Y member relationships: pIP231 and plasmid prophages P1 and P7. Plasmid 8:307–311

Cesarini G, Muesing MA, Polisky B (1982) Control of ColEI DNA replication: the *rop* gene product negatively affects transcription from the replication primer promoter. Proc Natl Acad Sci USA 79:6313–6317

Chabbert YA, Gerband GR (1974) Surveillance epidemiologique des plasmides responsable de la resistance au chloramphenicol de *Salmonella typhi*. Ann Microbiol (Paris) 125A:153–166
Chabbert YA, Scavizzi MR, Witchitz JL, Gerbaud GR, Bouanchaud DH (1972) Incompatibility groups and classification of *fi* resistance factors. J Bacteriol 112:666–675
Chang S, Cohen SN (1979) High frequency transformation of *Bacillus subtilis* protoplasts by plasmid DNA. Mol Gen Genet 168:111–115
Chaslus-Duncla E, Lafont J-P (1985) IncH plasmids in *Escherichia coli* strains isolated from broiler chicken carcasses. Appl Environ Microbiol 49:1016–1018
Chattoraj DK, Abeles AL, Yarmolinski M (1985) P1 maintenance: a paradigm of precise control. In: Helinski DR, Cohen SN, Clewell DB, Jackson D, Hollaender A (eds) Plasmids in bacteria. Plenum, New York
Chikami GK, Guiney DG, Schmidhauser TJ, Helinski DR (1985) Comparison of 10 IncP plasmids: homology in the regions involved in plasmid replication. J Bacteriol 162:656–660
Chopra I, Bennett PM, Lacey RW (1973) A variety of staphylococcal plasmids present as multiple copies. J Gen Microbiol 79:343–345
Coetzee JN, Datta N, Hedges RW (1972) R factors from *Proteus rettgeri*. J Gen Microbiol 72:543–552
Coetzee JN, Bradley DE, Fleming J, DuToit L, Hughes VM, Hedges RW (1985) Phage pilHα: a phage which absorbs to IncHI and IncHII plasmid-coded pili. J Gen Microbiol 131:1115–1121
Coetzee JN, Bradley DR, Hedges RW, Hughes VM, McConnell MM, DuToit L, Twee-huysen M (1986) Bacteriophages F° *lac h*, SR, SF: phages which absorb pili encoded by plasmids of the S-complex. J Gen Microbiol 132:2907–2917
Crosa JH, Falkow S (1981) Plasmids. In: Gerhart P, Murray RGE, Costilow RN, Nester EW, Wood WA, Kriegard NR, Phillips GB (eds) Manual of methods for general bacteriology. American Society for Microbiology, Washington, pp 266–282
Datta N (1975) Epidemiology and classification of plasmids. In: Schlessinger D (ed) Microbiology – 1974. American Society for Microbiology, Washington DC, pp 9–15
Datta N (1979) Plasmid classification: incompatibility groups. In: Timmis KN, Puhler A (eds) Plasmids of medical environmental and commercial importance. Elsevier, Amsterdam, pp 3–12
Datta N, Hedges RW (1971) Compatibility groups among *fi* R factors. Nature (Lond) 234:111–113
Datta N, Olarte J (1974) R factors in strains of *Salmonella typhi* and *Shigella dysenteriae* isolated during epidemics in Mexico: classification and compatibility. Antimicrob Agents Chemother 5:310–317
Datta N, Richards H, Datta C (1981) *Salmonella typhi* in vivo acquires resistance to both chloramphenicol and co-trimoxazole. Lancet 1:1181–1183
Eichenlaub R, Wehlmann H (1980) Amber-mutants of plasmid mini-F defective in replication. Mol Gen Genet 180:201–204
Eichenlaub R, Figurski D, Helinski DR (1977) Bidrectional replication from a unique origin in a mini-F plasmid. Proc Natl Acad Sci USA 74:1138–1141
Eichenlaub R, Wehlmann H, Ebbers J (1981) Plasmid mini-F encoded functions involved in replication and incompatibility. In: Levy SB, Clowes RC, Koenig EL (eds) Molecular biology, pathogenicity and ecology of bacterial plasmids. Plenum, New York, pp 327–336
Falkow S (1975) Infections multiple drug resistance. Pion, London
Figurski DH, Pohlman RF, Bechhofer DH, Prince AS, Kelton CA (1982) Broad host range plasmid RK2 encodes multiple *kil* genes potentially lethal to *Escherichia coli* host cells. Proc Natl Acad Sci USA 79:1935–1939
Fling ME, Walton L, Elwell LP (1982) Monitoring of plasmid-coded trimethoprim-resistant dihydrofolate reductase genes: detection of a new resistant enzyme. Antimicrob Agents Chemother 22:882–888
Freydman A, Maynell E (1969) Interactions between derepressed F-like R factors and wild type colicin B factors: superinfection, immunity and repressor susceptibility. Genet Res 14:315–332

Gaffney DR, Foster TJ (1978) Chloramphenicol acetyl transferases determined by R plasmids from gram-negative bacteria. J Gen Microbiol 109:351–358

Gellert M, O'Dea MH, Itoh T, Tomizawa J (1976) Novobiocin and coumermycin inhibit DNA supercoiling catalysed by DNA gyrase. Proc Natl Acad Sci USA 73:4474–4478

Grindley NDF, Grindley JN, Anderson ES (1972) R factor compatibility groups. Mol Gen Genet 119:287–297

Grindley NDF, Humphreys GO, Anderson ES (1973) Molecular studies of R factor compatibility groups. J Bacteriol 115:387–398

Grindley NDF, Grindley JN, Kelley WS (1978) Mutant plasmid with altered replication control. In: Schlessinger D (ed) Microbiology 1978. ASM, Washington DC, pp 71–73

Grindsted J, Saunders JR, Ingram LC, Sykes RB, Richmond MH (1972) Properties of an R factor which originated in *Pseudomonas aeruginosa* 1822. J Bacteriol 110:529–537

Gryczan TJ, Contente S, Dubnau D (1978) Characterization of *Staphylococcus aureus* plasmids introduced by transformation into *Bacillus subtilis*. J Bacteriol 134:318–329

Hansen JB, Olsen RH (1978) Isolation of large bacterial plasmids and characterization of the P2 incompatibility group plasmids pMG1 and pMG5. J Bacteriol 135:227–238

Hashimoto-Gotoh T, Inselburg J (1979) ColEI plasmid incompatibility; localization and analysis of mutations affecting incompatibility. J Bacteriol 139:608–619

Hedges RW (1974) R factors from *Providence*. J Gen Microbiol 81:171–181

Hedges RW, Datta N (1971) *fi*$^-$ R factors giving chloramphenicol resistance. Nature New Biol 234:220–221

Hedges RW, Datta N (1972) R124, an fi$^+$ R factor of a new compatibility class. J Gen Microbiol 71:403–405

Hedges RW, Datta N (1973) Plasmids determining I pili constitute a compatibility group. J Gen Microbiol 77:19–25

Hedges RW, Datta N, Coetzee JN, Dennison S (1973) R factors from *Proteus morganii*. J Gen Microbiol 77:249–259

Hedges RW, Rodriguez-Lemoine V, Datta N (1975a) R factors from *Serratia marcescens*. J Gen Microbiol 86:88–92

Hedges RW, Jacob AE, Barth PT, Grinter NJ (1975b) Compatibility properties of P1 and ϕAmp prophages. Mol Gen Genet 141:263–267

Helling RB, Lomax MI (1978) The molecular cloning of genes general procedures. In: Chakrabarty AM (ed) Genetic engineering. CRC, West Palm Beach, pp 1–30

Higgins NP, Peebles LC, Sugino A, Cozzarelli NR (1978) Purification of subunits of *Escherichia coli* DNA gyrase and reconstitution of enzymatic activity. Proc Natl Acad Sci USA 75:1773–1777

Holsters M, Silva B, Van Vlet F, Genetello C, DeBlock M, Dhaese P, Depicher A, Inze D, Engler G, Villarroel R, Van Montagu M, Schell J (1980) The functional organization of the nopaline *A. tumefaciens* plasmid pTiC58. Plasmid 3:212–230

Hu S, Ohtsubo E, Davidson N, Saedler H (1975) Electron microscope heteroduplex studies of sequence relations among bacterial plasmids. XII Identification and mapping of the insertion sequences *IS1* and *IS2* in F and R plasmids. J Bacteriol 122:764–775

Iordanescu S, Surdeanu M (1980) New incompatibility groups for *Staphylococcus aureus* plasmids. Plasmid 4:256–260

Iordanescu S, Surdeanu M, Della Latta P, Novick R (1978) Incompatibility and molecular relationships between small staphylococcal plasmids carrying the same resistance marker. Plasmid 1:468–479

Ippen-Ihler KA, Minkley EG Jr (1986) The conjugation system of F, the fertility factor of *Escherichia coli*. Annu Rev Genet 20:593–624

Ishiguro N, Sato G (1985) Nucleotide sequence of the gene determining plasmid-mediated citrate utilization. J Bacteriol 164:977–982

Ishiguro N, Oka Y, Hanzawa Y, Sato G (1979) Plasmids in *Escherichia coli* controlling citrate utilizing ability. Appl Environ Microbiol 38:956–964

Ishiguro N, Hirose K, Asagi M, Sato G (1981) Incompatibility of citrate utilization plasmids isolated from *Escherichia coli*. J Gen Microbiol 123:193–196

Ishiguro N, Sato G, Sasakawa C, Danbara H, Yoshikawa M (1982) Identification of citrate utilization transposon in Tn*3411* from a naturally occurring citrate utilization plasmid. J Bacteriol 149:961–968

Iyobe S, Hasuda K, Fuse A, Mitsuhaski S (1974) Demonstration of R factors from *Pseudomonas aeruginosa.* Antimicrob Agents Chemother 5:547–552
Jacoby GA (1974) Properties of R plasmids determining gentamicin resistance by acetylation in *Pseudomonas aeruginosa.* Antimicrob Agents Chemother 6:239–252
Jacoby GA (1978) An explanation for the apparent host specificity of *Pseudomonas* plasmid R91 expression. J Bacteriol 136:1159–1184
Jacoby GA (1984) Resistance plasmids of *Pseudomonas aeruginosa.* In: Bryan LE (ed) Antimicrobial drug resistance. Academic, Orlando, pp 497–514
Jobanputra RS, Datta N (1974) Trimethoprim R factors in enterobacteria from clinical specimens. J Med Microbiol 7:169–177
Jobling MG, Ritchie DA (1987) Genetic and physical analysis of plasmid genes expressing inducible resistance to tellurite in *Escherichia coli.* Mol Gen Genet 208:288–293
Johnson EM, Wohlheiter JA, Placek BP, Sleet RB, Baron LS (1976) Plasmid determined ability of *Salmonella tennessee* strain to ferment lactose and sucrose. J Bacteriol 125:385–386
Kamio Y, Tabuchi A, Itoh Y, Katagiri H, Terawaki Y (1984) Complete nucleotide sequence of mini-Rts1 and its copy mutant. J Bacteriol 158:307–312
Kawakami Y, Mikoshiba F, Nagosaki S, Matsumoto H, Tazaki T (1972) Prevalence of *Pseudomonas aeruginosa* strains possessing R factor in a hospital. J Antibiot (Tokyo) 25:607–609
Kline BC (1985) A review of mini-F plasmid maintenance. Plasmid 14:1–16
Kline BC, Lane HED (1980) A proposed system for nomenclature of incompatibility genes of the *Escherichia coli* sex factor plasmid F. Plasmid 4:231–232
Kline BC, Trawick J (1983) Identification and characterization of a second copy number control gene in mini-F plasmids. Mol Gen Genet 192:408–415
Kontomichalou P, Mitani M, Clowes RC (1970) Circular R factor molecules controlling penicillinase synthesis, replicating in *E. coli* under relaxed or stringent control. J Bacteriol 104:34–44
Kumar C, Novick RP (1985) Plasmid pT181 replication is regulated by two countertranscripts. Proc Natl Acad Sci USA 82:638–642
Lacatena RM, Cesareni G (1983) The interaction between RI and the primer precursor in the regulation of ColEI replication. J Mol Biol 170:635–650
Lane D, Gardner RC (1979) Second *Eco*R1 fragment capable of F self-replication. J Bacteriol 139:141–151
Lanka E, Lurz R, Furste JP (1983) Molecular cloning and mapping of *SphiI* restriction fragments of RP4. Plasmid 10:303–307
Levy SB (1984) Resistance to the tetracyclines. In: Bryan LE (ed) Antimicrobial drug resistance. Academic, Orlando, pp 191–240
Light J, Molin S (1982a) The sites of action of the two copy number control functions of plasmid R1. Mol Gen Genet 187:486–496
Loutit JS (1970) Investigation of the mating system of *Pseudomonas aeruginosa* strain 1. VI. Mercury resistance associated with the sex factor (FP). Genet Res 16:179–184
Maher D, Colleran E (1987) The environmental significance of thermosensitive plasmids of the H incompatibility group. In: Wise D (ed) Bioenvironmental systems, vol IV. CRC, Boca Raton, pp 1–35
Manis JJ, Kline BC (1977) Restriction endonuclease mapping and mutagenesis of the F sex factor replication region. Mol Gen Genet 152:175–182
Mendez B, Tachibana C, Levy SB (1980) Heterogeneity of tetracycline resistance determinants. Plasmid 3:99–108
Meynel E, Datta N (1966) The nature and incidence of conjugation factors in *E. coli.* Genet Res 7:134–140
Molin S, Nordstrom K (1980) Control of replication of plasmid R1 functions involved in replication copy number control, incompatibility and switch-off of replication. J Bacteriol 141:111–120
Moore RJ, Krishnapillai V (1982) Tn*7* and Tn*501* insertions into *Pseudomonas aeruginosa* plasmid R91-5: mapping of two transfer regions. J Bacteriol 149:276–283

Murotsu T, Matsubara T, Sugisaki H, Takanami M (1981) Nine unique sequences in a region essential for replication and incompatibility of the mini-F plasmid. Gene 15:257–271
Murotsu T, Tsutsui H, Matsubara K (1984) Identification of the minimal essential region for the replication origin of mini-F plasmid. Mol Gen Genet 196:373–378
Nakaya R, Nakamura A, Murata Y (1960) Resistance transfer agents in *Shigella*. Biochem Biophys Res Commun 3:654–659
Nordstrom K, Molin S, Aagaard-Hansen H (1980) Partitioning of plasmid R1 in *Escherichia coli*. II. Incompatibility properties of the partitioning system. Plasmid 4:332–349
Novick R (1967) Properties of a cryptic high frequency transducing phage in *Staphylococcus aureus*. Virology 33:155–166
Novick R (1976) Plasmid protein relaxation complexes in *Staphylococcus aureus*. J Bacteriol 127:1177–1187
Novick R (1987) Plasmid incompatibility. Microbiol Rev 51:381–395
Novick RP, Adler GK, Projan SK, Carlton S, Highlander S, Gruss A, Khan SA, Iordanescu S (1984) Control of pT181 replication. I. The pT181 copy control function acts by inhibiting the synthesis of a replication protein. EMBO J 3:2399–2405
Ogura T, Hiraga S (1983) Mini-F plasmid genes that couple host cell division to plasmid proliferation. Proc Natl Acad Sci USA 80:4784–4788
Ohtsubo H, Ohtsubo E (1978) Nucleotide sequence of an insertion element IS1. Proc Natl Acad Sci USA 75:615–619
Olsen RH, Shipley P (1973) Host range and properties of the *Pseudomonas aeruginosa* R factor R1822. J Bacteriol 113:772–780
Revel HR, Georgopoulos CP (1969) Restriction of nonglucosylated T-even bacteriophages by prophage P1. Virology 39:1–17
Richards H, Datta N (1979) Reclassification of incompatibility group L (IncL) plasmids. Plasmid 2:293–295
Roussel AF, Chabbert Y (1978) Taxonomy and epidemiology of gram-negative bacterial plasmids studied by DNA-DNA filter hybridization in formamide. J Gen Microbiol 104:269–276
Ruby C, Novick RP (1975) Plasmid interactions in *Staphylococcus aureus*: non-additivity of compatible plasmid DNA pools. Proc Natl Acad Sci USA 72:5031–5035
Sagai H, Kremery V, Hasuda K, Iyobe S, Knothe H, Mitsuhaski S (1975) R factor-mediated resistance to aminoglycoside antibiotics in *Pseudomonas aeruginosa*. Jpn J Microbiol 19:427–432
Sasatsu M, Misra TK, Chu L, Laddager R, Silver S (1985) Cloning and DNA sequence of a plasmid-determined citrate utilization system in *Escherichia coli*. J Bacteriol 164:983–993
Saul D, Lane D (1988) A replication region of the IncHI plasmid, R27, is highly homologous with the Rep FIA replicon of F. Molecular Microbiology 2:219–225
Scavizzi MR (1973) Nouveaux groupes d'incompatibilite des plasmides. Interet dans les epidemies de creche a *E. coli* 0111:B4. Ann Inst Pasteur Microbiol 124B:153–167
Scott JR (1984) Regulation of plasmid replication. Microbiol Rev 48:1–23
Scotland SM, Gross RJ, Cheasty T, Rowe B (1979) The occurrence of plasmids carrying genes for both enterotoxin production and drug resistance in *Escherichia coli* of human origin. J Hyg (Lond) 83:531–538
Shafferman A, Stalker DM, Tolun A, Kolter A, Helinski DR (1981) Structure-function relationships in essential regions for plasmid replication. In: Levy SB, Clowes RC, Konig EC (eds) Molecular biology, pathogenicity and ecology of bacterial plasmids. Plenum, New York, pp 259–270
Smith HR, Grindley NDF, Humphreys GO, Anderson ES (1973) Interaction of group H resistance factors with the F factor. J Bacteriol 115:623–628
Smith HW (1974) Thermosensitive transfer factors in chloramphenicol-resistant strains of *Salmonella typhi*. Lancet 2:281–282
Smith HW, Parsell Z, Green P (1978a) Thermosensitive antibiotic resistance plasmids in enterobacteria. J Gen Microbiol 109:37–47

Smith HW, Parsell A, Green P (1978b) Thermosensitive H1 plasmids determining citrate utilization. J Gen Microbiol 109:305–311
Stalker DM, Kolter R, Helinski DR (1982) Plasmid R6K DNA replication. I. Complete nucleotide sequence of an autonomously replicating segment. J Mol Biol 161:33–43
Summers A, Jacoby GA (1977) Plasmid-determined resistance to tellurium compounds. J Bacteriol 129:276–281
Tamm J, Polisky B (1983) Structural analysis of RNA molecules involved in plasmid copy number control. Nucleic Acid Res 11:6381–6397
Taylor DE (1983) Transfer-defective and tetracycline-sensitive mutants of the incompatibility group HI plasmid R27 generated by insertion of Transposon *7*. Plasmid 9:227–239
Taylor DE, Bradley DE (1987) Location on RP4 of a tellurite-resistance determinant not normally expressed in IncPα plasmids. Antimicrob Agents Chemother 31:823–825
Taylor DE, Brose EC (1985a) Characterization of incompatibility group HI1 plasmids from *Salmonella typhi* by restriction endonuclease digestion and hybridization of DNA probes for Tn*3*, Tn*9* and Tn*10*. Can J Microbiol 31:721–729
Taylor DE, Brose EC (1985b) Restriction endonuclease mapping of R27 (TP117) an incompatibility group HI subgroup 1 plasmid from *Salmonella typhimurium*. Plasmid 13:75–77
Taylor DE, Brose EC (1986) Location of plasmid-mediated citrate utilization in R27 and incidence in other H incompatibility group plasmids. Appl Environ Microbiol 52:1394–1397
Taylor DE, Grant RB (1976) Inhibition of bacteriophage lambda, T*1*, and T*7* development by R plasmids of the H incompatibility group. Antimicrob Agents Chemother 10:762–764
Taylor DE, Grant RB (1977a) Incompatibility and surface exclusion properties of H_1 and H_2 plasmids. J Bacteriol 131:174–178
Taylor DE, Grant RB (1977b) R plasmids of the S incompatibility group belong to the H2 incompatibility group. Antimicrob Agents Chemother 12:431–434
Taylor DE, Grant RB (1977c) Incompatibility and bacteriophage inhibition properties of N-1, a plasmid belonging to the H2 incompatibility group. Mol Gen Genet 153:5–10
Taylor DE, Levine JG (1979) Characterization of a plasmid mutation affecting maintenance, transfer and elimination by novobiocin. Mol Gen Genet 174:127–133
Taylor DE, Levine JG (1980) Studies of temperature-sensitive transfer and maintenance of H incompatibility group plasmids. J Gen Microbiol 116:475–484
Taylor DE, Summers AO (1979) Association of tellurium resistance and bacteriophage inhibition conferred by R plasmids. J Bacteriol 137:1430–1433
Taylor DE, Levine JG, Bradley DE (1981a) In vivo formation of a plasmid cointegrate expressing two incompatibility phenotypes. Plasmid 5:233–244
Taylor DE, Levine JG, Sibay G, Walter A (1981b) Genetic studies of H group plasmids by bacteriophage P1 transduction. Can J Microbiol 27:175–183
Taylor DE, Brose EC, Kwan S, Yan W (1985a) Mapping of transfer regions within incompatibility group HI plasmid R27. J Bacteriol 162:1221–1226
Taylor DE, Chumpitaz JC, Goldstein F (1985b) Variability of IncHI1 plasmids from *Salmonella typhi* with special reference to Peruvian plasmids encoding resistance to trimethoprim and other antibiotics. Antimicrob Agents Chemother 28:452–455
Taylor DE, Hedges RW, Bergquist PL (1985c) Molecular homology and incompatibility relationship between F and IncH1 plasmids. J Gen Microbiol 131:1523–1530
Timmis K, Andres L, Slocombe P (1978) Plasmid incompatibility: cloning of an IncFII determinant of R6-5. Nature 71:4556–4560
Timoney JF, Linton AH (1982) Experimental ecological studies on H2 plasmids in the intestines and faeces of the calf. J Appl Bacteriol 52:417–424
Timoney JF, Taylor DE, Shin DE, McDonough P (1980) pJT2: unusual H1 plasmid in a highly virulent lactose-positive and chloramphenicol-resistant *Salmonella typhimurium* strain from calves. Antimicrob Agents Chemother 18:480–482
Tolun A, Helinski DR (1981) Direct repeats of the plasmid *incC* region express F incompatibility. Cell 24:687–694

Tomizawa T, Som T (1984) Control of ColEI plasmid replication: enhancement of binding of RNAI and the primer transcript is reversible. Cell 40:527–535
Tomizawa T, Itoh T, Selzer G, Som T (1981) Inhibition of ColEI RNA primer formation by a plasmid-specified small RNA. Proc Natl Acad Sci USA 78:1421–1425
Tsutsui H, Fujiyama A, Murotsu T, Matsubara K (1983) Role of nine repeating sequences of the mini-F-genes for expression of F-specific incompatibility phenotype and copy number control. J Bacteriol 155:334–337
Watanabe T, Takano T, Arai T, Nishida H, Sato S (1966) Episome mediated transfer of drug resistance in *Enteribacteriaceae*. X Restriction and modification of phages of *fi*$^-$ R factors. J Bacteriol 92:477–486
Weisblum B, Graham MY, Gryczan T, Dubnau D (1979) Plasmid copy number control: isolation and characterization of high-copy-number mutants of plasmid pE194. J Bacteriol 137:635–643
Whiteley M, Taylor DE (1983) Identification of DNA homologies among H incompatibility group plasmids by restriction enzyme digestion and southern transfer hybridization. Antimicrob Agents Chemother 24:194–200
Willetts N, Wilkins B (1984) Processing of plasmid DNA during bacterial conjugation. Microbiol Rev 48:24–41
Witchitz JL, Chabbert YA (1971) Resistance transferable a la gentamicin. I. Expression du charactere de resistance. Ann Inst Pasteur 121:733–742
Wolfson JS, Hooper CD, Swartz MN, McHugh GL (1982) Antagonism of the B subunit of DNA gyrase eliminates plasmids pBR322 and pMG110 from *Escherichia coli*. J Bacteriol 152:338–344
Yakobson E, Guiney G (1983) Homology in the transfer origins of broad host range *IncP* plasmids: definition of two subgroups of P plasmids. Mol Gen Genet 192:436–438
Yan W, Taylor DE (1987) Characterization of transfer regions within the HII incompatibility group plasmid pHH1508a. J Bacteriol 169:2866–2868

CHAPTER 15

Clinical Laboratory Testing for Antimicrobial Resistance

F. D. SCHOENKNECHT

A. Introduction

After almost 50 years of clinical use of antibiotics and chemotherapeutic agents, many aspects of antibiotic susceptibility testing (AST) in the clinical laboratory are still actively discussed, under development, or undergoing rapid change. Browsing in the more than 1000 pages of *Antibiotics in Laboratory Medicine* in its second edition (LORIAN 1986), one feels overwhelmed by the magnitude and complexity of the clinical laboratory aspects of antibiotics and chemotherapeutic agents.

In this brief review, then, I will discuss only a few of the more important topics with which hospitals or clinical laboratories involved in AST are concerned. Going back to reviews of similar scope (SCHOENKNECHT and SHERRIS 1973, 1980), it is surprising that most of the topics discussed are still relevant and some of them will be covered again. Few entirely new issues have emerged. But shifts in emphasis and changes in the magnitude of some problems require a new consideration. Subjects that will not be covered include the following:

1. Testing of Antifungal Drugs. While there are three workable procedures described in a section of the latest edition of the American Society of Microbiology's (ASM) *Manual of Clinical Microbiology* (SHADOMI et al. 1985), the present state of affairs is still not satisfactory, partly due to lack of standardization (GALGIANI and STEVENS 1978; STILLER et al. 1983; GALGIANI 1984) and partly due to problems unique to fungi such as dimorphism and prolonged growth times. A subcommittee on antifungal susceptibility testing of the National Committee for Clinical Laboratory Standards (NCCLS) has been formed and has been operating since the end of 1985 (NCCLS 1985b).

2. Testing of Drugs Against Acid Fast Bacteria. Testing for these organisms is a procedure for larger reference, state and public health laboratories. The methods described in the latest edition of the ASM manual for clinical microbiology are widely in use and appear to work satisfactorily (SOMMERS and GOOD 1985; BAILEY et al. 1984). A semi-automated radiometric technique has also been in use for several years (SIDDIQI et al. 1981; SNIDER et al. 1981), and seems to be now the method of choice.

3. Serum Bactericidal Tests. There are differing opinions about the value of these tests. Lack of standardization again is a problem, although a document from the NCCLS is available now: *Methodology for the Serum Bactericidal Test* (NCCLS

1987a). Interested readers may also refer to the work and review by Reller and associates (Reller 1986; Stratton 1986).

4. Combination of Antibiotics. An excellent review and description of methods are available (Krogstad and Moellering 1986). In general these procedures are done as two dimensional or checkerboard tests and results are expressed involving fractional inhibitory concentrations (FIC) or fractional bactericidal concentrations (FBC). Editorial policy of the ASM journal *Antimicrobial Agents and Chemotherapy* encourages the use of this approach (Anonymous 1987).

5. Tolerance in Clinical Isolates. Several recent reviews by different workers have covered this topic from several points of view (Schoenknecht 1986; Tuomanen et al. 1986; Sherris 1986). Laboratory artifacts accounting for some reports of tolerance have been pointed out by Taylor et al. 1984, and many others.

B. Standardization of Test Procedures

I. Early Efforts

To a large extent, the value of AST as a reliable procedure to guide therapy, compare results over time and in different places, evaluate new drugs, monitor emergence of resistance and follow trends in nosocomial infections, depends on the use of methods that are expected or proved to have clinical relevance and which are reproducible. Recommendations for standardization of the principles to be followed towards these goals were spelled out already in 1961 in the Second Report of the Expert Committee on Antibiotics (WHO 1961). Ten years later the results of the investigations, conclusions and recommendations of an international collaborative study (ICS) were published (Ericsson and Sherris 1971). The minimal inhibitory concentration (MIC) determined by agar or broth dilution technics was proposed as the basic reference point. Mueller-Hinton (MH) medium, although not considered ideal, was selected as an interim reference medium because of generally good performance and reproducibility. This ICS group addressed many details for standardization of agar and broth dilution methods and of a disk diffusion technic, including inoculum strength or density, end point definition, a reference medium, the need for reference strains, and interpretative breakpoints. It also insisted on defining the limitations of the procedure. Reference laboratories were proposed that should have the responsibility of updating the procedures, monitoring standard strains for performance evaluation and developing quality control guidelines.

More than 15 years later this is a good point in time to review how well these goals have been reached, what remains to be done, and what problems, if any, have emerged. The first steps in the United States were the publication of a proposal by the FDA (Federal Register 1971) of a slightly modified Kirby-Bauer procedure (Ryan et al. 1970) and the establishment of a national antibiotic reference laboratory at the Centers for Disease Control (CDC). The actual drafting, publication and periodic updating of standard procedures fell to the National Committee for Clinical Laboratory Standards (NCCLS) through its newly founded subcommittee on susceptibility testing. These NCCLS standards have more and more become the means for achieving most of the goals outlined by the ICS.

II. Reports, Guidelines, and Standards by the National Committee for Clinical Laboratory Standards

I would like to briefly discuss the way these documents are developed and list the relevant individual standards currently available. The NCCLS is a nonprofit organization representing professional, industry and government interests and was incorporated in 1968. Microbiology is the subject of one of eight area committees dealing with various aspects of the clinical laboratory. The NCCLS publishes reports, guidelines and standards. A standard is "a document developed through the consensus process clearly identifying specific, essential requirements for materials, methods, or practices for voluntary use in an unmodified form. A standard may, in addition, contain discretionary elements. These discretionary elements are clearly identified."

A guideline "is a document developed through the consensus process describing criteria for a general operating practice, procedure, or material for the clinical laboratory community. A guideline can be used as written or modified by the user to fit specific needs." A "report is an NCCLS document that has not been subjected to consensus review and is released by the Board of Directors." Guidelines and standards pass through stages of "proposed" and "tentative" to the final "approved" document. The most widely used standard on AST concerned disk diffusion testing, and appeared in its third edition (NCCLS 1984).

Another important standard deals with dilution techniques (NCCLS 1985 d). It now recommends three interpretive categories: susceptible, moderately susceptible, and resistant. It also includes methods for testing clinically important fastidious organisms and provisions for more cost-effective quality control testing. In addition, the standard recommends testing at least five concentrations of a drug if MICs are reported out. If fewer than five concentrations are used, results should be reported as MIC categories.

Two documents, both in 1985, address the testing of anaerobic bacteria. One – the approved standard – describes the reference agar dilution procedure (NCCLS 1985 a), the other – a proposed guideline – details alternate methods, namely, limited agar dilution, broth microdilution, and broth disk dilution procedures suitable for routine use in the clinical laboratory (NCCLS 1985 c). The standard specifically encourages users to develop their own procedures and use them for routine testing after satisfactory studies comparing them with the reference agar dilution technique, which admittedly is too cumbersome and time consuming for routine testing in clinical laboratories.

In addition, NCCLS has begun to issue informational supplements, the first of which updates all the tables for the three approved standards mentioned above (NCCLS 1986 a). Its nine tables cover newly suggested groupings of drugs, MIC interpretive standards and quality control ranges, technical aspects like solvents and diluents for preparation of stock solutions and a scheme for preparing dilutions of antimicrobial agents, as well as acceptable MIC ranges for control strains.

Several additional proposed guidelines appeared in 1987 two of them dealing with bactericidal tests. One was titled Methodology for the Serum Bactericidal Test (NCCLS 1987 a), the other one covered methods for determining bactericidal activity of antimicrobial agents in artificial media (NCCLS 1987 b). Another guideline presents recommended data needed for the selection of appropriate interpretive standards and quality control guidelines for new antimicrobial agents (NCCLS 1987 c).

III. Culture Media for Antimicrobic Susceptibility Tests

For the past 20 years or so MH medium without much of a challenge continued to be the main culture medium used in the United States for all tests except for anaerobes and some fastidious bacteria. For anaerobes a special medium has been developed (WILKINS and CHALGREN 1976; SUTTER 1984), which is the culture base for the agar dilution reference technique. A broth version of this medium is also available in addition to alternates such as Schaedler, Brucella, or brain-heart infusion broth (NCCLS 1985 a, c; SUTTER et al. 1979). For fastidious aerobic and facultative bacteria various supplementations to MH broth or agar are necessary and recommended, including horse blood, sheep blood, hemoglobin, and factors V and X. For gonococci, however, GC agar base (Difco) with supplements should be used (NCCLS 1986 d).

Yet MH media are not without some problems. Medium dependent variability of test results with respect to sulfonamides, trimethoprim, aminoglycosides, tetracyclines and methicillin was, and to some extent still is, the most serious one. Peptones contain sulfonamide inhibitors (HARPER and CAWSTON 1945). Varying amounts of thymidine in different media affect the consistency of results with trimethoprim (BUSHBY and HITCHINGS 1968). Divalent cations, particularly calcium and magnesium, interfere with the uptake of gentamicin by *Pseudomonas aeruginosa*. The essential absence of these elements from unsupplemented MH broth lowers the MICs for these drugs with this species to the point of giving false results of susceptibility (TRAUB 1970). The varying amounts of these cations in different lots of MH agar can lead to considerable variations, for instance, in the interpretation of gentamicin susceptibility of *Pseudomonas aeruginosa* (GARROD and WATERWORTH 1969; D'AMATO et al. 1975; POLLOCK et al. 1978; KENNY et al. 1980). In addition, divalent cations will chelate with tetracyclines and reduce their activity (BRENNER and SHERRIS 1972). Finally, there is the well established beneficial influence of increased NaCl content on the expression of methicillin resistance by *Staph. aureus* (BARBER 1964; CHABBERT 1970).

Many studies and experiments have been directed to rectifying these problems. Interestingly enough, hardly any serious attempts at replacing MH media were made. Recently a proprietary broth formulation for fastidious bacteria was evaluated (BARRY et al. 1986) for microdilution ASTs. This clear medium, a modification of Schaedler broth, worked well when compared with the reference supplemented MH broth technique, as long as standard 100 mcl or 200 mcl test systems were used. Panels containing only 40 mcl in each well were less satisfactory.

A special NCCLS subcommittee tried to improve manufacturing and quality control of MH media for several years and finally, after extensive studies, selected one of the seven production lots submitted by seven major manufacturers. They called it the physical reagent standard (POLLOCK et al. 1986). This "golden pound" met best the current NCCLS midpoint standard and had the lowest variability. It served as reference for manufacturers to experimentally produce new production lots with as close a performance to the reference standard as possible. The difficulties encountered during these efforts can be best illustrated by the widely varying results of trimethoprim-sulfamethoxazole testing with the two quality control strains of *Streptococcus faecalis*: two of the seven lots gave no zone at all and two gave relatively small zones, presumably because of excessive thymine or thymidine content. Even after the new lots were produced, attempting to emulate the performance characteristics of the golden pound, four manufacturer's media had not reduced the number of drug-organism combinations with a greater than 1 mm difference between the mean zone diameters (POLLOCK et al. 1986).

Nevertheless, as a result of these NCCLS sponsored efforts, a proposed standard has been issued that outlines procedures for evaluating production lots of MH agar (NCCLS 1986 b). Quality control strains will continue to be an excellent and necessary means of monitoring the performance of media and for the detection of lot-to-lot or manufacturer-to-manufacturer variations. There are now well characterized strains of *Pseudomonas aeruginosa*, *Staph. aureus*, *Streptococcus faecalis*, *E. coli*, and *Bacteroides fragilis*, covering all organism-drug combinations for all AST procedures. Their reproducibility has been checked and found satisfactory for this purpose (COYLE et al. 1976). The details of their use and maintenance may be found in the respective NCCLS standards and the chapters dealing with various AST procedures in the current ASM Manual of Clinical Microbiology (WASHINGTON 1985; JONES et al. 1985; BARRY and THORNSBERRY 1985). To determine whether the MH agar has sufficiently low levels of thymine and thymidine, a *Streptococcus faecalis* (ATCC 29212) may be tested with trimethoprim-sulfamethoxazole disks (NCCLS 1984). Excessive amounts of these inhibiting compounds will result in smaller and less distinct zones. This may be remedied by the addition of lysed horse blood or thymidine phosphorylase. The best approach, though, is to secure media with low thymidine content from the manufacturer.

IV. Present State of Standardized AST

There is little doubt that procedural standardization has paid off and the performance of AST in the U.S. improved. Two reviews based on data from the College of American Pathologists (CAP) microbiology surveys covering the period from 1972 to 1983 make this point convincingly (JONES 1983; JONES and EDSON 1985). The surveys showed a trend toward use of the NCCLS standardized test methods, and documented greater compliance with the critical technical steps of the methods, for instance, the selecting of 3–5 colonies, standardization of the inoculum to 0.5 MacFarland turbidity standard, use of cotton swabs and MH agar, maintenance of 4 mm agar depths and verification of the pH of the agar. As a result, laboratory performance in proficiency tests has improved to an impressive 98% acceptable performance rate for dilution method results and 95.2% for disk diffusion results (JONES 1983).

V. Remaining Problems

However, other surveys focusing on problem drug-organism combinations such as methicillin resistance in *Staph. aureus* report less favorable results (PFALLER et al. 1987). Using questionnaires the authors surveyed the AST practices of 162 microbiology laboratories in the Veterans Administration system. Methicillin resistant *Staph. aureus* (MRSA) detection varied considerably but more importantly, fewer than 60% of the laboratories followed test guidelines as set by the NCCLS standards for key methodological variables. The authors do not have an answer for the lack of compliance but conclude that failure to adhere to established guidelines may lead to suboptimal detection of MRSA.

In spite of the considerable expense of time and efforts by manufacturers and the NCCLS subcommittee on behalf of media standardization, variability is still a problem and the procedures for verifying acceptable media in the individual clinical laboratory are cumbersome and time consuming. In addition to pH checking and tests for thymidine levels, checking the results of aminoglycoside tests with every new batch of MH medium is necessary. Cation supplementation has apparently not solved media related problems with *Pseudomonas aeruginosa* and netilmicin (BARRY et al. 1987b). The interpretive criteria in the NCCLS standards do not fit all organism-drug combinations equally well. JONES and EDSON (1985) list nine such problems involving mainly β-lactam drugs and a number of different species. The absence of any standards for testing of mycobacteria and fungi is another serious deficiency that hopefully will be corrected soon.

C. Relevance of Testing and Clinical Laboratory Correlation

Reproducibility and accuracy of laboratory tests intended to guide therapy was a prerequisite to determining clinical relevance. Standardization and appropriate quality control measures were the obvious answers to the former concern but questions of clinical relevance are much more difficult to solve. For one, the term "clinical relevance" may mean different things to different people: with respect to AST it might include rapid results versus those obtained by overnight incubation, quantitative versus qualitative results, properly interpreted reporting of results, or clinically useful and frequently updated panels of drugs to be tested. Of greatest concern, however, to most users, and to be discussed first, is the correlation between laboratory and clinical results, i.e., whether the results of in vitro tests really allow guidance of therapy and correlate well with the in vivo response to antibiotics.

Published opinions to this issue have been somewhat conflicting over the years, although most authorities do not any more seriously doubt the value and clinical usefulness of carefully conducted in vitro AST (MCCABE and TREADWELL

1986; MOELLERING 1985). Several reviews have appeared over the last 10 years (SANDERS WE JR and SANDERS CC 1982; MCCABE and TREADWELL 1986; WASHINGTON 1983) and most of the conclusions are still applicable: Therapy with drugs for which in vitro tests show resistance generally leads to treatment failure. This has been shown particularly well for bacteremias, enteric infections, relapsing urinary tract infections, tuberculosis and gonorrhoea. Success following antibiotic treatment with drugs showing in vitro susceptibility is most easily demonstrated in patients with less severe infections or without serious underlying diseases. There is no disagreement concerning the value of AST guiding therapy of subacute bacterial endocarditis. There is also agreement on the need for bactericidal drugs in the treatment of this condition, as well as for some other conditions such as sepsis due to *Pseudomonas aeruginosa*. Correlations are less convincing for anaerobic infections, probably because of their loculated and polymicrobial nature. Surgical drainage continues to be very important. Caution is also advised with laboratory tests guiding combination therapy.

Although somewhat interrelated, factors influencing laboratory-clinical correlation can be grouped into three major categories: (1) the nature and design of the test system, (2) host factors, and (3) problems with certain drugs and microorganisms.

I. Influence of the Nature and Design of the Test System

Antibiotic-susceptibility testing should be sufficiently reproducible; it has to satisfy the growth requirements of the test organisms and give readable results preferably within 24 h. Test conditions should not interfere with the activity of the drug and they should, if possible, approximate the condition under which the antimicrobic acts on the microorganism in vivo. Broth dilution tests appear to come closest to these requirements and are still considered the reference method against which other tests are measured. And yet even superficial reflection will show how remote a broth dilution AST is from the very complex situation of the in vivo interaction between antibiotic and bacteria.

There are practical limitations to simulation of the in vivo situation, and we will not consider here artificial culture media and protein binding. However, already the arbitrary choice of 18–24 h incubation appears to have been dictated more by the schedules of laboratories and technicians than based on the exigencies of microorganism-drug interactions. In fact, overnight incubation may not be the best standard and model, particularly when most therapeutic regimens of administration involve 6, 8, or 12 h intervals. Early read results, that is after less than 12 h of incubation, including some automated tests, could conceivably show better correlation.

A related problem is the action of subinhibitory concentrations on the microorganism. Victor Lorian has shown the various morphological changes occurring with low concentration of antibiotics in vivo and in vitro (LORIAN 1986). What is their clinical significance? Slower growth rates may shift the balance towards effecting the host's defenses. This leads to one of the most important differences between the laboratory AST and the in vivo situation, namely the choice of criteria for determining whether the microorganism is susceptible or resistant, the patient cured as a result of therapy or not. For broth dilution tests, our standard, absence of visual turbidity as determined with the naked eye, has been arbitrarily chosen as end point yielding MIC. But this does not mean absence of growth, since up to 10^5 or 10^6 bacteria/ml may be present without observable turbidity. In the patient, on the other hand, cultures negative for the offending pathogen in the blood, urine, etc., are often the indicators for successful therapy. In vitro determination of the MBC by subculturing onto antibiotic-free media tubes or wells without visible growth may give a more precise definition of "no growth" but this is applicable only with bactericidal drugs. For most clinical situations the inhibitory end point is quite sufficient as a guideline because inhibitory and bactericidal concentrations rarely differ much. There is also no doubt that many serious or life-threatening clinical infections are cured easily by therapy with bacteriostatic drugs, and – sadly – that in some situations even high doses of bactericidal drugs do not cure an infection due to an organism that is quite susceptible in vitro to the drugs used, i.e., neutropenic cancer patients. The host defenses obviously play an enormous role and one then could arrive at another definition of clinically relevant antibiotic susceptibility: infecting microorganisms are clinically susceptible to an antimicrobic when they are reduced in numbers or diminished in viability by the drug to a proportion and level manageable by the host's defenses.

In vitro AST has other limits: There are discrepancies between the doubling times of microorganisms in vivo and in vitro. For instance, the generation time of pneumococci in rabbit CSF in vivo is approximately 70 min. Logarithmic phase pneumococci in broth take only 20 min to double (DOROSHOW et al. 1981). The stage of disease has been shown to play a role in the effectiveness of penicillin when treating pneumococcal meningitis in dogs (PLORDE et al. 1965).

The relationship of the MIC to attainable levels of serum, urine, etc. on ordinary dosage schedules is widely accepted as an important criterion for defining resistance and susceptibility. However, whether peak, trough, or mean values are best for this purpose, and for which drugs, is often not clear to the user of AST results. One also should keep in mind that many infections involve tissue rather than blood and serum and ideally the relationship of MICs to attainable tissue levels should be used, a figure less easily obtained in the laboratory than blood levels.

Bactericidal test, especially in broth media, are plagued by technical problems and artifacts (TAYLOR et al. 1983), as well as by confusing events such as skipped tube and paradoxical phenomena (EAGLE and MUSSELMAN 1948; KIRBY 1945). They have given rise to a considerable literature on so-called tolerance, some of it laboratory artefact or of little clinical importance. Last not least the twofold dilution schedule of standard broth tests accounts for a considerable margin of error that may be a problem with AST of aminoglycosides and other drugs with only little difference between toxic and therapeutic concentrations.

Another issue of clinical relevance frequently discussed is the speed of result generation, or the turnaround time. The often voiced complaint and statement that clinical microbiology laboratories take usually a minimum of 48 h to isolate a pathogen and report species and antibiogram is simply not true. Many laboratories throughout the country routinely report the presence of *Staph. aureus*, Enterobacteriaceae and *Pseudomonas aeruginosa* and their susceptibility to antibiotics in 24 h or less from receipt of the blood sample, for instance. Both automated and traditional techniques, e.g., the disk diffusion test, allow for early reading and preliminary reports with good correlation to the final report (COYLE et al. 1984; SCHOENKNECHT et al. 1980). Comparability between early read and overnight MICs can be achieved, for instance, by inoculum manipulation (LAMPE et al. 1975). Automated systems also adjust the amount of antibiotic to which the test organism is exposed in order to facilitate earlier reading of results (THORNSBERRY 1985).

An issue to be discussed in this context is the choice of clinically useful panels of antibiotics to be routinely tested in a given hospital and how timely, especially in automated systems, they can be updated to keep pace with the rapid development and release of clinically applicable and desirable drugs. The disk diffusion test has proven in the author's laboratory to be the most flexible and rapidly adaptable system and will continue to be part of the laboratory's AST offering. Standards issued by the NCCLS, including the informational supplements (NCCLS 1986a), have in this author's opinion successfully addressed the difficult questions of which drugs to test for which organism and specimen and how to keep the large number of possible drugs to be tested to a reasonable level.

II. Influence of Host Factors

In an excellent series of papers over 20 years ago, WEINSTEIN and DALTON (1968) reviewed the host determinants of response to antimicrobial agents. Specifically they discussed age, pregnancy, genetic background, renal and hepatic function, electrolyte balance, nervous system abnormalities, metabolic disorders, indigenous microbial flora, allergy and immunodefense mechanisms. All of these are important factors. Additional problems have emerged: prosthetic devices, indwelling catheters and lines, monitoring devices, parenteral hyperalimentation, peritoneal and hemodialysis, as well as life-style related host factors such as drug abuse and/or the acquired immunodeficiency syndrome. Quite a few reviews have addressed one or the other of these newly recognized host changes (SCHIMPF 1980; PENNINGTON 1978; GRIECO 1980) and the latest edition of a current infectious disease text has an entire section with nine chapters on infections in special hosts (MANDELL et al. 1985). A detailed discussion of the various ways in which these factors affect the results of antibiotic and chemotherapy is impossible within the confines of this chapter, but a few examples may be helpful.

Advances in public health measures and medicine have not only extended the life expectancy of the population, but allowed many premature infants to survive. Complicated and invasive medical and surgical procedures are done routinely now on the very young and old. The sometimes unavoidable infectious complications pose particular challenges to the physician. Inherited disease with metabolic abnormalities may frustrate antibiotic therapy by specific interference with drug activity: large amounts of DNA from broken down white blood cells in bronchial secretions and pus of patients with mucoviscidosis and possibly also cystic fibrosis may inactivate aminoglycosides due to irreversible binding (BRYANT and HAMMOND 1974).

A very special group of abnormal hosts are patients iatrogenically rendered immunocompromised as an unavoidable by-product of modern therapeutic regimens, such as cancer chemotherapy, organ transplants or corticosteroid therapy of collagen vascular disease and some other entities. Ever since modern platelet transfusion techniques have dramatically reduced bleeding as a complication, infections have become the major limiting factor of medical treatment of solid and nonsolid neoplastic disease and other previously fatal conditions.

Much has been learned in the last ten years about such infectious complications, many of which are due to well known bacterial pathogens (GRIECO 1980; MANDELL et al. 1985). The frequent involvement of enteric gram negative rods, environmental gram negative rods, for instance *Pseudomonas aeruginosa*, *Serratia marcescens*, staphylococci and enterococci, makes empirical antibiotic therapy essential. The ability to predict which infections are most likely to accompany which type of immunodeficiency or compromised host status has also facilitated and encouraged empirical therapy. Thus, an increasing number of febrile neutropenic patients get antibiotic therapy without laboratory demonstration of the infecting agent throughout the course. To maximize the success of such treatment, antibiotic combinations are frequently used, although more recently with the advent of newer and third generation β-lactam compounds, monotherapy is again being evaluated (HATHORN et al. 1987).

Antibiotic susceptibility testing as a guide to antimicrobial therapy of infections in immunocompromised hosts poses some unique questions of relevance. Many leukemic patients during their induction period or during the aplastic phase of bone marrow transplants experience neutropenic episodes of 3 weeks and maybe longer with white cell counts in the range of 100 WBC per cmm or less. The resulting acute and life-threatening infections require immediate and thus empirical therapy. The results of AST in a given institution may be most beneficial if tabulated at 6 months intervals and made available to the medical staff in the form of collective antibiograms and frequency distributions of resistance and susceptibility of the hospital's major bacterial pathogens with respect to the antimicrobial agents in use. AST for individual patients often serves to confirm the validity of the empirical therapy already started or occasionally to change and improve drug therapy. There will be more need for determination of bactericidal end points, and, in general, an emphasis on quantitative data in the form of MICs or MBCs expressed in micrograms per milliliter. There has also been an increase in the requests for tests for synergistic combinations. Such data, plus therapeutic drug monitoring and serum bactericidal titers are considered valuable guides in a very difficult therapeutic situation.

Even more than for normal hosts the rule applies: Resistance to the drug in vitro predicts therapeutic failure, susceptibility demonstrated in vitro does not guarantee success in vivo. Understanding the nature of the underlying immune defect and the resulting risks for infection with certain s ecific microorganisms combined with the awareness of nosocomial infection patterns in the institution and antibiotic susceptibility distributions represent the best way to treat.

III. Influence of Reporting Methods

From these considerations it should be appreciated that the results of AST must be used and interpreted with the limitations and problems of the test conditions in mind, with knowledge of the clinical pharmacology of the drugs and based on clinical experience with infections in the human host. The laboratory can assist by doing more than just dispensing qualitative susceptibility data in the form of resistant, susceptible or intermediate categories or quantitative MIC values. A few comments will be made concerning possibilities and ways of improving the clinical relevance of AST reports.

The standardized disk diffusion test continues to be a major technique of AST in North America. Its flexibility, relative ease of performance, and nonincremental results appeal to many laboratories here and elsewhere. Accuracy and reproducibility are comparable to other approved AST procedures (Jones and Edson 1985). However, there is a current trend toward dilution tests. Diffusion tests are standardized for and work best with rapid growing bacteria like Enterobacteriaceae, *Pseudomonas* species and staphylococci. Dilution tests are less handicapped by slower growing and fastidious organisms including some of the increasingly encountered opportunistic pathogens. Results of diffusion tests are qualitative and actually include an interpretation, an advantage to many users and a limiting aspect to others. Breakpoints are based on comparison with standardized reference dilution tests, the consideration of attainable serum or urine levels with regular dosage schedules and, importantly, on the distributions among species known to contain clinically susceptible and resistant strains. Dilution tests with their quantitative results in micrograms per milliliter are in principle more satisfying and may be perceived by some users as more "scientific." However, this very point has also been one of their drawbacks. Physicians have to do their own interpretations and consult tables of blood and/or urine levels attainable with the drugs under consideration. In doing so they are often frustrated by the complexities involved: clinical pharmacology of the drug, peak or trough levels, protein binding, post-antibiotic effect, etc. Workers at the NIH Clinical Center have discussed these difficulties and tried various approaches to assist physicians. Nevertheless, "exasperation with MIC data has occasionally reached such levels that some physicians have ignored susceptibility reports and have treated patients on the basis of their assessment of a given pathogen's most probable antimicrobial agent susceptibility" (Witebsky et al. 1979). To remedy this situation, they adopted an economical microtitration based broth dilution system using only a few critical concentrations for each antibiotic and accompanying the MIC values in their report with one or two of seven interpretative categories in abbreviated form.

Eight years later the NIH group essentially is still using their system of AST and reporting of results. A published report on their experience is planned (Gill et al. 1989). Other institutions have similar policies. That is, they include qualitative categories, even when using dilution procedures and reporting out MICs in micrograms per milliliter (Jones 1982). The most recent NCCLS standard for dilution AST includes a table listing three MIC interpretive categories: susceptible, resistant, and moderately susceptible. This latter category indicates susceptibility

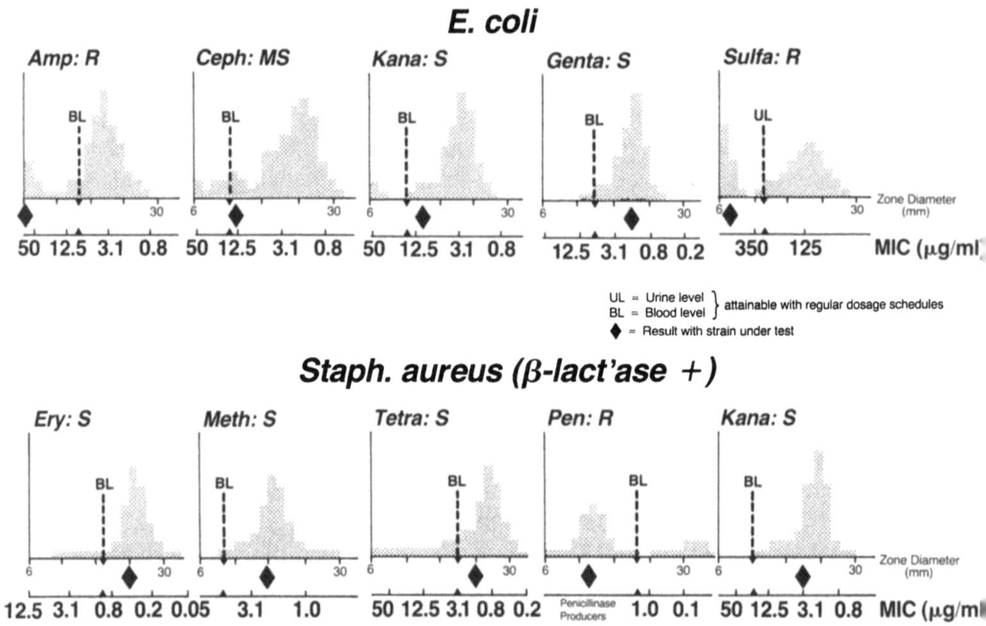

Fig. 1. Possible graphic presentation of a hospital's computer generated susceptibility histograms of *S. aureus* and *E. coli* plus attainable blood or urine levels on regular dosage schedules. The patient's test strain is superimposed as a symbol and the interpretive code entered as letters following each antimicrobic tested. (Adapted from SHERRIS 1977)

under certain conditions, namely inhibition only by blood levels achieved with maximum dosages indicated in the drug package insert literature. Some strains may also be treatable if the infection occurs in the urinary tract, where antimicrobial concentrations attained in the urine considerably exceed those obtained in blood, that is, lower urinary tract infections (NCCLS 1985 d).

One method of data presentation would attempt to communicate to the clinician as much as is feasible of the background information on which interpretation is based, together with the results on the individual patient's isolate, all in the form of a combination chart report (SHERRIS 1974, 1977). The report would present in graphical form the frequency distribution of the susceptibilities of strains within the particular species isolated and tested in the hospital over the last year or so, and their MIC's or MIC equivalents, interpretive breakpoints or the attainable blood or urine levels and superimposed or entered into such a preprinted form, the behavior or values of the clinical isolate in question, plus interpretive category, and possibly information about β-lactamase production (Fig. 1).

IV. Problems with Certain Organisms and Antibiotics

Standardized ASTs are quite satisfactory for most of the common bacterial clinical isolates and most correlation problems have either to do with the natural limitations of the test or with host factors. There are, nevertheless, a few organism-antibiotic combinations with particular problems that clinicians and laboratories need to be aware of. Most of these have been dealt with in previous publications and are outlined in the current versions of the NCCLS documents (SCHOENKNECHT and SHERRIS 1973, 1980; JONES 1983; NCCLS 1984, 1985d, 1986a).

1. Methicillin Resistant *Staphyloccocus aureus* (MRSA)

They are also called heteroresistant or intrinsically resistant. A small proportion of the population is resistant to the penicillinase resistant penicillins (PRPs), while the majority behaves like susceptible strains. After many years of studies the phenomenon of heteroresistant *S. aureus* has recently been elucidated (HARTMAN and TOMASZ 1981, 1986; ROSSI et al. 1985; UBUKATA et al. 1985; UTSUI and YOKOTA 1985). It appears that an altered target (PBP 2a or 2′) with extra low affinity for PRPs is the most important factor and that for many strains of MSRA this low affinity PBP is inducible by methicillin and other β-lactams. Certain in vitro features of the organism influence their detection: a slower growth rate requires longer incubation time, at least 24 h; larger colonies are formed at 30 ° rather than at 37 °C and in salt enriched media (2%–4%). The amount of this PBP produced is lower at pH 5.2 than at pH 7.0. It is also obvious that a dense inoculum such as recommended in the NCCLS standards and preferably prepared from overnight cultures (BAKER et al. 1983) can enhance chances to detect the smaller resistant proportion with their slower growth rate.

Workers at CDC have carefully outlined the in vitro aspects of reliable detection of these organisms (THORNSBERRY et al. 1983; MCDOUGAL and THORNSBERRY 1984; BAKER et al. 1983). The phenomenon of MRSA is further complicated by the recent discovery of the role of high level β-lactamase production in certain strains of *Staph. aureus* with marginal methicillin resistance. In other words, contrary to previous understanding, β-lactamase production *does* play a role in the methicillin resistance of some strains of *Staph. aureus* (MCDOUGAL and THORNSBERRY 1986). The following clues should alert the laboratory to the possibility of methicillin resistance in *Staph. aureus* (THORNSBERRY 1984):

1. Multiresistance and β-lactamase production.
2. Intermediate MIC values with PRPs turning to resistance upon prolonged incubation.
3. Cephalothin MIC's between 1 and 16 μg/ml.
4. Failure to show cross-resistance between PRPs.

2. Coagulase Negative Staphylococci (CNS)

Much of what has been outlined for MRSA should be applied to CNS as well, although less experimental work has been done with these. The number of clinical isolates of CNS showing methicillin resistance is much larger, reaching 60%–70% of the strains isolated and studied in larger institutions (SCHWALBE et al. 1987) *S. epidermidis* and *S. hemolyticus* appear to be the species most prone to methicillin and multiple resistance. Most authorities also agree that just as for MRSA, in vitro susceptibility to cephalosporins cannot be trusted. For clinical purposes they should be considered not treatable with these agents. However, there are conflicting reports on this subject and some workers claim an exception for cefamandole (MENZIES et al. 1987; RIGHTER 1987; FRONGILLO et al. 1986). Over- and underreporting of methicillin resistant staphylococci appears to be a problem (PEACOCK 1986; FLEMING et al. 1986). The use of vancomycin has dramatically increased and while *Staph. aureus* is still reliably treated with this drug, CNS have recently made headlines with the emergence of vancomycin resistance (SCHWALBE et al. 1987). Other species of CNS appear to be much more benign in their susceptibility patterns but even *Staph. saprophyticus*, generally considered very susceptible to most antimicrobics currently used, has been shown to produce a β-lactamase (LATHAM et al. 1984), which may be of clinical significance (LEE et al. 1987).

3. Antibiotic Resistant Pneumococci

For many years antibiotic susceptibility testing of pneumococci if carried out at all was done solely for the purpose of providing suggestions for alternate therapy, mainly tetracycline and erythromycin, in patients with penicillin allergy. Lessened susceptibility to penicillin (MIC 0.1–1.0 µg/ml) was first reported from Australia and New Guinea 20 years ago (HANSMAN and BULLEN 1967). The spread of pneumococci resistant to penicillin and many other antibiotics is well documented in a recent review (APPELBAUM 1987), including the emergence in South Africa of pneumococci with high level penicillin resistance (MIC of 2–8 µg/ml), causing serious, even fatal systemic infections. The mechanism of resistance, with the exception of chloramphenicol, does not involve antibiotic inactivating enzymes. Rather, a step-wise process mediated by at least four different genetic units is at work, which with regard to penicillin, results in different PBPs (ZIGHELBOIM and TOMASZ 1981), alteration of autolysin activity and tolerance (LIU and TOMASZ 1985; HANDWERGER and TOMASZ 1986).

Laboratory separation of susceptible from moderately resistant and resistant pneumococci by diffusion tests is better accomplished using one microgram oxacillin disks than penicillin disks (JACOBS et al. 1980; NCCLS 1986a). MIC testing is recommended to distinguish between resistant and partially resistant organisms. However, falsely susceptible MIC values have been encountered using a microtitration technique (SHANHOLTZER and PETERSON 1986).

4. Antibiotic Resistant Enterococci

Two problems require the special attention of the laboratory and clinician. One involves the reversal of the in vitro susceptibility of *Streptococcus faecalis* to trimethoprim-sulfamethoxazole (TMP-SMX) by folinic acid and the resulting false reports of susceptibility, since folinic acid is present in urine and serum in sufficient amounts to raise MICs and is absent in Mueller-Hinton broth (ZERVOS and SCHABERG 1985). Increases in the isolation of enterococci with high level aminoglycoside resistance is another matter of concern. Since its first description, this form of resistance has spread among clinical isolates of enterococci and now also involves aminoglycosides other than kanamycin and streptomycin (MEDERSKI-SAMORAJ and MURRAY 1983). This type of resistance affects only combined beta-lactam aminoglycoside therapy and is not detected by ordinary ASTs. It is best screened for on Mueller-Hinton agar plates containing appropriate amounts of the aminoglycoside (500 μg/ml or more).

5. Enteric Gram-Negative Rods with Chromosomally Mediated β-Lactamase

This mechanism for resistance was first described for cefamandole in *Enterobacter* species (FINDELL and SHERRIS 1976) and later on reported for other gram negative rods and other β-lactam antibiotics (GOOTZ et al. 1984; LAMPE et al. 1982; SEEBERG et al. 1983; SANDERS and SANDERS 1986, 1987). The enzymes involved are normally repressed chromosomally mediated Group 1 β-lactamases active against cephalosporins and, to a lesser degree, against penicillins. This type of resistance occurs either spontaneously when stably de-repressed hyperproducers of β-lactamase mutate from the wild strain at a frequency of 10^{-6} to 10^{-7} or as a result of an enzyme induction by certain β-lactam drugs, of which cefoxitin and imipenem are the most effective.

The clinical importance of this type of resistance has increased since the introduction of more β-lactam drugs. Multiply resistant mutants of various species of enterobacteriacae and *Pseudomonas aeruginosa* are blamed for therapy failures and severe outbreaks of nosocomial infections (SANDERS and SANDERS 1987). The situation is complicated by reports of unreliable detection of this type of resistance, particularly with AST techniques using lower inocula and/or shorter incubation times (SANDERS 1984; STONE and JUNGKIND 1983).

6. Non-β-lactamase Producing (NBLP) *Haemophilus influenza* and *Neisseria gonorrhoeae* Strains Resistant to β-lactams

Plasmid mediated β-lactamase production as the resistance mechanism in *Haemophilus influenza* and *Neisseria gonorrhoea* was recognized about ten years ago. The technical details of β-lactamase detection are fully described in the ASM Manual of Clinical Microbiology (LENNETTE et al. 1985). Non β-lactamase mediated resistance did not receive quite that attention, although in the case of gonococci, it preceded the acquisition of the TEM 1 β-lactamase by many years and was described not long after the discovery of enzyme inactivation of ampicillin by *H. influenza* (THORNSBERRY and KIRVEN 1974; PARR and BRYAN 1984; MARKOWITZ 1980). This form of resistance in contrast to the one mediated by β-lactamase production is of a low level type so far. From a laboratory point of view it raises two important issues. One, and a very obvious one, is the insufficiency of mere β-lactamase testing and the implications for the feasibility of rapid tests, non-culture methods, DNA probes, etc. Traditional standardized AST of these non β-lactamse producing strains avoids the problem. Concerned about the apparent rarity of such isolates of *H. influenza* in their pediatric patients, SMITH and colleagues (MENDELMAN et al. 1986) studied ampicillin resistant NBLP strains of *H. influenza* using an inoculum of 10^5 and 10^3 organisms with a 2 μg and the standard 10 μg ampicillin disk. The 2 μg ampicillin disk appeared to identify ampicillin resistant NBLP strains more reliably. It is to be hoped that the standard 10 μg disk, meticulous adherence to all details of NCCLS procedures, and maybe some breakpoint adjustment will result in reliable detection using the standard technique. Two disk methods in general are not desirable. Whether similar problems exist for gonococci is not quite clear. Penicillin resistant NBLP *N. gonorrhoea* have PBPs with reduced affinity for penicillin (DOUGHERTY et al. 1980). Such strains are also likely to be resistant to other antibiotics. Another laboratory problem is the occasional increased susceptibility to vancomycin with some strains, since it will make them nondetectable with the commonly employed vancomycin containing screening media (BRORSON et al. 1973). Laboratories should be well aware of these and related problems since chromosomally mediated resistant *N. gonorrhoea* are increasing in North America and elsewhere (CENTERS FOR DISEASE CONTROL 1984).

D. DNA Probes for AST

> "It is our earnest hope that clinical laboratories may begin to routinely attempt genetic cross and agar gel electrophoresis."
> (ELWELL and FALKOW 1986)

How realistic is this expectation? Have DNA probes and related molecular biology techniques found their way into clinical laboratories for the purpose of detecting resistance to antibiotics? Table 1 lists reports about the use of DNA probes toward this end, as published in the last three years or so in major journals covering infectious disease, antimicrobial agents and chemotherapy and clinical microbiology. Most of these studies employed probes for epidemiological purposes: screening for drug resistance in hospitals, monitoring classes of β-lactamases in nosocomial isolates or the study of resistance mechanisms.

Only one study – involving the detection of African and Asian strains of penicillinase producing *Neisseria gonorrhoea* (PPNG) – can be called a clinical diagnostic attempt. And even so, it is more of a field study, since the clinical material was batched and sent to a central reference laboratory (PERINE et al. 1985).

In order to better understand the potential value and the limitations of DNA hybridization applied to AST, it is useful to briefly discuss traditional ways of generating such information in the clinical laboratory and the convention of interpretation and use of the results by the clinician. Practically all tests require growth of the organism in pure culture in the presence of the antibiotic under question and then measuring the degree of inhibition. Results are being expressed either quantitatively as MICs in micrograms per milliliter and/or as interpretive categories. For disk diffusion tests, results are given in the form of interpretive categories only: *Sensitive*. Implies that the organism is readily inhibited by the concentrations of antibiotic attainable in the blood. *Moderately Susceptible*. This category includes strains that may be inhibited by attainable concentrations of certain antimicrobial agents, e.g., β-lactams, using higher dosages or in body sites where the drugs are physiologically concentrated. *Intermediate*. This category provides a buffer zone which should prevent small uncontrolled technical factors from causing major discrepancies in interpretation. Results in that category may have to be followed up with dilution tests. *Resistant*. Such strains are not inhibited

Table 1. Use of DNA probes for the determination of antimicrobial resistance in clinical isolates

bes for the ection of	Antimicrobials and microorganisms involved	Purpose	Labeling system	Reference
)-adenyl ransferase	Aminoglycosides Enteric gram negative rods	Hospital epidemiology	^{32}P	GOOTZ et al. (1985)
-MDa cryptic nd 4.4 MDa -lactamase lasmid	Penicillinase producing *N. gonorrhoeae*	Clinical epidemiological field study	^{32}P	PERINE et al. (1985)
M-1 -lactamase	β-lactams Enteric gram-negative rods	Epidemiology of β-lactamases in nosocomial infections	^{32}P	COOKSEY et al. (1985)
loramphenicol cetyl ransferase	Chloramphenicol *Haemophilus parainfluenzae* *Haemophilus ducreyi*	Study of resistance mechanism	^{3}H	ROBERTS et al. (1980)
inoglycoside nodifying nzymes	Aminoglycosides *S. aureus*	Study and survey of nosocomial isolates	^{32}P	DICKGIESSER and KREISWIRTH (1986)
M-1 and EM-2 -lactamases	β-Lactams Gram negative rods (*E. coli, P. aeruginosa, Proteus* spp., *H. influenzae, Aeromonas* and *Achromobacter* spp.)	Study of urinary tract infections	Biotin-11-dUTP	CARTER et al. (1987)

by drug concentrations achieved in blood or tissue with normal dosages (NCCLS 1984, 1985 d). As one can see, this information takes into consideration attainable blood and urine levels, concentration of the drug by the kidneys, technical factors, and the toxicity of the drug.

Many laboratories have followed a trend toward determining and reporting MICs but still accompany the quantitative results by interpretive categories since uninterpreted MIC data have not always been well received or used by clinicians (WITEBSKY et al. 1979). Depending on the method used and the laboratory setting – hospital, clinic, or commercial laboratory – such tests can be completed once a pure culture is available, in 5–18 h for rapid growers and may cost between $ 5 and $ 20 per antibiogram of 10–12 antibiotics. This methodology has been very successful in day-to-day diagnostic work, for epidemiological investigations and many research applications. It lends itself equally well for doing volume work and for single tests at odd times, stat work, etc. The methodology is standardized nationwide and quality control by federal and state agencies and professional organizations is well established.

DNA hybridization in contrast does not necessarily require growth of the organism nor is pure culture an absolute requirement. Typically the organisms to be tested, e.g., colony, microorganism in body fluids, urethral pus, etc. is lysed to release the DNA which in turn is applied or spotted onto nitrocellulose paper.

Reacting this target DNA with labeled DNA or RNA (the probe) the presence of complementary DNA in the specimen can be detected. This so-called spot or dot blot technique is quite simple and relatively quick. More involved in time and effort but more specific is the Southern blot technique (SOUTHERN 1975), which allows the detection of specific DNA fragments and sequences. This requires the use of specific restriction endonucleases in order to cut the test organisms' DNA. The resulting fragments are electrophoretically separated by size on agar gel and then transferred to nitrocellulose paper (Southern transfer) for the hybridization with the probe or probes.

Commercially prepared diagnostic probes for the identification of microorganisms are beginning to be available (e.g., adenovirus II, CMV, EB virus, hepatitis B, HSV, chlamydia, mycoplasma). Detection is either by autoradiography using radiolabeled probes (mostly ^{32}P) or more recently by non-isotopic labeling techniques (LANGER et al. 1981). These latter techniques hold great promise since they eliminate the problems of instability, disposal and licensing requirements associated with radioactive labels. They are constantly being improved and specificity and sensitivity appear to be quite satisfactory for clinical laboratory purposes. Research laboratories may continue to resort to isotope labels, which can be more readily manipulated, for instance, by extending the autoradiography time for increased sensitivity.

A recent evaluation of DNA probes for the detection of PPNG strains in urethral exudates of men with urethritis comes closest to a clinical diagnostic application of this technique and may serve as an illustration of the details involved, inherent limitations and advantages of its use (PERINE et al. 1985). Two probes were actually used: one employing the gonococcal cryptic plasmid to specifically detect *Neisseria gonorrhoea* in the uretheral exudate, the other utilizing the 4.4 megadalton β-lactamase plasmid to determine penicillin resistance by β-lactamase production. Three points are worth making at this stage. First, once a nonculture method is chosen for identification of a pathogen, a nonculture technique is required for the detection of resistance to antibiotics. Having to follow up with cultures just for the purpose of AST diminishes some of the advantages of identification by noncultural DNA probe techniques.

Second, the probe is very specific and resistance by mechanisms other than β-lactamase production will not be detected. Even some other β-lactamases, and there are quite a few, will not be detected. In other words, one needs to choose a very specific enzyme like the gonococcal TEM β-lactamase that is responsible for most resistance in this species. Lastly, β-lactamases do occur in other microorganisms, for instance, *Hemophilus* species. Their possible coexistence with PPNG in female cervical and/or urethral exudates makes this technology much more suitable for the study of male urethral discharge.

The exudate was collected with a cotton swab or wire loop and transferred to a 1 cm spot on nitrocellulose paper. After air drying, the strip was mailed to the reference laboratory for analysis. This approach, pioneered by MOSELEY et al. (1980) in a study of enterotoxigenic *E. coli* and diarrhea in Bangladesh, is ideally suited for field work in third world countries where culture based laboratory work is not feasible. The results, of course, are not immediately available under these conditions, but are still useful for determining therapeutic policies in this outpatient setting. They were comparable to those obtained with conventional techniques. Preparation of the radioactive probe, including the isolation of the plasmids and the nick translation technique for labeling the DNA with ^{32}P and finally hybridization by Southern transfer are probably still the domain of larger and reference laboratories. Commercially available probes will hopefully eliminate or simplify this part of the effort.

A very recent study demonstrates the successful use of a non-isotopic spot hybridization technique for the detection of the most common plasmid mediated β-lactamases (TEM 1 and TEM 2) in gram negative bacteria (CARTER et al. 1987). The authors labeled a plasmid fragment representing part of the TEM 1 β-lactamase gene with a commercial biotin preparation. Hybridization was analyzed using a commercially available streptavidine detection system. As expected, the probe proved to be very specific and using an inoculum of $3–4 \times 10^6$ cells gave optimum positive discrimination. Seventy-two percent of ampicillin resistant *E. coli* strains gave a positive hybridization reaction. This figure is in agreement with the assessment by other means of TEM β-lactamases in urinary tract isolates of *E. coli*. Spot hybridization has been shown to be a reliable and quick method suitable for volume work in clinical laboratories (GOOTZ et al. 1985).

In summary then, regarding DNA probes there are still some reservations:

- DNA probe techniques for AST are still in the beginning stages.
- They have been mainly used to analyze mechanisms of resistance and for epidemiological and/or surveillance work in hospitals and field studies.
- So far, DNA probes are practical only for the detection of resistance factors with identifiable structural genes, for instance, plasmid mediated resistance to aminoglycosides or β-lactamase production.
- The many different β-lactamases in Enterobacteriaceae alone require concentration on one or two of the clinically most important ones, e.g., TEM 1 and TEM 2.
- The presence of similar resistance mechanisms in many normal flora species limits DNA probes to cultures or clinical specimens from normally sterile sites such as the urethra.
- Another source of false resistant results is due to the failure of some species to phenotypically express their resistance. All the probe is detecting is the presence of a gene specifying resistance, usually by coding for an inactivating enzyme.

However, on the positive side: in a few carefully selected clinical situations, DNA probes can be used with confidence.

- Single plasmid screens and agar gel electrophoretic methods (HOLMES and QUIGLEY 1981; MEYERS et al. 1976; BIRNBOIM and DOLY 1979) could be performed in many clinical laboratories, and the outlays for gel phoresis equipment, UV light sources, polaroid cameras, etc. are modest.
- Commercial probes and detection kits are available.
- New non-isotypic techniques are beginning to be utilized.
- Technical details are adequately outlined in laboratory manuals and chapters (TOMPKINS 1985; ELWELL and FALKOW 1986; MANIATIS et al. 1983).

E. Conclusions

In vitro susceptibility testing has come a long way and is now well standardized for most antibiotics and clinically important regular bacterial isolates. The available reference procedures should make it much easier to study automated equipment, innovative procedures, and new drugs, and to establish the degree of clinical-laboratory correlation and the predictive value of the tests.

Physicians and laboratory workers need to be aware of factors that negatively influence good clinical laboratory correlation, such as problems with certain organism-antibiotic combinations, the limitations of the test conditions, and host factors.

Careful attention by the laboratory to the report format of results and the means of interpretation to physicians are essential. This may include periodic distribution to the hospital staff of institutional susceptibility patterns of the most commonly encountered microorganisms, lists of MIC breakpoints applicable to the treatment of systemic infections with ordinary dosage schedules and the blood and urine levels of the more commonly used antibiotics attainable with such regimens. Otherwise utilization of the test results by physicians will continue to be suboptimal.

In vitro tests cannot replace adequate knowledge of clinical pharmacology of the drugs, of basic principles of medical microbiology and infectious disease, and of the role of host factors.

Future developments, including DNA probe technology, will require even better understanding of these factors and their influence on the value and meaning of antibiotic susceptibility test.

For all these reasons, clinical correlation of AST is best when resistance is detected. Although there is good correlation with the results of antimicrobial therapy when susceptibility is reported, success cannot be guaranteed based on a report of susceptibility alone with the same degree of confidence as failure is assured for therapy with a drug for which in vitro tests show resistance. In fact, rather than call it AST, it probably would have been better to call the procedure antibiotic resistance test.

Acknowledgement. I wish to thank Drs. John C. Sherris, Steve Lory and Fred Tenover for helpful suggestions and critique.

References

Anonymous (1987) Instructions of authors. Antimicrob Agents Chemother 31:i–xi
Appelbaum PC (1987) World-wide development of antibiotic resistance in pneumococci. Eur J Clin Microbiol 6:367–377
Bailey WC, Bass JB, Hawkins JE, Kubica GP, Wallace RS (1984) Drug susceptibility testing for mycobacteria. Am Thorac Soc News 10:9–10
Baker CN, Thornsberry C, Hawkinson RW (1983) Inoculum standardization in antimicrobial susceptibility testing: evaluation of overnight agar cultures and the rapid inoculum standardization system. J Clin Microbiol 17:450–457
Barber M (1964) Naturally occurring methicillin-resistant staphylococci. J Gen Microbiol 35:pp 183–190

Barry AL, Thornsberry C (1985) Susceptibility tests: diffusion test procedures. In: Lennette EH, Balows A, Hausler WJ Jr, Shadomy HJ (eds) Manual of clinical microbiology, 4th edn. American Society for Microbiology, Washington DC, p 978
Barry AL, Cotton JL, Jones RN, Packer RR (1986) Evaluation of a proprietary broth medium for microdilution susceptibility testing of nutritionally fastidious bacteria. J Clin Microbiol 24:701–704
Barry AL, Gavan TL, Ayers LW, Fuchs PC, Gerlach EH, Thornsberry C (1987a) Quality control limits for microdilution susceptibility tests with norfloxacin. J Clin Microbiol 25:165–166
Barry AL, Miller GH, Thornsberry C, Hare RS, Jones RN, Lorber RR, Ferraresi R, Cramer C (1987b) Influence of cation supplements on activity of netilmicin against *Pseudomonas aeruginosa* in vitro and in vivo. Antimicrob Agents Chemother 31:1514–1518
Bell SM, Plowman O (1980) Mechanisms of ampicillin resistance in *Haemophilus influenzae* from respiratory tract. Lancet i:279–280
Bennett PM, Heritage J, Hawkey PM (1986) An ultra-rapid method for the study of antibiotic resistance plasmids. J Antimicrob Chemother 18:421–424
Birnboim HC, Doly J (1979) A rapid alkaline extraction procedure for screening recombinant plasmid DNA. Nucleic Acid Res 7:1513–1523
Boissinot M, Mercier J, Levesque RC (1987) Development of natural and synthetic DNA probes for OXA-2 and TEM-1 beta-lactamases. Antimicrob Agents Chemother 31:728–734
Brenner VC, Sherris JC (1972) Influence of different media and bloods on the results of diffusion antibiotic susceptibility tests. Antimicrob Agents Chemother 1:116–122
Brorson JE, Holmberg I, Nygren B, Seeberg S (1973) Vancomycin-sensitive strains of *Neisseria gonorrhoeae*. A problem for the diagnostic laboratory. Br J Venereal Dis 49:452–453
Bryant RE, Hammond D (1974) Interaction of purulent material with antibiotics used to treat *Pseudomonas* infections. Antimicrob Agents Chemother 6:702–707
Bushby SRM, Hitchings GH (1968) Trimethoprim a sulphonamide potentiator. Br J Pharmacol 33:72
Carter GI, Towner KJ, Slack RCB (1987) Detection of TEM beta-lactamase genes by non-isotopic spot hybridisation. Eur J Clin Microbiol 6:406–409
Centers for Disease Control (1984) Chromosomally mediated resistant *Neisseria gonorrhoeae* – United States. MMWR 33:408–410
Chabbert YA (1970) Detection of methicillin and cephalothin-resistant staphylococci. In: Watt PJ (ed) The control of chemotherapy, E and S. Livingstone, Edinburgh, p 17
Cooksey RC, Clark NC, Thornsberry C (1985) A gene probe for TEM type beta-lactamases. Antimicrob Agents Chemother 28:154–156
Coyle MB, Lampe MF, Aitken CL, Feigl P, Sherris JC (1976) Reproducibility of control strains for antibiotic susceptibility testing. Antimicrob Agents Chemother 10:436–440
Coyle MB, McGonagle LA, Plorde JJ, Clausen CR, Schoenknecht FD (1984) Rapid antimicrobial susceptibility testing of isolates from blood cultures by direct inoculation and early reading of disk diffusion test. J Clin Microbiol 20:473–477
D'Amato RF, Thornsberry C, Baker CN, Kirven LA (1975) Effect of calcium and magnesium ions on the susceptibility of *Pseudomonas* species to tetracycline, gentamicin, polymyxin B, and carbenicillin. Antimicrob Agents Chemother 7:596–600
Dickgiesser N, Kreiswirth BN (1986) Determination of aminoglycoside resistance in *Staphylococcus aureus* by DNA hybridization. Antimicrob Agents Chemother 29:930–932
Doroshow CA, Drake TA, Sande MA (1981) Dynamics of bacterial killing in experimental pneumococcal meningitis by moxalactam (abstr). 21st ICAAC, Chicago
Dougherty TJ, Koller AE, Tomasz A (1980) Penicillin-binding proteins of penicillin-susceptible and intrinsically resistant *Neisseria gonorrhoeae*. Antimicrob Agents Chemother 18:730–737
Eagle H, Musselman AD (1948) The rate of bactericidal action of penicillin in vitro as a function of its concentration, and its paradoxically reduced activity at high concentrations against certain organisms. Am J Exp Med 88:99–131

Easmon CSF (1985) Gonococcal resistance to antibiotics. J Antimicrob Chemother 16:409–412
Elwell LP, Falkow S (1986) The characterization of R plasmids and the detection of plasmid-specified genes. In: Lorian V (ed) Antibiotics in laboratory medicine (2nd ed). Williams and Wilkins, Baltimore, p 683
Ericsson HM, Sherris JC (1971) Antibiotic sensitivity testing. Report of an international collaborative study. Acta Pathol Microbiol Scand [B] [Suppl] 217:1–90
Ernst JD, Sander MA (1984) In vitro susceptibility testing and the outcome of treatment of infection. In: Root RK, Sande MA (eds) New dimensions in infectious diseases. Churchill Livingstone, New York, p 293
Federal Register (1971) Proposed rule making. Antibiotic susceptibility discs. Department of Health, Education and Welfare, Washington DC, vol 36, p 6899
Findell CM, Sherris JC (1976) Susceptibility of *Enterobacter* to cefamandole: evidence for a high mutation rate to resistance. Antimicrob Agents Chemother 9:970–974
Fleming DW, Helgerson SD, Mallery BL, Foster LR, White MC (1986) Methicillin-resistant *Staphylococcus aureus*: how reliable is laboratory reporting? Infection Control 7:164–167
Frongillo RF, Donati L, Federico G, et al. (1986) Clinical comparative study of the activity of cefamandole in the treatment of serious staphylococcal infections caused by methicillin-susceptible and methicillin-resistant strains. Antimicrob Agents Chemother 29:789–796
Galgiani JN (1984) Why not standardize antifungal susceptibility testing. Antimicrob Newslett 1:40
Galgiani JN, Stevens DA (1978) Turbidimetric studies of growth inhibition of yeasts with three drugs: inquiry into inoculum-dependent susceptibility testing, time of onset of drug effect, and implications for current and newer methods. Antimicrob Agents Chemother 13:249–254
Garrod LP, Waterworth PM (1969) Effect of medium composition on the apparent sensitivity of *Pseudomonas aeruginosa* to gentamicin. J Clin Path 22:534
Gill VJ, Witebsky FG, MacLouwry JD (1989) Multi-category interpretive reporting of susceptibility testing with selected antimicrobial concentrations: ten years of laboratory and clinical experience. Clin Lab Med 9 (2, June 1989)
Gootz TD, Jackson DB, Sherris JC (1984) Development of resistance to cephalosporins in clinical strains of *Citrobacter* spp. Antimicrob Agents Chemother 25:591–595
Gootz TD, Tenover FC, Young SA, Gordon KP, Plorde JJ (1985) Comparison of three DNA hybridization methods for detection of the aminoglycoside 2″-O-adenylyltransferase gene in clinical bacterial isolates. Antimicrob Agents Chemother 28:69–73
Grieco MH (ed) (1980) Infections in the abnormal host. Yorke Medical Books
Handwerger S, Tomasz A (1986) Alterations in penicillin-binding proteins of clinical and laboratory isolates of pathogenic *Streptococcus pneumoniae* with low levels of penicillin resistance. J Infect Dis 153:83–89
Hansman D, Bullen MM (1967) A resistant pneumococcus. Lancet II:264–265
Harper GJ, Cawston WC (1945) The in vitro determination of the sulphonamide sensitivity of bacteria. J Path Bacteriol 57:59
Hartman BJ, Tomasz A (1981) Altered penicillin binding proteins in methicillin-resistant strains of *Staphylococcus aureus*. Antimicrob Agents Chemother 19:726–735
Hartman BJ, Tomasz A (1986) Expression of methicillin resistance in heterogeneous strains of *Staphylococcus aureus*. Antimicrob Agents Chemother 29:85–92
Hathorn JW, Rubin M, Pizzo PA (1987) Empirical antibiotic therapy in the febrile neutropenic cancer patient: clinical efficacy and impact of monotherapy. Antimicrob Agents Chemother 31:971–977
Holmes DS, Quigley M (1981) A rapid boiling method for the preparation of bacterial plasmids. Anal Biochem 114:193–197
Jacobs MR, Gaspar MN, Robins-Browne RM, Koornhof HJ (1980) Antimicrobic susceptibility testing of pneumococci. 2. Determination of optimal disc diffusion test for detection of penicillin G resistance. J Antimicrob Chemother 6:53–64

Jones RN (1982) The antimicrobial susceptibility test: rapid and overnight, agar and broth, automated and conventional, interpretation and trend analysis. In: Lorian V (ed) Significance of medical microbiology in the care of patients. Williams and Wilkins, Baltimore, p 341
Jones RN (1983) Antimicrobial susceptibility testing (AST): A review of changing trends, quality control guidelines, test accuracy, and recommendation for the testing of β-lactam drugs. Diagn Microbiol Infect Dis 1:1–24
Jones RN, Edson DC (1985) Antibiotic susceptibility testing accuracy. Arch Pathol Lab Med 109:595–601
Jones RN, Barry AL, Gavan TL, Washington JA II (1985) Susceptibility tests: microdilution and macrodilution broth procedures. In: Lennette EH, Balows A, Hausler WJ Jr, Shadomy HJ (eds) Manual of clinical microbiology, 4th ed. American Society for Microbiology, Washington DC, p 972
Joshi JH, Schimpff SC (1985) Infections in the compromised host. In: Mandell GL, Douglas RG Jr, Bennett JE (eds) Principles and practice of infectious diseases, 2nd edn. Wiley, New York, p 1644
Jouvenot M, Deschaseaux ML, Royez M, Mougin C, Cooksey RC, Michel-Briand Y, Adessi GL (1987) Molecular hybridization versus isoelectric focusing to determine TEM-type beta-lactamases in gram-negative bacteria. Antimicrob Agents Chemother 31:300–305
Kenny MA, Pollock HM, Minshew BH, Casillas E, Schoenknecht FD (1980) Cation components of Mueller-Hinton agar affecting testing of *Pseudomonas aeruginosa* susceptibility to gentamicin. Antimicrob Agents Chemother 17:55–62
Kim KS (1987) Effect of antimicrobial therapy for experimental infections due to Group B streptococcus on mortality and clearance of bacteria. J Infect Dis 155:1233–1241
Kirby WMM (1945) Bacteriostatic and bacteriolytic actions of penicillin on sensitive and resistant staphylococci. J Clin Invest 24:165–169
Krogstad DJ, Moellering RC (1986) Antimicrobial combinations. In: Lorian V (ed) Significance of medical microbiology in the care of patients, 2nd edn. Williams and Wilkins, Baltimore, p 537
Lampe MF, Aitken CL, Dennis PG, Forsythe PS, Patrick KE, Schoenknecht FD, Sherris JC (1975) Relationship of early readings of minimal inhibitory concentrations to the results of overnight tests. Antimicrob Agents Chemother 8:429–433
Lampe MF, Allan BJ, Minshew BH, Sherris JC (1982) Mutational enzymatic resistance of *Enterobacter* species to beta-lactam antibiotics. Antimicrob Agents Chemother 21:655–660
Langer PR, Waldrop AA, Ward DC (1981) Enzymatic synthesis of biotin-labeled polynucleotides: novel nucleic acid affinity probes. Proc Natl Acad Sci USA 78:6633–6637
Latham RH, Zeleznik D, Minshew BH, Schoenknecht FD, Stamm WE (1984) *Staphylococcus saprophyticus* β-lactamase production and disk diffusion susceptibility testing for three β-lactam antimicrobial agents. Antimicrob Agents Chemother 26:670–672
Lee W, Carpenter RJ, Phillips LE, Faro S (1987) Pyelonephritis and sepsis due to *Staphylococcus saprophyticus*. J Infect Dis 155:1079–1080
Lennette EH, Balows A, Hausler WJ Jr, Shadomy HJ (1985) Manual of clinical microbiology, 4th edn. American Society for Microbiology, Washington DC
Liu HH, Tomasz A (1985) Penicillin tolerance in multiply drug-resistant natural isolates of *Streptococcus pneumoniae*. J Infect Dis 152:365–372
Lorian V (1982) The antibacterial range: an approach to the assessment of in vitro activity of antibiotics. In: Lorian V (ed) Significance of medical microbiology in the care of patients. Williams and Wilkins, Baltimore, p 370
Lorian V (1986) Effect of low antibiotic concentrations on bacteria: effects on ultrastructure, their virulence, and susceptibility to immunodefenses. In: Lorian V (ed) Antibiotics in laboratory medicine, 2nd edn. Williams and Wilkins, Baltimore, p 596
Mandell GL, Douglas RG Jr, Bennett JE eds (1985) Principles and practice of infectious diseases, 2nd edn. Wiley, New York
Maniatis T, Fritsch EF, Sambrook J (1983) Molecular cloning: a laboratory manual. Cold Spring Harbor Laboratory, New York

Markowitz SM (1980) Isolation of an ampicillin-resistant, non-β-lactamase-producing strain of *Haemophilus influenzae*. Antimicrob Agents Chemother 17:80–83

Mayer KH, Hopkins JD, Gilleece ES, Chao L, O'Brien TF (1986) Molecular evolution, species distribution, and clinical consequences of an endemic aminoglycoside resistance plasmid. Antimicrob Agents Chemother 29:628–633

McCabe WR, Treadwell TL (1986) In vitro susceptibility tests: correlations between sensitivity testing and clinical outcome in infected patients. In: Lorian V (ed) Antibiotics in laboratory medicine, 2nd edn. Williams and Wilkins, Baltimore, p 925

McDougal LK, Thornsberry C (1984) New recommendations for disk diffusion antimicrobial susceptibility tests for methicillin-resistant (heteroresistant) staphylococci. J Clin Microbiol 19:482–488

McDougal LK, Thornsberry C (1986) The role of β-lactamase in staphylococcal resistance to penicillinase-resistant penicillins and cephalosporins. J Clin Microbiol 23:832–839

Mederski-Samoraj BD, Murray BE (1983) High-level resistance to gentamicin in clinical isolates of enterococci. J Infect Dis 147:751–757

Mendelman PM, Chaffin DO, Clausen C, et al. (1986) Failure to detect ampicillin-resistant, Non-β-lactamase-producing *Haemophilus influenzae* by standard disk susceptibility testing. Antimicrob Agents Chemother 30:274–280

Menzies RE, Cornere BM, MacCulloch D (1987) Cephalosporin susceptibility of methicillin-resistant, coagulase-negative staphylococci. Antimicrob Agents Chemother 31:42–45

Meyers JA, Sanchez D, Elwell LP, Falkow S (1976) Simple agarose gel electrophoretic method for the identification and characterization of plasmid deoxyribonucleic acid. J Bacteriol 127:1529–1537

Mickelsen PA, Plorde JJ, Gordon KP, Hargiss C, McClure J, Schoenknecht FD, Condie F, Tenover FC, Tompkins LS (1985) Instability of antibiotic resistance in a strain of *Staphylococcus epidermis* isolated from an outbreak of prosthetic valve endocarditis. J Infect Dis 152:50–58

Moellering RC Jr (1985) Anti-infective therapy. In: Mandell GL, Douglas RG Jr, Bennett JE (eds) Principles and practice of infectious diseases, 2nd edn. Wiley, New York, p 153

Moseley SL, Huq I, Alim ARMA, So M, Samadpour-Motalebi M, Falkow S (1980) Detection of enterotoxigenic *Escherichia coli* by DNA colony hybridization. J Infect Dis 142:892–898

National Committee for Clinical Laboratory Standards (1984) Performance standards for antimicrobial disk susceptibility tests. vol 4/16, 3rd edn. NCCLS, Villanova

National Committee for Clinical Laboratory Standards (1985a) Reference agar dilution procedure for antimicrobial susceptibility testing of anaerobic bacteria, vol 5/2. NCCLS, Villanova

National Committee for Clinical Laboratory Standards (1985b) Antifungal susceptibility testing; Committee Report, vol 5/17. NCCLS, Villanova

National Committee for Clinical Laboratory Standards (1985c) Alternative methods for antimicrobial susceptibility testing of anaerobic bacteria, vol 5/18. NCCLS, Villanova

National Committee for Clinical Laboratory Standards (1985d) Methods for dilution antimicrobial susceptibility tests for bacteria that grow aerobically, vol 5/22. NCCLS, Villanova

National Committee for Clinical Laboratory Standards (1986a) Performance standards for antimicrobial susceptibility testing, vol 6/21. NCCLS, Villanova

National Committee for Clinical Laboratory Studies (1986b) Evaluating production lots of dehydrated Mueller-Hinton agar, vol 6/22. NCCLS, Villanova

National Committee for Clinical Laboratory Standards (1987a) Methodology for the serum bactericidal test, vol 7/1. NCCLS, Villanova

National Committee for Clinical Laboratory Standards (1987b) Methods for determining bactericidal activity of antimicrobial agents, vol 7/2. NCCLS, Villanova

National Committee for Clinical Laboratory Standards (1987c) Development of in vitro susceptibility testing criteria and quality control parameters, vol 7/4. NCCLS, Villanova

National Committee for Clinical Laboratory Standards (1987 d) Quality assurance for commercially prepared microbiological culture media; tentative standard. NCCLS, Villanova

Obbink DJG, Ritchie LJ, Cameron FH, Mattick JS, Ackerman VP (1985) Construction of a gentamicin resistance gene probe for epidemiological studies. Antimicrob Agents Chemother 28:96–102

Parr TR Jr, Bryan LE (1984) Mechanism of resistance of an ampicillin-resistant, β-lactamase-negative clinical isolate of *Haemophilus influenzae* type b to β-lactam antibiotics. Antimicrob Agents Chemother 25:747–753

Peacock JE Jr (1986) Methicillin-susceptible "methicillin-resistant *Staphylococcus aureus*": a sheep in wolves' clothing. Infection Control 7:161–163

Pennington JE (1978) Infection in the compromised host. Recent advances and future directions. In: Weinstein L, Fields BN (eds) Seminars in infectious disease, vol I. Stratton Intercontinental Medical Book Corporation, New York, p 142

Perine PL, Totten PA, Holmes KK, Sng EH, Ratnam AV, Widy-Wersky R, Nsanze H, Habte-Gabr E, Westbrook WG (1985) Evaluation of a DNA-hybridization method for detection of African and Asian strains of *Neisseria gonorrhoeae* in men with urethritis. J Infect Dis 152:59–63

Pfaller MA, Wakefield DS, Hammons GT, Massanari RM (1987) Variation from standards in *Staphylococcus aureus* susceptibility testing. Am J Clin Pathol 88:231–235

Plorde JJ et al. (1965) Studies on the pathogenesis of meningitis. V. Action of penicillin in experimental pneumococcal meningitis. J Lab Clin Med 65:71–80

Pollock HM, Minshew BH, Kenny MA, Schoenknecht FD (1978) Effect of different lots of Mueller-Hinton agar on the interpretation of the gentamicin susceptibility of *Pseudomonas aeruginosa*. Antimicrob Agents Chemother 14:360–367

Pollock HM, Barry AL, Gavan TL, Fuchs PC, Hansen S, Thornsberry CL, Frankel H, Forsythe SB (1986) Selection of a reference lot of Mueller-Hinton agar. J Clin Microbiol 24:1–6

Reller LB (1986) The serum bactericidal test. Rev of Infect Dis 8:803–808

Righter J (1987) Treatment of coagulase-negative staphylococcal infections: dilemmas for laboratory and clinician. J Antimicrob Chemother 20:459–462

Roberts MC, Swenson CD, Owens LM, Smith AL (1980) Characterization of chloramphenicol-resistant *Haemophilus influenzae*. Antimicrob Agents Chemother 18:610–615

Rossi L, Tonin E, Cheng YR, Fontana R (1985) Regulation of penicillin-binding protein activity: description of a methicillin-inducible penicillin-binding protein in *Staphylococcus aureus*. Antimicrob Agents Chemother 27:828–831

Ryan KJ, Schoenknecht FD, Kirby WMM (1970) Disc sensitivity testing. Hosp Pract 5:91

Sanders CC (1984) Failure to detect resistance in antimicrobial susceptibility tests: a "very major" error of increasing concern. Antimicrob Newslett 1:27–31

Sanders WE Jr, Sanders CC (1982) Do in vitro antimicrobial susceptibility tests accurately predict therapeutic responsiveness in infected patients? In: Lorian V (ed) Significance of medical microbiology in the care of patients. Williams and Wilkins, Baltimore, p 325

Sanders CC, Sanders WE Jr (1986) Type I beta-lactamases of gram-negative bacteria: interactions with beta-lactam antibiotics. J Infect Dis 154:792–800

Sanders CC, Sanders WE Jr (1987) Clinical importance of inducible beta-lactamases in gram-negative bacteria. Eur J Clin Microbiol 6:435–437

Schimpff SC (1980) Infection prevention during granulocytopenia. In: Remington JS, Swartz MN (eds) Current clinical topics in infectious diseases. McGraw-Hill, New York, p 85

Schoenknecht FD (1986) Bacterial tolerance to antimicrobial agents. Clinical Microbiology Newsletter 8:72–74

Schoenknecht FD, Sherris JC (1973) New perspectives in antibiotic susceptibility testing. In: Dyke SC (ed) Recent advances in clinical pathology, series 6. Churchill Livingstone, Edinburgh, pp 275–292

Schoenknecht FD, Sherris JC (1980) Recent trends in antimicrobial susceptibility testing. Lab Med 11:824–832

Schoenknecht FD, Washington II JA, Gavan TL, Thornsberry C (1980) Rapid determination of minimum inhibitory concentrations of antimicrobial agents by the autobac method: a collaborative study. Antimicrob Agents Chemother 17:824–833
Schwalbe RS, Stapleton JT, Gilligan PH (1987) Emergence of vancomycin resistance in coagulase-negative staphylococci. N Engl J Med 316:927–931
Seeberg AH, Tolxdorff-Neutzling RM, Wiedemann B (1983) Chromosomal β-lactamases of *Enterobacter cloacae* are responsible for resistance to third-generation cephalosporins. Antimicrob Agents Chemother 23:918–925
Shadomy S, Espinel-Ingroff A, Cartwright RY (1985) Laboratory studies with antifungal agents: susceptibility tests and bioassays. In: Lennette EH, Balows A, Hausler WJ Jr, Shadomy HJ (eds) Manual of clinical microbiology, 4th edn. American Society for Microbiology, Washington DC, pp 991–999
Shanholtzer CJ, Peterson LR (1986) False susceptible penicillin G MIC's for *Streptococcus pneumoniae* with a commercial microdilution system. Am J Clin Pathol 85:626–629
Sherris JC (1974) General considerations in in vitro susceptibility testing – a summation. In: Balows A (ed) Current techniques for antibiotic susceptibility testing. Thomas, Springfield, pp 123–137
Sherris JC (1977) The antibiotic sensitivity test. Variability. Interpretation. Rapid versus overnight. Agar versus broth. In: Lorian V (ed) Significance of medical microbiology in the care of patients. Williams and Wilkins, Baltimore, p 170
Sherris JC (1986) Problems in vitro determination of antibiotic tolerance in clinical isolates. Antimicrob Agents Chemother 30:633–637
Siddiqi SH, Libonati JP, Middlebrook G (1981) Evaluation of a rapid radiometric method for drug susceptibility testing of *Mycobacterium tuberculosis*. J Clin Microbiol 13:908–912
Snider DE Jr, Good RC, Kilburn JO, Laskowski LF, Lusk RH, Marr JJ, Reggiardo Z, Middlebrook G (1981) Rapid drug susceptibility testing of *Mycobacterium tuberculosis*. Am Rev Respir Dis 123:402–406
Sommers HM, Good RC (1985) Mycobacterium. In: Lennette EH, Balows A, Hausler WJ Jr, Shadomy HJ (eds) Manual of clinical microbiology, 4th edn. American Society for Microbiology, Washington DC, pp 216–248
Southern EM (1975) Detection of specific sequences among DNA fragments separated by gel electrophoresis. J Mol Biol 98:503–517
Spencer RC, Wheat PF (1986) Novel mechanisms for determining antibiotic susceptibilities. J Antimicrob Chemother 17:404–407
Stiller RL, Bennett JE, Scholer HJ, Wall M, Polak A, Stevens DA (1983) Correlation of in vitro susceptibility test results with in vivo response: flucytosine therapy in a systemic candidiasis model. J Infect Dis 147:1070–1077
Stone LL, Jungkind DL (1983) False-susceptible results from the MS-2 system used for testing resistant *Pseudomonas aeruginosa* against two third-generation cephalosporins, moxalactam and cefotaxime. J Clin Microbiol 18:389–394
Stratton CW (1986) Standardization of the serum bactericidal test and its relationship to levels of antimicrobial agents. Eur J Clin Microbiol 5:61–66
Sutter VL, Barry AL, Wilkins TD, Zabransky RJ (1979) Collaborative evaluation of a proposed reference dilution method of susceptibility testing of anaerobic bacteria. Antimicrob Agents Chemother 16:495–502
Taylor PC, Schoenknecht FD, Sherris JC, Linner EC (1983) Determination of minimum bactericidal concentrations of oxacillin for *Staphylococcus aureus*: influence and significance of technical factors. Antimicrob Agents Chemother 23:142–150
Tenover FC (1986) Studies of antimicrobial resistance genes using DNA probes. Antimicrob Agents Chemother 29:721–725
Tenover FC, Gootz TD, Gordon KP, Tompkins LS, Young SA, Plorde JJ (1984) Development of a DNA probe for the structural gene of the 2″-O-adenyltransferase aminoglycoside-modifying enzyme. J Infect Dis 150:678–687
Thornsberry C (1984) Methicillin-resistant (hetero-resistant) staphylococci. Antimicrob Newslett 1:43–47

Thornsberry C (1985) Automated procedures for antimicrobial susceptibility tests. In: Lennette EH, Balows A, Hausler WJ Jr, Shadomy HJ (eds) Manual of clinical microbiology 4th edn. American Society for Microbiology, Washington DC, p 1015

Thornsberry C, Kirven LA (1974) Ampicillin resistance in *Haemophilus influenzae* as determined by a rapid test for beta-lactamase production. Antimicrob Agents Chemother 6:653–654

Thornsberry C, McDougal LK (1983) Successful use of broth microdilution in susceptibility test for methicillin-resistant (heteroresistant) staphylococci. J Clin Microbiol 18:1084–1091

Tompkins LS (1985) DNA methods in clinical microbiology. In: Lennette EH, Balows A, Hausler WJ Jr, Shadomy HJ (eds) Manual of clinical microbiology, 4th edn. American Society for Microbiology, Washington DC, p 1023

Totten PA, Holmes KK, Handsfield HH, Knapp JS, Perine PL, Falkow S (1983) DNA hybridization technique for the detection of *Neisseria gonorrhoeae* in men with urethritis. J Infect Dis 148:462–471

Traub WH (1970) Susceptibility of *Pseudomonas aeruginosa* to gentamicin sulphate in vitro: lack of correlation between disc diffusion and broth dilution sensitivity data. Appl Microbiol 20:98

Tuomanen E, Durack DT, Tomasz A (1986) Antibiotic tolerance among clinical isolates of bacteria. Antimicrob Agents Chemother 30:521–527

Ubukata K, Yamashita N, Konno M (1985) Occurrence of a β-lactam-inducible penicillin-binding protein in methicillin-resistant staphylococci. Antimicrob Agents Chemother 27:851–857

Utsui Y, Yokota T (1985) Role of an altered penicillin-binding protein in methicillin- and cephem-resistant *Staphylococcus aureus*. Antimicrob Agents Chemother 28:397–403

Washington JA II (1983) Discrepancies between in vitro activity of and in vivo response to antimicrobial agents. Diagn Microbiol Infect Dis 1:25–31

Washington JA II (1985) Susceptibility tests: agar dilution. In: Lennette EH, Balows A, Hausler WJ Jr, Shadomy HJ: manual of clinical microbiology, 4th edn. American Society for Microbiology, Washington DC, p 967

Weinstein L, Dalton AC (1968) Host determinants of response to antimicrobial agents. N Engl J Med 279:467–473, 524–531, 580–588

Wilkins TD, Chalgren S (1976) Medium for use in antibiotic susceptibility testing of anaerobic bacteria. Antimicrob Agents Chemother 10:926–928

Witebsky FG, MacClowry JD, French SS (1979) Broth dilution minimum inhibitory concentrations: rationale for use of selected antimicrobial concentrations. J Clin Microbiol 9:589–595

World Health Organization (1961) Standardization of methods for conducting microbic sensitivity tests. Second Report of the Expert Committee on Antibiotics. Technical Report Series, No 210, pp 1–24

Zervos MJ, Schaberg DR (1985) Reversal of the in vitro susceptibility of enterococci to trimethoprim-sulfamethoxazole by folinic acid. Antimicrob Agents Chemother 28:446–448

Zighelboim S, Tomasz A (1981) Multiple antibiotic resistance in South African strains of *Streptococcus pneumoniae*: mechanism of resistance to β-lactam antibiotics. Rev Infect Dis 3:267–276

CHAPTER 16

The Molecular Epidemiology of Antimicrobial Resistance

D. M. SHLAES and C. A. CURRIE-MCCUMBER

A. Introduction

Endemic antibiotic resistance is a problem worldwide. Six task forces have recently been organized to address this global problem in a quantitative way. Condensed reports from these task forces were recently published in the *Reviews of Infectious Diseases* (LEVY et al. 1987). It is clear that large amounts of a variety of antibiotics, but especially of tetracyclines, broad spectrum penicillins and sulfamethoxazole-trimethoprim, are being used throughout the world (COL and O'CONNOR 1987). In many countries, this usage is uncontrolled, and widespread underdosing from use of over-the-counter combinations obtained without prescription is the rule.

From worldwide surveys, about 80% of *E. coli* and *Shigella* from most centers reporting to the task force were resistant to sulfonamides. Over 80% of *S. aureus* strains were resistant to penicillin, almost all of which could be attributed to the penetration of this species by a single beta-lactamase gene. The resistance of *E. coli* to ampicillin has been more variable, and ranged from 17% to 72%. Surveys in the US revealed an increasing prevalence of beta-lactamase producing *H. influenzae* from blood and cerebrospinal fluid isolates. The same was true for *N. gonorrhoeae*. Aminoglycoside resistance has also become widespread among Enterobacteriaceae worldwide. In some countries, aminoglycoside resistance is being seen in surveillance cultures and urinary isolates obtained from outpatients. Resistance to chloramphenicol, trimethoprim and other agents was also shown to be widespread, and, for some agents, apparently increasing resistance over time was noted (O'BRIEN et al. 1987).

Clearly, the problem of antibiotic resistance is global, and its cost to society is yet to be determined. Bacterial resistance makes the use of more costly antibiotics necessary, and may prolong or complicate the treatment of infected patients. In some countries, newer agents are not easily available, and patients remain essentially untreated for infections caused by highly resistant strains.

This chapter addresses the mechanism of spread of antibiotic resistance among human populations. The genetic mechanisms of spread among bacteria have been addressed by other authors in this volume (TAYLOR, this volume). We hope to show how spread of resistance determinants among bacterial species contributes to spread among humans. Suggestions for attempts at limiting the emergence and dissemination of antibiotic resistance will be presented.

Dissemination of antibiotic resistance should be distinguished from maintenance of the "resistance reservoir." From the studies of LEVY (1986), ourselves

(CURRIE-MCCUMBER et al. submitted; SHLAES et al., submitted), and others (CHASLUS-DANCLA et al. 1987), it is becoming clear that although antibiotic selective pressure may be required for establishing the reservoir of resistance, such pressure may no longer be required for its maintenance. The role of antibiotic selective pressure in establishing a reservoir of resistance, and the factors that are important in maintaining the reservoir, will be discussed in this chapter.

In general, the dissemination of antibiotic resistance within and between human populations occurs by one of three mechanisms: (1) The spread of a resistant strain (epidemic or endemic); (2) the spread of a bacterial plasmid encoding antibiotic resistance among several bacterial species or genera (plasmid epidemic or endemic): or (3) the spread of a specific resistance determinant among different plasmids or bacterial chromosomes (endemic resistance). More than one mechanism may operate simultaneously within a human population. A variety of factors influence this spread. They include antimicrobial selective pressure, the virulence of the resistant strain, the presence of a reservoir of the resistance determinant, a vector for spread, the presence of a susceptible host or host population, specific host risk factors and mixing of host populations. Examples of these mechanisms of spread will be presented, and the role of these factors in influencing the spread of resistance will be discussed.

The goal of this chapter is to present a limited review of the English language literature dealing with the epidemiology of antibiotic resistance among human populations emphasizing key points. We will begin with a brief discussion of the methods used to track antibiotic resistance, and then proceed to review examples where these methods have been used to track the spread of antimicrobial resistance.

B. Plasmids as Strain Markers

I. Brief Review of Methods

Resistance plasmids are valuable markers for the comparison of bacterial strains responsible for nosocomial infections as well as outbreaks in the community setting. As methods used in molecular biology have been simplified, plasmid analysis has been applied increasingly to investigate epidemiologic problems. Techniques used to evaluate outbreaks include plasmid "fingerprinting," DNA-DNA hybridization, heteroduplex analysis and Southern blot hybridization.

In contrast to phage typing, serotyping and biotyping, plasmid fingerprinting, which includes agarose gel electrophoresis and restriction endonuclease analysis, can be used to identify epidemic strains of bacteria, as well as epidemic plasmids that have transferred through different species. Hybridization techniques are useful in studying the evolution of plasmids during outbreaks and in demonstrating the presence and spread of transposons.

In the past decade, plasmid DNA isolation techniques have been simplified (WACHSMUTH 1986). Preparation times have been reduced from days to hours and the volume of broth culture required has been greatly reduced. Several protocols and their modifications can be found in the literature, most notably those described by KADO and LIU (1981), BIRNBOIM and DOLY (1979), HOLMES and QUIGLEY (1981) and MEYERS et al. (1976). In general, the outer bacterial cell membrane is disrupted, the cell wall is removed and internal membranes are lysed by one or more of the following: EDTA, lysozyme and detergent. The chromosome is denatured by alkaline pH, and precipitated along with cellular debris by centrifugation. Plasmid DNA is precipitated by adding cold ethanol, freezing and centrifugation. The DNA is electrophoresed through agarose gels, stained with ethidium bromide, and visualized under ultraviolet transillumination.

Plasmid DNA can be further purified by cesium chloride ultracentrifugation or other procedures which utilize ribonuclease and phenol extraction, and then can be cleaved by restriction endonucleases. Restriction enzymes recognize specific nucleotide sequences in DNA molecules and cut within that site. Identical plasmids would generate identical fragments, which can be separated on agarose gels producing a specific restriction endonuclease digestion profile.

Gene probing involves transferring denatured DNA from agarose gels to nitrocellulose or nylon membranes by the Southern blotting technique (SOUTHERN 1975). Colonies or bacterial suspensions can also be lysed, the DNA denatured and fixed onto filters or membranes (GRUNSTEIN and HOGNESS 1975; MASS 1983). Upon exposure to labelled denatured probe DNA, complementary single strands join and hybrids are detected by autoradiography or other methods depending on the method used to tag the probe.

II. Plasmids as Strain Markers

Many gram-negative bacilli bear plasmids that can serve as epidemiological markers in single species outbreaks. Numerous studies appear in the literature which illustrate the usefulness of plasmid profiling. These methods have been helpful in elucidating epidemics involving: *K. pneumoniae*, *S. marcescens*, *E. cloacae*, *S. typhimurium*, *P. stuartii*, *Acinetobacter* spp., *P. aeruginosa*, *P. cepacia*, *Ewingella americana*, *L. pneumophila*, and others (JOHN and TWITTY 1986). Species in which R plasmid fingerprinting may not be particularly useful include *S. typhi* and *Shigella* spp. for reasons that will be discussed later.

The majority of intergeneric and single species nosocomial outbreaks have involved *K. pneumoniae*. ELWELL et al. (1978) found a 60 MDa R plasmid in *K. pneumoniae* and *E. cloacae* in burn patients in 1978. This study utilized a rapid plasmid DNA isolation technique and DNA-DNA hybridization, and represented the first study of its kind in which molecular technology was applied. Most studies prior to this had identified R plasmids based on their drug resistance markers.

Agarose gel electrophoresis of plasmid DNA was first used by O'CALLAGHAN et al. (1978) to resolve differences in three different strains of *K. pneumoniae* involved in outbreaks in a nursery. HARDY et al. (1980) found 8 kanamycin resistant strains of *K. pneumoniae* to contain six plasmids that were the same size in each strain.

Strains of multiply resistant *K. pneumoniae* isolated during an epidemic in the neonatal ICU at Vanderbilt University-affiliated hospitals in 1978 were shown to contain the same plasmid as strains responsible for nosocomial infections on adult wards beginning in 1973 (RUBENS et al. 1981; MCKEE et al. 1982). This was followed by another epidemic of infections with *K. pneumoniae* one year later (JOHN et al. 1983). This time, however, the R plasmids were shown to be different than those previously observed, even though it was suggested epidemiologically that the sequential outbreaks in neonates may have been related. Another similar outbreak occurred in the NICU at the Nashville General Hospital in 1983. Plasmid profiling revealed that this was a separate outbreak, rather than an extension of the earlier epidemics at Vanderbilt.

Because *Serratia* species also acquire and stably maintain a wide variety of R plasmids, plasmid analysis has been a useful tool in examining intergeneric and single species outbreaks involving these bacteria (JOHN and MCNEILL 1981; AMBROSIO et al. 1979; BIDWELL et al. 1981; BRYAN et al. 1980; ECHOLS et al. 1984; NEWPORT et al. 1985; SHLAES and CURRIE 1983; LEE et al. 1984). An epidemic strain of *S. marcescens* contained a conjugative 45 MDa plasmid, which was consistently detected in *S. marcescens* and 4 other species during a study at the Seattle VA from 1976–1978 (TOMPKINS et al. 1980). JOHN et al. observed plasmid diversity throughout three outbreaks over a 7 year period at the Medical University Hospital and Veterans Administration Medical Center in Charleston, SC (JOHN and MCNEILL 1981; BRYAN et al. 1980; NEWPORT et al. 1985; JOHN and MCNEILL 1980). *Hae*II restriction fragments of a conjugative R plasmid, isolated from *Serratia* involved in an outbreak in their NICU, were almost identical to those fragments generated by a *Serratia* plasmid isolated 5 years earlier at the VAMC.

MARKOWITZ et al. (1983) tested the ability of plasmid typing to evaluate two separate outbreaks of *E. cloacae* on a burn unit. The first major outbreak of *E. cloacae*, resistant to sulfadiazine and mafenide acetate, occurred in 1976. These isolates were compared to strains collected during another smaller outbreak in 1982, in which susceptibility patterns were variable or dissimilar to the earlier *E. cloacae* isolates. Agarose gel electrophoresis revealed uniform patterns of 4 plasmid bands (ranging from 2–66 MDa) in the epidemic strains (1976) and no such patterns in the silver sulfadiazine, mafenide acetate sensitive strains isolated in 1982, thus separating the two epidemics. This study also suggested that silver sulfadiazine resistance is associated with a 55 MDa plasmid.

Plasmid profiling is also useful in studying the epidemiology of outbreaks caused by most *Salmonella* spp., the major exception being *S. typhi*. BRUNNER et al. (1983) compared plasmid analysis with phage typing, resistance pattern determination and biotyping to study a limited epidemic of *S. typhimunium* infections in a large geographic area. They concluded that characterization of plasmids is as useful as phage typing and more accurate than the other typing methods. Single plasmid patterns were associated with different lysotypes. Holmberg et al. has also shown that plasmid typing is at least as reliable as phage typing and that both are superior to antimicrobial susceptibility testing (HOLMBERG et al. 1984). Others (OLSVIK et al. 1985; NAKAMURA et al. 1986; SPIKA et al. 1987) have used plasmid typing methods to show the transmission of *Salmonella* from animals to humans, an occurrence which creates tremendous problems in the food industry, not to mention the potential health hazard for humans.

In 1981, plasmid fingerprinting was used to trace a national outbreak of salmonellosis caused by *S. muenchen*. The organism was sensitive to multiple antibiotics and there was no phage typing or other system for distinguishing individual strains or clones. Thus plasmid profiling proved to be a sensitive indicator of a common-source outbreak (TAYLOR et al. 1982).

Although *S. typhi* remains an important enteric pathogen in many parts of the world, and outbreaks have been caused by antibiotic resistant *S. typhi*, these organisms are usually susceptible to antibiotics. Studies (MURRAY et al. 1985; TAYLOR et al. 1985) have shown a general absence of R factors in strains isolated from outbreaks, indicating that they probably do not successfully persist in nature. Plasmid profiling, therefore, would be of limited usefulness as an epidemiologic tool in tracking these strains. MURRAY et al. (1985) found R plasmids in 8 of 100 isolates from an outbreak in Chile and in 3 of 50 from Thailand. When these plasmids were transferred to *E. coli*, subsequent transfer frequencies were the same as those seen for the *Salmonella* parents. When plasmid-bearing and cured *S. typhi* strains were compared, further slowing of an already slow growth rate was observed with some plasmids. In addition, some plasmids appeared unstable in their *S. typhi* hosts.

In strains in which R plasmids have been demonstrated, variations in restriction patterns have occurred (TAYLOR et al. 1985). Modular evolution involving sequential deletion and stepwise acquisition of transposons has been proposed as a mechanism to explain this variability.

While not necessarily helpful in the endemic situation, fingerprinting techniques can be useful when attempting to differentiate epidemic strains of *Shigella* spp. bearing multiple plasmids (TACKET et al. 1984; FROST et al. 1985). PRADO et al. (1987) examined total plasmid content in 75 strains of *S. sonnei* isolated worldwide; 89% of the 57 strains from Houston, Mexico City and Guadalajara had identical or nearly identical plasmid profiles, which remained constant over 5 years. This study exemplifies an important limitation in plasmid fingerprinting, in that it would be very difficult to identify a common source of infection when examining strains bearing multiple endemic plasmids. If however the usual profile was well defined for a given locale, the authors felt the identification of a distinctly different plasmid pattern would still be helpful when investigating an outbreak.

Pseudomonas spp. have also been studied for plasmid patterns with variable outcome. Plasmid DNA from *Pseudomonas* spp. can be difficult to obtain consistently by standard lysis methods. Perhaps this explains the shortage of epidemiologic studies incorporating plasmid fingerprinting. JACOBY (1984) classifed many *P. aeruginosa* plasmids with known molecular sizes into 13 incompatibility groups. JOHN and TWITTY (1986) followed a multiply resistant serotype 12 strain which originated on a burn unit in 1979, for 4 years. Two large, nonconjugal plasmids were detected consistently among a number of the more than 100 strains evaluated. Antibiograms, serotypes and plasmid profiles were compared by MAYO et al. (1986), and used to determine a common source for corneal infection in contact lens wearers. Again, plasmid profiling did not appear to add much to serotyping.

In contrast to the above work, OGLE et al. (1987) used DNA restriction fragments from the exotoxin A gene to probe more than 100 different strains of *P. aeruginosa*. Isolates with variable colonial morphology, serotype and biotype were identical by Southern blot hybridization and isolates indistinguishable by serotyping, biotyping and antibiograms were differentiated by this method. These data suggest that previous epidemiological tools may have led to erroneous conclusions, but this will certainly require further confirmation from other laboratories and other epidemiologic circumstances.

III. Molecular Epidemiology in Gram-Positive Cocci

ZERVOS et al. (1987) documented nosocomial acquisition of enterococci with high-level (>2000 μg/ml) resistance to gentamicin, using plasmid content as an epidemiological marker. Transmission appeared to be due to patient-to-patient transfer as well as interhospital spread. A strain of gentamicin-resistant *S. faecalis* found in patients clustered in the surgical care units at the University of Michigan Hospital was in fact identical to an isolate from the surgical intensive care unit at the Ann Arbor Veterans Administration Medical Center. Presumably, this was mediated by transient hand-carriage of personnel who rotated between the two hospitals, or by patients who were transferred between hospitals. Presently, 16% of all enterococci isolated at the University of Michigan Hospital, and 55% of strains at the VA in Ann Arbor, show high level resistance to gentamicin. Prior studies by the same investigators (ZERVOS et al. 1986a, b) of transconjugants suggested plasmid heterogeneity, as at least seven different restriction endonuclease profiles were observed, indicating that resistance to gentamicin in *S. faecalis* is expressed on a variety of physically distinct conjugative and nonconjugative plasmids. Significant risk factors appeared to be: prior antimicrobial therapy, perioperative antibiotic prophylaxis, prior surgical procedures and longer hospitalization (ZERVOS et al. 1986a).

Plasmid analysis has been shown to be superior to bacteriophage typing and other typing methods for the epidemiological investigation of outbreaks due to antibiotic-resistant *Staphylococcus aureus* (MRSA) (MCGOWAN et al. 1979; RHINEHART et al. 1987; ARCHER and MAYHALL 1983) and *S. epidermidis* (SCHABERG and ZERVOS 1986; ARCHER et al. 1984; PARISI and HECHT 1980). It has been our experience that plasmid profiling was easier, more rapid and more specific than bacteriophage typing in evaluating an outbreak of MRSA at the Cleveland Clinic Foundation (CCF) (Fig. 1). Between December 1983 and December 1984 there was an outbreak of MRSA centered mainly on a vascular surgery service. Organisms isolated before and during the outbreak were characterized by bacteriophage typing and plasmid profiling; phage typing was discrepant in 9 (56%) of the 17 repeated analyses compared with one (3.4%) of the 29 for plasmid profiling. We found that the epidemic strain was introduced into the hospital from the community 15 months before the outbreak, and was probably transmitted by the hands of health care personnel. The index case was an employee who was subsequently a patient at another hospital in NE Ohio. At the time this individual was hospitalized, the latter institution was experiencing an outbreak of MRSA infection involving strains of the bacteriophage type as those eventually isolated at CCF. Plasmid analysis of the outlying hospital's MRSA isolates, whose phage types were identical to those of the isolates at CCF, revealed that they were identical to each other but different from the index case and CCF outbreak strains. Therefore, the outbreak strain did not appear to originate in the outlying hospital, but

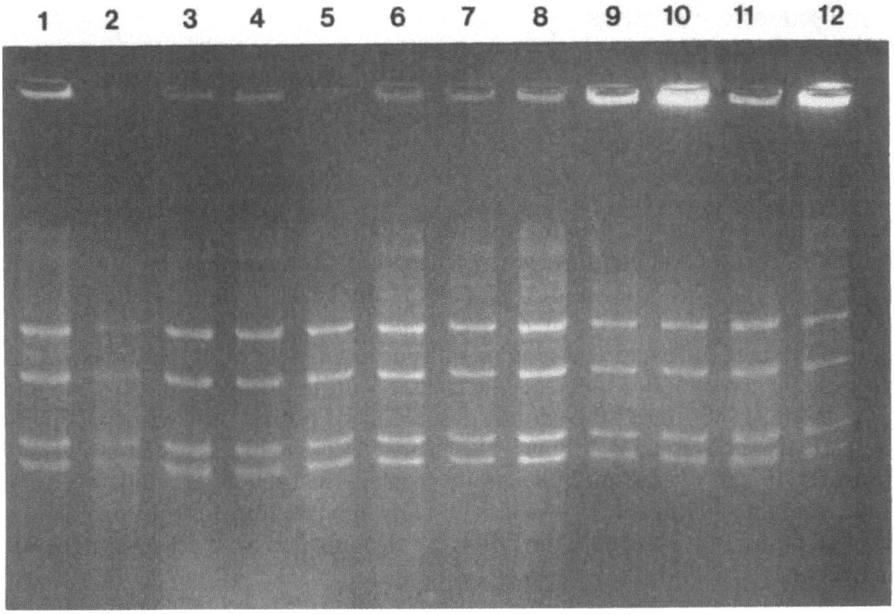

Fig. 1. *Eco*RI digestions of plasmid DNA from epidemic methicillin-resistant *Staphylococcus aureus* from the Cleveland Clinic outbreak. (RHINEHART et al. 1987)

rather was introduced from the community. This study again demonstrates the potential to generate misleading information when using bacteriophage typing as the sole means to investigate outbreaks of *Staphylococcus* (RHINEHART et al. 1987).

ARCHER and MAYHALL (1983) assessed the use of four epidemiological markers to follow an outbreak of nosocomial infection caused by a single strain of MRSA: antibiogram, phage type, production of aminoglycoside-modifying enzyme and plasmid pattern. Again, phage typing and use of antibiotic resistance patterns were unreliable. While the epidemic strain did produce a unique phosphotransferase, the detection of the enzymes require specialized procedures not readily available to clinical laboratories. Further, the investigators noted that many gentamicin resistant staphylococci of the same or different species may produce the same aminoglycoside modifying enzymes. Plasmid pattern analysis therefore proved to be the method of choice: it is rapid and inexpensive; plasmid patterns are usually stable and can differentiate isolates with similar antibiograms. Others (MCGOWAN et al. 1979; SARAVOLATZ et al. 1982; LOCKSLEY et al. 1982; SCHAEFLER et al. 1981) have also used plasmid analysis to study infections caused by *S. aureus*.

C. Epidemic Plasmids

R factors can also be transferred to a variety of different genera, adding to the pool of multiresistant organisms. These so called "epidemic plasmids" appear to be increasing in prevalence in nosocomial infections, and plasmid profiling and hybridization techniques have been invaluable in unraveling these outbreaks. The urinary tract and/or urine catheter bags are likely sites of conjugation, and Schaberg et al. have shown that multiresistant enteric isolates from clinical cases readily undergo conjugation in vitro when they are incubated in sterile urine (SCHABERG et al. 1977). GRIFFIN et al. (1985) found closely related IncC plasmids (120 MDa) in clinical isolate of *E. coli*, *S. marcescens*, *P. vulgaris*, and *M. morganni*. The index plasmid was able to transfer in vitro between these species, indicating the likelihood of interspecific transfer within the hospital. NAGANO and TAKAHASHI (1985) found that nondisposable urine bottles were associated with dissemination of resistant strains of Enterobacteriaceae in the Chiba University Hospital. In some cases, multiple strains bearing the same R plasmids were isolated from the same bottle. In addition to many opportunities for the introduction of contaminants, it was determined that the cleaning and disinfection system was inadequate.

A 65 MDa conjugative multiple resistance epidemic plasmid which contained a transposon conferring trimethoprim and streptomycin resistance was isolated and characterized by DATTA et al. (1979). It was first found during an outbreak of hospital infection in a urological ward caused by *K. pneumoniae* and later in *Citrobacter koseri* and *E. coli*. The plasmid in the latter two strains showed slight variations in their genetic or physical properties. The transposon appeared identical to Tn*7*, which had been previously identified in unrelated plasmids in bacteria from other European and Australian hospitals. The plasmid was involved in numerous hospital outbreaks of multiple serotypes of *K. pneumoniae* in Britain (CASEWELL et al. 1977).

MARKOWITZ et al. (1980) found a common 71 Mdalton conjugative gentamicin-resistance plasmid among different serotypes of multiply resistant *K. pneumoniae* collected during sequential outbreaks in an NICU. Restriction endonuclease analysis indicated this plasmid was disseminated in epidemic strains and in bowel flora, implicating the gastrointestinal tract of patients as the reservoir for gentamicin-resistant *K. pneumoniae* and personnel hands as a potential mode of transmission.

COURTNEY et al. (1980) used restriction endonuclease digestion followed by Southern blotting and DNA-DNA hybridization to compare 6 isolates of multiply resistant *K. pneumoniae*, which had appeared during a 2 year period on different wards of a Louisville Hospital. All strains were of a different serotype but were shown to bear identical R plasmids.

The Brigham and Women's Hospital reported finding trimethoprim resistance among species of Entrobacteriaceae which was spread by a single, stable conjugative plasmid encoding type II dihyrofolate reductase (DHFR) (MAYER et al. 1985). Thirty-seven of 42 trimethoprim-resistant (tmp^r) isolates from six species of gram-negative bacilli transferred tmp^r by conjugation. The species included *E. coli*, *K. pneumoniae*, *E. cloacae*, *E. gergoviae*, *C. freundii*, *P. stuartii* and

Acinetobacter calcoaceticus. Restriction profiling showed identical patterns in strains resistant to either trimethoprim alone or both trimethoprim and sulfamethoxazole. The plasmid had a molecular size of 52.5 kb. Another plasmid type (present in 21 of the 32 donors), which in addition mediated a β-lactamase, was 4 kb larger, and shared many restriction fragments with the smaller plasmid. DNA hybridization probes detected the type II DHFR gene on these plasmids but no genes for trimethoprim-resistant DHFR were detected on the chromosome, indicating that the spread of tmp^r in this hospital occurred by the transfer of one plasmid without transposition.

In another study, workers at the Brigham and Women's Hospital observed the resurgence of an endemic plasmic (pBWHI) in a new species using plasmid fingerprinting, restriction endonuclease digestion and computer assisted analysis (O'Brien et al. 1980; Mayer et al. 1986). The conjugative 92 kb Inc M plasmid originally appeared in 1975 in a urease negative strain of *K. pneumoniae*. It encoded resistance to chloramphenicol, sulfonamide, gentamicin, tobramycin, and beta-lactamases. Subsequently, it spread serially, causing successive outbreaks in new strains of *K. pneumoniae* and nine other species of Enterobacteriaceae, representing forty-nine different biotypes. This plasmid underwent various molecular changes during the first 6 years of its appearance; however, these variations did not seem to account for shifts in species distribution. The latest outbreak occurred in 1981 on a burn unit and involved an uncommon ornithine decarboxylase-negative strain of *E. cloacae*. In addition to harboring pBWHI, this strain was chromosomally resistant to topical silver salts and cephalosporins, commonly used antibiotics on the unit. This outbreak illustrates re-establishment and further dissemination of an endemic plasmid in a new host species facilitated by the presence of genes which allow that strain to occupy a particular clinical niche.

Rubens et al. (1979) described the transposition of genes encoding for aminoglycoside resistance, from a small nonconjugative plasmid to a large conjugative plasmid which had coexisted in clinical isolates of *S. marcescens*. The resultant multiresistance plasid became disseminated among other Enterobacteriaceae and caused an epidemic of nosocomial infection at the Vanderbilt Medical Center. This experience indicates that large, conjugative plasmids can acquire resistance transposons and serve as a means of dissemination of resistance during an outbreak.

D. Endemic Antibiotic Resistance

I. The Spread of Resistant Strains

The spread of a resistant strain among a population usually constitutes an epidemic or outbreak. This situation has been discussed earlier in this chapter. However, we think it is worth mentioning here that some strains may establish themselves endemically within a population in the absence of person to person spread within that population. The best example of this is *Pseudomonas aeruginosa*. *Pseudomonas* has a number of virulence properties that allow ready colonization of susceptible host populations. Once colonization or infection occurs, selection of antibiotic resistant variants of the colonizing strain can occur through antibiotic selective pressure. Although epidemic spread of antibiotic resistant clones of *Pseudomonas* has been described as related to personnel carriage or from a common environmental source (SHOOTER et al. 1969; FARMER et al. 1982; GUSTAFSON et al. 1983; RATNAM et al. 1986; LEVIN et al. 1984; PEDERSON et al. 1986), endemic antibiotic resistant *Pseudomonas* appears to result from selection of resistant variants of already colonizing strains. OLSON et al. (1984) looking prospectively at an intensive care unit population, were unable to demonstrate a common source or significant clustering of *Pseudomonas aeruginosa* colonization or infection (PEDERSON et al. 1986). This was in spite of an overall colonization rate of 37%. In addition, they demonstrated that, with antimicrobial therapy, previously colonized patients became colonized with resistant subpopulations of the same serotype. These resistant subpopulations were later lost or replaced by different, susceptible serotypes of *Pseudomonas*, but only after transfer out of the intensive care setting.

Our own experience with *Pseudomonas aeruginosa* on an intermediate care ward illustrates some similarities to the above studies. We carried out a prospective study of these wards over a six month period, culturing for gentamicin-resistant *Pseudomonas* using selective media (MACARTHUR et al. 1988). Thus, we were unable to follow patients for the development of resistance with time as Olson et al. were able to do. In our study, 21% of patients were culture positive for *Pseudomonas aeruginosa* at least once. The most common serotype was 011, accounting for 26% of colonized patients. Of the colonized patients, 37% were already on the wards at study initiation, 34% were colonized at the time of transfer from other hospital areas to the intermediate care wards, and 29% became colonized during their stay on the wards. Like OLSON et al. (1984, 1985), we were unable to demonstrate statistically significant clustering by either serotyping or plasmid profiling. Even a careful review of patients acquiring their colonization after admission to the ward did not demonstrate cross infections. It may be that those patients culture negative at the time of transfer were already colonized with susceptible strains and that resistant strains emerged during their admission. An analysis of risk factors for colonization was consistent with this hypothesis, since one would predict that antibiotic usage might therefore be a risk factor. However, only limited ambulatory status and length of stay were risk factors for colonization. In addition, not all these risk factors appeared independent and some could be shown to be additive. Thus, spread of resistant *Pseudomonas aeruginosa* appeared related to prior colonization, which in turn was probably related to host specific risk factors.

II. Endemic Resistance Resulting from the Spread of R Plasmids Between Strains

Endemic antibiotic resistance can also result from the dissemination of R plasmids between bacterial strains. This can occur interspecifically or intergenerically. We would like to focus on four illustrative examples from four different types of patient populations taken from our own experience. The four populations emphasize differences in mechanisms of resistance and their spread.

1. The Intensive Care Unit

Around 1981, 20% of gram-negative bacilli isolated from samples submitted for culture from the combined coronary care-medical intensive care unit of the Cleveland VA Medical Center were resistant to gentamicin. We carried out a prospective study over a six month period culturing all patients at regular intervals and at various sites for gentamicin resistant gram-negative bacilli in an attempt to understand the overall extent of this problem and the mechanisms contributing to this apparently high prevalence of resistance on the unit. A total of 147 patients were studied and 12 (8.2%) were colonized at least once with 20 strains of gentamicin-resistant gram-negative bacilli. Four environmental strains were also isolated. None of these strains could be shown to be cross-infecting. Seven of the isolates were non-*Proteae* members of Enterobacteriaceae. All seven carried R plasmids. Transmission of these R plasmids, from an index patient or from the environment, to three other patients was suggested. This transmission involved five different species of Enterobacteriaceae (SHLAES et al. 1986). Thus, about one-third of the gentamicin-resistant gram-negative bacilli isolated during this prospective study could be explained by transmission of plasmids encoding gentamicin resistance between patients on the unit.

2. The Intermediate Care Ward

Intermediate care wards are becoming increasingly prevalent in the United States. This is the natural result of current US hospital reimbursement policies. These wards care for patients who do not have physician and nursing care requirements that would justify acute hospital ward care, but are too ill to be placed in a nursing home or domicilary unit. Since these patients are more ill than the nursing home population, one might except more frequent transfers between the intermediate care areas and the acute care areas. Therefore, some relationship between the resistant strains or their R plasmids might be expected.

The Cleveland VA Medical Center has an intermediate care unit made of two wards located 20 miles from the acute care hospital facility. Of the gram-negative bacilli isolated from patient cultures submitted to the clinical microbiology laboratory 35% were resistant to gentamicin. Again, a similarly designed six month prospective study was performed (SHLAES et al. 1988). Fifteen patients, accounting for 10% of the population studied and for 30% of all patients colonized with gentamicin-resistant Enterobacteriaceae, were colonized with 22 strains including 10 different species all carrying the identical 60 kb conjugative plasmid (Fig. 2). This plasmid, pDS1134, encodes ANT (2″) and the OHIO-1 β-lactamase. One of the colonized individuals was a nurse with a positive hand culture for *K. pneumoniae* located on the ward where 9 of the 15 patients were also located. At first glance, this seemed to be an outbreak of the 60 kb plasmid occurring on the intermediate care wards. However, on closer examination of the epidemiology, we found that of the 15 patients, five were on the ward at the initiation of the study, six were transferred to the intermediate care wards from acute care wards already colonized with strains bearing this plasmid and only one patient during the 6 month prospective study apparently acquired his plasmid by cross-transmission

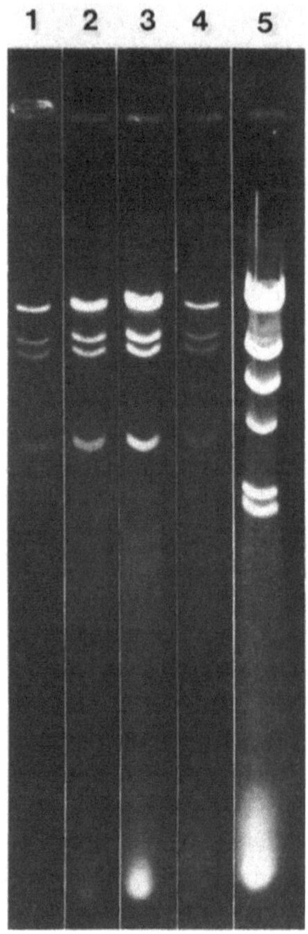

Fig. 2. *Eco*RI digestion of purified plasmid DNA from *E. coli* transconjugants of the following parental strains; *Lane 1*, *C. freundii*, patient 3; *lane 2*, *P. stuartii*, patient 4; *lane 3*, *M. morganii*, patient 1; *lane 4*, *K. pneumoniae*, nurse hand culture; *lane 5*, *Hin*dIII digestion of bacteriophage lambda DNA as a molecular weight standard. (SHLAES et al. 1988)

from his roommate, who was heavily colonized. In fact, two of these patients rapidly lost their colonization after transfer to the intermediate care wards.

Examination of an endemic strain on the same wards revealed similar results (SHLAES et al., submitted). A multiply resistant *Serratia liquefaciens* was isolated from 15 patients on the intermediate care wards. This strain was characterized by the presence of a 26 kb cryptic plasmid. Of these patients, seven were present on the wards at the initiation of the study, five were transferred from acute care areas already colonized with the strain and only three acquired colonization during their admission on the wards. Of the latter three, two apparently acquired their strain from another, colonized patient. Thus, this strain dissemination has the same epidemiologic characteristics as the dissemination of the plasmid, pDS1134, discussed above.

For the majority of colonized new admissions, the strain is brought into the wards from the acute care areas. Spread of the resistant strain or the plasmids pDS1134 was infrequent on the intermediate care wards. This epidemiology is to be contrasted to that occurring in the intensive care area, where about 30% of the endemic aminoglycoside resistance could be accounted for by cross-transmission of R plasmids from patient to patient.

For the intermediate care population, using multivariate methods of analysis, antibiotic use could not be shown to be a risk factor for colonization with gentamicin-resistant Enterobacteriaceae. Other risk factors, such as colonization at other sites, use of urinary drainage devices, presence of diabetes, history of a previous urinary tract infection, length of stay, and diminished ambulatory status were all more important depending on the site of colonization examined as the dependent variable. This is similar to the epidemiology of *Pseudomonas aeruginosa* in the same patient population, where antibiotic usage is a more important risk factor for colonization with resistant strains (MacArthur et al. 1988). These data suggest that, at least for Enterobacteriaceae, once a reservoir of resistance has been established, antibiotic usage is less important for maintaining that reservoir than other factors. This is a point we will address in more detail later.

3. The Nursing Home

Given our experience in other patient areas, we were not surprised to find that 35% of gram-negative bacilli isolated from specimens submitted by the Cleveland VA Medical Center nursing home care unit were also resistant to gentamicin and multiple other antibiotics. We assumed that it was likely that plasmids mediating gentamicin resistance were at least part of the problem.

To study this on the nursing home, we were only able to carry out a single point prevalence study (Shlaes et al. 1986). Thus, for a single two week period in time, all 86 inpatients, multiple environmental sites and patient care personnel were cultured for gentamicin-resistant gram-negative bacilli. These strains were subjected to the same analysis utilized in our previous studies. The results for the nursing home population, however, were quite different.

Twenty-six (30%) of the 86 patients were colonized with gentamicin-resistant gram-negative bacilli. Of the 49 strains isolated, none were able to transfer gentamicin resistance by conjugation. 21 strains could be analyzed for plasmid content. Only two plasmids could transform an *E. coli* recipient to gentamicin resistance. Thus, on the nursing home, although gentamicin resistance was fairly common among gram-negative rods colonizing these patients, it was rarely plasmid mediated. A review of antibiotic usage on the unit during the six months preceding the study revealed that no gentamicin had been used but 27 courses of trimethoprim-sulfamethoxazole and 19 courses of ampicillin had been prescribed. Retrospectively, conjugative ampicillin resistance, always due to the TEM β-lactamase, was discovered in a number of isolates, and this was always linked to sulfonamide resistance on the same plasmid.

In addition, cross-colonization with either resistant strains or R plasmids accounted for 57% of the strains that could be analyzed by plasmid profiling (SHLAES et al. 1986). Geographic clustering was obvious in the two nursing home unit wards. Although this was only a point prevalence study, it suggests that, at least in our nursing home, cross-transmission is a frequent occurrence, and that both transmission of resistant strains as well as R plasmids account for the majority of resistant strains observed. Transmission by health care personnel hands is the most likely explanation for the geographic clustering we observed.

The findings on the nursing home appear to contrast with those on the intermediate care wards where cross-transmission was infrequent. They also suggest that patients transferred to our nursing home are less likely to be a reservoir of gentamicin-resistance plasmids than patients transferred to our intermediate care wards. Thus, nursing home patients are less likely to reintroduce these plasmids to the acute care areas when transferred back than are intermediate care patients.

4. The Discharged Patient

Recently, we had the opportunity to study patients discharged within one week of having had a positive culture from any site for *Serratia* spp. resistant to an aminoglycoside antibiotic as determined from cultures submitted to the clinical microbiology laboratory (CURRIE-MCCUMBER CA et al., submitted). Three patients were followed weekly after discharge and 22 others were studied retrospectively from 3 weeks to 182 days after discharge. In addition, 26 cohabitants, most of whom were the primary caregivers for the study patients, were also followed. Of the 25 discharged patients, 11 retrospectively studied were culture positive for up to six months post-discharge. Two of the three prospectively followed patients remained culture positive for 5 and 6 months respectively. Only one of 26 cohabitants became colonized with the index strain, and this was only transient. For this small cohort of patients, only use of a Foley catheter ($P = 0.006$) and hospital use of gram-negative β-lactam antibiotics ($P = 0.06$) could be shown to be related to culture positivity at home by multivariate analysis (stepwise multiple regressions).

Twenty of the 25 resistant gram-negative strains isolated from the patients were *Serratia*, reflecting, probably, the entry criteria. Twenty-two Enterobacteriaceae were examined for R plasmids. Four *Serratia* carried the 93 kb conjugative endemic VA gentamicin-resistance plasmid (see below). Four other non-conjugative gentamicin-resistance plasmids were isolated. Fourteen *Serratia* and one *E. cloacae* carried the same, cryptic, nonconjugative 26 kb plasmid. No evidence of extra-*Serratia* spread of an R plasmid was detected outside the hospital.

These data demonstrate that patients colonized with resistant Enterobacterioaceae while inpatients can be colonized for prolonged periods as outpatients, even in the absence of antibiotic selective pressure. These patients may pose a finite but small risk for dissemination to their caregivers at home. They may also be a risk for other hospital patients upon readmission and will also contribute to levels of endemic antibiotic resistant flora in the outpatient community as a whole.

III. The Contribution of Stable R Plasmids to Endemic Resistance

A number of others have also studied the contribution of R plasmid dissemination to endemic resistance although, in most cases, this was done through retrospective rather than prospective analysis. In some cases, wide geographic dissemination of stable plasmids has been demonstrated. As described earlier, an epidemic of multiresistant *Serratia marcescens* infection occurring during the years 1973–1979 at the Seattle VA Hospital was studied retrospectively. The epidemic strain and a number of other enteric species isolated during the outbreak were shown to possess the identical plasmid (pLST1000), a 60 kb conjugative plasmid encoding ANT(2″), as well as β-lactamase production and sulfonamide resistance. The mechanism of spread of the plasmid could not be discerned from the published data. Subsequently, it has been shown that this is a highly stable plasmid with a worldwide distribution (O'BRIEN et al. 1985).

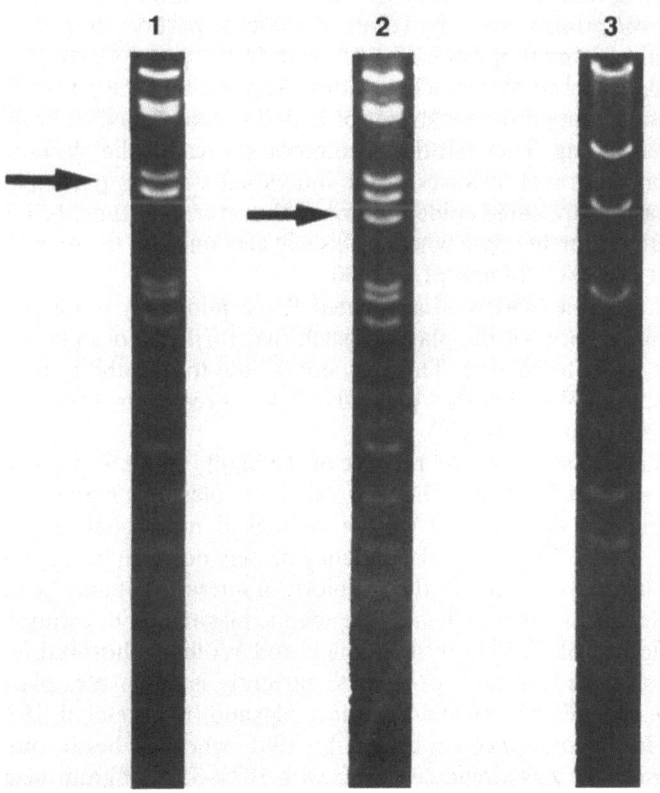

Fig. 3. *Eco*RI restriction endonuclease digestions of purified plasmid DNA from pSCL14 (MVAMC) and pDS3 (Schering-Parkland Memorial, Dallas). *Lane 1*, pSCL14; *lane 2*, pDS3; *lane 3*, *Hin*dIII digestion of bacteriophage lambda DNA for molecular weight standards. *Arrows* indicate the presence of a 7.3 kb doublet in pDS3 and the 6.4 kb fragment seen in pSCL14 but missing from pDS3. (SHLAES et al. 1987)

Another widespread, stable plasmid, also encoding ANT(2″) is pSCL14. This plasmid was first isolated in 1975 during an outbreak of multiply resistant *K. pneumoniae* at the Minneapolis VA Medical Center (SADOWSKI et al. 1979). The index strain was introduced to the hospital by a nursing home patient. The plasmid has remained endemic at that institution since that time and is widespread in multiple species of Enterobacteriaceae (LEE et al. 1986). We found the same plasmid in multiple species of Enterobacteriaceae during our prospective studies at the Cleveland VA (SHLAES and CURRIE-MCCUMBER 1986). More recently, we have discovered the plasmid at Parkland Memorial Hospital in Dallas, Texas (Fig. 3) (SHLAES et al. 1987). The Dallas patient, from whom the plasmid was recovered, had not been outside of Dallas and had not been in a VA medical center as far as we could determine. This is consistent with the idea that pSCL14 is another, highly stable, widely distributed R plasmid encoding ANT(2″).

Another stable plasmid that may be widely disseminated has been described by Rudy and Murray, and encodes resistance to trimethoprim-sulfamethoxazole (RUDY and MURRAY 1984). This plasmid encodes ampicillin and streptomycin resistance as well, is conjugative and is 38.4 Mdalton in size. The plasmids were isolated from *E. coli* strains from the stools of students participating in a placebo controlled trial of trimethoprim-sulfamethoxazole for prophylaxis of travelers' diarrhea during travel to Mexico. The authors showed that the plasmid had disseminated among many different strains of *E. coli* as determined by both plasmid content and serotyping. They felt that a common source for the plasmid was unlikely based on the travel histories of the individual students participating. Although this plasmid appeared epidemic among the returning students, it is impossible to say without further data whether this will also turn out to be a widespread, stable plasmid like pSCL14 and pLST1000.

These highly stable, widely disseminated R plasmids may represent an end-stage evolutionary form of the plasmid, such that further molecular rearrangements are less likely to survive. This may contribute to our ability to recognize them as they spread. Whether they play other roles as reservoirs for resistance determinants is not clear (see below).

It is of interest to speculate on the role of the highly stable R plasmids in this regard. Some authors have hypothesized that these plasmids may be the source of a new resistance determinant for an ecological niche such as a hospital (O'BRIEN et al. 1985). The stable plasmid may or may not then be responsible for endemic or epidemic resistance to the antibiotic of interest, but may be the source of the determinant for other endemic or epidemic plasmids. For example, before the introduction of pLST1000 into Brigham and Women's hospital in Boston, gentamicin resistance was rare. pLST1000 currently is still a rare plasmid, but pBWH1 is the endemic gentamicin-resistance plasmid (MAYER et al. 1986).

Likewise, in our own medical center, by 1981, when we began our studies, gentamicin resistance was already endemic with 10%–35% of gram-negative bacilli from different locations within the hospital resistant to this agent. In 1975, the Minneapolis VA experienced an outbreak caused by gentamicin-resistant *K. pneumoniae* bearing a 93 kb plasmid encoding ANT(2″) (probably encoded by *aad*B). The same plasmid and its closely related congeners have existed at that medical center since then (LEE et al. 1986), and has been endemic at our own medical center since at least 1981 (LEE et al. 1986). A survey of gentamicin resistance plasmids at our medical center in 1981 revealed wide dissemination of ANT(2″) among a large group of closely related plasmids (SHLAES et al. 1983).

One wonders if it is possible that these highly stable conjugative plasmids "brought" the ANT(2″) gene to the Brigham and Women's Hospital and the Minneapolis VA Medical Center, respectively, during the 1970s.

IV. The Role of Antibiotic Usage in the Selection and Dissemination of Antibiotic Resistance

Antibiotic usage appears to play a key role in the selection and dissemination of resistant strains within a population over time (LEVY et al. 1987; LEVY 1986; SPIKA et al. 1987; MCGOWAN 1983; DUPONT and STEELE 1987; MURRAY and RENSIMER 1983; STEEL and SKOLD 1985). This principal has been reaffirmed in both animals and humans in countless studies. A recent potential challenge to this principal was related to the aminoglycoside amikacin. This derivative of kanamycin has only a small number of amino or hydroxyl groups available for modification by aminoglycoside modifying enzymes, the principal mechanism of resistance to aminoglycosides among the Enterobacterioaceae (PRICE et al. 1981). Among these potential sites, only one enzyme in gram-negatives was known to modify amikacin, AAC(6′), and only about one-third of Enterobacteriaceae producing the enzyme were resistant to clinically achievable levels of the drug (PRICE et al. 1981). A number of hospitals with endemic resistance to gentamicin responded to this by discontinuing the use of all aminoglycosides other than amikacin. Before changing antibiotic usage, a baseline study was performed to assess rates of aminoglycoside resistance. The hospitals then prospectively followed resistance rates and mechanisms of resistance during the period of amikacin usage. The studies have reported results for about 5 years of usage. In general, there was a decrease in gentamicin resistance especially among certain species of Entrobacteriaceae. No increase in amikacin resistance was observed (BETTS et al. 1984). In fact, in one of the participating hospitals, use of amikacin led to significant decreases in amikacin resistance (LARSON et al. 1986). Another hospital, not participating in the prospective trial, however, did report increased amikacin resistance and increased numbers of Enterobacteriaceae producing AAC(6′) during periods when amikacin usage was high (LEVINE et al. 1985). In a retrospective survey of 26 hospitals in 6 different geographic areas of the United States, we found different results (HARE et al., in preparation). The hospitals were divided into those using $\geq$20% of their total aminoglycosides as amikacin and those using $<$20%. For the amikacin using hospitals, gentamicin resistance was decreased, but amikacin resistance was increased (Table 1). Furthermore, the frequency of strains resistant to all aminoglycosides was higher in the amikacin using hospitals. A careful examination of the mechanisms of resistance in the aminoglycoside resistant strains collected from these hospitals revealed increased frequencies of AAC(6′) in the hospitals that used more amikacin. This was frequently combined in the same strains with the gentamicin-modifying enzymes (ANT(2″) or AAC(3) which led to pan-aminoglycoside resistance (Table 2). We also showed that these resistance mechanisms could be transferred from about 40% of the multiply aminoglycoside

Table 1. Aminoglycoside resistance and hospital amikacin usage for 515 aminoglycoside resistant strains of gram-negative bacilli

Antibiotic	Amikacin usage Resistance (%)	
	≧20%	<20%
Gentamicin	88.0[a]	94.1
Tobramycin	93.7[a]	88.2
Netilmicin	60.0[b]	36.8
Amikacin	31.4[b]	4.4

[a] $P<0.05$ [b] $P<0.005$

Table 2. Enzymatic mechanisms of aminoglycoside resistance and amikacin usage for 515 aminoglycoside resistant gram-negative bacilli

Mechanism	Amikacin usage (%)	
	≧20%	<20%
AAC(6′)	10.3	2.0
AAC(6′) + AAC(3) or ANT(2″)	39.3	12.9

resistant strains by conjugation. Thus, in our study, involving 595 aminoglycoside resistant isolates from around the United States, we were able to demonstrate a significant correlation between amikacin usage and amikacin resistance, and were able to show plasmid mediated pan-aminoglycoside resistance in amikacin-using centers as well.

Although one would expect to see differences in patterns of resistance from center to center, it may be that our more global retrospective look at aminoglycoside use and resistance provided a more realistic picture of the relationship between amikacin usage and resistance. These studies and others raise the question of why the relationship between antibiotic use and resistance is not seen more universally.

The link between the antibiotic used and the resistance eventually observed is not always obvious. For example, it has been argued that the use of antibiotics that will never be applied to human populations in animal feed will not lead to the transmission of relevant resistance to human populations. This is clearly in error. Two recent examples of this come from France. In France, apramycin was recently introduced into animal feed. Apramycin is an aminoglycoside not released for use in humans. It is modified by the AAC(3)-IV enzyme which is usually plasmid mediated. This enzyme also mediates resistance to gentamicin, tobramycin, and netilmicin, antibiotics that are frequently used in the treatment of infections in humans. An outbreak of multiply resistant *Salmonella typhimurium* associated with resistant strains of *E. coli* occurring in calves has recently been reported (CHASLUS-DANCLA et al. 1986). These strains were frequently resistant to multiple aminoglycosides including apramycin, as well as to other agents such as ampicillin, chloramphenicol and trimethoprim, agents not fed to animals. This illustrates that the use of apramycin, a non-human agent, nevertheless selects for a mechanism of resistance which also yields cross resistance to other aminoglycosides, and therefore represents a potential threat to the human population. It also illustrates that selection by one drug can select plasmids encoding multiple resistance determinants, including those for agents not related to the selecting agent. Another recent example of the latter is the selection of trimethoprim resistance plasmids experimentally in populations of chickens (CHASLUS-DANCLA et al. 1987). The chickens studied were fed chloramphenicol, streptomycin, neomycin, and tetracycline every 10–11 days. An epidemic plasmid encoding resistance to trimethoprim and ampicillin occurred in the flock, and was maintained over time in the apparent absence of specific selective pressure. In this case, the epidemic plasmid was also isolated from *E. coli* contaminating the food source for the flock. Similar results have been documented for macrolide-lincosamide-streptogramin B resistance in gram-positive cocci during a tylosin feeding experiment in pigs (Christy and Dunny 1984).

We believe the distinction that must be recognized is that between selection of the resistant clone and its maintenance within a population. Although antibiotic selection may be required for establishing a reservoir of resistance within a population, that reservoir may include unselected resistance phenotypes. In addition, it is likely that after the reservoir has been established by selection other factors then become more important in maintaining the reservoir.

A number of authors have attempted to address the distinction between antibiotic selection and maintenance of the reservoir of resistance. In a classic study of tetracycline resistant *E. coli* in chickens, Levy showed that after having been exposed to the antibiotic and becoming colonized with the resistant strains, the chickens would maintain their colonization for prolonged periods of time in the absence of antibiotic selective pressure. Only by mixing the colonized chickens with a noncolonized population could the resistance determinant be eliminated (Levy et al. 1976). The more recent study quoted above also demonstrated the dissemination of a plasmid encoding resistance to antibiotics to which the chickens had not been exposed apparently from food contaminated with strains carrying the plasmid (Chaslus-Dancla et al. 1987). This plasmid was maintained in the flock without selective pressure. Early studies have demonstrated the survival of antibiotic resistant *E. coli* and their ability to transfer R plasmids to gut flora in the absence of antibiotic selective pressure (Hartely and Richmond 1975; Petrocheilou et al. 1976). Our own studies, examining specific populations over defined time periods in a prospective manner, have frequently failed to find that antibiotics were a significant risk factor for colonization with resistant Enterobacteriaceae or even, specifically, R plasmid bearing strains (Shlaes and Currie 1983; Shlaes et al., submitted). This again emphasizes the importance of other factors in the maintenance of antibiotic resistant populations of bacteria after the resistant clone has been introduced.

References

Ambrosio RE, van Wyk AJ, deKlerk HC (1979) Antibiotic resistant *Serratia marcescens* infection in a hospital. S Afr Med J 55:584–587

Archer GL, Mayhall CG (1983) Comparison of epidemiological markers used in the investigation of an outbreak of methicillin-resistant *Staphylococcus aureus* infection. J Clin Microbiol 18:395–399

Archer GL, Vishniavsky N, Stiver HG (1982) Plasmid pattern analysis of *Staphylococcus epidermidis* isolates from patients with prosthetic valve endocarditis. Infect Immun 35:627–632

Archer GL, Karchmer AW, Vishniavsky N, Johnston JL (1984) Plasmid pattern analysis for the differentiation of infecting from non-infecting *Staphylococcus epidermidis*. J Infect Dis 149:913–920

Betts RF, Valenti WM, Chapman SW et al. (1984) Five year surveillance of aminoglycoside usage in a university hospital. Ann Intern Med 100:219–222
Bidwell JL, Reeves RS, Bullock DW (1981) Diversity of R plasmids in epidemic *Serratia* marcescens from the south west of England. In: Grassi GG, Sabath LD (eds) New trends in antibiotics: research and therapy. Elsevier/North Holland, Amsterdam, pp 268–270
Birnboim HC, Doly J (1979) A rapid alkaline extraction procedure for screening recombinant plasmid DNA. Nucleic Acids Res 7:1513–1523
Brunner F, Margadant A, Peduzzi R, Piffaretti J-C (1983) The plasmid pattern as an epidemiologic tool for *Salmonella typhimurium* epidemics: comparison with the lysotype. J Infect Dis 148:7–11
Bryan CS, Parker E, Schoenlein PV, Northey J, Ely B, John JF (1980) Plasmid mediated antibiotic resistance in a changing hospital environment: efficacy of control measures. Am J Infect Control 8:65–71
Casewell MW, Webster M, Dalton MT, Phillips I (1977) Gentamicin resistant *Klebsiella aerogenes* in a urological ward. Lancet II:444–446
Chaslus-Dancla E, Martel JL, Carlier C et al. (1986) Emergence of aminoglycoside 3-*N*-acetyltransferase IV in *Escherichia coli* and *Salmonella typhimurium* isolated from animals in France. Antimicrob Agents Chemother 29:239–243
Chaslus-Dancla E, Gerbaud G, Lagorce M et al. (1987) Persistence of an antibiotic resistance plasmid in intestinal *Escherichia coli* of chickens in the absence of selective pressure. Antimicrob Agents Chemother 31:784–788
Christie PJ, Dunny GM (1984) Antibiotic selection pressure resulting in multiple antibiotic resistance and localization of resistance determinants to conjugative plasmids in streptococci. J Infect Dis 149:74–82
Col NF, O'Connor RW (1987) Estimating worldwide current antibiotic useage: report of task force 1. Rev Infect Dis 9 [Suppl 3]:S232–S243
Courtney MA, Miler JR, Summersgill J, Melo J, Raff MJ, Streips UN (1980) R-factor responsible for outbreak of multiple resistant *Klebsiella pneumoniae*. Antimicrob Agents Chemother 18:926–929
Datta N, Hughes VM, Nugent ME, Richards H (1979) Plasmids and transposons and their stability and mutability in bacteria isolated during an outbreak of hospital infection. Plasmid 2:182–196
DuPont HL, Steele JH (1987) Use of antimicrobial agents in animal feeds: implications for human health. Rev Infect Dis 9:447–460
Echols RM, Palmer DL, King RM, Long GW (1984) Multidrug resistant *Serratia marcescens* bacteriuria related to urologic instrumentation. South Med J 77:173–177
Elwell LP, Inamine JM, Minshew BH (1978) Common plasmid specifying tobramycin resistance found in two bacteria isolated from burn patients. Antimicrob Agents Chemother 13:312–317
Farmer JJ, Weinstein RA, Zierdt CH, Brokopp CD (1982) Hospital outbreaks caused by *Pseudomonas aeruginosa*: importance of serogroup p11. J Clin Microbiol 16:226–270
Frost JA, Willshaw GA, Barclay EA, Rowe B (1985) Plasmid characterization of drug-resistant *Shigella dysenteriae* I from an epidemic in Central Africa. J Hyg (Camb) 94:163–172
Griffin HG, Foster TJ, Falkiner FR, Carre ME, Coleman DC (1985) Molecular analysis of multiple resistance plasmids transferred from gram negative bacteria isolated in a urological unit. Antimicrob Agents Chemother 28:413–418
Grunstein M, Hogness DS (1975) Colony hybridization: a method for the isolation of cloned DNAs that contain a specific gene. Proc Natl Acad Sci USA 72:3961–3965
Gustafon TL, Band JD, Hutcheson RH, Schaffner W (1983) *Pseudomonas* folliculitis: an outbreak and review. Rev Infect Dis 5:1–8
Hardy DJ, Legeai RJ, O'Callaghan RJ (1980) *Klebsiella* neonatal infections: mechanism of broadening aminoglycoside resistance. Antimicrob Agents Chemother 18:542–548
Hartely CL, Richmond MH (1975) Antibiotic resistance and the survival of *E. coli* in the alimentary tract. Br Med J [Clin Res] iv:71–74

Holmberg SD, Wachsmuth KI, Hickman-Brenner FW, Cohen ML (1984) Comparison of plasmid profile analysis, phage typing and antimicrobial susceptibility testing in characterizing *Salmonella typhimurium* isolates from outbreaks. J Clin Microbiol 19:100–104

Holmes DS, Quigley M (1981) A rapid boiling method for the preparation of bacterial plasmids. Anal Biochem 114:193–197

Jacoby GA (1984) Resistance plasmids of *Pseudomonas aeruginosa*. In: Bryan LE (ed) Antimicrobial drug resistance. Academic, Orlando, pp 497–514

John JF, McNeill WF (1980) Plasmid diversity in multi-resistant *Serratia marscens* isolates from hospitals. In: Nelson JD, Grassi C (eds) Current chemotherapy and infectious disease. Proceeding of the 11th International Congress of Chemotherapy and the 19th Interscience Conference on Antimicrobial Agents and Chemotherapy, vol 1. American Society for Microbiology, Washington DC, pp 28–30

John JF, McNeill WF (1981) Characteristics of *Serratia marcescens* containing a plasmid coding for gentamicin resistance in nosocomial infections. J Infect Dis 143:810–817

John JF Jr, Twitty JA (1986) Plasmids as epidemiologic markers in nosocomial gram-negative bacilli: experience at a university and review of the literature. Rev Infect Dis 8:693–704

John JF, McKee KT, Twitty JA, Schaffner W (1983) Molecular epidemiology of sequential nursery epidemics caused by multiresistant *Klebsiella pneumoniae*. J Pediatr 102:825–830

Kado CI, Liu ST (1981) Rapid procedure for detection and isolation of large and small plasmids. J Bacteriol 145:1365–1373

Larson TA, Garrett CR, Gerding DN (1986) Frequency of aminoglycoside 6′-*N*-acetyltransferase among *Serratia* species during increased use of amikacin in the hospital. Antimicrob Agents Chemother 30:176–178

Lee SC, Gerding DN, Cleary PP (1984) Plasmid macroevolution in a nosocomial environment: demonstration of a persistent molecular polymorphism and construction of a cladistic phylogeny on the basis of restriction data. Mol Gen Genet 194:173–178

Lee SC, Gerding DN, Cleary PP (1986) Hospital distribution, persistence, and reintroduction of related gentamicin R plasmids. Antimicrob Agents Chemother 29:654–659

Levin MH, Weinstein RA, Nathan C et al. (1984) Association of infection caused by *Pseudomonas aeruginosa* serotype 011 with intravenous abuse of pentazocine mixed with tripelennamine. J Clin Microbiol 20:758–762

Levine JF, Maslow MJ, Leibowitz RE et al. (1985) Amikacin-resistant gram negative bacilli: correlation of occurrence with amikacin use. J Infect Dis 151:295–300

Levy SB (1986) Ecology of antibiotic resistance determinants. Banbury report 24: antibiotic resistance genes: ecology, transfer and expression. Cold Spring Harbor Laboratory, pp 17–30

Levy SB, Fitzgerald GB, Macone AB (1976) Spread of antibiotic resistant plasmids from chicken to chicken and from chicken to man. Nature 260:40–42

Levy SB, Burke JP, Wallace CK (eds) (1987) Antibiotic use and antibiotic resistance worldwide. Rev Infect Dis 9 [Suppl 3]:S231–S316

Locksley RM, Cohen ML, Quinn TC, Tompkins LS, Coyle MB, Kirihara JM, Counts GW (1982) Multiply antibiotic resistant *Staphylococcus aureus*: introduction, transmission and evolution of nosocomial infection. Ann Intern Med 97:317–324

Maas R (1983) An improved colony hybridization method with significantly increased sensitivity for detection of single genes. Plasmid 10:296–298

MacArthur RD, Lehman MH, Currie-McCumber CA, Shlaes DM (1988) The epidemiology of resistant *Pseudomonas aeruginosa* on an Intermediate Care Ward. Am J Epidemiol 128:821–827

Markowitz SM, Smith SM, Williams DS (1983) Retrospective analysis of plasmid patterns in a study of burn unit outbreaks of infection due to *Enterobacter cloacae*. J Infect Dis 148:18–23

Markowitz SM, Veazey JM, Macrina FL, Mayhall CG, Lamb VA (1980) Sequential outbreak of infection due to *Klebsiella pneumoniae* in a neonatal intensive care unit: implication of conjugative R plasmid. J Infect Dis 142:106–112

Mayer KH, Fling ME, Hopkins JD, O'Brien TF (1985) Trimethoprim resistance in multiple genera of Enterobacteriaceae at a U.S. hospital: spread of the type II dihydrofolate reductase gene by a single plasmid. J Infect Dis 151:783–789
Mayer KH, Hopkins JD, Gilleece ES, Chao L, O'Brien TF (1986) Molecular evolution, species distribution, and clinical consequences of an endemic aminoglycoside resistance plasmid. Antimicrob Agents Chemother 29:628–633
Mayo MS, Cook WL, Schlitzer RL, Ward MA, Wilson LA, Ahearn DG (1986) Antibiograms, serotypes and plasmid profiles of *Pseudomonas aeruginosa* associated with corneal ulcers and contact lens wear. J Clin Microbiol 24:372–376
McGowan JE (1983) Antimicrobial resistance in hospital organisms and its relation to antibiotic use. Rev Infect Dis 5:1033–1048
McGowan JE, Terry PM, Huang T-SR, Houk CL, Davies J (1979) Nosocomial infections with gentamicin-resistant *Staphylococcus aureus*: plasmid analysis as an epidemiologic tool. J Infect Dis 140:864–872
McKee KT, Cotton RB, Stratton CW, Lavely GB, Wright PF, Shenai JP, Evans ME, Melly MA, Farmer JJ, Karzon DT, Schaffner W (1982) Nursery epidemic due to multiply resistant *Klebsiella pneumoniae*: epidemiologic setting and impact on perinatal health care delivery. Infect Control 3:150–156
Meyers JA, Sanchez D, Elwell LP, Falkow S (1976) Simple agarose gel electrophoretic method for the identification and characterization of plasmid deoxyribonucleic acid. J Bacteriol 127:1529–1537
Murray BE, Rensimer ER (1983) Transfer of trimethoprim resistance from fecal *Escherichia coli* isolated during a prophylaxis study in Mexico. J Infect Dis 147:724–728
Murray BE, Levine MM, Cordano AM et al. (1985) Survey of plasmids in *Salmonella typhi* from Chile and Thailand. J Infect Dis 151:551–555
Nagano Y, Takahashi S (1985) Stored urine as a reservoir of gentamicin-resistant bacteria and as a site of conjugative R plasmid transfer. J Hosp Infect 6:245–251
Nakamura M, Sato S, Ohya T, Suzuki S, Ikeda S (1986) Plasmid profile analysis in epidemiological studies of animal *Salmonella typhimurium* infection in Japan. J Clin Microbiol 23:3605
Newport MT, John JF, Michel YM, Levkoff AH (1985) Endemic *Serratia marcescens* infection in a neonatal intensive care nursery associated with gastrointestinal colonization. Pediatr Infect Dis 4:160–167
O'Brien TF, Ross DG, Guzman MA, Medeiros AA, Hedges RW, Botstein D (1980) Dissemination of an antibiotic resistance plasmid in hospital patient flora. Antimicrob Agents Chemother 17:537–543
O'Brien TF, Pla MdP, Mayer KH et al. (1985) Intercontinental spread of a new antibiotic resistance gene on an epidemic plasmid. Science 230:87–88
O'Brien TF and members of task force 2 (1987) Resistance of bacteria to antibacterial agents: report of task force 2. Rev Infect Dis 9 [Suppl 3]:S244–S260
O'Callagahan RJ, Rousset KM, Harkess NK, Murray ML, Lewis AC, Williams WL (1978) Analysis of increasing antibiotic resistance of *Klebsiella pneumoniae* relative to changes in chemotherapy. J Infect Dis 138:293–298
Ogle JW, Janda JM, Woods DE, Vasil ML (1987) Characterization and use of a DNA probe as an epidemiological marker for *Pseudomonas aeruginosa*. J Infect Dis 155:119–126
Olson B, Weinstein RA, Nathan C et al. (1984) Epidemiology of endemic *Pseudomonas aeruginosa*: why infection control efforts have failed. J Infect Dis 150:808–816
Olson B, Weinstein RA, Nathan C et al. (1985) Occult aminoglycoside resistance in *Pseudomonas aeruginosa*: epidemiology and implications for therapy and control. J Infect Dis 152:769–774
Olsvik O, Sorum H, Birkness K, Wachsmuth K, Fjolstad M, Lassen J, Fossum K, Feeley JC (1985) Plasmid characterization of *Salmonella typhimurium* transmitted from animals to humans. J Clin Microbiol 22:336–338
Parisi JT, Hecht DW (1980) Plasmid profiles in epidemiological studies of infections by *Staphylococcus epidermidis*. J Infect Dis 141:637–643

Pederson SS, Koch C, Hoiby N, Rosendal K (1986) An epidemic spread of multiresistant *Pseudomonas aeruginosa* in a cystic fibrosis centre. J Antimicrob Chemother 17:505–516

Petrocheilou V, Grinsted J, Richmond MH (1976) R-plasmid transfer in vivo in the absence of antibiotic selection pressure. Antimicrob Agents Chemother 10:753–761

Prado D, Murray BE, Cleary TG, Pickering LK (1987) Limitations of using the plasmid pattern as an epidemiological tool for clinical isolates of *Shigella sonnei*. J Infect Dis 155:314–316

Price KE, Kresel PA, Farchione LA et al. (1981) Epidemiological studies of aminoglycoside resistance in the USA. J Antimicrob Chemother 8 [Suppl A]:89–105

Ratnam S, Hogan K, March SB, Butler RW (1986) Whirlpool-associated folliculitis: report of an outbreak and review. J Clin Microbiol 23:655–659

Rhinehart E, Shlaes DM, Keys TF, Serkey J, Kirkley B, Kim C, Currie-McCumber CA, Hall G (1987) Nosocomial clonal dissemination of methicillin-resistant *Staphylococcus aureus*. Arch Intern Med 147:521–524

Rubens CE, McNeill WF, Farrar WE (1979) Evolution of multiple antibiotic resistance plasmids mediated by transposable plasmid deoxyribonucleic acid sequences. J Bacteriol 140:713–719

Rubens CE, Farrar WE, McGee ZA, Schaffner W (1981) Evolution of a plasmid mediating resistance to multiple antimicrobial agents during a prolonged epidemic of nosocomial infections. J Infect Dis 143:170–181

Rudy RP, Murray BE (1984) Evidence for an epidemic trimethoprim-resistance plasmid in fecal isolates of *Escherichia coli* from citizens of the United States studying in Mexico. J Infect Dis 150:25–29

Sadowski PL, Peterson BC, Gerding DN, Clearly PP (1979) Physical characterization of ten R plasmids obtained from an outbreak of nosocomial *Klebsiella pneumoniae* infections. Antimicrob Agents Chemother 15:616–624

Saravolatz LD, Markowitz N, Arking L, Pohlod D, Fisher E (1982) Methicillin-resistant *Staphylococcus aureus*: epidemiologic observations during a community acquired outbreak. Ann Intern Med 96:11–16

Schaberg DR, Zervos M (1986) Plasmid analysis in the study of the epidemiology of nosocomial gram positive cocci. Rev Infect Dis 8:705–712

Schaberg DR, Highsmith AK, Wachsmuth IK (1977) Resistance plasmid transfer by *Serratia* marcescens in urine. Antimicrob Agents Chemother 11:449–450

Schaefler S, Jones D, Perry W et al. (1981) Emergence of gentamicin and methicillin resistant *Staphylococcus aureus* strains in New York City hospitals. J Clin Microbiol 13:754–759

Shlaes DM, Currie CA (1983) Endemic gentamicin resistant R factors on a spinal cord injury unit. J Clin Microbiol 18:236–241

Shlaes DM, Currie-McCumber CA (1986) Dissemination of a plasmid determining multiple antibiotic resistance between two Veterans Administration Medical Centers. Infect Control 7:362–364

Shlaes DM, Vartian C, Currie CA (1983) Variability in DNA sequence of closely related nosocomial gentamicin-resistance plasmids. J Infect Dis 148:1013–1018

Shlaes DM, Currie-McCumber CA, Eanes M et al. (1986a) Gentamicin-resistance plasmids in an intensive care unit. Infect Control 7:355–361

Shlaes DM, Lehman MH, Currie-McCumber CA et al. (1986b) Prevalence of colonization with antibiotic resistant gram negative bacilli in a nursing home care unit. The importance of cross-colonization as documented by plasmid analysis. Infect Control 7:538–545

Shlaes DM, Currie-McCumber CA, Yessayan A (1987) The VA ANT(2″) plasmid in Dallas. Letter. Antimicrob Agents Chemother 31:1155

Shlaes DM, Currie-McCumber C, Lehman MH (1988) Introduction of a plasmid encoding the Ohio-I β-lactamase to an intermediate care ward by patient transfer. Infect Control Hosp Epidemiol 9:317–319

Shooter RA, Cooke EM, Gaya H et al. (1969) Food and medicaments as possible sources of hospital strains of *Pseudomonas aeruginosa*. Lancet I:227–229

Southern EM (1975) Detection of specific sequences among DNA fragments separated by gel electrophoresis. J Mol Biol 98:503–517
Spika JS, Waterman SH, Soo Hoo GW et al. (1987) Chloramphenicol-resistant *Salmonella newport* traced through hamburger to dairy farms. A major persisting source of human salmonellosis in California. N Engl J Med 316:565–570
Steen R, Skold O (1985) Plasmid-borne or chromosomally mediated resistance by Tn7 is the most common response to ubiquitous use of trimethoprim. Antimicrob Agents Chemother 27:933–937
Tacket CO, Shahid N, Huq MI, Alim ARMA, Cohen ML (1984) Usefulness of plasmid profiles for differentiation of *Shigella* isolates in Bangladesh. J Clin Microbiol 20:300–301
Taylor DN, Wachsmuth IK, Shangkuan YH et al. (1982) Salmonellosis associated with marijuana: a multistate outbreak traced by plasmid fingerprinting. N Engl J Med 306:1249–1253
Taylor DE, Chumpitaz JC, Goldstein F (1985) Variability of Inc HII plasmids from *Salmonella typhi* with special reference to Peruvian plasmids encoding resistance to trimethoprim and other antibiotics. Antimicrob Agents Chemother 28:452–455
Tompkins LS, Plorde JJ, Falkow S (1980) Molecular analysis of R factors from multiresistant nosocomial isolates. J Infect Dis 141:625–636
Wachsmuth K (1986) Molecular epidemiology of bacterial infections: examples of methodology and of investigations of outbreaks. Rev Infect Dis 8:682–692
Zervos MJ, Dembinski S, Mikesell T, Schaberg DR (1986a) High level resistance to gentamicin in *Streptococcus faecalis*: risk factors and evidence for exogenous acquisition of infection. J Infect Dis 153:1075–1083
Zervos MJ, Mikesell TS, Schaberg DR (1986b) Heterogeneity of plasmids determining high level resistance to gentamicin in clinical isolates of *Streptococcus faecalis*. Antimicrob Agents Chemother 30:78–81
Zervos MJ, Kauffman CA, Therasse PM, Bergman AG, Mikesell TS, Schaberg DR (1987) Nosocomial infection by gentamicin-resistant *Streptococcus faecalis*. Ann Intern Med 106:687–691

CHAPTER 17

Microbial Persistence or Phenotypic Adaptation to Antimicrobial Agents: Cystic Fibrosis as an Illustrative Case

L. E. BRYAN

A. Introduction

This chapter considers adaptive changes which allow microorganisms to persist despite apparently effective antimicrobial therapy by in vitro testing. Such changes are normally manifest mainly during the course of therapy but in some instances may be stable beyond its termination. Even in the latter circumstances when bacterial colonization continues, isolates expressing lower susceptibility are often replaced by more susceptible organisms.

Clearly the above changes are of consequence where therapeutic response is slow or where it is unsuccessful. The greatest probability of this is under clinical conditions where there is some type of impairment of host defenses or foreign or necrotic material is present at the infection site. Perhaps the best example is the colonization of lungs with *Pseudomonas aeruginosa* in patients with cystic fibrosis. The purpose of this review will be principally to draw attention to those factors which contribute to the persistence of *P. aeruginosa* in cystic fibrosis as a reasonably well studied example of microbial persistence. These same factors in part or in entirety may contribute to other clinical examples of therapeutic failure or slow response.

Factors contributing to microbial persistence or phenotypic adaptation to antimicrobial agents are as follows:

1. *Host related*
   a) Limited antibiotic entry to a tissue or tissue fluid compartment
   b) Antagonism of the action of antimicrobial agents by local physiological factors
   c) Inactivation of antibiotics by normal bacterial flora, other colonizing bacteria or other pathogens
   d) Inability of host defenses to clear residual quantities of bacteria after a course of antibiotics which has been partially successful
2. *Bacterially related*
   a) Acquisition of additional genetic material such as a plasmid. In general while this is an important cause of resistance, it is not an important cause of persistence
   b) Mutations reducing antibiotic susceptibility which may be associated with other properties placing the organism at a selective disadvantage in the absence of antibiotics

c) Gene regulation modifying drug entry or drug inactivation or the activity of targets of antimicrobial agents
d) Expression of extracellular or cell surface products as part of the adaptation to host defenses which in turn may modify drug binding to the microbe
e) The rate of bacterial growth in vivo may be lowered reducing susceptibility to certain drugs

B. Cystic Fibrosis and Microbial Persistence

The natural history of most patients with cystic fibrosis is that they will undergo pulmonary colonization with *P. aeruginosa* (HOIBY 1982) and in many instances *Pseudomonas cepacia*. Colonization with *Staphylococcus aureus* and *Haemophilus influenzae* is also an almost universal finding but does not present the problem of severe persistent colonization that *P. aeruginosa* and perhaps *P. cepacia* represent (BLESSING et al. 1979).

Therapeutic attempts to eradicate *Pseudomonas* colonization using repeated courses of intravenous antimicrobial agents active by in vitro susceptibility testing against sputum isolates have been unsuccessful. However, there seems to be little question that the use of such repeated courses of therapy does reduce the rate of pulmonary damage and prolonged patient survival.

It is likely that pulmonary damage associated with *P. aeruginosa* colonization is due to a combination of the destructive processes of products and toxins elaborated by *P. aeruginosa* (VASIL 1986; WOODS and SOKOL 1985), tissue damage secondary to host defenses such as polymorphonuclear phagocytes and damage mediated through immunopathology associated with deposited immune complexes (HOIBY and SCHIOTZ 1982). There is no universal agreement on how these mechanisms produce pulmonary damage. It seems clear that if an understanding of the processes of microbial persistence which allow the continuation of *P. aeruginosa* colonization were achieved that more effective mechanisms to diminish or eradicate the organism might be undertaken.

The question of why *P. aeruginosa* is able to persist within the pulmonary environment must be considered. This question is difficult to answer particularly when persistence occurs in spite of what seems effective antimicrobial therapy by virtue of the usual clinical testing methods. There is no adequate immunological explanation to explain failure of eradication of the organism. Acute exacerbations of infection frequently occur. Total numbers of *P. aeruginosa* present in the bronchoaveolar exudate are elevated. However, there is evidence to suggest that these exacerbations may actually be the result of underlying viral or mycoplasma infections (WANG et al. 1984; WRIGHT et al. 1976). Even so except in very late stage cystic fibrosis, antimicrobial therapy results in clinical improvement of the patients with acute exacerbation of pulmonary infection. There is no clear correlation between clinical improvement and response of *P. aeruginosa* (BEAUDRY et al. 1980; STEPHENS et al. 1983; MCLAUGHLIN et al. 1983; GOLD et al. 1985). In a large percentage of cases total numbers of *P. aeruginosa* declined during the course of antimicrobial therapy and may even be eradicated for short periods of time. If numbers are depressed at the end of the antibiotic treatment period they normally return to pretreatment levels within a few days to a few weeks.

C. Factors Associated with Persistence of *P. aeruginosa* During Antimicrobial Therapy in Cystic Fibrosis

I. Host-Related Factors

1. Drug Entry to Bronchoalveolar Spaces

Studies have shown that entry of the aminoglycoside tobramycin, for example, or the β-lactam ticarcillin may not be adequate to exceed concentrations needed to inhibit growth of *P. aeruginosa* as determined by conventional susceptibility testing. Thus, in our own study the sputum concentration of tobramycin frequently did not reach concentrations adequate to inhibit the growth of *P. aeruginosa* particularly if the organism were tested under conditions incorporating the antagonistic effects of local physiology (see below) (RABIN et al. 1980). These observations were also true for the β-lactam ticarcillin. In response much higher levels of intravenous tobramycin (12–16 mg kg^{-1} day^{-1}) were administered with doses of ticarcillin up 100 mg/kg every 4 h. Even with these very large doses only short term suppression of *P. aeruginosa* could be achieved within the lungs.

Determination of bronchoalveolar concentrations of antibiotics is beset with numerous difficulties. In particular technical problems with assay methods and variation in composition of the sample are particular difficulties. Important factors influencing in vivo concentrations include the degree of mucosal inflammation, method of collecting samples, timing of samples relative to dosing, pooling of samples and averaging concentrations, methods of homogenization, diluent used in assay procedures and the use of bioassay versus radioenzymatic or immunoassay (LEVY 1986). Even so the view is widely held that entry of aminoglycosides and β-lactams probably by passive diffusion into bronchial-alveolar secretions is relatively poor.

A partial explanation of reduced pulmonary antibiotic activity lies in the fact that the pharmacokinetics of at least some drugs is different in patients with cystic fibrosis. It appears that the rate of renal excretion is greater, for example, ceftazidime (LEEDER et al. 1984; REED et al. 1987), methicillin (YAFFE et al. 1977) and cloxacillin (SPINO et al. 1984), and the total body clearance is greater with tobramycin (LEVY et al. 1984) and cloxacillin (SPINO et al. 1984).

The result of these observations is that only relatively small changes in susceptibility to either tobramycin or ticarcillin, for example, are needed to allow the organism to persist. Some of these changes in susceptibility are low enough that they would not be detected unless a selection was made for low level resistance of *P. aeruginosa* from the sputum of patients undergoing treatment. Additionally, as noted below some of the adaptive processes resulting in lower levels of resistance may not be stable.

Penetration of ciprofloxacin into the respiratory tract does not seem to be a limiting factor in its efficacy. Bronchial and sputum concentrations seem relatively high ranging from a 0.8 to 1.1 ratio to that found in serum (SHALIT et al. 1987). In contrast to the situation with several β-lactams and aminoglycosides, ciprofloxacin pharmacokinetics do not markedly differ between individuals who have or do not have cystic fibrosis (BLUMER et al. 1985; LEBEL et al. 1986).

2. Antagonism of the Action of Antibiotics

Aminoglycosides which have been a mainstay of treatment in cystic fibrosis for several years are severely antagonized by the exudate present in bronchoaveolar spaces. Aminoglycosides are cationic antibiotics and bind to phosphate residues within the lipopolysaccharide portion of the outer membrane of *P. aeruginosa*. This process destablizes the outer membrane following for the drug to pass through the outer membrane not only by the normal porin channels but through disorganization of the outer membrane. Divalent cations such as magnesium and calcium are in competition with aminoglycosides for binding to the phosphate residues within the outer membrane. The concentration of particularly calcium interferes with binding of the aminoglycosides and reduces its activity on *P. aeruginosa* (BRYAN 1984). Furthermore, because of the cationic nature of the aminoglycosides they may also bind to polyanionic material present in the form of DNA liberated from disrupted polymorphonuclear leukocytes or bacteria or to exopolysaccharide of the organism itself. These effects have been shown to modify the activity of aminoglycosides and when taken into account in susceptibility testing methods better correlations with drug efficacy have been achieved (RABIN et al. 1980). Finally, the slightly acidic pH within the bronchoaveolar environment also reduces the activity of aminoglycosides due to the requirement for an electrical potential within the bacterial cell for them to be transported into the bacterial cell (BRYAN 1984). β-Lactams are not strongly affected by these competitive and antagonistic factors but as noted later their activity may be reduced when the rate of growth of bacteria is reduced.

Another important factor not effectively taken into account in testing susceptibility of bacteria in cystic fibrosis to antibiotics is the inoculum effect. Counts of *P. aeruginosa* may frequently reach 10^8 to 10^9/ml of exudate. These are far higher numbers than used in conventional susceptibility testing and can reduce susceptibility to many β-lactams. Susceptibility is especially reduced to compounds susceptible to slow hydrolysis by β-lactamases.

3. Inactivation of Antibiotics in Bronchoalveolar Exudate

The colonizing flora of most cystic fibrosis patients is complex. It comprises *P. aeruginosa*, *S. aureus*, *H. influenzae* and frequently *P. cepacia*. Many of the more recent beta-lactams including antipseudomonal beta-lactams are relatively resistant to hydrolysis by β-lactamases (BUSH and SYKES 1984; FISHER 1984). Although there is a paucity of good data it is improbable that there is a substantial loss of recent β-lactams particularly cephalosporins activity in the extracellular environment due to β-lactamases from any of the above organisms. Compounds such as ceftazidime are hydrolyzed very poorly by most plasmid-mediated and the *Pseudomonas* chromosomal β-lactamases. In order to contribute to resistance under these conditions a large quantity of β-lactamase must be present, the permeation of the drug must be poor and significant hydrolysis occurs at low (periplasmic) concentrations (Vu and Nikaido 1985; Godfrey and Bryan 1984). While these conditions may exist in the periplasm of *P. aeruginosa*, they do not exist in the extracellular bronchoalveolar environment. Under these circumstances concentration of β-lactamases is low and drug concentration is high relative to periplasmic concentrations. Hence extensive β-lactam degradation seems unlikely.

4. Inability of Host Defenses to Clear Residual Quantities of Bacteria After a Course of Antibiotics

Ineffective host defense may contribute to resistance of especially *P. aeruginosa* in cystic fibrosis. Pulmonary secretions within this disease are dehydrated and most studies of mucociliary clearance have shown that it is impaired (Wood et al. 1985; Mathews and Drotar 1984). *Pseudomonas* infection itself appears to result in a factor in serum that reduces the ability of aveolar macrophages to phagocytose and kill *Pseudomonas*. Otherwise immunologic and other pulmonary defenses appear normal (Mathews and Drotar 1984). It would appear that antimicrobial agents are able to significantly reduce the flora in some instances to levels which are less or in some cases far less than 1% of the original counts. In circumstances where there was no impairment of pulmonary defenses the residual organisms would be readily removed. In the case of cystic fibrosis it is likely that the residual population which is able to resist the action of antimicrobial agents through various changes reducing its antibiotic susceptibility (see next section) is able to persist. This relatively resistant population can then serve as the source for the organism to return to prior levels of colonization. In some instances this may occur during the course of antimicrobial therapy in which case the organisms may be recognized as resistant. In other instances the residual population may serve as the source of susceptible revertants which re-establish the colonizing population once the antimicrobial agent is removed. Under these circumstances the "resistance" may not be easily recognized.

II. Bacterially Related Factors

1. Acquisition of "New" Genetic Material

While the acquisition of new genetic information contributes to microbial persistence to antimicrobial agents it is not, in my view, the common cause. This is in decided contrast to the situation where one is examining resistance in the normal host or resistance that is present at the time of initiation of therapy in epidemiological surveys of resistance. Under these conditions a selection is made for stable forms of resistance and for relatively higher levels of resistance. Plasmid mediated resistance mechanisms for the most part do not likely produce a severe impairment of the microbes capability to grow. Therefore strains which have plasmids frequently are carried for long periods of time even if there is a gradual loss of the plasmid containing strains from a population. Examination of isolates which arise from treatment failures of cystic fibrosis in our experience have not demonstrated that the mechanism of resistance is plasmid mediated (Schryvers et al.

1987). However PRINCE (1986) has reported that β-lactamase production occurs in the majority of isolates of *P. aeruginosa* from CF patients. *P. aeruginosa* isolates specify a chromosomally inducible β-lactamase and nearly all (if not all) strains could be stated to produce β-lactamase. The actual role of this enzyme and even that of some plasmid-specified enzymes in resistance to a particular β-lactamase-resistant β-lactam is open to question. For example, in the series reported by PRINCE (1986) 90% of strains resistant to imipenem produced β-lactamase but this is not a recognized mode of resistance to imipenem in *P. aeruginosa* presently. It is probably fair to conclude that plasmid-specified β-lactamase may be a cause of persistence but there is a lack of evidence to support this as a common cause of persistence. The chromosomal enzyme likely contributes a greater role (see next section).

2. Mutation

Mutational forms of resistance are much more common under circumstances of microbial persistence in cystic fibrosis. Frequently such mutations while associated with antimicrobial resistance are also associated with some phenotypic change which impairs the competitive capabilities of the organism. This has recently been shown, for example, in a patient under treatment with tobramycin and ceftazidime (SCHRYVERS et al. 1987). During the course of treatment strains were isolated which constitutively expressed high level production of β-lactamase. These strains showed resistance to a very wide range of β-lactam antibiotics in keeping with the patterns seen with such types of isolates from nosocomial infections (SANDERS and SANDERS 1983). In these mutants the β-lactamase expressed was a much increased quantity of the normally expressed inducible β-lactamase. The enzyme which has been associated with a pI of about 8.4 showed four or more isozymes with pIs varying from 7.0 to 8.4. When growth rates of the strains expressing the constitutive β-lactamase were compared with sensitive isolates present at the initiation of therapy, it was apparent that there was a reduction of the growth rate in the case of the mutants. When a mixture of susceptible and resistant strains were placed together in broth, the susceptible strain consistently outgrew the resistant and gradually became predominant in the population under nonselective circumstances. Essentially identical results were obtained with laboratory derived mutants of the originally susceptible strains showing the same constitutive β-lactamase expression (SCHRYVERS et al. 1987).

The process of either induction of the β-lactameas or as described above mutation resulting in its constitutive expression clearly illustrate the process of microbial persistence. These strains have undergone an adaptive change which allows them to survive in the presence of an unfavorable circumstance, i.e., treatment with modern antipseudomonal β-lactams. However, that adaptive change does place the organism at a selective disadvantage in the absence of antimicrobial agents. Therefore, the strain is likely to disappear once antimicrobial agents are removed. Under these circumstances unless very careful surveillance is carried out the actual resistance may be missed and the failure to eradicate colonized *P. aeruginosa* will be said to be associated with no change in susceptibility to the antimicrobial agents.

The aminoglycosides gentamicin and tobramycin have been widely used in the therapy of *P. aeruginosa* pulmonary infections in cystic fibrosis. However, the outcome of treatment has been a temporary reduction in numbers of the organism or temporary eradication followed by recolonization to prior levels within a few days to a few weeks. In some instances this has been associated with long-term carriage of aminoglycoside resistance. However, in many other instances resistance in the usual sense has not been shown to account for the therapeutic failure or it has been of temporary duration. Exhaustive studies of the mechanisms of resistance to account for therapeutic failure in cystic fibrosis have not been carried out. However, it has been repeatedly shown that *P. aeruginosa* can develop so-called "small-colony phenotypes." These small colony forms which have reduced growth rates show broad resistance to aminoglycoside antibiotics. They are resistant principally because they do not transport the antimicrobial agents inside the cell (see Chap. 2). In order to adapt to the presence of the aminoglycoside antibiotics, however, the cell has reduced its capability to grow in unselected conditions, i.e., where no antibiotics are present. Therefore, these isolates would be expected to be uncommonly detected following the end of therapy.

3. Gene Regulation Modifying Drug Entry or Drug Inactivation or the Activity of Targets of Antimicrobial Agents

With the exception of inducible β-lactamases there is very little information concerning a microbe's capability to control specific gene functions which would modify susceptibility to antimicrobial agents (see Chap. 6 and 7). It remains possible that there are subtle ways to modulate the structure of lipopolysaccharide, the number or function of outer membrane porins, the relative prevalence of penicillin binding proteins, the contributions of electrical potential compared to pH gradients to drive intracellular transport of various compounds, etc. In view of the fact that many of the mutational changes noted produce deleterious effects on cell growth rate, it is unlikely that gene regulation mechanisms producing these changes would ever be detected. It seems highly likely that the gene control mechanism would revert to "normal" state as soon as the organism was studied under unselected growth conditions. Control of the many factors contributing to the level of antibiotic susceptibility is, for the most part, poorly understood and needs further study.

In CF patients treated with co-trimoxazole, thymidine-dependent *Staphylococcus aureus* have been frequently defected (GILLIGAN et al. 1987; HOWDEN 1981; SPARHAM et al. 1978). Co-trimoxazole inhibits the synthesis of tetrahydrofolate and reduces the synthesis of thymine. Resistance may be achieved to this compound to some degree by the acquisition of thymidine from the growth medium thereby partly bypassing the site of inhibition. Such strains frequently manifest reduced growth rates and abnormal biochemical reactions. They are likely to disappear upon removal of the antibiotic.

4. Expression of Extracellular or Cell Surface Products as Part of the Adaptation to Host Defenses Which in Turn May Modify Drug Binding to the Microbe

It has been recognized for some time that *P. aeruginosa* strains isolated from patients with cystic fibrosis have a much greater prevalence of production of a mucoid exopolysaccharide containing large quantities of polysaccharide alginate. This substance which has antiphagocytic activities is also a polyanion. Although TANNENBAUM et al. (1984) reported a failure to detect tobramycin binding to alginate in physiological buffer, more sensitive assay procedures have confirmed that such binding does occur at low levels (NICHOLS et al. 1987).

Aminoglycoside diffusion through alginate is reduced (SLACK and NICHOLS 1982) but apparently not enough to modify antibiotic activity in microcolonies. However, some studies have shown that mucoid strains are somewhat less sensitive to aminoglycoside and β-lactam antibiotics (GOVAN and FYFE 1978). These small differences in susceptibility are likely to be a result of the reduced growth rate associated with alginate rather than binding of the drug by alginate.

5. The Rate of Bacterial Growth In Vivo May Be Lower, Reducing Susceptibility to Certain Drugs

Micro-organisms growing in vivo would in almost all circumstances grow significantly slower than in growth medium. Susceptibility to antimicrobial agents may depend upon the rate of growth. This is particularly striking for β-lactam antibiotics. Early studies on the action of penicillin showed bactericidal activity of that compound depends on cell growth (HOBBY et al. 1942). More recent studies have established that in general the rate of killing of *E. coli* is directly proportional to the rate of growth (TUOMANEN et al. 1986). The rate of death is faster for some β-lactams than others (e.g. cefonicid kills faster than CGP17520) but any given drug kills *E. coli* at some rate per generation (COZENS et al. 1986).

The reason for a reduced rate of killing with reduced growth rate is not known. Reasons speculated include the frequency with which a cell-wall component is incorporated to the cell wall or relationship of synthesis of a particular protein relative to growth rate. TUOMANEN et al. (1986) have pointed out that binding of penicillin to PBPs 1a/1b decreased in proportion to growth rate.

TUOMANEN et al. (1986) have also pointed out that bacteria become phenotypically tolerant to β-lactams not only in vitro but also in vivo in animals. Thus these effects are likely to contribute to response in human infections. Organisms which are suppressed but not killed may serve to maintain colonization in the host when antibiotics are withdrawn.

References

Beaudry PH, Marks MI, McDougall D (1980) Is anti-*Pseudomonas* therapy warranted in acute respiratory exacerbations in children with cystic fibrosis. Acta Pediatr 97:144–147

Blessing J, Walker J, Mayberry B (1979) *Pseudomonas cepacia* and multiphilia in the cystic fibrosis patient (abstr). Am Rev Respir Dis 119:262

Blumer JL, Stern RC, Myers CM, Klinger JD, Reed MD (1985) Pharmacokinetics and pharmacodynamics of ciprofloxacin in cystic fibrosis (Abstr 5-40-14). Proceedings of the 14th International Congress of Chemotherapy, Kyoto, p 178

Bryan LE (1984) Mechanisms of action of aminoglycoside antibiotics. In: Root RK, Sande MA (eds) New dimensions in antimicrobial therapy. Churchill Livingston, New York, pp 17–36

Bush K, Sykes RB (1984) Interaction of beta-lactam antibiotics with beta-lactamases as a cause for resistance. In: Bryan LE (ed) Antimicrobial drug resistance. Academic, Orlando, pp 1–32

Cozens RM, Tuomanen E, Tosch W, Zak O, Suter J, Tomasz A (1986) Evaluation of the bactericidal activity of beta-lactam antibiotics on slowly growing bacteria cultured in the chemostat. Antimicrob Agents Chemother 29:797–802

Fisher J (1984) Beta-lactams resistant to hydrolysis by the beta-lactamase. In: Bryan LE (ed) Antimicrobial drug resistance. Academic, Orlando, pp 33–80

Gilligan PH, Gage PA, Welch DF, Muszynski MJ, Wait KR (1987) Prevelance of thymidine-dependent *Staphylococcus aureus* in patients with cystic fibrosis. J Clin Microbiol 25:1258–1261

Godfrey AJ, Bryan LE (1984) Resistance of *Pseudomonas aeruginosa* to new beta-lactamase – resistant beta-lactams. Antimicrob Agents Chemother 26:485–488

Gold R, Overmeyer A, Knie B, Fleming AC, Levinson H (1985) Controlled trial of cetazidime versus ticarcillin and tobramycin in the treatment of acute respiratory exacerbations in patients with cystic fibrosis. Pediatr Infect Dis 4:172–177

Govan JRW, Fyfe JAM (1978) Mucoid *Pseudomonas aeruginosa* and cystic fibrosis: resistance of a mucoid form to carbenicillin, flucloxacillin and tobramycin and the isolation of mucoid variants in vitro. J Antimicrob Chemother 4:233–240

Hobby GL, Meyer K, Chaffee E (1942) Observation on the mechanism of penicillin. Proc Soc Exp Biol Med 50:281–585

Hoiby N (1982) Microbiology of lung infections in cystic fibrosis patients. Acta Paediatr Scand [Suppl] 301:33–54

Hoiby N, Schiotz PO (1982) Immune complex mediated tissue damage in the lungs of cystic fibrosis with *Pseudomonas aeruginosa* infections. Acta Paediatr Scand [Suppl] 301:63–73

Howden R (1981) A new medium for isolation of *Staphylococcus aureus* including thymine requiring strains from sputum. Med Lab Sci 38:29–33

LeBel M, Bergeron MG, Balle F, Fiset C, Chasse G, Bigonesse P, Rivard G (1986) Pharmacokinetics and pharmacodynamics of ciprofloxacin in cystic fibrosis patients. Antimicrob Agents Chemother 30:260–266

Leeder JS, Spino M, Isles AF, Tesoro AM, Gold R, MacLeod SM (1984) Ceftazidime disposition in acute and stable cystic fibrosis. Clin Pharmacol Ther 36:355–362

Levy J (1986) Antibiotic activity in sputum. J Pediatr 108:841–846

Levy J, Smith AL, Koup JR, Williams-Warren J, Ramsey B (1984) Disposition of tobramycin in patients with cystic fibrosis: a perspective controlled study. J Pediatr 105:117–124

Mathews LW, Drotar D (1984) Cystic fibrosis – a challenging long-term chronic disease. Pediatr Clin North Am 31:133–152

McLaughlin FJ, Matthews WJ, Strieder DJ (1983) Clinical and bacteriological reponses to three antibiotic regimens for acute exacerbations of cystic fibrosis: ticarcillin-tobramycin, azlocillin-tobramycin and azlocillo-placebo. J Infect Dis 147:559–567

Prince A (1986) Antibiotic resistance of *Pseudomonas* species. J Pediatr 108:830–834

Rabin HR, Harley FL, Bryan LE, Elfring G (1980) Evaluation of a high dose tobramycin and ticarcillin treatment protocol in cystic fibrosis based on improved susceptibility criteria and antibiotic pharmacokinetics. In: Sturgess J (ed) Perspectives in cystic fibrosis. Canadian Cystic Fibrosis Foundation, Toronto, pp 370–375

Reed MD, Stern RC, O'Brien CA, Crenshaw DA, Blumer JL (1987) Randomized double-blind evaluation of ceftazidime dose ranging in hospitalized patients with cystic fibrosis. Antimicrob Agents Chemother 31:698–702

Sanders CC, Sanders WE (1983) Emergence of resistance during therapy with the newer beta-lactam antibiotics: role of inducible beta-lactamases and implications for the future. Rev Infect Dis 5:639–648

Schryvers AB, Ogunarriwo J, Godfrey AJ, Chamberland S, Rabin HR, Bryan LE (1987) Mechanism of persistence of *Pseudomonas aeruginosa* during treatment of lung infection in cystic fibrosis patients with third generation cephalosporins. Antimicrob Agents Chemother 31:1438–1439

Shalit I, Stutman HR, Marks MI, Chartrand SA, Hilman BC (1987) Randomized study of two dosage regimens of ciprofloxacin for treating chronic bronchopulmonary infection in patients with cystic fibrosis. Am J Med [Suppl 4a] 82:189–195

Slack MPE, Nichols WS (1982) Antibiotic penetrations through bacterial capsules and exopolysaccharides. J Antimicrob Chemother 10:368–372

Sparham PD, Lobban DI, Speller CE (1978) Isolation of *Staphylococcus aureus* from sputum in cystic fibrosis. J Clin Pathol 31:913–918

Spino M, Chai RP, Isles AF (1984) Cloxacillin absorption and disposition in cystic fibrosis. J Pediatr 105:829–835

Stephens D, Garey N, Isles AF (1983) Efficacy of inhaled tobramycin in the treatment of pulmonary exacerbations in children with cystic fibrosis. Pediatr Infect Dis 2:209–211

Tannenbaum CS, Hastie AT, Higgins ML, Kuppers F, Weinbaum G (1984) Inability of purified *Pseudomonas aeruginosa* exopolysaccharide to bind selected antibiotics. Antimicrob Agents Chemother 25:673–675

Tuomanen E, Cozens R, Tosch W, Zak O, Tomasz A (1986) The rate of killing of *Escherichia coli* by beta-lactam antibiotics strictly proportional to the rate of bacterial growth. J Gen Microbiol 132:1297–1304

Vasil ML (1986) *Pseudomonas aeruginosa*: biology, mechanisms of virulence, epidemiology. J Pediatr 108:800–805

Vu H, Nikaido H (1985) Role of beta-lactam hydrolysis in the mechanism of resistance of a beta-lactamase constitutive *Enterobacter cloacae* strain to extended spectrum beta-lactams. Antimicrob Agents Chemother 27:393–398

Wang EL, Prober CG, Manson B, Corey M, Levison H (1984) Association of respiratory viral infections with pulmonary deterioration in patients with cystic fibrosis. N Engl J Med 311:1653–1658

Wood RE, Wanner A, Hirsch J (1985) Tracheal-mucociliary transport in patients with cystic fibrosis and its stimulation by terbutaline. Am Rev Respir Dis 111:733–739

Woods DE, Sokol PA (1985) The use of transposon mutants to assess the role of exo-enzyme S in the chronic pulmonary disease due to *Pseudomonas aeruginosa*. Eur J Clin Microbiol 4:163–169

Wright PF, Khawk T, Oxman MN, Shwachman H (1976) Evaluation of the safety of amantidine. HCL and the role of respiratory viral infection in children with cystic fibrosis. J Infect Dis 134:144–149

Yaffe SJ, Gerbracht LM, Mosovich LL, Mattar ME, Danish M, Jusko WJ (1977) Pharmacokinetics of methicillin in patients with cystic fibrosis. J Infect Dis 135:828–831

CHAPTER 18

Microbes Causing Problems of Antimicrobial Resistance

L. E. BRYAN

A. *Staphylococcus* Species

The mainstay of therapy for both *Staphylococcus aureus* and coagulase negative staphylococci has been β-lactam antibiotics. Resistance to penicillin, normally the result of an inducible β-lactamase, is common in both groups. The β-lactamase is plasmid-specified and resistances to other compounds particularly heavy metals are frequently part of the same plasmid (reviewed by BRUNTON 1984). For practical purposes the widespread distribution of these enzymes and plasmids has rendered penicillin and other staphylococcal penicillinase-susceptible β-lactams ineffective for primary therapy of staphylococcal infections. Plasmids specifying β-lactamase belong to more than one incompatibility group (see Chap. 14, Taylor, this volume) and have been reported to also specify gentamicin resistance (COHEN et al. 1982).

Plasmids are common in staphylococci and range from about 2 to 35 megadaltons in size with 13 incompatibility groups described. Transfer may be by transduction, transformation, conjugation or phage-mediated conjugation. Generally small plasmids specify resistance to one antibiotic with resistance to more drugs associated with larger plasmids (Chap. 14, Taylor, this volume; SCHABERG and ZERBOS 1986).

Strains of staphylococci resistant to penicillinase-resistant beta-lactams are termed methicillin resistant. Methicillin resistant *Staphylococcus aureus* (MRSA) have increased in frequency over the past several years especially in hospitals and particularly large hospitals. For example, in one survey the number of hospitals reporting MRSA increased over four fold between 1975 and 1980 (BOYCE and CAUSEY 1982). Infections with MRSA in medical school associated tertiary referral hospitals of greater than 600 beds rose significantly between 1974 and 1981 (HALEY et al. 1982). MRSA have appeared endemically or as major outbreaks. Patient risk factors to develop MRSA infections include: length of stay; previous therapy with multiple antibiotics or with β-lactamase-resistant β-lactams or cephalosporins; and surgical wound infections. Community outbreaks of MRSA are uncommon but do occur especially in drug users (reviewed in ALDRIDGE 1985).

The mechanism of methicillin resistance is partly understood. MRSA posses an additional penicillin binding protein (PBP), PBP 2a or PBP 2′, which has low affinity for a wide range of β-lactams. Even when other PBPs have bound β-lactam, PBP 2′ continues to be active extensively compensating for the inhibited PBPs. Some morphological effects on the cell particularly increased size were still observed in MRSA treated with β-lactams. In most cases PBP 2′ is inducible by penicillins or cephalosporins. However, penicillinase plasmid-negative strains appear to constitutively produce PBP 2′ (UBUKATA et al. 1985; HARTMAN and TOMASZ 1984; ROSSI et al. 1985). Recently evidence has been provided that the constitutive strains and minority of strains show homogeneous (HOMO) resistance. The HOMO phenotype involves expression of methicillin resistance relatively independently of temperature, pH and salt concentration. The much more common HETERO phenotype results from a small fraction of the population expressing resistance to penicillinase-resistant β-lactams (including most cephalosporins) under usual antibiotic susceptibility testing conditions. If tested at 30° to 35 °C or with hypertonic growth medium a larger fraction of the population expresses resistance. These strains possess a plasmid specifying penicillinase and those producing the most β-lactamase also are the most resistant to penicillinase-resistant β-lactams, cephalosporins and imipenem. It appears that similar regulatory genes may govern expression of PBP 2′ and β-lactamase (BOYCE and MEDEIROS 1987). Thus when large quantities of β-lactamase are induced it seems more of PBP 2′ is induced and resistance to non-hydrolyzable drug is increased.

The mechanism of MRSA makes it clear that resistance is expressed to a wide range of cephalosporins and imipenem in addition to penicillinase-resistant β-lactams. Thus HETERO MRSA should not be treated with β-lactams even though they may appear susceptible when tested at 37 °C and with no increased NaCl in the medium. Effective detection of MRSA can be achieved by the use of 2% NaCl in Mueller-Hinton broth with incubation at 35 °C for 24 h or 6 μg/ml oxicillin or nafcillin or 10 μg/ml methicillin in Mueller-Hinton agar containing 4% sodium chloride. Cephamandole is frequently more active on MRSA in vitro but the significance clinically is unknown. At the present time (late 1987) vancomycin is the drug of choice for MRSA. Resistance to vancomycin is very uncommon although tolerance has rarely been noted.

Gentamicin resistance has been recognized increasingly commonly in *S. aureus* particularly in hospitals. Several outbreaks of gentamicin resistance have been reported. The experience with gentamicin resistance suggests a common evolution for many of the plasmids involved (SCHABERG et al. 1985). These plasmids are self-transferrable and show structural relationships. Another important suggestion has also developed from the study of gentamicin resistant *S. aureus* and *Staphylococcus epidermidis*. It seems probable that *S. epidermidis* serves as a reservoir for resistance which can be transferred to *S. aureus*. Evidence for this probability is based on similar resistance patterns and aminoglycoside modifying enzyme in outbreaks, similar restriction endonuclease patterns of plasmids, interspecies transfer of resistance in vitro or on skin as well as other structural similarities (reviewed in SCHABERG and ZERV 1986). Interestingly, intergeneric transfer of several resistances among different genera of gram-positive cocci has been shown on several occasions (reviewed in SCHABERG and ZERVOS 1986).

Tolerance to β-lactam antibiotics refers to that circumstance where the antibiotic concentration (minimal bactericidal concentration, MBC) needed to produce extensive killing (greater than 99% or greater than 99.9%) is many times (usually ≧32-fold) that needed to cause growth inhibition (minimal inhibitory concentration, MIC). Mechanistically this seems due to reduced activity of the cell wall lytic enzymes. The demonstration of tolerance to β-lactams depends upon testing conditions including growth medium, pH, incubation time, inoculum and temperature. Tolerance has clearly accounted for episodes of clinical failure although its role in a specific clinical circumstance may be difficult to assess (reviewed in PARR and BRYAN 1984a).

Resistance to a variety of other antibiotics has been reported with variable frequency. Resistance to erythromycin, clindamycin, fusidic acid, rifampicin, tetracycline and novobiocin has been recognized as a cause of clinical failure particularly when these agents are used alone. Vancomycin resistance remains extremely rare. Trimethoprim resistance in *S. aureus* has been reported with increasing frequency recently and in one study 10% of *S. aureus* were resistant and 17% of *S. epidermidis*. *S. aureus* to *S. epidermidis* transfer of trimethoprim resistance has also been reported (ARCHER et al. 1986).

Coagulase negative staphylococci comprise a group of species of which the most common pathogen in *S. epidermidis* and most comments which follow refer principally to the latter organism. Infections with these organisms have been increasingly detected over the past several years including an increased frequency of bacteremia. In general they remain low grade pathogens and are usually found in patients with prostheses. Infections are difficult to treat due in part both to the antibiotic resistance of *S. epidermidis* and the presence of a foreign body.

The incidence of resistance to specific antibiotics varies with location and time. However, resistance to several has posed significant problems. These include a high incidence of resistance to penicillin-labile β-lactams, penicillinase-resistant β-lactams (methicillin resistance) and gentamicin. It is probable that methicillin resistance will have a similar explanation in *S. epidermidis*. Certainly cephalosporins and imipenem should not be considered for therapy of methicillin-resistant isolates. Again, vancomycin is the agent of choice in most circumstances where "blind" therapy must be initiated. Aminoglycosides are frequently used in association with vancomycin. Cefamandole is the most active cephalosporin in vitro but the clinical meaning is not known. Netilmicin has been reported to be the most active aminoglycoside but this likely reflects its more limited use.

Resistance to vancomycin is very uncommon. Rifampicin is usually highly active but resistance is a clear risk to develop during therapy if this drug is used alone. The pattern of susceptibility to erythromycin and chloramphenicol is unpredictable. Several centers have reported increased frequencies of resistance to trimethoprim. The combination of the latter with widespread sulfonamide resistance suggests resistance to co-trimoxazole will be more common (DAVIES and STONE 1986; ARCHER et al. 1986).

Several more drugs are under evaluation as antistaphylococcal agents. These include quinolones especially ciprofloxacin, teichoplanin and coumermycin.

B. *Streptococcus* Species

I. *Streptococcus pneumoniae*

Penicillin resistance in *S. pneumoniae* has been described since 1967 (HANSMAN and BULLEN 1967). Since then there have been reports of frequent penicillin resistance often coupled with resistance to other agents. Isolates have been from both children and adults and from hospital or community based investigations (JACOBS et al. 1978; LINARES et al. 1983; CASAL 1982; LATORRE et al. 1985; PEREZ et al. 1987). Penicillin resistance may be present alone or associated with other resistance. Tetracycline resistance has been common and there have been some reports of high frequency of chloramphenicol resistance (LATORRE et al. 1985; PEREZ et al. 1987). Resistance to erythromycin and clindamycin has been generally of low frequency. Co-trimoxazole resistance occurs and was reported as 79.2% of strains in a Spanish study (PEREZ et al. 1987). Low level aminoglycoside resistance is a species characteristic.

Penicillin remains the drug of choice as some penicillin resistance still responds to therapy with the drug. Most of the "resistant" strains have MIC values of 0.1 to 1 µg/ml and are more correctly considered as intermediate in resistance. Resistance levels of greater than or equal to 1 µg/ml are still uncommon in almost all strains (e.g. 3% in a recent study from Spain (PEREZ et al. 1987).

Penicillin resistance is associated with reduced penicillin binding affinity for penicillin and changes in penicillin binding patterns. Additional lower molecular weight bands in the region of PBP 1a of *S. pneumoniae* are likely derived from PBP 1a or, at least, are antigenically related. In the case of PBP 1c, some reduction in the amount of protein may occur in mutants with higher levels of resistance. PBP 2 seems to show mainly a decrease in affinity for penicillin without an associated loss in the quantity of the protein (HANDWERGER and TOMASZ 1986; HAKENBACK et al. 1986).

II. *Streptococcus pyogenes*

Resistance to penicillin is extremely rare. Tetracycline resistance has been reported commonly and chloramphenicol and sulfonamide resistance, although less common, still occur frequently. Erythromycin resistance (MLS type) has been described on several occasions but its overall frequency generally remains low. The small MLS type resistance plasmid pAC1 is from *S. pyogenes* and can transfer to other streptococci and *S. aureus* (SCHABERG and ZERBOS 1986). Several other plasmids specifying erythromycin resistance have been described (CLEWELL 1981).

III. *Streptococcus faecalis*[1]

Intrinsic resistance occurs to many commonly used antibiotics including aminoglycosides, penicillins, cephalosporins and clindamycin. Acquired resistance to erythromycin, chloramphenicol and tetracycline is common. High level streptomycin, kanamycin and gentamicin resistance has been increasingly detected. Enterococci also show relatively poor susceptibility to many recently introduced cephalosporins. Use of the latter may select for the emergence of infections due to *S. faecalis* because of their low susceptibility to this group of compounds.

Beta-lactamase activity has been described in a small number of *S. faecalis* isolates. In two strains studied the β-lactamase was similar but specified different plasmids which were both transferable. Among β-lactams to which resistance was

[1] Now termed *Enterococcus fecalis*

specified were penicillin, ampicillin and piperacillin. In both cases β-lactamase was linked to erythromycin and gentamicin resistance and in one case was also linked to streptomycin, tetracycline and chloramphenicol resistance (MURRAY et al. 1986).

Therapy for serious *S. faecalis* infections particularly endocarditis normally involves the use of a β-lactam and an aminoglycoside. The combination of the two apparently overcomes the low level of aminoglycoside resistance secondary to the fermentative metabolism of these organisms. However, in the last several years high level of resistance to streptomycin, kanamycin and gentamicin has been described. This level of resistance prevents therapy with the aminoglycosides. High level resistance to streptomycin is both ribosomal and enzymatic whereas that due to gentamicin is enzymatic only. Several different enzyme activities have been described giving rise to resistance to the above drugs as well as amikacin and tobramycin (MEDERSKI-SAMORAI and MURRAY 1983; HORODNICEANU et al. 1979; KROGSTAD et al. 1978; COURVALIN et al. 1980).

The high level aminoglycoside resistance and the more uncommon β-lactamase seem to be plasmid specified. Recently, LEBLANC et al. (1986) have shown that the relatively common resistance to erythromycin, kanamycin and streptomycin among human and animal sources of *S. faecalis* had homology with R-plasmid pJH1 which specifies these same resistances. Furthermore, in a set of plasmids examined in more detail these resistances were inherited as a unit on a 9–11 kilobase (kb) pair segment of DNA. The erythromycin resistance is transposable by a unit essentially identical to Tn*917*. This transposon specifies erythromycin resistance and is a conjugative transposon (resistance transfer occurs in the absence of plasmid DNA) like Tn*916* which specifies tetracycline resistance. The phenomenon also occurs in other streptococci (A, B, F and G) and in *S. pneumoniae* (CLEWELL 1981).

Plasmids in *S. faecalis* fall into two general categories. MLS-type resistance is usually on a 20–30 kb pair "broad-host" range plasmid which does not transfer in broth. Larger plasmids (greater than 45 kb) usually encode for several resistances, have a narrow host range, are pherome responsive and transfer in both broth and on filter matings (reviewed in SCHABERG and ZERBOS 1986).

Resistance transfer between streptococci and staphylococci occurs, suggesting that resistance determinants may be widely distributed among gram-positive cocci in this manner. Courvalin et al. have suggested that a gentamicin modifying enzyme in *S. faecalis* originated in *S. aureus* (COURVALIN et al. 1980).

Intrinsically penicillin-resistant *Streptococcus faeceium* strains have a slow reacting PBP5. Those strains which demonstrated this PBP were relatively more resistant to penicillin and were inhibited with a penicillin concentration saturating the low affinity PBP5. A *S. faeceium* mutant deficient in PBP5 production had a similar level of susceptibility to penicillin. It seems probable that the slow reacting PBP5 found in *S. faeceium* is responsible both for their natural intrinsic insusceptibility and when overproduced for greater resistance to penicillin. Low level β-lactam resistance is widespread among *S. faecalis* and the preceding seems the most likely explanation (FONTANA et al. 1983, 1985).

IV. *Haemophilus influenzae*

A problem of major significance was the emergence of β-lactamase mediated ampicillin resistance in approximately 1974 at several international locations. Since that time there has been a steady progression in the incidence of ampicillin resistant isolates in several parts of the world. However, it is worth noting that the incidence of resistant strains does vary considerably depending upon geographical location and among types. In general resistant levels in most locations range between 15% and 30% (WILLIAMS and MOOSDEEN 1986; BRUNTON et al. 1986). Occasionally higher levels of resistance have been reported such as a resistance level of 41% in blood and CSF strains from Spain (CAMPOS et al. 1984).

The most common basis for resistance has been plasmid specified β-lactamase activity. The most frequent β-lactamase has been the TEM enzyme although at least one additional enzyme (ROB-1) has been reported (RUBIN et al. 1981; MEDEIROS et al. 1986).

Beta-lactamase inhibitors including clavulanic acid and sulbactam inhibit the β-lactam hydrolytic activity of the TEM β-lactamase. A combination of these inhibitors with susceptible β-lactams restores the activity of these drugs. In addition the TEM type β-lactamase does not have significant activity for many modern cephalosporins which show high activity on *Haemophilus influenzae* including, for example, cefuroxime, ceftriaxone, cefotaxime, and several others. Chloramphenicol has frequently been combined with ampicillin to treat meningitis due to *H. influenzae* in the past. This combination remains effective on ampicillin resistant isolates because the incidence of chloramphenicol resistance is low in most parts of the world. Chloramphenicol resistance is due to a chloramphenicol acetyl transferase. Although chloramphenicol and ampicillin resistance specified by a single plasmid has been described (BRYAN 1978; SMITH 1983) this combination has remained rare.

β-Lactam resistance not associated with β-lactamase has been described on several occasions and shown to account for therapeutic failure. At least some of this resistance is due to reduced affinity of penicillin binding proteins for ampicillin and other β-lactams (PARR and BRYAN 1984b; MENDELMAN et al. 1984). Strains demonstrating β-lactam resistance due to modification of penicillin binding proteins have a wider spectrum of β-lactam resistance than that associated with β-lactamase but in many instances it is of a lower level. However, some level of resistance is almost always expressed to the therapeutically most active cephalosporins, for example, cefotaxime. To date this has not been of a level which has resulted in clinical failure. It is probable that an additional mutation or mutations would be necessary to raise the level of resistance to a drug like cefotaxime to a high enough level to be therapeutically ineffective. However, it has been shown in laboratory mutants that the potential through mutation to reach relatively high levels of resistance exists in *Escherichia coli* (HEDGE and SPRATT 1985). It is therefore predictable that more resistant isolates may emerge with wider distribution of the low level resistant mutants associated with defective penicillin binding proteins.

Resistance to other antibiotics occurs with reasonable frequency although again this varies with time and location. Resistant levels of 10% for tetracycline and 28% for sulfonamides have been reported from Britain, for example (WILLIAMS and ANDREWS 1974). Rifampicin resistance has been reported to occur after rifampicin prophylaxis (MURPHY et al. 1981; NICOLLE et al. 1982). Again, resistance to co-trimoxaxole has been variable with most locations reporting a low incidence of resistance. However, with a worldwide increase in trimethoprim resistance and a significant base of sulfonamide resistance within *H. influenzae* it is likely that there will be a progressive increase in co-trimoxacole resistance among isolates.

Plasmids have been widely reported in *H. influenzae*. These tend to fall into two groups. In the first group the size of the plasmids have varied from 30 to 41 megadaltons and specified single or multiple resistance to ampicillin, chloramphenicol, tetracycline and kanamycin. The second group of plasmids are smaller in the range of 3–7 megadaltons and specify ampicillin resistance. The larger plasmids can transfer among *Haemophilus* species whereas the smaller plasmids are not self-transferable. Ampicillin resistance is specified by the Tn*A* sequence in both the large and small plasmids. There seems to be an extensive relationship between the small *β*-lactamase plasmids of *H. influenzae*, *Haemophilus ducreyi* and *Neisseria gonorrhoeae*. Current evidence is consistent with the view that the small *β*-lactamase plasmids of both *N. gonorrhoeae* and *Haemophilus* species originated by the insertion of Tn*A* into cryptic replicons found commonly in *Haemophilus parainfluenzae*. Presumably the plasmids were then transferred to *H. influenzae* and *N. gonorrhoeae*. However, evidence suggests that the sulfonamide resistance plasmids detected in *H. ducreyi* may have originated from the *Enterobacteriaceae*.

Haemophilus parainfluenzae, a common commensal may act as a reservoir of antibiotic resistance plasmids for *Haemophilus influenzaes* (BRUNTON et al. 1986). Evidence is consistent with the view that *H. parainfluenzae* may transfer this resistance to *H. influenzae* and *N. gonorrhoeae* as noted. However, it is also important to note that it has been extremely difficult to demonstrate direct plasmid transfer from *H. parainfluenzae* to *N. gonorrhoeae* (reviewed in BRUNTON et al. 1986).

The conjugative plasmids of *Haemophilus influenzae* have a guanine plus cytosine content similar to that of the *Haemophilus* chromosome. These plasmids seem to share a high degree of homology, indicating they are related (see ALBRITTON 1984; BRUNTON 1984).

V. *Neisseria gonorrhoeae*

Benzylpenicillin has been the most extensively used therapy for gonorrhoea. In the middle 1950s therapeutic failure with penicillin was observed with increasing frequency. Since that time a significant number of strains have been isolated which show reduced susceptibility to penicillin. Until approximately 1976 the majority of these strains showed low level resistance and rarely had MIC values in excess of 2 µg/ml. Most gonococcal genital infections due to such isolates still could be effectively treated, for example with 4.8 million units of penicillin used with 1 gram of oral probenicid. In 1976 isolates of *N. gonorrhoeae* producing *β*-lactamase and resistant to penicillin and ampicillin appeared in the Far East and England. These isolates have now been recognized from many parts of the world and occur both endemically and epidemically at many international locations. More recently in the last few years there have been increased reports of chromosomally mediated penicillin resistance expressed at relatively high levels and associated with a high frequency of therapeutic failure (FARUKI et al. 1985). In addition plasmid mediated resistance to tetracycline and chromosomally mediated resistance to erythromycin and trimethoprim sulfomethoxazole have been increasingly noted. In particular an increase in high-level plasmid-specified tetracycline resistance has been noted (MMWR 1986; KNAPP et al. 1987). Tetracycline remains widely used in clinical practise for coverage of both *Chlamydia trachomatis* and *N. gonorrhoeae*.

Spectinomycin has been used widely to treat penicillinase producing strains and in many instances chromosomally mediated β-lactam resistant isolates. Once again, resistance to this drug has been reported, with increased frequency resulting in approximately 8% therapeutic failures in one recent study (BOSLEGO et al. 1987). Spectinomycin resistance can occur both as a result of the chromosomal mutation affecting ribosomal structure or the presence of adenylylating enzymes which can inactivate spectinomycin. To date most evidence favors the former mechanism as the major cause of resistance in *N. gonorrhoeae* although more information is necessary to make a definite conclusion. Penicillinase producing strains remain susceptible to many of the recently introduced cephalosporins. For example, ceftriaxone is highly effective after a single dose for *N. gonococcal* infections (ZAJDOWICZ et al. 1983; HANDSFIELD and MURPHY 1983).

Penicillinase producing isolate of *N. gonorrhoeae* are resistant both to penicillin and ampicillin. Resistance is specified by means of the TEM β-lactamase normally specified by a 3.4–4.7 megadalton plasmid. These plasmids contain a partial Tn*A* sequence which includes the information for the β-lactamase. The difference between the 3.4 and 4.7 megadalton plasmids is due to the insertion of a 1.3 megadalton sequence which is also found in *H. ducreyi*. There is some evidence that this 1.3 megadalton sequence may be an insertion element. In addition to small plasmids specifying β-lactamase it is common to detect a 2.7 megadalton cryptic plasmid in isolates of *N. gonorrhoeae*. A conjugative plasmid of 24.5 megadaltons is also widely distributed in *N. gonorrhoeae* and is capable of mobilizing the small plasmids. Its host range, which includes *N. gonorrhoeae*, has been reported to also include *N. cinerea* (reviewed in BRUNTON et al. 1986 and ALBRITTON 1984).

There have been reports of penicillinase producing *N. gonorrhoeae* from essentially all parts of the world. Interestingly a decline in the prevelance of these strains has been reported among US military personnel in the Republic of Korea (BOSLEGO et al. 1987).

C. Gram-Negative Aerobic Bacilli

I. Gastrointestinal Pathogens

1. *Shigella*

Resistance to a variety of antimicrobial agents is widespread but the frequency in any given locale and in an individual species varies significantly. The major problem results from R plasmids, which were first described in bacteria in *Shigella* in 1959.

Multiresistant strains of *S. dysenteriae* have been described from several countries as outbreaks. Strains arising in Central America, Bangladesh, India, and Sri Lanka carried B incompatibility plasmids and specified chloramphenicol and tetracycline resistance and in some cases streptomycin and sulfonamide resistance. *S. dysenteriae* from African countries also included ampicillin resistance and was encoded by incompatibility group X plasmids and group I_1 plasmids which specified ampicillin, sulfonamide, trimethoprim, tetracycline, chloramphenicol and streptomycin resistances. Streptomycin and sulfonamide resistance often reside on a nonconjugative plasmid.

Overall among the other species of *Shigella*, resistance to tetracycline, chloramphenicol, sulfonamides, streptomycin, kanamycin and more recently co-trimoxazole (sulfametoxazole and trimethoprim) is frequently detected. However, as pointed out by Murray the extent and incidence varies substantially. Resistance to streptomycin, tetracyclines, ampicillin and chloramphenicol rose steadily from 1974 to 1982 in Great Britain. During this time period resistance to sulfonamides was uniformally high and a clear but small rise in trimethoprim resistance occurred from 1979 to 1982 (ROWE and THRELFALL 1984; MURRAY 1986).

In summary antimicrobial resistance is common among isolates of *Shigella* and when therapy is warranted it should be accompanied by antimicrobial susceptibility testing.

2. *Salmonella*

Chloramphenicol is a major drug used in the treatment of typhoid fever. Outbreaks of chloramphenicol-resistant *Salmonella typhi* have been reported on several occasions. These have been due to plasmids of incompatibility group H_1 and include isolates from outbreaks in Mexico and India as well as isolates from sporadic resistance in Chile and Southeast Asia and endemic resistance from Thailand. Other resistances specified with H_1 plasmids include tetracycline, streptomycin and sulfonamide (ROWE and THRELFALL 1984).

Among the nontyphoid *Salmonella* serotypes, antimicrobial resistance can be a problem. In the U.S. in a survey of 211 nationwide hospitals for the period of 1975 to 1984 resistance to ampicillin (14%–24%) and tetracycline (18%–31%) was most common with resistance to co-trimoxazole (3%–7%) and chloramphenicol (2%–6%) being lower (LORIAN 1986).

Outbreaks of resistance in nontyphoid *Salmonella* have been reported among several serotypes from many countries of South America, the Middle East, Africa, and the Indian subcontinent. Most outbreaks have been associated with plasmids of the F_1me incompatibility group. Resistance to ampicillin, chloramphenicol, tetracycline, streptomycin and sulfonamides has been most common but resistance to kanamycin, trimethoprim and gentamicin also occurs. Many cases from outbreaks were characterized by the severity of the enteritis produced (ROWE and THRELFALL 1984).

Based on reports from various areas of the world it appears that co-trimoxazole resistance frequency is rising (MURRAY 1986). Resistance among different serotypes may vary markedly within a single country. This may be due to use of the drug for animal rearing or in certain countries due to drugs used for human infections (MURRAY 1986; ROWE and THRELFALL 1984).

In most cases of nontyphoid *Salmonella* enteritis antimicrobial therapy is not warranted unless complications occur.

3. *Vibrio cholerae*

Transferable resistance in *V. cholerae* was detected from strains isolated in the Philippines as early as 1964. Subsequently there have been several reports from Algeria, Tanzania, Bangladesh, and Zaire of further resistance. Many have been in the E1 Tor biotype. All plasmids belong to the C-incompatibility group.

Tetracycline is the drug of choice when antimicrobial agents are used for *Cholera*. Many resistant isolates have specified tetracycline resistance but resistance to chloramphenicol, sulfonamide, trimethoprim and ampicillin has been a common part of the phenotype (DUPONT et al. 1985; ROWE and THRELFALL 1986).

4. Enterotoxigenic *E. coli*

Information on resistance is less available as the susceptibility testing of these organisms is less common. However, resistance does occur and seems more prevalent to ampicillin, tetracyclines and sulfonamides. Resistance to chloramphenicol seems generally low and co-trimoxazole resistance may be on the increase. Linkage between both heat-labile (LT) and heat-stable (ST) toxin production and antibiotic resistance is regonized to occur in some circumstances. Resistance in strains of *E. coli* following doxycycline prophylaxis for traveller's diarrhea has been reported (MCCONNEL et al. 1979; STIEGLITZ et al. 1980; MURRAY 1986; ESCHEVERIA et al. 1978; SACK et al. 1978).

5. *Campylobacter* Species

Antimicrobial therapy is not indicated for most cases of enteritis due to *Campylobacter jejuni*. Erythromycin is usually considered the drug of choice for therapy but resistance has been detected, for example, 8% in a recent study. Resistance to trimethoprim is extremely common but is uncommon to ampicillin, fluoroquinolones, several new cephalosporins (cefpirome, cefotaxime, ceftazidime) furazolidone and the rifamycin compound ansamycin (VAN DER AUWER and SCORNEAUX 1985). Plasmid-mediated resistance has only been shown to occur for tetracycline and kanamycin resistance. Studies with the latter have shown that aminoglycoside resistant determinants *aph*A-1 and *aph*A-3 may have arisen from *Enterobacteriaceae* and gram-positive organisms respectively. Plasmids are common in *C. jejuni* and *E. coli* but only tetracycline resistance correlated with the presence of plasmids (TENOVER et al. 1985; TAYLOR et al. 1983; OUELLETTE et al. 1987).

Recently *Campylobacter pylori* (*pyloridis*) has been correlated with gastritis and may play an etiological role in this common disease. Although the organism shows in vitro susceptibility to penicillin G, ampicillin, some cephalosporins, aminoglycosides, erythromycin, tetracycline and rifampicin in vitro, its eradication in vivo has been difficult. This may be due to the relatively hostile environment posed by the stomach in the form of low acidity and gastric mucus. Bismuth subcitrate combined with amoxycillin has been somewhat more active and shows syngerism with oxolinic acid, rifampixin and several β-lactams (VAN CAEKENBERGAG and BREYSSENS 1987; LAMBERT et al. 1986).

6. *Yersinia enterocolitica*

Resistance to erythromycin and to many β-lactams is frequent on a species basis. All strains have been reported to produce at least one β-lactamase. Several newer β-lactams, however, do possess excellent activity including cefotaxime, ceftriaxone, imipenem, and ceftazidime. Most isolates are susceptible to several aminoglycosides, tetracyclines and chloramphenicol (HORNSTEIN et al. 1985; BRYAN 1982).

7. *Aeromonas* Species

Aeromonas hydrophilia, *A. caviae* and *A. sobria* are resistant to many of the older penicillins and cephalosporins. However, newer cephalosporins including cefotaxime, gentamicin, chloramphenicol, tetracyclines and co-trimoxazole are usually very active. *A. hydrophilia* is generally less susceptible than the other two strains (MOTYL et al. 1985).

II. Nosocomial Gram-Negative Bacteria

As a group antimicrobial resistance has been a major problem. This has been especially so with *Klebsiella* species and *Pseudomonas aeruginosa*. Resistance problems among *Serratia*, *Enterobacter*, *Proteus*, *Providencia*, *E. coli*, *Citrobacter*, *Morganella* and *Acinetobacter* have also occurred commonly.

1. *Pseudomonas aeruginosa*

Pseudomonas aeruginosa remains an important opportunistic pathogen causing in particular pulmonary and septicemic infections of a severe nature. The resistance problem in this organism arises in three major ways – intrinsic resistance, adaptive resistance produced by mechanisms of persistence and by acquisition of new genetic material in the form of plasmids and transposons.

The most common plasmids in *P. aeruginosa* are host restricted for host range, are of very large molecular weight and belong to the P-2 incompatibility group. However, plasmids of other groups do occur albeit at a lower frequency. These plasmids have been shown to specify a wide range of β-lactamase and aminoglycoside modifying enzymes and resistance to tetracycline, sulfonamides, chloramphenicol and mercury boron, tellurium and other agents. Some plasmids like the P-1 group do have a wide host range which includes *P. aeruginosa* and may serve to transmit resistance genes to and from *P. aeruginosa* (JACOBY 1984; BRYAN 1982).

Plasmid mediated resistance has been most of the problem in outbreaks of resistance usually associated with high concentrations of drug such as by topical use or in the urinary tract (LOWBURY et al. 1972; HOLDER 1976).

Intrinsic resistance in *P. aeruginosa* to many antibiotics results from the combination of poor permeability of the outer membrane and chromosomally mediated enzymatic resistance (BRYAN 1979). Thus, resistances to many of the older β-lactams is due to the presence of an inducible chromosomally specified β-lactamase (SABATH and ABRAHAM 1964). The same seems true for widespread kanamycin resistance due to a chromosomally specified aminoglycoside phosphorylating enzyme. In addition it has been shown that *P. aeruginosa* has two sizes of F-porin pore diameter. The majority are of small diameter and low permeability (WOODRUFF et al. 1986). Thus many antimicrobials that use the porin mediate pathway such as chloramphenicol and tetracycline have poor activity. The low penetration rate for many β-lactams enhances β-lactam resistance through a combination of that effect and the chromosomally specified β-lactamase. On the other hand most aminoglycosides are active because they bind and partially disrupt the phosphate-rich outer membrane of *P. aeruginosa*. In this manner their penetration rate is improved. Polymyxin activity is also facilitated by the phosphate-rich LPS of the *P. aeruginosa* outer membrane.

The third form of resistance seen with *P. aeruginosa* is particularly under circumstances where host defenses are compromised. A set of adaptive changes may occur that cause reduced antimicrobial susceptibility and may also be associated with reduced growth rates. These changes are effective for producing therapeutic failure, slow response or recurrence of the infection. Many of the adaptive changes are unstable and in the absence of the antibiotics such as under routine isolation procedures in many microbiology laboratories the susceptible revertants may overgrow the resistant isolates and the presence of the latter may not be detected. Because this form of resistance has clearly different properties seen from that associated with plasmid-specified resistance, it is better thought of as an independent process. For this reason the processes involved have been termed mechanism of persistence. Such mechanisms are often found due to decreased drug entry (aminoglycosides, fluoroquinolones), constitutive expression of normally inducible enzymes (β-lactams) and modified targets (β-lactams) (see Chap. 17).

Other species of *Pseudomonas* show severe intrinsic resistance to several antibiotics particularly *P. cepacia* and *P. multiphilia*.

2. Enteric Bacilli

Pneumonic, urinary, septicemic, neurological and other infections involving intensive care, urology, burn, neurosurgical, pediatric and geriatric hospital units have been major problems of antimicrobial resistance. This has been especially so with species of *Klebsiella*, *Serratia*, *Providencia*, *Enterobacter*, *Proteus*, *Acinetobacter* and *Citrobacter*. As with *Pseudomonas* intrinsic resistance is of importance particularly for certain organisms like *Providencia* and *Acinetobacter*. Plasmid acquired resistance plays a role in all but seems especially important for *Klebsiella* with frequent spread to *Serratia*, *E. coli*, *Enterobacter*, *Proteus* and *Citrobacter*.

Outbreaks of resistant bacteria likely result from a single type of resistant bacterium which may frequently colonize the gut and spread to other body sites. The isolate may be transmitted to other patients. However, molecular methods have now shown that the related plasmids appear in different genera during these outbreaks thus confirming plasmid spread among strains (see Chap. 16). Many examples have been shown to support this process. One example involved multiply-resistant isolates from a urological unit. These involve *Serratia marcescens*, *Proteus* (*Morganella*) *morganii*, *Proteus vulgaris*, *E. coli* and *Enterobacter* species. The first four species harbored an IncC plasmid of 120 megadaltons shown by hybridization studies to be very closely related. The 160 megadalton plasmid of *Enterobacter* was not related (GRIFFIN et al. 1985).

Many of the plasmid-mediated outbreaks of multiple resistance can be controlled by improved infection control and better use of antibiotics. Reduction or elimination of the use of antibiotics from a unit or reduction of use of topical agents has been shown to have effectively controlled such resistance (PRICE and SLEIGH 1970; LOWBERRY et al. 1972).

Resistance to β-lactams, aminoglycosides, tetracycline, chloramphenicol, sulfonamides and trimethoprim are frequently specified. Plasmids specifying these resistance has been of several different incompatibility groups.

Resistance of enteric bacilli has been only of limited importance outside of hospitals. Resistance occurring within the course of a treatment occurs occasionally perhaps most commonly with nalidixic acid due to a mutation affecting DNA gyrase.

The pattern of resistance of bacteria from a mean of 242 hospitals in the U.S. from 1971 to 1982 has been reported by ATKINSON and LORIAN (1984). Among *E. coli*, *P. mirabilis* and *K. pneumoniae* no major population shift in resistance percentage has occurred. A trend to decreasing susceptibility to gentamicin and perhaps tobramycin has been noted from about 1977 to 1982 for *P. aeruginosa*. Thus, there has not been an overall trend to higher resistance in a large population sample of these isolates. However, this study does not reflect on the importance of the outbreaks which occur in hospitals and individual hospital units and which pose major problems for a limited time. Such isolates represent a relatively small fraction of the huge numbers of enteric bacteria isolated annually in the United States and subjected to susceptibility testing.

III. Mycobacteria

The nomenclature used to describe resistance in mycobacteria includes the following categories. Primary resistance includes those strains of mycobacteria which are naturally resistant or when resistance has been acquired from another individual. Initial resistance is the isolation of a resistant strain from an individual who claims not to have had chemotherapy. Acquired resistance is that situation in which there has been a history of unsuccessful chemotherapy. Initial resistance includes both primary resistance and undisclosed acquired resistance.

Among isolates of *Mycobacterium tuberculosis* there is a higher level of primary drug resistance in developing countries than in the so-called developed countries. However, the incidence of resistance in the community does not seem to represent a major problem to control of tuberculosis. The reason for this statement is that the incidence of primary resistance even in developing countries is not seriously high and the rate of further development of resistance appears relatively slow. In addition it is also clear that drug resistance to isoniazid or to isoniazid and streptomycin does not normally result in failure of the drug regimen of isoniazid rifampicin and ethambutol or to the same three drugs plus pyrazinamide.

In developing countries it is particularly difficult to get a true esimate of the level of primary resistance. Under conditions where testing criteria have been adequate and where true histories of previous treatment have been obtained in Madras some reliable resistance levels have been reported. In 1957 the resistance level to isoniazid was 4% and streptomycin 4% and 1% to combined drugs. In 1975 the resistance level to isoniazid was 7% to streptomycin 15% and to both 4% (MITCHISON 1984).

There is also some evidence that highly isoniazid-resistant *M. tuberculosis* are of slightly reduced pathgenicity in man. In some circumstances it is also felt that there is a probability of resistant strains reverting to sensitive strains or to have overgrowth of resistant strains by sensitive strains.

In the event of failure of therapy particularly to isoniazid, resistance is common. It has been reported that the situation is different for a relapse where organisms are usually susceptible. In both circumstances this is an indication for susceptibility testing. The other major indication for susceptibility testing is for epidemiological surveys for resistance.

It is clear that high levels of acquired resistance to antituberculous drugs do exist in some developing countries. It has been suggested that a high prevelance of resistance is an indication of inadequate arrangements for treatment in that community. Levels of primary or initial resistance have been reported, for example, as 9.3% to any antituberculous drug in Tanzania to 20.4% to any drug in India. On the other hand, acquired resistance levels have been reported as about 62% from Hong Kong and 81.7% from the UK to any antituberculous drug (MITCHISON 1984).

In the case of leprosy there has been a marked increase in the prevelance of dapsone resistance over a 30-year period. This would seem to be due to the use of monotherapy. It has been estimated that about 10% of newly diagnosed patients in some centers may have resistant strains (MITCHISON 1984).

In the case of mycobacteria other than *M. tuberculosis* and *Mycobacterium leprae* there is widespread antimicrobial resistance. Most of this resistance is natural resistance and not acquired resistance. An agent which has become important particularly in AIDS patients is the *Mycobacterium avium–Mycobacterium intracellurare* complex. This group demonstrates resistance in vitro to most antituberculous drugs. If treatment is required the combination of isoniazid, ethambutol and rifampicin for 18–24 months plus streptomycin for the first 2–3 months is often used for pulmonary disease. The drugs clofazimine and ansamycin have shown promise by in vitro testing but have been generally unsuccessful clinically. However, evaluation of these drugs is incomplete at this time. *Mycobacterium scrofulaceum* shows resistance to isoniazid, streptomycin, ethambutol and paraaminosalysilic acid (PAS). *M. kansasii* is frequently susceptible to rifampicin and shows only low resistance to isoniazid, ethambutal and streptomycin. Among *M. fortuitum – chelonae* complex, *M. simiae*, *M. ulcerans* and *M. haemophilum* resistance to several drugs is common (WOODS and WASHINGTON 1987).

IV. *Bacteroides* Species

Bacteroides fragilis and members of the *B. fragilis* group of anaerobes are important pathogens from clinical materials. In general members of the *B. fragilis* group are somewhat more resistant to antimicrobial agents than *B. fragilis* itself. β-lactamase activity principally of a cephalosporinase type is widespread among *B. fragilis* and members of the *B. fragilis* group. These cephalosporinases probably associated with relatively poor antibiotic permeability account for widespread resistance to many β-lactams including ampicillin and benzylpenicillin. *B. gracilis* is a recently recognized important pathogen in deep tissue infections. It shows extensive β-lactam resistance but that is not associated with the presence of β-lactamase.

Several β-lactam antibiotics do show high levels of activity on *B. fragilis* and the *B. fragilis* group. These include particularly cefoxitin and imipenem. The combination of ampicillin and sulbactam also seems highly active on this group of organisms.

Several non-β-lactam antibiotics have substantial activity on *B. fragilis* and the *B. fragilis* group of organisms. These include metronidazole, chloramphenicol and clindamycin. Resistance to metronidazole is highly uncommon and this drug has been shown to have good efficacy clinically. Resistance to clindaymicin has been reported more recently. Plasmid specified transferable clindamycin resistance has been described. WEXLER and FINEGOLD (1987) have recently pointed out that of 30 patients with pulmonary and orofacial infections due to oral bacteroides, about one-third of isolates showed high level resistance. This group of isolates plus another third which showed a low level of resistance were reported to be unlikely to respond to clindamycin therapy. In general resistance to chloramphenicol is low although the susceptibility level tends to be very close to the breakpoint for determining susceptibility to this organism.

Recently transferable cefoxitin resistance has been reported in isolates of *B. fragilis* specifying a β-lactamase capable of hydrolyzing cefoxitin. This form of resistance remains relatively limited (CUCHURAL et al. 1983). More recently PIDDOCK and WISE (1987) have also described *Bacteroides* species which appear to have reduced affinity of two penicillin binding proteins and perhaps a change in outer membrane protein. It is likely in the case of *B. gracilis* that either or both of the latter two mechanisms account for β-lactam resistance due to the failure to detect β-lactamase in these organisms.

Tetracycline resistance has been reported to be widespread among *B. fragilis* and in general is no longer considered as a drug of choice for infections due to this group of bacteria. Anaerobic bacteria are intrinsically resistant to aminoglycosides because of their markedly reduced transport of the compound resulting from reduced rates of electron transport and reduced magnitude of electrical potential (BRYAN and KWAN 1981).

V. *Legionella pneumophila*

Erythromycin with or without rifampicin has been used widely in the treatment of infections due to this organism. Susceptibility testing using a pneumonia model in guinea pigs has shown rifampicin, erythromycin, doxycycline, trimethoprim, sulfamethoxazole and ciprofloxacin to be effective. β-Lactam antibiotics and gentamicin in the animal model were not active (Edelstein et al. 1984). More recently susceptibility testing using monocyte associated *L. pneumophila* has more or less paralleled these results although gentamicin was found effective. In addition the latter study also showed that several fluoroquinolone antibiotics appeared to have activity as well (Havlichek et al. 1987).

VI. Miscellaneous Bacteria

In general there are a large number of other microorganisms for which antimicrobial resistance has not been a problem. Tetracycline is widely used to treat mycoplasma and ureaplasma and for the most part these organisms remain susceptible. A small number of strains resistant to tetracycline have been described in the case of *Ureaplasma urealyticum*. However, these strains remain susceptible to erythromycin. *Chlamydia trachomatis* although not widely tested for susceptibility remains clinically responsive to tetracyclines and erythromycin. Chlorhexidine and povodone-iodine are effective disinfectants for this organism. Significant resistance among *Chlamydia trachomatis* has not yet been reported. *Gardnerella vaginallis* is frequently treated with metronidazole. It is also susceptible to ampicillin, erythromycin and several other β-lactams. Antimicrobial resistance has not been reported as a problem among isolates of *Brucella*, *Francicella tularensis*, *Yersinia pestis*, *Pasteurella multiceda* and *Bordetella pertussis*.

References

Albritton WL (1984) Resistant plasmids of *Haemophilus* and *Neisseria*. In: Bryan LE (ed) Antimicrobial drug resistance, chap. 18. Academic, Orlando, pp 515–529

Aldridge KE (1985) Methicillin resistance *Staphylococcus aureus*: clinical and laboratory features. Infect Control 6:461–465

Archer GL, Coughter JP, Johnston JL (1986) Plasmid-encoded trimethoprim resistance in Staphylococci. Antimicrob Agents Chemother 29:733–740

Atkinson BA, Lorian V (1984) Antimicrobial agents susceptibility patterns of bacteria in hospitals from 1971–1982. J Clin Microbiol 20:791–796

Boslego JW, Tramont EC, Takfuji ET, Diniega BM, Mitchell BS, Small JW, Khan WN, Stein DC (1987) Effective spectinomycin use on the prevalence of spectinomycin-resistant and penicillinase-producing *Neisseria gonorrhoeae*. N Engl J Med 317:272–278

Boyce JM, Causey WA (1982) Increasing occurrence of methicillin-resistance *Staphylococcus aureus* in the United States. Infect Control 3:377–383

Boyce JM, Medeiros AA (1987) Role of beta-lactamase in expression of resistance by methicillin-resistant *Staphylococcus aureus*. Antimicrob Agents Chemother 31:1426–1428

Brunton J (1984) Antibiotic resistance plasmids of streptococci, staphylococci and *Bacteroides*. In: Bryan LE (ed) Antimicrobial drug resistance, chap 19. Academic, Orlando, pp 530–565

Brunton J, Clare D, Meier MA (1986) Molecular epidemiology of antibiotic resistance plasmids of *Haemophilus* species and *Neisseria gonorrhoeae*. Rev Infect Dis 8:713–724

Bryan LE (1978) Transferable chloramphenicol and ampicillin resistance in strain *Haemophilus influenzae*. Antimicrob Agents Chemother 14:154–156
Bryan LE (1979) Resistance to antimicrobial agents: the general nature of the problem and the basis of resistance. In: Doggett RG (ed) *Pseudomonas aeruginosa*, chap 9. Academic, Press, New York, pp 219–271
Bryan LE (1982) Bacterial resistance and susceptibility to chemotherapeutic agents. Cambridge University Press, Cambridge, Chaps 4, 6, pp 104–134, 161–191
Bryan LE, Kwan S (1981) Mechanisms of resistance of anaerobic bacteria and facultative bacteria grown anaerobically. J Antimicrob Chemother 8 [Suppl D]:1–8
Campos J, Garcia-Tornel F, Sanfeliu I (1984) Susceptibility studies of multiply resistant *Haemophilus influenzae* isolated from pediatric patients and contacts. Antimicrob Agents Chemother 25:706–709
Casal J (1982) Antimicrobial susceptibility of *Streptococcus pneumoniae*: serotype distribution of penicillin-resistant strains in Spain. Antimicrob Agents Chemother 22:222–225
Clewell DB (1981) Plasmids, drug resistance and gene transfer in the genus *Streptococcus*. Microbiol Rev 45:409–436
Cohen ML, Wong ES, Falkow S (1982) Common R-plasmids in *Staphylococcus aureus* and *Staphylococcus epidermidis* during a nosocomial *Staphylococcus aureus* outbreak. Antimicrob Agents Chemother 21:210–215
Courvalin P, Carlier C, Collatz E (1980) Plasmid mediated resistance to aminocyclotol antibiotics in group D streptococci. J Bacteriol 143:541–551
Cuchural GJ, Tally FP, Jacobus MV, Marsh PK, Mayhew JW (1983) Cefoxitin inactivation by *Bacteroides fragilis*. Antimicrob Agents Chemother 24:936–940
Davies AJ, Stone JW (1986) Current problems of chemotherapy of infections with coagulase-negative staphylococci. Eur J Clin Microbiol 5:277–281
Dupont M-J, Jouvenot M, Couetdic G, Michel-Briand Y (1985) Development of plasmid-mediated resistance in *Vibrio cholera* during treatment with trimethoprim-sulfamethoxazole. Antimicrob Agents Chemother 27:280–281
Edelstein P, Calarco L, Yasui V (1984) Antimicrobial therapy of experimentally induced Legionnaire's disease in guinea pigs. Am Rev Respir Dis 130:849–856
Escheverria P, Ulyango CV, Ho MT, Verheaert L, Komalarinia S, Orskov F (1978) Antimicrobial resistance and enterotoxin production among isolates of *Escherichia coli* in the Far East. Lancet II:589–592
Faruk H, Kohmescher RN, McKinney WP, Sparling PF (1985) A community-based outbreak of infection with penicillin-resistant *Neisseria* gonorrhoeae not producing penicillinase (chromosomally mediated resistance). N Engl J Med 313:607–611
Fontana R, Cerini R, Longoni P, Grossato A, Canepari P (1983) Identification of a streptococcal penicillin binding protein that reacts very slowly with penicillin. J Bacteriol 155:1340–1350
Fontana R, Grossato A, Rossi L, Cheng YR, Satta G (1985) Transition from resistance to hypersusceptibility to β-lactam antibiotics associated with loss of a low affinity penicillin binding protein in a *Streptococcus faeceium* mutant highly resistant to penicillin. Antimicrob Agents Chemother 28:678–683
Griffin HG, Foster TJ, Falkiner FR, Carr ME, Coleman DC (1985) Molecular analysis of multiple-resistance plasmids transferred from gram-negative bacteria isolated in a urological unit. Antimicrob Agents Chemother 28:413–418
Hakenback R, Ellerbrok H, Briese T, Handwerger S, Tomasz A (1986) Penicillin-binding proteins of penicillin-susceptible and -resistant pneumococci. Immunological relatedness of altered proteins and changes in peptides carrying the β-lactam binding site. Antimicrob Agens Chemother 30:553–558
Haley RW, Hightower AW, Khabbaz RF (1982) The emergence of methicillin resistant *Staphylococcus aureus* infections in United States hospitals. Possible role of a house staff – patient transfer circuit. Ann Intern Med 97:297–308
Handsfield HH, Murphy VL (1983) Comparative study of ceftriaxone and spectinomycin for treatment of uncomplicated gonorrheae in men. Lancet II:67–70

Handwerger S, Tomasz A (1986) Alterations in kinetic properties of penicillin-binding proteins of penicillin-resistance *Streptococcus pneumoniae*. Antimicrob Agents Chemother 30:57–63

Hansman D, Lullen MM (1967) A resistance pneumococcus. Lancet II:264–265

Hartman BJ, Tomasz A (1984) Low-affinity penicillin-binding protein associated with beta-lactam resistance in *Staphylococcus aureus*. J Bacteriol 258:513–516

Havlichek D, Saravolatz L, Pohlad D (1987) Effective quinolones and other antimicrobial agents on cell-associated *Legionnella pneumophilia*. Antimicrob Agents Chemother 31:1529–1534

Hedge PJ, Spratt BG (1985) Resistance to β-lactam antibiotics by remodelling the active site of an *E. coli* penicillin binding protein. Nature 318:478–480

Holder IA (1976) Gentamicin resistant *Pseudomonas aeruginosa* in a burns unit. J Antimicrob Chemother 2:309–316

Hornstein MJ, Jupeau AM, Scavizzi MR, Philippon AM, Grimont PAD (1985) In vitro susceptibility of 126 clinical isolates of *Yersinia enterocolitica* to 21 β-lactam antibiotics. Antimicrob Agents Chemother 27:806–811

Horodniceanu T, Bougueleret L, El-Sohl M, Bieth G, Delbos F (1979) High-level, plasmid-borne resistance to gentamicin and *Streptococcus faecalis* subsp. *Zymogenes*. Antimicrob Agents Chemother 16:686–689

Jacobs MR, Koornhof HJ, Robins-Browne RM, Stevenson CM, Vermaak ZA, Frieman I, Miller B, Wicomb MA, Isaacson M, Ward JI, Austrian R (1978) Emergence of multiply resistant pneumococci. N Engl J Med 299:735–740

Jacoby GA (1984) Resistant plasmids of *Pseudomonas aeruginosa*. In: Bryan LE (ed) Antimicrobial drug resistance, chap 17. Academic, Orlando, pp 497–514

Knapp JS, Zenilman JM, Biddle JW (1987) Frequency and distribution in the United States of strains of *Neisseria gonorrhoeae* with plasmid-mediated, high-level resistance to tetracycline. J Infect Dis 155:819–822

Krogstad DJ, Korfhagen TR, Moellering RC Jr, Wennersten C, Swartz MN, Perzynski S, Davies J (1978) Aminoglycoside-inactivating enzymes in clinical isolates of *Streptococcus faecalis*: an explanation for resistance to antibiotic synergism. J Clin Invest 62:480–486

Lambert T, Megraud F, Gerbaud G, Courvalin P (1986) Susceptibility of *Campylobacter plyoridis* to 20 antimicrobial agents. Antimicrob Agents Chemother 30:510–511

Latorre C, Juncosa T, Sanfeliui (1985) Antibiotic resistance and serotypes of 100 *Streptococcus pneumoniae* isolated in a children's hospital in Barcelona Spain. Antimicrob Agents Chemother 28:357–359

LeBlanc DJ, Inamine JM, Lee LN (1986) Broad geographical distribution of homologous erythromycin, kanamycin and streptomycin resistance determinants among group D streptococci of human and animal origins. Antimicrob Agents Chemother 29:549–555

Linares J, Garau J, Dominguez C, Perez JL (1983) Antibiotic resistance and serotypes of *Streptococcus pneumoniae* from patients with community-acquired pneumococcal disease. Antimicrob Agents Chemother 23:545–547

Lorian V (1986) *Salmonella* susceptibility patterns in hospitals from 1975 through 1984. J Clin Microbiol 23:826–827

Lowbury EJL, Babb JR, Roe E (1972) Clearance from a hospital of gram-negative bacilli that transfer carbenicillin-resistance to *Pseudomonas aeruginosa*. Lancet II:941–945

McConnell MM, Willshaw GA, Smith HR, Scotland SM, Rowe B (1979) Transposition of ampicillin resistance to an enterotoxin plasmid in an *Escherichia coli* strain of human origin. J Bacteriol 139:346–355

Medeiros AA, Levesque R, Jacoby G (1986) An animal source for the ROB-1 β-lactamase of *Haemophilus influenzae* type B. Antimicrob Agents Chemother 29:212–215

Mederski-Samoraj BD, Murray BE (1983) High-level resistance to gentamicin in clinical isolates of Enterococci. J Infect Dis 147:751–757

Mendelman PM, Chaffin DO, Stull TL, Rubens CE, Mack KD, Smith AL (1984) Characterization of non-β-lactamase mediated ampicillin resistance in *Haemophilus influenzae*. Antimicrob Agents Chemother 26:235–244

Mitchison DA (1984) Drug resistance in *Mycobacteria*. Br Med Bull 40:84–90
MMWR (1986) Plasmid-mediated tetracycline-resistant *Neisseria gonorrhoeae* – Georgia, Mass, Oregon. MMWR 35:304–306
Motyl MR, McKinley, Janda JM (1985) In vitro susceptibilities of *Aeromonas hydrophilia*, *Aeromonas sobria* and *Aeromonas caviae* to 22 antimicrobial agents. Antimicrob Agents Chemother 28:151–153
Murphy TV, McCraken GH Jr, Zweighaft TC, Hansen EJ (1981) Emergence of rifampin-resistant *Haemophilus influenzae* after prophylaxis. J Pediatr 99:406–409
Murray BE (1986) Resistance of *Shigella*, *Salmonella* and other selected enteric pathogens to antimicrobial agents. Rev Infect Dis 8 [Suppl 2]:S172–S181
Murray BE, Church DA, Wanger A, Zscheck K, Levison ME, Ingerman MJ, Abrutyn E, Mederski-Samoraj B (1986) Comparison of two β-lactamase-producing strains of *Streptococcus faecalis*. Antimicrob Agents Chemother 30:861–864
Nicolle LE, Postl B, Kotelewetz E, Albritton W, Harding GKM, Bougault A-M, Ronald AR (1982) Emergence of rifampin-resistant *Haemophilus influenzae*. Antimicrob Agents Chemother 21:498–500
Ouellette M, Gerbaud G, Lambert T, Courvalin P (1987) Acquisition by a *Campylobacter* like strain of *aph* A-1. A kanamycin resistance determinant from members of the family *Enterobacteriaceae*. Antimicrob Agents Chemother 31:1021–1026
Parr T Jr, Bryan LE (1984a) Non-enzymatic resistance to beta-lactam antibiotics and resistance to other cell wall synthesis inhibitors. In: Bryan LE (ed) Antimicrobial drug resistance, chap 3. Academic, Orlando, pp 81–111
Parr TR Jr, Bryan LE (1984b) Mechanism of resistance of an ampicillin-resistant β-lactamase negative clinical isolate of *Haemophilus influenzae* type B to β-lactam antibiotics. Antimicrob Agents Chemother 25:747–753
Perez JL, Linares J, Bosch J, Lopez De Goicoechea MJ, Martin R (1987) Antibiotics resistance of *Streptococcus pneumoniae* in childhood carriers. J Antimicrob Chemother 19:279–280
Piddock LJV, Wise R (1987) Cefoxitin resistance in *Bacteroides* species: evidence indicating two mechanisms causing decreased susceptibility. J Antimicrob Chemother 19:161–170
Price DJE, Sleigh JD (1970) Control of infection due to *Klebsiella aerogenes* in a neurosurgical unit by withdrawal of all antibiotics. Lancet ii:1213–1215
Rossi L, Tonin E, Cheng YR, Fontana R (1985) Regulation of penicillin-binding protein activity: description of a methicillin-inducible penicillin-binding protein in *Staphylococcus aureus*. Antimicrob Agents Chemother 27:828–831
Rowe B, Threlfall EJ (1984) Drug resistance in gram-negative aerobic bacilli. Br Med Bull 40:68–76
Rubin LG, Medeiros AA, Yolken RH, Moxon ER (1981) Ampicillin treatment failure of apparently β-lactamase negative *Haemophilus influenzae* type B meningitis due to a novel β-lactamase. Lancet II:1008–1010
Sabath LD, Abraham EP (1964) Synergistic action of penicillins and cephalosporins against *Pseudomonas pyocyanea*. Nature 204:1066–1069
Sack DA, Kaminsky DC, Sack B, Itotio JN, Arthur RR, Kapikian AZ, Orscov F, Orscov I (1978) Prophylactic doxycycline for traveller's diarrhea. N Engl J Med
Schaberg DR, Zerbos MJ (1986) Intergeneric and interspecies gene exchange in gram-positive cocci. Antimicrob Agents Chemother 30:817–822
Schaberg DR, Power RG, Betzold J, Forbes BA (1985) Conjugative R-plasmids in antimicrobial resistance of *Staphylococcus aureus* causing nosocomial infections. J Infect Dis 152:43–49
Smith AL (1983) Antibiotic resistance in *Haemophilus influenzae*. Pediatr Infect Dis 2:352–355
Stieglitz H, Fonesca R, Olarte J, Kupersztoch-Ponrtnoy YM (1980) Linkage of heat-stable enterotoxin activity and ampicillin resistance in a plasmid isolated from a *Escherichia coli* of human origin. Infect Immun 30:617–620
Taylor DE, Garner RS, Allan BJ (1983) Characterization of tetracycline resistance plasmids from *Campylobacter jejuni* and *Campylobacter coli*. Antimicrob Agents Chemother 24:930–935

Tenover FC, Williams S, Gordon KP, Nolan C, Plorde JJ (1985) Survey of plasmids and resistance factors in *Campylobacter jejuni* and *Campylobacter coli*. Antimicrob Agents Chemother 27:37–41
Ubukata K, Yamshita N, Kono M (1985) Occurrence of a Beta-lactam inducible penicillin-binding protein in methicillin-resistant staphylococci. Antimicrob Agents Chemother 17:851–857
Van Caekenbergag DL, Breyssens J (1987) In vitro synergistic activity between bismith subcitrate and various antimicrobial agents against *Campylobacter pyloridis* (*C. pylori*). Antimicrob Agents Chemother 31:1429–1430
Van der Auwer P, Scorneaux B (1985) In vitro susceptibility of *Campylobacter jejuni* to 27 antimicrobial agents and various combinations of β-lactams with clavulanic acid or sulbactam. Antimicrob Agents Chemother 28:37–40
Wexler HM, Finegold SM (1987) Antimicrobial resistance in *Bacteroides*. J Antimicrob Chemother 19:143–146
Williams JD, Andrews J (1974) Sensitivity of *Haemophilus influenzae* to antibiotics. Br Med J [Clin Res] 1:134–137
Williams JD, Moosdeen F (1986) Antibiotic resistance in *Haemophilus influenzae*: epidemiology mechanisms and therapeutic possibilities. Rev Infect Dis 8 [Suppl 5]:S555–S561
Woodruff WA, Parr TR, Hancock REW, Hanne LF, Nicas TI, Iglewski BH (1986) Expression in *Escherichia coli* and function of *Pseudomonas aeruginosa* outer membrane porin protein F. J Bacteriol 186:473–479
Woods GL, Washington JA (1987) Mycobacteria other than *Mycobacterium* tuberculosis: review of microbiologic and clinical aspects. Rev Infect Dis 9:275–294
Zajdowicz TR, Sanches PL, Berg SW, Kerbs SBJ, Newquist RL, Harrison WO (1983) Comparison of ceftriazone with cefoxitin in the treatment of penicillin-resistant to gonnoccal urethritis. Br J Venereal Dis 59:176–178

Subject Index

Handbook of Experimental Pharmacology

Springer-Verlag
Berlin Heidelberg
New York London
Paris Tokyo Hong Kong

Volume 51
Uric Acid

Volume 52
Snake Venoms

Volume 53
Pharmacology of Ganglionic Transmission

Volume 54: Part 1
Adrenergic Activators and Inhibitors I

Part 2
Adrenergic Activators and Inhibitors II

Volume 55
Psychotropic Agents

Part 1
Antipsychotics and Antidepressants

Part 2
Anxiolytics, Gerontopsychopharmacological Agents and Psychomotor Stimulants

Part 3
Alcohol and Psychotomimetics, Psychotropic Effects of Central Acting Drugs

Volume 56, Parts 1 + 2
Cardiac Glycosides

Volume 57
Tissue Growth Factors

Volume 58
Cyclic Nucleotides

Part 1
Biochemistry

Part 2
Physiology and Pharmacology

Volume 59
Mediators and Drugs in Gastrointestinal Motility

Part 1
Morphological Basis and Neurophysiological Control

Part 2
Endogenous and Exogenous Agents

Volume 60
Pyretics and Antipyretics

Volume 61
Chemotherapy of Viral Infections

Volume 62
Aminoglycoside Antibiotics

Volume 63
Allergic Reactions to Drugs

Volume 64
Inhibition of Folate Metabolism in Chemotherapy

Volume 65
Teratogenesis and Reproductive Toxicology

Volume 66
Part 1: **Glucagon I**

Part 2: **Glucagon II**

Springer

Handbook of Experimental Pharmacology

Springer-Verlag
Berlin Heidelberg
New York London
Paris Tokyo Hong Kong

Volume 67
Part 1
Antiobiotics Containing the Beta-Lactam Structure I

Part 2
Antibiotics Containing the Beta-Lactam Structure II

Volume 68, Parts 1 + 2
Antimalarial Drugs

Volume 69
Pharmacology of the Eye

Volume 70
Part 1
Pharmacology of Intestinal Permeation I

Part 2
Pharmacology of Intestinal Permeation II

Volume 71
Interferons and Their Applications

Volume 72
Antitumor Drug Resistance

Volume 73
Radiocontrast Agents

Volume 74
Antieliptic Drugs

Volume 75
Toxicology of Inhaled Materials

Volume 76
Clinical Pharmacology of Antiangial Drugs

Volume 77
Chemotherapy of Gastrointestinal Helminths

Volume 78
The Tetracycline

Volume 79
New Neuromuscular Blocking Agents

Volume 80
Cadmium

Volume 81
Local Anesthetics

Volume 82
Radioimmunoassay in Basic and Clinical Pharmacology

Volume 83
Calcium in Drug Actions

Volume 84
Antituberculosis Drugs

Volume 85
The Pharmacology of Lymphocytes

Volume 86
The Cholinergic Synapse

Volume 87
Part 1
Pharmacology of the Skin I

Part 2
Pharmacology of the Skin II

Volume 88
Drugs for the Treatment of Parkinson's Disease

Volume 89
Antiarrhythmic Drugs

Volume 90
Part 1
Catecholamines I

Part 2
Catecholamines II

Springer

MIX
Papier aus verantwortungsvollen Quellen
Paper from responsible sources
FSC® C105338

If you have any concerns about our products,
you can contact us on
ProductSafety@springernature.com

In case Publisher is established outside the EU,
the EU authorized representative is:
Springer Nature Customer Service Center GmbH
Europaplatz 3, 69115 Heidelberg, Germany

Printed by Libri Plureos GmbH
in Hamburg, Germany